Movement Disorder Surgery

The Essentials

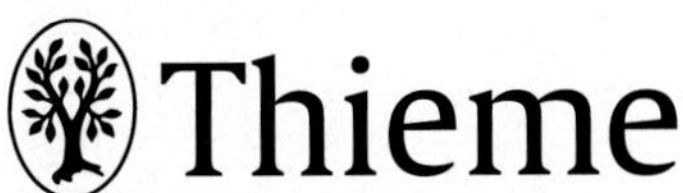

Movement Disorder Surgery

The Essentials

Roy A. E. Bakay, MD
A. Watson Armour III and Sarah Armour Presidential Chair
Residency Research Director
Department of Neurological Surgery
Rush University Medical Center
Chicago, Illinois

Thieme
New York • Stuttgart

To Mark, Scott, Jacqueline, and Candace.

Thieme Medical Publishers, Inc.
333 Seventh Ave.
New York, NY 10001

Executive Editor: Kalen Conerly
Associate Editor: Ivy Ip
Vice President, Production and Electronic Publishing: Anne T. Vinnicombe
Production Editor: Print Matters, Inc.
Vice President, International Marketing and Sales: Cornelia Schulze
Chief Financial Officer: Peter van Woerden
President: Brian D. Scanlan
Compositor: The Manila Typesetting Co.
Printer: Maple-Vail Book Manufacturing Group

Library of Congress Cataloging-in-Publication Data

Movement disorder surgery : the essentials / [edited by] Roy A.E. Bakay.
     p. ; cm.
  Includes bibliographical references and index.
  ISBN 978-1-58890-397-6 (alk. paper)
  1. Movement disorders–Surgery. I. Bakay, Roy A. E.
  [DNLM: 1. Movement Disorders–surgery. 2. Deep Brain Stimulation. 3. Stereotaxic Techniques. WL 390 M9348 2008]
  RD594.M72 2008
  616.8'3–dc22
                        2007050268

Printed in the United States

5 4 3 2 1

ISBN 978-1-58890-397-6

Contents

Preface . . . . **ix**

Contributors . . . . **xi**

1   History of Surgery for Movement Disorders 1
Philip L. Gildenberg

The Pre-stereotactic Era (1890–1954) 1
The Early Stereotactic Era (1947–1968) 3
The Latent Period (1968–1992) 6
Reintroduction of Ablative Stereotactic Surgery (1992–1999) 7
Implanted Stimulators (1997–present) 7

2   Rationale for Movement Disorder Surgery 12
*Cameron C. McIntyre, Christopher R. Butson, Benjamin L. Walter, and
Jerrold L. Vitek*

Anatomy and Physiology of the Basal Ganglia and Thalamus 13
Pathophysiological Basis of Movement Disorders 15
Therapeutic Mechanisms of Movement Disorder Surgery 18

3   Setting Up a Movement Disorder Surgery Practice 25
Brian Harris Kopell, Kenneth Baker, and Nicholas M. Boulis

Capital Expenses 25
Building a Program 32
The Business of a Movement Disorder Surgery Practice 38
Conclusion 46

4   Selection of Centers, Disorders, and Patients for Movement Disorder Surgery 48
Leo Verhagen Metman

Selection of a Center 48
Selecting Disorders 50
Selecting Patients 52
Future Perspectives 55

5   Preparation for Movement Disorder Surgery 58
Ron L. Alterman and Michele Tagliati

Presurgical Evaluation 58
Preoperative Preparation 61
Surgical Preparation 61
Conclusion 67

6   Anesthesia for Movement Disorder Surgery **70**
Robert E. Gross, Klaus Mewes, and Ghaleb A. Ghani

Preoperative Evaluation 70
Peri- and Intraoperative Anesthetic Approaches 72
Postoperative Anesthetic Issues 80
Anesthetic Complications 80
Conclusion 80

7   Stereotactic Surgery with Microelectrode Recordings **83**
Diane K. Sierens, Scott Kutz, Julie G. Pilitsis, and Roy A. E. Bakay

Operative Techniques and Patient Positioning 83
Microelectrode Recording 87
Conclusion 110

8   Stereotactic Surgery without Microelectrode Recording **115**
Marwan I. Hariz and Nathalie Vayssiere

Stereotactic Imaging 115
Electrophysiological Testing and Intraoperative Target Adjustment 116
Advantages and Disadvantages of Surgery without Microelectrode Recording 120
Postoperative Stereotactic Magnetic Resonance Imaging 120
Conclusion 121

9   Implantation of Multiple Electrodes and Robotic Techniques **126**
Alim Louis Benabid, Bradley Wallace, Dominique Hoffmann, Stephan Chabardes,
Sylvie Grand, and Jean FranÁois LeBas

Materials 126
X-ray Intraoperative Setup 128
Method 129
Results 135
Discussion 136

10   Frameless Functional Stereotactic Approaches **140**
Jaimie M. Henderson

STarFix Platform 140
NeXframe 140
Conclusion 147

11   Deep Brain Stimulation for Tremor **153**
Jorge L. Eller and Kim J. Burchiel

Stereotactic Frame Placement 157
Anatomical Targeting 157
Surgical Exposure and Trajectory 157
Physiological Targeting 158
Deep Brain Stimulation Lead Placement and Anchoring 158
Internal Pulse Generator Placement 158
Deep Brain Stimulation Programming 158
Efficacy of Deep Brain Stimulation in the Treatment of Tremor 162
Complications Associated with Deep Brain Stimulator Placement 162
Conclusion 163

12   Deep Brain Stimulation for Dystonia **166**
Brian Harris Kopell, Craig I. Horenstein, and Ali R. Rezai

Classification of Dystonia 166

History of Treatment for Dystonia ... 167
Deep Brain Stimulation for Dystonia ... 168
Results of Deep Brain Stimulation for Dystonia ... 175
Complications ... 182
Intermittent Pulse Generator Programming Considerations ... 183
Conclusion ... 183

13 Deep Brain Stimulation Programming ... **187**
Erwin B. Montgomery Jr.

Basic Electrophysiology ... 187
Deep Brain Stimulation Electronics ... 190
Importance of Regional Anatomy in Deep Brain Stimulation Effects ... 199
Strategies of Deep Brain Stimulation Management ... 206
Future of Deep Brain Stimulation ... 208

14 Avoiding Complications and Correcting Errors in Movement Disorder Surgery ... **214**
Philip A. Starr

Operative Complications ... 214
Long-Term Hardware-Related Complications ... 219
Rare but Spectacular Complications ... 222
Deep Brain Stimulation and Magnetic Resonance Imaging ... 222
Troubleshooting the Lead that Doesn't Work ... 222
Cognitive Decline in Parkinson Disease Patients ... 224
Complications Unique to Lesioning Surgery ... 225

15 Efficacy and Complications of Deep Brain Stimulation for Movement Disorders ... **227**
Erich O. Richter, Clement Hamani, and Andres M. Lozano

Efficacy of Deep Brain Stimulation Surgery ... 227
Complications of Deep Brain Stimulation Surgery ... 229
Conclusion ... 230

16 Gamma Knife ... **237**
Ronald F. Young

Indications and Controversies ... 237
Target Selection and Identification ... 238
Dose and Distribution ... 242
Results and Complications ... 242

17 The Future of Treatment for Advanced Parkinson Disease ... **247**
Shivanand P. Lad, Eleonora M. Lad, Roy A. E. Bakay, and Jeffrey H. Kordower

Advances in Deep Brain Stimulation ... 247
Biological Therapies for Parkinson Disease ... 247
Cellular Therapies for Parkinson Disease ... 248
Neurotrophic Factor Therapies for Parkinson Disease ... 251
Challenges for Future Treatments for Parkinson Disease ... 251

Index ... **258**

Preface

Why write a textbook on deep brain stimulation for movement disorders? While there are a number of books on surgical treatment of movement disorders by experts for experts, they simply do not cover topics completely. By focusing here solely on deep brain stimulation, the scope can be reduced, and readers can obtain in a simple tome a complete, overall appreciation for the state of the art. Now that the field is maturing, the knowledge base is starting to solidify, and enough experience has been gathered that reasonable, authoritative discussions can be made within this somewhat esoteric subspecialty of stereotactic and functional neurosurgery. The field has undergone a dramatic increase in interest because of the ability to reach intracranial targets to effect therapeutic benefits with great accuracy and safety. Stereotactic philosophies, approaches, and techniques are being incorporated into general neurosurgery continuously. Now with deep brain stimulation, there is a technique that is totally unique and extremely powerful. The brain is an electrical organ, and therefore it is reasonable that electrical stimulation can be therapeutic. We now have the tools and the delivery system to be able to effectively alter any type of brain function, provided we understand the basic circuitry and know where tipping points reside. Movement disorder is the tip of the iceberg but the leading edge from which multiple therapies will eventually emerge. Thus stereotactic and functional neurosurgery is no longer the crossroads but has leaped out into the forefront of neurosurgery practice. This methodology clearly will be an important part of the future therapeutic armamentarium of neurosurgery.

One of the most important aspects of this text is the unique nature of many of the chapters. Nearly half are so unusual that they would not be found as chapters in any other stereotactic and functional textbooks. The purpose of this book is to provide an encyclopedic template for students, residents, fellows, and even practicing physicians on how to go about practicing functional neurosurgery for movement disorders. The purpose is education – we want to make you a better practitioner.

To that end, each chapter includes supplemental material in the form of "Editor's Comments". These passages are designed to provide the reader with additional information on a topic, and in some instances offer a different perspective. (It is also hoped that the Editor's Comments will supply some continuity between chapters.) The Editor's Comments were added for the sake of interest, and the reader must remember that the individual contributors are the experts who were asked to write the specific chapters. Theirs represents the primary database, the primary subject matter, upon which this book rests. Additionally, suggestions for further reading and research are presented via URL's to pertinent websites.

The introductory chapters are to provide an overall historical perspective and to give a state of the art understanding as to the exact mechanism(s) of action deep brain stimulation entails. This is essential material for one in the field and forms the basis for everything else that is written. The chapter on setting up a practice details successful techniques that have been used to establish movement disorder centers, both private and academic. There are, in addition, pearls regarding what the key elements are for a movement disorder center from both neurosurgical and neurological perspectives. Also, the communications and the infrastructure are discussed. In no other text will you read about how to appropriately bill patients for your services. The two chapters on patient evaluations are again from both the neurosurgeon's and the neurologist's perspectives. The neurologist is the expert in diagnosis and is, in most situations, the gatekeeper for the functional neurosurgeon. These are the primary persons who will take care of the patient before surgery and after surgery. Because of the two different perspectives there may be some degree of overlap in these chapters, but in my opinion this is a useful thing . Finally, the preparatory steps of getting the patient ready for the operating room are discussed.

The next seven chapters make up the keystone to surgical intervention. A truly unique chapter on anesthesia for functional neurosurgery is provided so that the patient can be comfortable and safely operated on. There is a wealth of information that is shared by both a neurosurgeon and an anesthesiologist. Chapter 7 provides a comprehensive approach, from start to finish, of operations for deep brain stimulation using microelectrode recordings. It is meant to be extremely comprehensive and technique-rich. Subtle nuances are discussed in detail to provide even the expert additional information as to approaches to the most common targets currently used for deep brain stimulation: the thalamus, the subthalamus, and the globus pallidus. The electrophysiology is extensively reviewed, and illustrations are provided to help even the novice begin to understand the approach and rationale of at least one highly experienced surgical team. Chapter 8 compares and contrasts operative techniques involving microelectrode recording to surgery without the use of microelectrode recordings. This clearly is a separate way of performing surgery that requires somewhat different expertise and philosophy. These differences are discussed within both the chapter and in the editorial comments. Chapter 9, by Dr. Alim Louis Benabid, discusses his pioneering technique using multiple electrodes and a robotic device. From a pioneer in this field, his insights are invaluable. Two chapters provide additional specialized technical information specific to tremor and dystonia. Each of these are distinct movement problems that need to be dealt with somewhat differently from Parkinson disease, and those differences become obvious throughout these chapters. One of the new frontiers that didn't even reach the level of interest to be included in the initial plan of the book now grounds a chapter on frameless stereotactic approaches. Frameless stereotaxis has taken off dramatically. Chapter 10 presents an unprecedented discussion of the many new directions in which stereotactic and functional neurosurgery is headed.

The next set of chapters are designed to assist in getting through the postoperative phase—with special focus on properly programming the neurostimulator, avoiding and treating the complications of surgery, and summarizing anticipated results. Once the patient has been properly operated on, they have to be programmed, and Chapter 13 outstandingly covers programming and the very basic aspects of electrophysiology in a way that should be understood by all. The methodology that is proposed is straightforward and extremely useful. Chapter 14, on pre-

venting complications, is absolutely essential reading. This chapter summarizes the way in which to maximize surgical benefit and minimize and problems. It takes a great deal of expertise to be able to discuss complications in a reasonable manner. A rather complete review of the outcomes of DBS surgery for movement disorders, covering both efficacy and safety, is detailed in Chapter 15. This type of review is essential to understand where problems lie so that future approaches may be able to avoid some of the same pitfalls. Finally, Chapter 16 addresses radiosurgery for movement disorders. This option should be kept in mind for certain select patients.

The last chapter discusses some of the future options that may be available both for deep brain stimulation but also in terms of other adjuvant therapy. Deep brain stimulation is really quite primitive at this time and simply provides a constant stimulation at a single location. Different types of electrical activity at different times of the day with different activities may then need a more robust way of controlling movements to replicate what is done naturally. In addition, there may be multiple areas that need stimulation. One could envision an electrode to assist certain symptomatologies and another in a different place to assist others. Stimulation technology will evolve, and will evolve rather quickly, with appropriate competition and clinical success. Deep brain stimulation is not the only cutting edge technology. Soon there may be no disease, no symptom, and no target that is not treated by nerve stimulation. Cellular therapy and gene therapy are fully discussed. These may be adjuvants to deep brain stimulation in the future or may potentially replace it in the very distant future.

The one thing that is quite sure is that nothing stands still. Undoubtedly, some of the information in these chapters is outdated simply by virtue of time, even though that time period is relatively short. As this book goes to press, the Web sites have been checked and are working appropriately. In a rapidly moving field, some of these had changed from the initial writing to the page proofs, and it is quite likely that they will have changed yet again by the time the reader attempts to access them. Similarly, recommendations and equipment evaluations have been based on current experience and will change with advances in the field. I offer special thanks to Dr. Diane Sierens for proofreading many of the chapters and comments. Finally, I would like to thank all of my multiple fellows—from Dr. Philip Starr, my first, to Dr. Julie Pilitsis, my most recent. Each of them has taught me a number of lessons and I am indebted to them all as well as the residents that I have taught throughout the years. Enjoy your journey.

Contributors

Ron L. Alterman, MD
Associate Professor
Department of Neurosurgery
Mount Sinai School of Medicine
New York, New York

Roy A. E. Bakay, MD
A. Watson Armour III and Sarah Armour Presidential Chair
Residency Research Director
Department of Neurological Surgery
Rush University Medical Center
Chicago, Illinois

Kenneth Baker, PhD
Department of Neurosurgery
Cleveland Clinic Foundation
Cleveland, Ohio

Alim Louis Benabid, MD, PhD
Joseph Fourier University
University Hospital
Grenoble, France

Nicholas M. Boulis, MD
Center for Neurological Restoration
Cleveland Clinic Foundation
Cleveland, Ohio

Kim J. Burchiel, MD, FACS
John Raaf Professor and Chairman
Department of Neurological Surgery
Professor
Department of Anesthesiology and Perioperative
Medicine
Oregon Health and Science University
Portland, Oregon

Christopher R. Butson, PhD
Research Associate
Department of Biomedical Engineering
Cleveland Clinic Foundation
Cleveland, Ohio

Stephan Chabardes, MD
Joseph Fourier University
University Hospital
Grenoble, France

Jorge L. Eller, MD
Assistant Professor
Department of Neurological Surgery
Oregon Health and Science University
The Portland VA Medical Center
Portland, Oregon

Ghaleb A. Ghani, MB, BCh
Associate Professor
Department of Aneshtesiology
Emory University School of Medicine
Division of Anesthesiology
Emory University Hospital
Atlanta, Georgia

Philip L. Gildenberg, MD, PhD
Houston Stereotactic Concepts
Houston, Texas

Sylvie Grand, MD, PhD
Joseph Fourier University
University Hospital
Grenoble, France

Robert E. Gross, MD, PhD
Assistant Professor
Department of Neurosurgery
Emory University School of Medicine
Division of Neurosurgery
Emory University Hospital
Atlanta, Georgia

Clement Hamani, MD, PhD
University of Toronto
Toronto Western Hospital
Toronto, Ontario, Canada

Marwan I. Hariz, MD, PhD
Edmond J. Safra Chair of Functional Neurosurgery
Institute of Neurology
University College London
Honorary Consultant
Unit of Functional Neurosurgery
National Hospital for Neurology and Neurosurgery
London, United Kingdom

Jaimie M. Henderson, MD
Director
Division of Stereotactic and Functional Neurosurgery
Stanford University Medical Center
Stanford, California

Dominique Hoffmann, MD
Joseph Fourier University
University Hospital
Grenoble, France

Craig I. Horenstein, MD
Department of Neurosurgery
Center for Neurological Restoration
Cleveland Clinic Foundation
Cleveland, Ohio

Brian Harris Kopell, MD
Assistant Professor
Departments of Neurosurgery and Psychiatry
Medical College of Wisconsin
Froedert Memorial Lutheran Hospital
Milwaukee, Wisconsin

Jeffrey H. Kordower, PhD
Department of Neurological Sciences
Rush University Medical Center
Chicago, Illinois

Scott Kutz, MD
North County Neurosurgery
DePaul Medical Group
Bridgeton, Missouri

Eleonora M. Lad, MD
Department of Neuroscience
Finch University of Health Sciences
Chicago, Illinois

Shivanand P. Lad, MD, PhD
Department of Neurosurgery
Stanford University Medical Center
Stanford, California

Jean FranÁois LeBas, MD, PhD
Professor
Department of Neuro-Radiology
Joseph Fourier University
University Hospital
Grenoble, France

Andres M. Lozano, MD, PhD, FRCSC
Senior Scientist
Division of Brain Imaging and Behaviour Systems—Neuroscience
Toronto Western Research Institute
Toronto Western Hospital
Toronto, Ontario, Canada

Cameron C. McIntyre, PhD
Associate Staff
Department of Biomedical Engineering
Cleveland Clinic Foundation
Cleveland, Ohio

Klaus Mewes, PhD
Assistant Professor
Department of Neurosurgery
Emory University School of Medicine
Atlanta, Georgia

Erwin B. Montgomery Jr., MD
Clinical Science Center
University of Wisconsin Hospital and Cinics
Madison, Wisconsin

Julie G. Pilitsis, MD, PhD
Assistant Professor
Director of Functional Neurosurgery
Division of Neurosurgery
UMASS Memorial Medical Center
Worcester, Massachusetts

Ali R. Rezai, MD
Co-Chairman
Center for Neurological Restoration
Cleveland Clinic Foundation
Cleveland, Ohio

Erich O. Richter, MD
Neurosurgeon
Georgia Neurological Institute
Macon, Georgia

Diane K. Sierens, MD
Assistant Professor
Department of Neurological Surgery
University of Illinois College of Medicine
Rockford Health System
Division of Neurological Surgery
Rockford, Illinois

Philip A. Starr, MD, PhD
Associate Professor in Residence
Department of Neurological Surgery
University of California, San Francisco
San Francisco, California

Michele Tagliati, MD
Associate Professor
Department of Neurology
Mount Sinai School of Medicine
Division of Movement Disorders
Mount Sinai Hospital
New York, New York

Nathalie Vayssiere, PhD
CNRS Research Engineer
Centre de Recherche Cerveau et Cognition—CerCo
University of Toulouse
FacultÈ de Medicine de Rangueil
Toulouse, France

Leo Verhagen Metman, MD, PhD
Department of Neurological Sciences
Rush University Medical Center
Chicago, Illinois

Jerrold L. Vitek, MD, PhD
Co-Chairman
Center for Neurological Restoration
Cleveland Clinic Foundation
Cleveland, Ohio

Bradley Wallace, MD, PhD
Joseph Fourier University
University Hospital
Grenoble, France

Benjamin L. Walter, MD
Associate Staff
Department of Neurology
Neurological Institute
Cleveland Clinic Foundation
Cleveland, Ohio

Ronald F. Young, MD
Medical Director
Gamma Knife Center
Northwest Hospital
Seattle, Washington
Co-Medical Director
Neuroscience Gamma Knife Center
Los Robles Hospital
Thousand Oaks, California

1 History of Surgery for Movement Disorders

Philip L. Gildenberg

The history of surgery for movement disorders can be divided into five stages: the pre-stereotactic era (1890–1954), the early stereotactic era prior to the introduction of L-dopa (1947–1968), the latent period (1968–1992), reintroduction of ablative stereotactic surgery (1992–1999), and the use of implanted stimulators (1997–present). There is overlap between the various periods, particularly between the first two, because open ablative, resection craniotomy, or laminectomy was performed for several years until stereotactic surgery had time to demonstrate its superiority, by both improved results and safety. Not much happened for several years after the introduction of L-dopa, around 1968, until it became well established that medication was not the ultimate answer for Parkinson disease (PD). Reports of success of pallidotomy were reintroduced. The patients, however, were different from those in the first stereotactic phase because they were much later in their disease and had the complications of the medication added to their parkinsonian symptoms. The use of implanted stimulators for movement disorders was introduced gradually. Original observations were made as early as 1980, but it was not until 1998 that deep brain stimulation for movement disorders became common in Europe. In 2001 it was approved for widespread use in the United States. Even so, ablation procedures are still performed for various reasons, not the least of which is economic.

■ The Pre-stereotactic Era (1890–1954)

The groundwork for surgery for movement disorders began in the last part of the nineteenth century. The concept of localized activity of the cerebral cortex was based on electrical stimulation studies such as those of Fritsch and Hitzig[1] and such clinical observations as Jackson's[2] observation of a loss of motor or sensory function associated with cerebral lesions and Broca's[3] similar observation of a loss of speech. The functions of the basal ganglia were not well appreciated because of the difficulty in experimental manipulation of such subcortical structures.

The father of functional neurosurgery was also the father of the scientific approach to surgery for movement disorders, Sir Victor Horsley. As early as 1890, he performed extirpation of the motor cortex for treatment of athetosis.[4] In 1909, he obtained relief of postscarlatina hemiathetosis in a 15-year-old boy by resecting the upper-extremity portion of the contralateral precentral gyrus, but paresis and dyspraxia ensued.[5] In subsequent reports[6] he acknowledged improvement in other types of movement disorders, but at the expense of paralysis or severe paresis, which usually improved gradually, often as the abnormality returned. In the absence of other treatment, however, it was considered to be a reasonable trade-off to exchange paresis for involuntary movements despite a mortality rate of up to 15%.

One might speculate that it was his frustration at these imperfect results that led him to physiological experiments on subcortical structures. In 1908, he and Clarke reported on physiologic observations following production of lesions in the dentate nucleus of the monkey.[7] This paper is a classic in every sense and should be read in the original by anyone interested in the history of stereotactic surgery. The literary quality of the writing is rarely seen in scientific publications today. After defining the need for more information about the connections between cerebellum and cortex, the authors state, "An essential preliminary, therefore, to further progress was to find some method which would satisfy these conditions, viz., a means of producing lesions [of the cerebellar nuclei] which should be accurate in position, limited to any desired degree in extent, and involving as little injury as possible to other structures." This remains the goal of stereotactic surgery even today.

The paper has four sections. "Rectilinear topography" describes how they created the first stereotactic atlas by sectioning the rhesus monkey brain in a fashion to provide anatomical slices that related to the skull anatomy. "Stereotaxic instrument," the section most quoted, describes the original stereotaxic apparatus, based on a Cartesian coordinate system that was the basis for the development of a human stereotactic apparatus 40 years later. "Electrolysis" presents the description of a controlled lesion made with direct current that has yet to be matched. "Excitation" was perhaps the first report of mechanical and electrical stimulation of a subcortical structure. The authors determined that faradic stimulation was superior to direct current stimulation, unipolar was more practical than bipolar, and that the cerebellar nuclei appeared to be more excitable than cerebellar cortex, both of which were not as excitable as certain areas of the cerebral cortex. All of this information was new and all was important in the subsequent development of surgery for movement disorders. With this experimental breakthrough, the first part of the twentieth century provided the laboratory information regarding the extrapyramidal system that later became the basis for movement disorder surgery.

Even so, in the absence of understanding about the cerebral extrapyramidal system, attempts at treating movement disorders, especially PD, involved a variety of other structures. Foerster[8] performed posterior rhizotomy for the treatment of spasticity and rigidity as early as 1908. Sympathetic ramisection and ganglionectomies were reported from the 1920s[9,10] to as late as 1949.[11] Posterolateral cordotomy was employed during the 1930s,[12] and even thyroidectomy was used.[13]

In the 1930s attention returned to ablation of the cerebral cortex and the pyramidal system (**Fig. 1.1**). In 1932, Bucy and Buchanan[14] presented their first report on a series

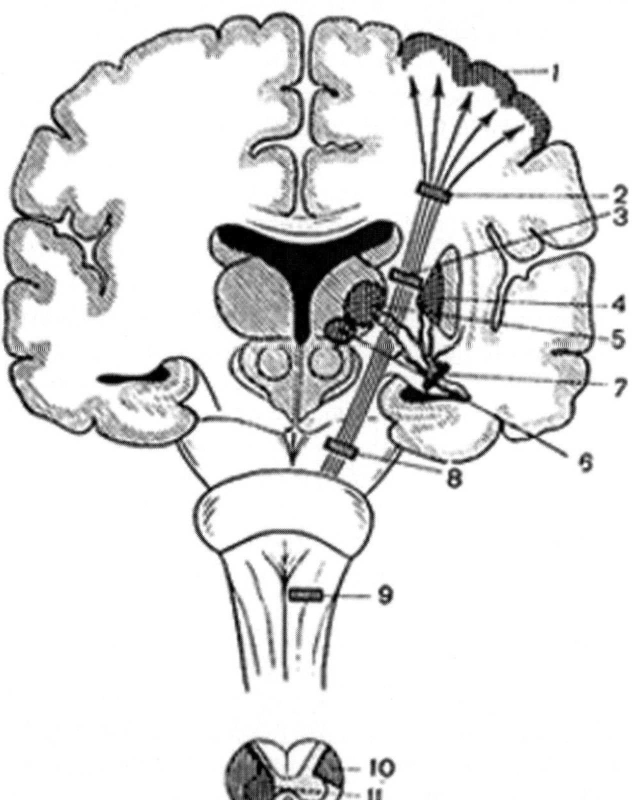

Fig. 1.1 Evolution of surgical operations for movement disorders. 1, Extirpation of premotor and motor areas of cortex (Horsley,[4] Bucy[16]); 2, Section of pyramidal tract in the semioval center (pyramidotomy) (Polenov[18]); 3, Section of pyramidal tract in the internal capsule (Browder[19]); 4, Surgical or stereotactic pallidotomy (Meyers,[32] Spiegel and Wycis,[58] Cooper[47]); 5, Ventrolateral thalamotomy (Hassler and Riechert,[39] Cooper et al[49]); 6, Subthalamotomy (Spiegel and Wycis[66]); 7, Clipping of anterior choroidal artery (Cooper[61]); 8, Section of pyramidal tract in peduncle (pedunculotomy) (Walker[25]); 9, Section of rubrospinal and tegmental tracts in medulla oblongata (bulbotomy) (Burdenko and Klosovski[24]); 10, Section of pyramidal tract in dorsal part of spinal cord lateral column (Putnam[21]); 11, Section of lateral column of the spinal cord (Oliver[22]). (From Kandel EI Functional and Stereotactic Neurosurgery. New York, London: Plenum; 1989.) Reprinted by permission.

of ablation of Brodmann areas 4 and 6, the primary motor cortex and adjacent tissue, for the treatment of athetosis. The resection area was extended somewhat for the treatment of parkinsonian tremor.[15] Even much later, after it was clearly demonstrated that PD symptoms could be controlled by extrapyramidal lesions, Bucy[16] (as well as Gillingham et al[17]) insisted that, regardless of the primary target, it was necessary to include some of the pyramidal system for the procedure to be successful. In 1937, Polenov[18] interrupted the pyramidal fibers in the internal capsule, as did Browder[19] in 1948.

As late as 1951, Takebayashi[20] reported the undercutting of the precentral cortex for the treatment of PD. The pyramidal tract was also attacked at the level of the cervical spinal cord, when Putnam[21] modified his extrapyramidal cervical cordotomy to section the posterolateral quadrant, and Oliver[22] cut the lateral column to include the pyramidal tract to treat tremor.

It was during the 1930s and 1940s that the extrapyramidal pathways became the target of choice for treatment of movement disorders. One of the first efforts was high cervical anterolateral cordotomy for management of choreoathetosis reported by Putnam[23] in 1933. In 1937, Burdenko[24] sectioned the rubrospinal and tegmental tracts in the medulla.

Approaching the extrapyramidal tracts at intracranial levels, even prior to the acceptance of stereotactic localization, was more challenging, and the two dominant figures reporting these procedures were Walker and Meyers. Walker[25] incised the lateral two thirds of the contralateral pedicle to a depth of 6 to 7 mm for the management of first hemiballismus and later PD,[26] and in Europe Guiot and Pecker[27] made a similar but shallower incision, also for PD.

Meyers, on the other hand, selected mainly intracerebral targets. As early as 1939, he performed a transventricular craniotomy approach to extirpate the contralateral head of the caudate nucleus in hemiparkinsonism in a patient who had failed cortical undercutting[28] (**Fig. 1.2**). This was particularly adventurous given that Dandy[29] had, less than a decade before, decreed—erroneously[30]—that the basal ganglia should not be disturbed, assuming that a lesion there would cause unconsciousness. This was based on observations of stroke that involved the anterior cerebral artery. The patient did well for 4 years with no significant deficit, which opened the door to even more adventurous procedures on the basal ganglia for movement disorders. When extirpation of the head of the caudate proved to be insufficient in many patients, Meyers[31] added section of the anterior internal capsule, section of the ansa lenticularis (ansotomy), and even encroachment on the putamen. Slightly over 60% of patients had some benefit, but although the operative mortality decreased from 16%, it was never reduced below 10%, even in the latter part of the series. Meyers eventually considered the risk:benefit ratio to be insufficient to justify such procedures, and indicated that it "became apparent that open surgery at the level of the

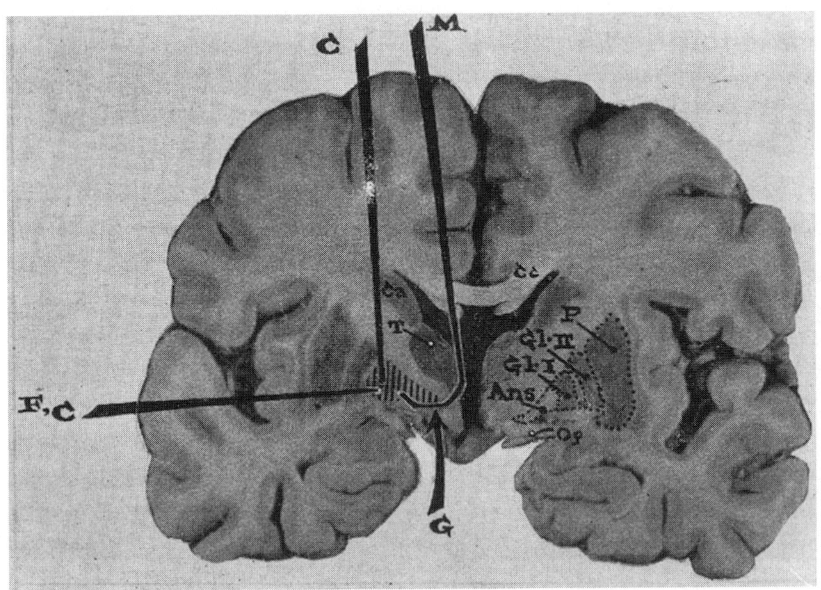

Fig. 1.2 Diagram of open surgical approaches to extrapyramidal structures. Frontal section at level of foramen of Monro, showing ansa lenticularis (Ans) and other pallidofugal elements interrupted in ansotomy for the relief of contralateral hemiparkinsonian tremor. M, approach employed by Meyers via corpus callosum (Cc), lateral and third ventricles; C, approach used by Cooper[47] and Fenelon[114] to globus pallidus; G, approach employed by Guiot and Brion[115] via perforated substance in neighborhood of optic tract (Op); Ca, body of caudate nucleus; T, thalamus; P, putamen; GI I, globus pallidus, crus I (medial segment); GI II, globus pallidus, crus II (lateral segment). (From Meyers R. Historical background and personal experiences in the surgical relief of hyperkinesia and hypertonus. In: Fields W, ed. Pathogenesis and Treatment of Parkinsonism. Springfield, IL: Chas C Thomas; 1958:229–270.) Reprinted by permission.

basal ganglia had a very limited applicability to the problem of paralysis agitans."[31] He did, however, confirm that lesions in the basal ganglia would not cause unconsciousness, that tremor could be abolished without paralysis, and that rigidity could be significantly reduced without paresis or postoperative spasticity, hyperreflexia, dyspraxia, abnormal postures or circumduction. Consequently, he prepared the way for the use of stereotactic surgery to target the basal ganglia and associated pathways for the treatment of movement disorders.

■ The Early Stereotactic Era (1947–1968)

The stage had been set for the introduction of human stereotactic surgery. A concept of potential subcortical targets had been developed from laboratory research, particularly on the extrapyramidal system. A basic concept of the pathophysiology of movement disorders had been obtained from extrapyramidal surgery, which demonstrated that such surgery was possible without disruption of voluntary movements or consciousness.[28,32] Intraoperative x-ray was introduced, with rapid (at that time 30 minute) film processing and sufficient resolution to demonstrate such structures as pineal calcification or the foramen of Monro on ventriculography. Surgical experience on the limbic system had derived from prefrontal lobotomy.[33,34] Indeed, the motivation for the development of human stereotactic surgery was Spiegel's desire to obtain the benefits of prefrontal lobotomy without the risk of devastating neurological deficit.[35]

Human stereotactic surgery was introduced when Spiegel et al[36] published a brief account in *Science* describing a technique to produce accurate lesions in specific sub-

cortical targets within the human brain. The frame was a modification of the Horsley-Clarke apparatus that had been described 40 years earlier.[7] The electrode holder was mounted on a system to move translationally in each of three planes corresponding to the three Cartesian coordinates. The major technical advance was that it used internal landmarks within the brain for targeting, rather than skull derived landmarks, which would have proven too inaccurate to use in humans.[37] Consequently, they called this new field "stereoencephalotomy." Despite the original plan to treat psychiatric disorders, the first recorded case involved alcohol injection into the pallidum and dorsomedian nucleus in a patient with Huntington chorea, producing significant clinical benefit.[36]

Originally, Spiegel and Wycis[38] used as their landmarks the calcified pineal gland and the foramen of Monro. It was not long, however, before Hassler and Riechert[39] and Talairach et al[40] advocated using the intercommissural line, which immediately became the standard. During the first 2 decades, numerous surgeons visited Spiegel and Wycis and came away with plans to develop their own stereotactic programs. There was no commercially available apparatus, so each surgeon designed his own (**Fig. 1.3**). A great deal of innovation was demonstrated. Leksell[41] produced the first arc-centered device in 1948. Hécaen et al[42] in Paris designed an apparatus that involved insertion of electrodes through a grid system. Riechert and Wolff[43] in Germany introduced a phantom base to adjust their offset arc-centered electrode. Bailey and Stein[44] used a pointing device mounted at the burr hole. Relatedly, Uchimura and Narabayashi,[45] who did not have access to the Western literature in Japan, independently invented a translational type of stereotactic apparatus.

Originally, the lesion was made with the injection of alcohol in hopes of sparing the fibers *en passage*. Spiegel et al[36] soon modified their technique to utilize the same

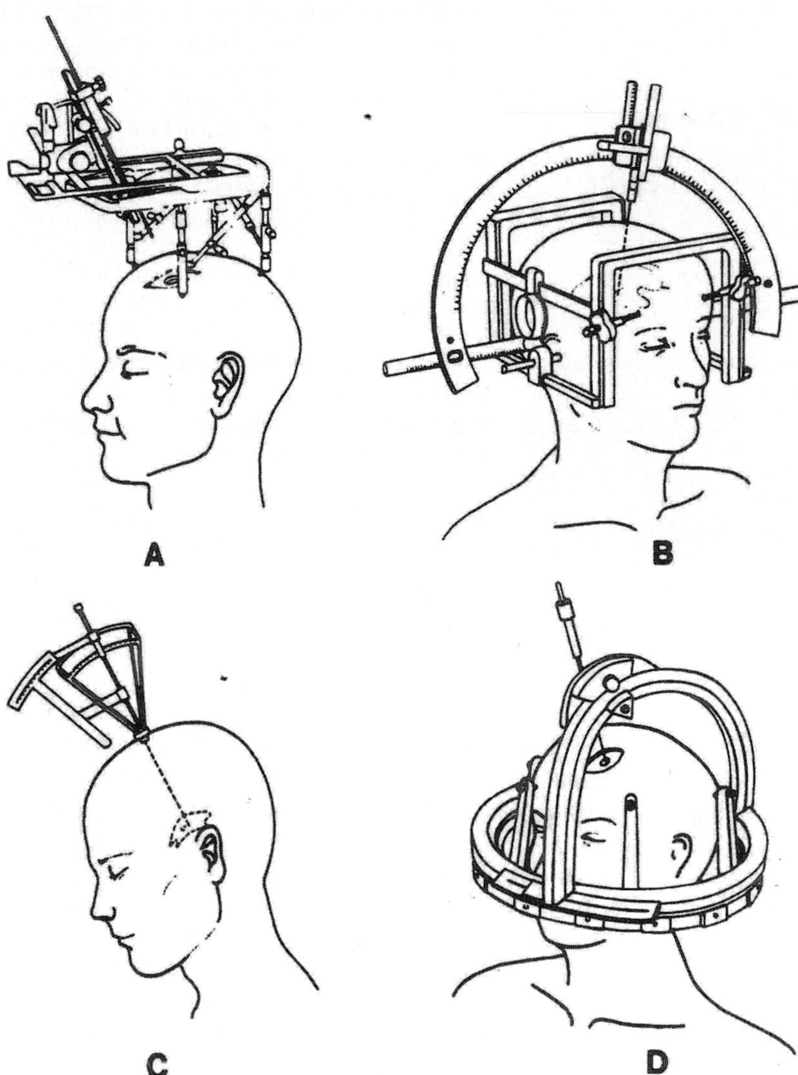

Fig. 1.3 The four basic types of stereotactic apparatus. **(A–C)** developed within the first decade of stereotactic surgery, and **(D)** with the advent of image guided surgery in 1979. **(A)** translational system (Spiegel-Wycis Model V[116]); **(B)** arc centered system (Leksell[41]); **(C)** burr-hole mounted apparatus; **(D)** system of interlocking arcs.

direct current that Horsley and Clarke[7] had described in their 1908 paper. Other techniques were soon developed. Narabayashi and Okuma[46] developed an oil–procaine or oil–procaine–wax mixture. Cooper[47] employed alcohol injection but soon realized that it diffused uncontrollably; he then combined the alcohol with a thickening agent. When that proved also to be poorly controlled,[48] he and colleagues tried to produce a cavity that would contain the alcohol by temporarily inflating a balloon,[49] which still failed to control the extent of the lesion.[48] Obrador developed a mechanical device, a leukotome, with a wire that could be extended to the side to make a lesion by rotating the central shaft.[50] Hassler and Riechert[39] utilized a radio frequency current to heat the tissue adjacent to the electrode tip, and similar devices eventually became the standard means of making a lesion.[51]

An interesting side story concerns Cooper and Lee's[52] plan to use a cryoprobe, a closed cannula through which liquid nitrogen flowed in a controlled fashion to freeze the surrounding tissue. Cooper had coincidentally hired an en-

gineer by the name of Arnold St. J. Lee who had previously worked in Spiegel's laboratory and was the fourth author on the original stereotactic paper.[36] Cooper persisted in use of the cryoprobe even after radio frequency heating became the standard for safe and reliable lesioning.

The first few decades of stereotactic surgery provided a cornucopia of innovation and human experimentation. There were no experimental models for most motor disorders, so it was necessary to develop hypotheses from the logic of what was known about motor control and then try the new procedures in patients. Despite the risks, these patients had few options. All were severely disabled. There were few if any effective medications. The morbidity and mortality rates of open surgery were unacceptable. Movement disorders continued to be the major indication for stereotactic surgery, and eventually most movement disorder surgery involved stereotaxis. The mortality rate decreased from 15% in the pre-stereotactic era[53] to 2% within a year[54] and less than 1% by the second year.[55]

Neurophysiological observations made in the operating room while the electrode was inserted provided the best opportunity to define the pathophysiology of the diseases being treated. Observations on each group of patients led to refinements and improved choice of targets for the next group. It was a period of rapidly advancing knowledge and therapy. Things did not advance in a linear fashion, however. Observations were most often subjective and reports were anecdotal. The selection of a particular target often depended on the success with the prior patient, rather than statistical analyses. Even though such an approach would be looked down upon today, it promoted the rapid, thorough, and empirical development of techniques, some of which have since been validated.

It must be recognized that the progression of PD that existed then was not the same as we see today. Prior to the introduction of L-dopa, patients became disabled more rapidly and presented for surgery much earlier in their disease. There was no medication-induced dyskinesia to be treated. Because tremor was the most obvious symptom and could be quantitated (albeit subjectively) better than bradykinesia or dystonia, most reports of that era discuss only relief of tremor. There were still many patients with postencephalitic parkinsonism in the patient pool, so the average age of the patients tended to be younger than it is now. Consequently, one must be cautious in comparing results from those days with present-day figures.

Although there were a variety of targets for movement disorders, most involved interruption of the extrapyramidal circuit at the globus pallidus, the thalamus, or the pathways in between, and occasionally the subthalamic nucleus (STN) for PD. The literature at the advent of stereotactic surgery used the Walker[56] nomenclature for the thalamic nuclei, and that continued to be most frequently used in the United States. The Europeans, however, adopted Hassler's[57] system when it became available, which identified smaller subnuclei on the basis of subtle differences in cytoarchitecture.

The original target for all movement disorders was in the globus pallidus. In addition, the original intention was to interrupt as many of the emerging fibers as possible, to obtain the greatest extrapyramidal denervation as possible. Lesions involved the emerging fibers of the ansa lenticularis, and the procedure was named pallidoansotomy or pallidothalamotomy.[58] Spiegel,[35] however, was reluctant to interrupt this system in parkinsonian patients. In experimental animals, such lesions may cause hypokinesis, and he feared that the akinesia of PD would be made worse by surgery. It was only after Hassler and Riechert[39] and Talairach et al[59] treated parkinsonism by lesions in the ventrolateral thalamic nucleus in 1951 that stereotactic surgery was considered as a treatment of PD. Spiegel and Wycis[60] began to treat PD, but they primarily targeted the pallidum, however, as did Narabayashi and Okuma[46] and most others.

In 1953, Cooper[61] attempted a nonstereotactic craniotomy to perform Walker's section of the cerebral peduncle in a patient with PD but encountered an interesting "surgical accident." He inadvertently cut a vessel as he exposed the midbrain, and he stopped the procedure as soon as he had controlled the bleeding. The patient awoke with no neurological deficit, and the tremor and rigidity were abolished. In retrospect, Cooper determined that it had been the anterior choroidal artery that had been damaged, so he thereafter advocated purposefully ligating that vessel as a form of treatment. Although there was significant improvement reported in 16% of 55 patients thus treated, the operative mortality rate was 13.3%, and there was a significant morbidity rate as well. Cooper[47] assumed that the benefit was from infarction of the globus pallidus and later advocated injecting that target with alcohol, although by that time the pallidum was already a favorite target of stereotacticians.

When Cooper switched to injecting alcohol into the pallidum in ~1955, he did not use a stereotactic apparatus, but only a needle guide that directed the needle through the temporal lobe somewhat upward toward the globus pallidus.[47] Around 1957, after a patient on whom he had an excellent result died of other causes, the autopsy revealed the lesion not to be in the pallidum but in the ventrolateral thalamus, which then became his target of choice.[49] By that time, however, Hassler and Hess[62] had already defined that thalamic target. In addition Cooper et al[63] advocated pulvinotomy for treatment of spasticity, which was never documented by others.

Athetosis, dyskinesia, and rigidity responded well to pallidotomy. Intention tremor and essential tremor were treated with lesions in the ventrolateral nucleus,[64] according to the Walker nomenclature. This target included Hassler's ventrointermedius (Vim) nucleus, the area eventually identified as the best target for tremor of any etiology.[65] Although poststroke hemiballismus was produced by a small infarction in the STN, it might be treated by making larger STN[66] or thalamic lesions.[67]

When Hassler began to divide the thalamic ventrolateral region into subnuclei in 1954,[57] he and Riechert refined their ventrolateral target to conform to the new nomenclature; they advocated making the lesion for PD in the ventralis oralis posterior for tremor and another in the ventralis oralis anterior for rigidity.[39] However, as time went on, the ideal target for tremor was defined more narrowly within the ventrolateral region, leading to the identification of the Vim subnucleus as the generally accepted target for tremor. Many surgeons followed Riechert and Hassler when they moved their lesion to the thalamus for all parkinsonian manifestations.

Some surgeons, however, continued to advocate pallidotomy. Both studies of Spiegel and Wycis[35] and Leksell and colleagues[68] noted that a lesion placed somewhat more ventral and posterior than the usual pallidoansotomy target might produce increased improvement in rigidity and bradykinesia. In the late 1950s, Spiegel and Wycis and colleagues[69,70] moved their lesion to H Forel field, to interrupt

Editor's Comments

The father of functional neurosurgery is Sir Victor Horsley, who introduced surgery not directed at lesions but at symptoms of epilepsy, trigeminal neuralgia, and movement disorders, including PD, chorea, and dystonia.[118] And of course, he and Clarke introduced the stereotactic frame and stereotactic concept of placing neuroanatomy into a Cartesian coordinate system. He was a man far ahead of his time and it would be 40 years and two World Wars later before Spiegel and Wycis performed the first true stereotactic surgery on a patient.

This early era of functional neurosurgery was marked by trial and error, with an empirical emphasis due to the rudimentary understanding of the neuroanatomy and neuropathophysiology of the motor system. Speigel and Wyclis would lead the scientific study of functional neurosurgery and leave the groundwork for today's practice. In contrast, Irving Cooper would perform a great number of operations and establish very little but succeeded in the popularization of functional neurosurgery in the press. Unfortunately, Cooper was unable to clearly articulate or quantitatively analyze his results. He was probably as honest as his recollection and ego would allow. His reputation was diminished when he promoted anterior choroidal artery ligation as a safe and effective means of treating PD and let his colleagues discover on their own that this procedure is extremely variable in its efficacy and produces an unacceptable mortality rate of ~13%. And, to some, it took on an air of dishonesty.

He never adopted stereotactic techniques but continued to rely on freehand or aiming devices, which led to highly variable results. His "serendipitous" finding that the thalamus was a better target than the globus pallidus represented a targeting error of over a centimeter. How can any of his results be trusted based on the accuracy of this type of targeting? Although he is credited for moving to a target that was better for tremor, the ventrolateral thalamus had already been identified as a better target for tremor by Hassler and Riechert based on a more scientific approach. Many of Cooper's results in the surgical treatment of spasticity, epilepsy, and dystonia remained largely unreproducible. His major contribution was an extremely large surgical experience stimulating interest in several surgical treatments for a variety of movement disorders. However, his superficial analysis of the data, his nonstandardized reporting, and his "enthusiastic" clinical assessment along with a lack of confirmation of targets undoubtedly resulted in unscientific observations for which there can be very little reliability. His observations may be starting points for investigations but they certainly could not be used to prove anything.

Cooper's contribution pales in comparison with that of Spiegel and Wycis who developed true stereotactic techniques with the first clinically usable functional stereotactic frame, publication of a stereotactic atlas, establishment of a journal dedicated to functional and stereotactic neurosurgery, and organized multiple scientific meetings. They trained and inspired generations of functional neurosurgeons. They did not perform large volumes of cases as did Cooper; however, they conducted the surgical investigations in ways that would reliably advance the field. This team of a neurologist and a neurosurgeon that treated every case as a unique opportunity to advance the field should be an example to all of us.

---

the most pallidofugal fibers with the smallest lesion, and they observed further improvement in rigidity and bradykinesia, as well as significant improvement in tremor.

In the early 1960s the intraoperative microelectrode was introduced, not as a localization tool but as a means for studying human neurophysiology, especially the thalamic target for tremor.[71] The use of stereotactic surgery for movement disorders became consolidated during the 1960s, with further study of pathophysiology of the diseases under treatment, ever enlarging series documenting the role of various procedures, and the gradual spread of stereotactic techniques through the neurosurgical community.

Stereotactic surgery had grown from a curiosity to an important procedure during a 20-year period. Spiegel estimated in 1965[72] that 25,000 cases had been done throughout the world, and by 1969[73] that number had grown to 37,000. All the activity came to an abrupt halt at about that time with the introduction of L-dopa for PD control.

■ The Latent Period (1968–1992)

When L-dopa became widely used in 1968, it was thought that it would control PD to the exclusion of stereotactic surgery.

It was not immediately apparent that medical management would have its failures and its complications. Neurologists stopped referring PD patients for stereotactic surgery, and the lines of referral were broken. Many neurosurgeons abandoned stereotaxis, so there were fewer resources to treat other motor disorders. Even when it was realized that L-dopa therapy eventually had diminishing benefit and produced significant dyskinesia, the potential benefit of surgery in this new group of patients was uncertain, especially because many of the symptoms were side-effects of the medication and not symptoms of the primary disease. Because PD had originally been the major indication for movement disorder stereotactic surgery, the field dwindled and was confined to several academic centers. Those few centers that continued to perform stereotactic surgery for other movement disorders continued to see some PD patients, but not with enough regularity to document the benefits. In this vacuum, the focus was redirected to the treatment of the disease process, rather than treating symptoms.

In the early 1980s, it was observed that individuals taking "angel dust," an illicit recreational drug containing MPTP (1-methyl-4-pheryl-1,2,3,6-tetra-hydropyridine) developed a syndrome similar to PD. It was further discovered that MPTP caused a deficit in dopamine, which produced a syndrome similar to PD in experimental animals.[74]

This gave the first laboratory model of this disease, which facilitated and hastened new developments in the treatment of this disease.

In 1985, Backlund et al[75] reported on the first clinical trials of autologous transplantation of adrenal medulla tissue into the head of the caudate nucleus in two patients. The response was modest, and the report was cautious but suggested that further investigation might be warranted. In 1987, Madrazo and his group[76] reported on an additional two patients with perhaps somewhat more encouraging results. Later that year, they reported enthusiastic results in 18 patients,[77] which attracted considerable interest. Soon after, several series were done at several different institutions,[78,79] but with mixed results.[80] In addition, this group of patients with end-stage PD was fragile and tolerated adrenalectomy poorly, and often there was a paucity of medullary tissue in the exhausted adrenal gland.[81] There were significant complications of consciousness and mentation with the craniotomy approach,[82] which generally did not occur with stereotactic injection of the tissue.[83] Despite some encouragement, the long-term results were inadequate, and within 3 years this procedure was no longer performed.

Transplantation of fetal tissue was developing quietly at about the same time. A 1984 symposium was devoted to consideration of the use of embryonic tissue for treatment of central nervous system (CNS) disorders, including movement disorders.[84] The scientific basis for such a move had been documented both experimentally[79] and in initial clinical trials involving at first two patients[85] and then a European consortium.[86] The organization of such surgery is extremely difficult because it is necessary to coordinate the implantation surgery with availability of fetal tissue, sometimes from more than one source, identification and removal of the appropriate tissue, processing of the tissue, and implantation.[78] In addition, late problems may involve an excessive dopamine effect with dyskinesia.[87] At present, initial studies have begun to see whether stem cells might be a more satisfactory source for tissue transplantation for PD.[88] During the latent period, several patients were still referred to those few centers still doing stereotactic surgery for movement disorders, utilizing the same techniques that had been developed prior to 1968, but little new information emerged.

■ Reintroduction of Ablative Stereotactic Surgery (1992–1999)

The field of stereotactic surgery for PD was reawakened by Laitinen and colleagues,[89,90] who reviewed Leksell's old pallidotomy cases and cautiously reintroduced around 1990 the same technique and target for this new group of patients, those suffering not only from PD, but also from the severe side effects of L-dopa–related medication. Se-

vere bradykinesia, severe medication-induced dyskinesia, profound akinesia, and sudden on–off medication effects all responded to varying degrees to stereotactic ventral posterior pallidotomy. Thus the old procedure treated not only the disease but the medication effects as well.

This report prompted an enthusiastic rush back to stereotactic ablative procedures to treat late-stage PD, and many pallidotomy series were reported over the following 5 years.[91-93] Many of the movement disorder neurologists who referred such patients were also involved with neurophysiological laboratory investigations using microelectrode recording, so those techniques were reintroduced into the operating room, this time more to verify localization than to investigate the pathophysiology. In one survey, half the neurosurgeons performing pallidotomy used microelectrodes, but the other half did not.[94] There is a suggestion that the use of microelectrode recording may improve targeting,[92] but there is also concern that it may increase complications, especially bleeding at the electrode site.[95]

The resurgence in stereotactic activity also led to a renewal of investigation into new targets. Improvements in imaging during the latent years permitted more accurate direct visualization of anatomical structures. Lesions have been placed in the STN[96] and the zona incerta[97] with some success.

The coincidental resurgence in activity in ablative surgery for movement disorders and also the spread of stereotactic radiosurgery have converged. Although the gamma knife was originally invented for functional stereotactic surgery, it was rarely used for that purpose. It has recently been suggested that pallidotomy lesions made with the gamma knife have results comparable to conventional stereotactic surgery, with the effect developing gradually over several months,[98] although that view is still controversial.[99]

■ Implanted Stimulators (1997–present)

During the latent period for treatment of movement disorders by stereotactic ablative techniques, implanted stimulators were introduced for the management of pain.[100] The first target for stimulation was the dorsal surface of the spinal cord.[101] However, it soon became apparent that similar pain relief might be obtained by stimulating the area around the third ventricle, which was subsequently identified as a source of endorphins.[102,103]

The first procedure involving an implanted stimulator for treatment of a movement disorder was the insertion of a high cervical, very high frequency spinal cord stimulator for spasmodic torticollis, which occured in 1971.[104] The first report of the use of brain stimulation for movement disorders was by Bechtereva et al[105] in 1975, although she did not have an implantable stimulator available. Her parkinsonian patients came to the laboratory daily for several weeks, during which time she noted considerable, albeit temporary, improvement. The first report (which received insufficient attention) of chronic implantation of deep brain stimulators specifically for treatment of movement disorders was by Brice and McLellan[106] in 1980, who used thalamic stimulators in two patients for management of tremor in multiple sclerosis.

In the mid-1980s, Siegfried and Lippitz[107] and Benabid et al[108] observed improvement in tremor in patients in whom they had implanted thalamic deep brain stimulators for the treatment of pain, although neither study reported these observations until some years later. Both groups subsequently advocated insertion of stimulators for the treatment of PD and dyskinesias. Siegfried and Lippitz[107] stimulate the thalamus and pallidum. Based on laboratory evidence that stimulation of the STN may improve the motor disorder of PD,[109] Benabid's group[110] have concentrated on stimulating the STN. In a reversal of the usual trend, this has led to renewed interest in lesioning the STN, with some success.[111]

Editor's Comments

Those who are ignorant of history are destined to repeat the mistakes of the past. In other words, history provides us with important information on how to proceed in the future. The first and foremost lesson is that becoming a master of a specific technology without moving that technology forward will ultimately result in the obsolescence of that technology. There are multiple examples of this in the history of functional neurosurgery for movement disorders. Being masterful at performing a procedure is only part of the goal. The main emphasis must be in understanding the process and how to push the process forward for greater safety and efficacy, while at the same time preparing for emerging technology. Thus, although it may have been nice to be the "king of pallidotomy," it should be remembered that the pallidotomy kingdom had a very short reign. Ten years ago thousands of pallidotomies were performed, but these have been all but completely replaced by more advanced technology.

The histories of the frame and stereotactic surgery are closely intertwined, but the frame is only the starting place for stereotactic surgery. The ability to registrate in Cartesian coordinates is not restricted to the use of a frame; therefore, frameless technology is the wave of the future. Imaging techniques have always driven the stereotactic field, and the newest and most advanced imaging techniques should be incorporated into the use of functional neurosurgery. This is a time of tremendous interest in the study of the brain and represents great new opportunity for movement disorder neurosurgery. It is absolutely critical in advancing the understanding of the anatomy and electrophysiology of the normal and pathological states. From the frontiers of basic research will come the knowledge for translational clinical investigations. An excellent example is represented in the development of DBS for the STN and the basic monkey electrophysiological studies that led to this novel treatment paradigm. It is unlikely in the future that the reverse will be true. Funding and regulatory agencies will not allow the "cowboy" approach of the past.

And finally, no amount of technological improvement will save the ultimate fate of stereotactic and functional neurosurgery if it is not practiced scientifically. In this regard, it is imperative to be able to scientifically understand functional procedures and outcomes. Any thorough review of the giants of the past will reveal that there are many concepts that they firmly held which proved to be erroneous.[118] Experience is great for developing skills, but it is terrible in blinding us

to the realities and weakness of our own technology. We remember far more about our successes than our failures. We want to excuse the failures of the past with observations of improvements in the present. No one can remember all of these subtleties in the degree of improvement or lack thereof in individual patients. We can have the impression that tremors improve to a greater extent than bradykinesia, but without standardized assessment instruments we cannot make those evaluations quantitative. Without careful records subtleties are lost in the big picture. Although there is a need to experiment and to gain experience, at some point the technology must be put under the scrutiny of a randomized, unbiased assessment.

Bias is all around us. Patients come to us because they want to succeed, and following surgery they are therefore reluctant to deny success even in the face of adversity. Furthermore, patients want to please their surgeon, especially if they find him or her amiable and enthusiastic about the procedure. Surgeons certainly hope for a successful procedure and want to see their patients improve. Furthermore, it is not the individual patient that forms our opinions as much as the group. Thus we can accept that Mr. Smith and Mr. Jones did not get better if there are dozens of others who did get better. In several ways, neurologists, especially if they are an active part of the surgical program, may also be biased toward wanting to see improvements in the patients they refer for surgery. They too do not want to be wrong about the utility of the procedure. Against this background is the tremendous effect of placebo in all medical interventions. This effect is especially powerful in surgical interventions and it is even more so in movement disorders where the symptoms are quite fluctuant and subject to emotional response. Only blinded evaluations of patients randomized in their treatment can completely overcome the effects of bias and placebo.

The technical aspects of movement disorder surgery performed today will be of little value in the future, but the scientific principles will continue to be vital to our future.

Our field will ultimately rise or fall based on the application and deductions of evidence-based medicine. In the future, studies will have to include rigorous, prospective, randomized trials that employ standardized measures performed by experts in a blinded manner that will determine the safety and efficacy of procedures. We have to continuously prove our value.

The effects of moderately high frequency stimulation are nearly the same as making a lesion; hence the targets for stimulation are, for the most part, the same as for lesions in the pallidum and thalamus. In addition, Velasco et al[112] stimulated the prelemniscal radiations with success, a target just lateral to the old campotomy target.[70] The use of implanted stimulators has become commonplace in Europe over the past 5 years and is becoming popular in the United States since approval for use of stimulation was obtained in 2002. The results of stimulation appear to be comparable to lesion production, though with theoretically less risk.

Activity in surgical management of movement disorders is in resurgence. The future holds much promise for progress and innovation, especially as we continue to learn about the pathophysiology of the underlying diseases.

References

1. Fritsch G, Hitzig E. Über die elektrische Erregbarkeit des Grosshirns. Arch Anat Physiol Swiss Med 1870;37:300–332
2. Walker AE. The development of the concept of cerebral localization in the nineteenth century. Bull Hist Med 1957;31:99–121
3. Broca P. Perte de la parole, ramollissement chronique et destruction partielle du lobe antérieur gauche du cerveau [Translation in Wilkins RH. Neurosurgical Classics, American Association of Neurological Surgeons, 1992, pp 63–68]. Bull Soc Anthrop, Paris 1861;2:235–238
4. Horsley V. Remarks on the surgery of the central nervous system. BMJ 1890;2:1286–1292
5. Horsley V. The function of the so-called motor area of the brain. BMJ 1909;2:125–132
6. Horsley V. The Linacre Lecture on the function of the so-called motor area of the brain. BMJ 1909;21:125–132
7. Horsley V, Clarke RH. The structure and functions of the cerebellum examined by a new method. Brain 1908;31:45–124
8. Foerster O. Über eine neue operativ Methode der behandlung spastischer Lahmungen durch Resektion hinterer Ruckenmarkswurzeln. Z Orthop Chir 1908;22:202–223
9. Hunter JI. Influence of sympathetic nervous system in genesis of rigidity of striated muscle in spastic paralysis. Surg Gynecol Obstet 1924;39:721–743
10. Rees CE. Observations following sympathetic ganglionectomy in case of postencephalitic parkinsonian syndrome. Am J Surg 1933;21:411–415
11. Gardner WJ, Williams GH. Interruption of the sympathetic nerve supply to the brain: effect on Parkinson's syndrome. Arch Neurol Psychiatry 1949;61:413–421
12. Rizatti E, Moreno G. Cordotomia laterale posteriore nella cura della ipertonic extrapyramidali postencefalitische. Schizofreni 1936;5:117
13. Meyerson A, Berlin DD. Case of postencephalitic Parkinson's disease treated by total thyroidectomy. N Engl J Med 1934;210:1025–1026
14. Bucy PC, Buchanan DN. Athetosis. Brain 1932;55:479–492
15. Bucy PC, Case TJ. Tremor physiologic mechanism and abolition by surgical means. Arch Neurol Psychiatry 1939;41:721–746
16. Bucy PC. The surgical treatment of abnormal involuntary movements. J Neurosurg Nurs 1970;2:31–39
17. Gillingham FJ, Watson WS, Donaldson AA, Naughton JAL. The surgical treatment of parkinsonism. BMJ 1960;2:1395–1402
18. Polenov AL. New developments in surgery of central nervous system. Vestn Khir 1937;49:223–227
19. Browder J. Section of the fibers of the anterior limb of the internal capsule in Parkinsonism. Am J Surg 1948;75:264–268
20. Takebayashi H. T-tomy, a new technique in extrapyramidal surgery. Med J Osaka Univ 1951;2:4–8
21. Putnam TJ. Relief from unilateral paralysis agitans by section of pyramidal tract. Arch Neurol Psychiatry 1938;40:1049–1054
22. Oliver LC. Surgery in Parkinson's disease: complete section of the lateral column of the spinal cord for tremor. Lancet 1950;i:847–848
23. Putnam TJ. Treatment of athetosis and dystonia by section of the extrapyramidal motor tracts. Arch Neurol Psychiatry 1933;29:504–521
24. Burdenko NN, Klosovski BN. Bulbectomy, Report I: Ceasing of hyperkinetic phenomena by cutting the extrapyramidal tract in the medulla oblongata. Vopr Neirokhir 1937;1:5–16
25. Walker AE. Cerebral pedunculotomy for the relief of involuntary movements; hemiballismus. Acta Psychiatr Neurol Scand 1949;24:723–729
26. Walker AE. Cerebral pedunculotomy for the relief of involuntary movements: parkinsonian tremor. J Nerv Ment Dis 1952;116:766–775
27. Guiot G, Pecker J. Tractotomie mesencephalique anterieure pour tremblement parkinsonien. Rev Neurol 1949;81:387–391
28. Meyers R. Surgical procedure for postencephalitic tremor, with notes on the physiology of premotor fibers. Arch Neurol Psychiatry 1940;44:455–459
29. Dandy WE. Changes in our conceptions of localization of certain functions in the brain. Am J Physiol 1930;93:643–647
30. Meyers R. Dandy's striatal theory of the "center of consciousness": surgical evidence and logical analysis indicating its improbability. Arch Neurol Psychiatry 1951;65:659–671
31. Meyers R. Historical background and personal experiences in the surgical relief of hyperkinesia and hypertonus. In: Fields W, ed. Pathogenesis and Treatment of Parkinsonism. Springfield, IL: Chas C Thomas; 1958:229–270
32. Meyers R. The modification of alternating tremors, rigidity and festination by surgery of the basal ganglia. Assoc Nerv Ment Dis 1942;20:602–665
33. Freeman W, Watts JW. Psychosurgery: Intelligence, Emotional and Social Behavior following Prefrontal Lobotomy for Mental Disorders. Springfield, IL: Chas C Thomas; 1942
34. Moniz E. Prefrontal leucotomy in the treatment of mental disorders. Am J Psychiatry 1994;151(Suppl 6)236–239
35. Spiegel EA. Guided Brain Operations. Basel: Karger; 1982
36. Spiegel EA, Wycis HT, Marks M, Lee AS. Stereotaxic apparatus for operations on the human brain. Science 1947;106:349–350
37. Gildenberg PL. The birth of stereotactic surgery: a personal retrospective. Neurosurgery 2004;54:199–208
38. Spiegel EA, Wycis HT. Stereoencephalotomy, Part I. New York: Grune & Stratton; 1952
39. Hassler R, Riechert T. Indikationen und Lokalisationsmethode der gezielten Hirnoperationen. Nervenarzt 1954;25:441–447
40. Talairach J, David M, Tournoux P, Corredor H, Kvasina T. Atlas d'anatomie stereotaxique. Paris: Masson, 1957
41. Leksell L. A stereotaxic apparatus for intracerebral surgery. Acta Chir Scand 1949;99:229–233
42. Hécaen H, Talairach J, David M, Dell MD. Coagulations limitées du thalamus dans les algies du syndrome thalamique. Rev Neurol (Paris) 1949;81:917–931

43. Riechert T, Wolff M. Über ein neues Zielgeraet zur intrakraniellen elektrischen Abteilung und Ausschaltung. Arch Psychiat Z Neurol 1951;186:225–230

44. Bailey P, Stein SN. A stereotaxic apparatus for use on the human brain. AMA Scientific Exhibit, Atlantic City, NJ; 1951

45. Uchimura Y, Narabayashi H. Stereoencephalotom. Psychiat Neurol Jap 1951;52:265

46. Narabayashi H, Okuma T. Procaine oil blocking of the globus pallidus for the treatment of rigidity and tremor of parkinsonism. Proc Jpn Acad 1953;29:310–318

47. Cooper IS. Chemopallidectomy: an investigative technique in geriatric parkinsonians. Science 1955;121:217

48. Gildenberg PL. Studies in stereoencephalotomy, VIII: Comparison of the variability of subcortical lesions produced by various procedures (radio-frequency coagulation, electrolysis, alcohol injection). Confin Neurol 1957;17:299–309

49. Cooper IS, Bravo G, Riklan M, Davidson N, Gorek E. Chemopallidectomy and chemothalamectomy for parkinsonism. Geriatrics 1958;13:127–147

50. Obrador S. A simplified neurosurgical technique for approaching and damaging the region of the globus pallidus in Parkinson's disease. J Neurol Neurosurg Psychiatry 1957;20:47–49

51. Cosman ER, Nashold BS Jr, Bedenbaugh P. Stereotactic radiofrequency lesion making. Appl Neurophysiol 1983;46:160–166

52. Cooper IS, Lee A St J. Cryostatic congelation. J Nerv Ment Dis 1961;133:259–263

53. Meyers R. Surgical experiments in the therapy of certain "extrapyramidal diseases". Acta Psychiat Neurol 1951;26:1–42

54. Spiegel EA, Wycis HT, Baird HW III. Long-range effects of electropallido-ansotomy in extrapyramidal and convulsive disorders. Neurology 1958;8:734–740

55. Riechert T. Long-term follow-up of results of stereotaxic treatment of extrapyramidal disorders. Confin Neurol 1962;22:356–363

56. Walker AE. Normal and pathological physiology of the thalamus. In: Schaltenbrand G, Walker AE, eds. Stereotaxy of the Human Brain. Stuttgart, New York: Georg Thieme Verlag; 1982:181–217

57. Hassler R. Architectonic organization of the thalamic nuclei. In: Schaltenbrand G, Walker AE, eds. Stereotaxy of the Human Brain. Stuttgart, New York: Georg Thieme Verlag; 1982:140–180

58. Spiegel EA, Wycis HT. Pallido-thalamotomy in chorea. Arch Neurol Psychiat Chicago 1950;64:495–496

59. Talairach J, De Ajuriaguerra J, David M. Etudes stéréotaxiques et structures encephaliques profondes chez l'homme. Presse Med 1952;28:605–609

60. Spiegel EA, Wycis HT. Ansotomy in paralysis agitans. AMA Arch Neurol Psychiatry 1954;71:598–614

61. Cooper IS. Ligation of the anterior choroidal artery for involuntary movements of parkinsonism. Psychiatr Q 1953;27:317–319

62. Hassler R, Hess WR. Experimentelle und anatomische Befunde Über die Drehbewegungen und die nervösen Apparate. Arch Psychiatr Nervenkr 1954;192:488–526

63. Cooper IS, Amin I, Chandra R, Waltz JM. A surgical investigation of the clinical physiology of the LP- pulvinar complex in man. J Neurol Sci 1973;18:89–110

64. Cooper IS. Neurosurgical alleviation of intention tremor of multiple sclerosis and cerebellar disease. N Engl J Med 1960;263:441–444

65. Ohye C, Maeda T, Narabayashi H. Physiologically defined VIM nucleus: its special reference to control of tremor. Appl Neurophysiol 1976;39:285–295

66. Spiegel EA, Wycis HT. Sterencephalotomy, Part II. New York: Grune & Stratton; 1962

67. Andy OJ. Diencephalic coagulation in the treatment of hemiballism. Confin Neurol 1962;22:346–350

68. Svennilson E, Torvik A, Lowe R, Leksell L. Treatment of parkinsonism by stereotactic thermolesions in the pallidal region: a clinical evaluation of 81 cases. Acta Psychiatr Neurol Scand 1960;35:358–377

69. Spiegel EA, Wycis HT, Szekely EG, Adams J, Flanagan M, Baird HW. Campotomy in various extrapyramidal disorders. J Neurosurg 1963;20:871–881

70. Spiegel EA, Wycis HT, Szekely EG, Soloff L, Adams J, Gildenberg PL. Stimulation of Forel's field during stereotaxic operations in the human brain. Electroencephalogr Clin Neurophysiol 1964;16:537–548

71. Albe-Fessard D, Arfel G, Guiot G, Hardy J, Hertzog E, Aleonard P. Identification et délimitation précise de certaines structures souscorticales de l'homme par l'electro-physiologie. CR Acad Sci (Paris) 1961;243:2412–2414

72. Spiegel EA. Methodological problems in stereoencephalotomy. Confin Neurol 1965;26:125–132

73. Spiegel EA. History of human stereotaxy (stereoencephalotomy). In: Schaltenbrand G, Walker AE, eds. Stereotaxy of the Human Brain: Anatomical, Physiological and Clinical Applications. Stuttgart, New York: Georg Thieme Verlag; 1982:3–10

74. Bakay RA, Fiandaca MS, Barrow DL, Schiff A, Collins DC. Preliminary report on the use of fetal tissue transplantation to correct MPTP-induced Parkinson-like syndrome in primates. Appl Neurophysiol 1985;48:358–361

75. Backlund EO, Granberg PO, Hamberger B, Knutsson E, Martensson A, Sedvall G. Transplantation of adrenal medullary tissue to striatum in parkinsonism: first clinical trials. J Neurosurg 1985;62:169–173

76. Madrazo I, Drucker-Colin R, Diaz V. Open microsurgical autograft of adrenal medulla to the right caudate nucleus in two patients with intractable Parkinson's disease. N Engl J Med 1987;316:831–834

77. Drucker-Colin R, Madrazo I, Diaz V. Open microsurgical autograft of adrenal medulla to caudate nucleus of patients with Parkinson's disease. Schmitt Neurological Sciences Symposium, Rochester, NY; June 30–July 3, 1987

78. Bakay RA, Barrow DL. Neural transplantation for Parkinson's disease. J Neurosurg 1988;69:807–810

79. Bakay RA, Herring CJ. Central nervous system grafting in the treatment of parkinsonism. Stereotact Funct Neurosurg 1989;53:1–20

80. Penn RD, Goetz CG, Tanner CM, et al. The adrenal medullary transplant operation for Parkinson's disease: clinical observations in five patients. Neurosurgery 1988;22:999–1006

81. Stoddard SL, Tyce GM, Ahlskog JE, Zinsmeister AR, Carmichael SW. Decreased catecholamine content in parkinsonian adrenal medullae. Exp Neurol 1989;104:22–27

82. Jankovic J, Grossman R, Goodman C, et al. Clinical, biochemical, and neuropathologic findings following transplantation of adrenal medulla to the caudate nucleus for treatment of Parkinson's disease. Neurology 1989;39:1227–1234

83. Gildenberg PL, Pettigrew LC, Merrell R, et al. Transplantation of adrenal medullary tissue to caudate nucleus using stereotactic techniques. Stereotact Funct Neurosurg 1990;54–55:268–271

84. Proceedings of the Colloquium on the Use of Embryonic Cell Transplantation for Correction of CNS Disorders. Chestnut Hill, Mass., June 27–29, 1983. Appl Neurophysiol 1984;47:1–76

85. Lindvall O, Rehncrona S, Brundin P, et al. Human fetal dopamine neurons grafted into the striatum in two patients with severe Parkinson's disease: a detailed account of methodology and a 6-month follow-up. Arch Neurol 1989;46:615–631

86. Hitchcock ER, Clough CG, Hughes RC, Kenny BG. Transplantation in Parkinson's disease: stereotactic implantation of adrenal medulla and foetal mesencephalon. Acta Neurochir Suppl (Wien) 1989;46:48–50

87. Freed CR, Greene PE, Breeze RE, et al. Transplantation of embryonic dopamine neurons for severe Parkinson's disease. N Engl J Med 2001;344:710–719

88. Freed CR. Will embryonic stem cells be a useful source of dopamine neurons for transplant into patients with Parkinson's disease? Proc Natl Acad Sci U S A 2002;99:1755–1757

89. Laitinen LV, Bergenheim AT, Hariz MI. Ventroposterolateral pallidotomy can abolish all parkinsonian symptoms. Stereotact Funct Neurosurg 1992;58:14–21

90. Laitinen LV, Bergenheim AT, Hariz MI. Leksell's posteroventral pallidotomy in the treatment of Parkinson's disease. J Neurosurg 1992;76:53–61

91. Goetz CG, Diederich NJ. There is a renaissance of interest in pallidotomy for Parkinson's disease. Nat Med 1996;2:510–514

92. Lozano A, Hutchison W, Kiss Z, Tasker R, Davis K, Dostrovsky J. Methods for microelectrode-guided posteroventral pallidotomy. J Neurosurg 1996;84:194–202

93. Vitek JL, Bakay RA. The role of pallidotomy in Parkinson's disease and dystonia. Curr Opin Neurol 1997;10:332–339

94. Favre J, Taha JM, Nguyen TT, Gildenberg PL, Burchiel KJ. Pallidotomy: a survey of current practice in North America. Neurosurgery 1996;39:883–892

95. Hariz MI. Safety and risk of microelectrode recording in surgery for movement disorders. Stereotact Funct Neurosurg 2002;78: 146–157

96. Patel NK, Heywood P, O'Sullivan K, McCarter R, Love S, Gill SS. Unilateral subthalamotomy in the treatment of Parkinson's disease. Brain 2003;126:1136–1145

97. Nandi D, Chir M, Liu X, et al. Electrophysiological confirmation of the zona incerta as a target for surgical treatment of disabling involuntary arm movements in multiple sclerosis: use of local field potentials. J Clin Neurosci 2002;9:64–68

98. Young RF. Gamma knife radiosurgery as an alternative form of therapy for movement disorders. Arch Neurol 2002;59:1660–1662

99. Okun MS, Vitek JL, Delong MR. Not our knife: gamma knife surgery for Parkinson disease. Arch Neurol 2002;59:1334–1335

100. Shealy CN, Mortimer JT, Reswick JB. Electrical inhibition of pain by stimulation of the dorsal columns: preliminary clinical report. Anesth Analg 1967;46:489–491

101. Nashold BS Jr, Somjen G, Friedman H. The effects of stimulating the dorsal columns of man. Med Prog Technol 1972;1:89–91

102. Long DM, Hagfors N. Electrical stimulation in the nervous system: the current status of electrical stimulation of the nervous system for relief of pain. Pain 1975;1:109–123

103. Richardson DE, Akil H. Pain reduction by electrical brain stimulation in man, I: Acute administration in periaqueductal and periventricular sites. J Neurosurg 1977;47:178–183

104. Gildenberg PL. Treatment of spasmodic torticollis by dorsal column stimulation. Appl Neurophysiol 1978;41:113–121

105. Bechtereva NP, Bondartchuk AN, Smirnov VM, Meliutcheva LA, Shandurina AN. Method of electrostimulation of the deep brain structures in treatment of some chronic diseases. Confin Neurol 1975;37:136–140

106. Brice J, McLellan L. Suppression of intention tremor by contingent deep-brain stimulation. Lancet 1980;1:1221–1222

107. Siegfried J, Lippitz B. Chronic electrical stimulation of the VL–VPL complex and of the pallidum in the treatment of movement disorders: personal experience since 1982. Stereotact Funct Neurosurg 1994;62:71–75

108. Benabid AL, Pollak P, Gervason C, et al. Long-term suppression of tremor by chronic stimulation of the ventral intermediate thalamic nucleus. Lancet 1991;337:403–406

109. Delong MR. Primate models of movement disorders of basal ganglia origin. Trends Neurosci 1990;13:281–285

110. Benabid AL, Pollak P, Gross C, et al. Acute and long-term effects of subthalamic nucleus stimulation in Parkinson's disease. Stereotact Funct Neurosurg 1994;62:76–84

111. Alvarez L, Macias R, Guridi J, et al. Dorsal subthalamotomy for Parkinson's disease. Mov Disord 2001;16:72–78

112. Jimenez F, Velasco F, Velasco M, et al. Subthalamic prelemniscal radiation stimulation for the treatment of Parkinson's disease: electrophysiological characterization of the area. Arch Med Res 2000;31:270–281

113. Kandel EI. Functional and Stereotactic Neurosurgery. New York, London: Plenum; 1989.

114. Fenelon F. Essais de traitement ceurochirurgical du syndrome parkinsonien par intervention directe sur les voies extrapyramidales immédiatement sous striopallidales (anse lenticulaire): Communication suivie de projection du film d'un opérés pris avant at après l'intervention. Rev Neurol (Paris) 1950;83:437–440

115. Guiot G, Brion S. Traitment neurochirurgical de syndrome choreoathetosique et parkinsoniens. Sem Hop Paris 1952;49:2095–2099

116. Spiegel EA, Wycis HT, Goode R. Studies in stereoencephalotomy, V: A universal stereoencephalotome (Model V) for use in man and experimental animals. J Neurosurg 1956;13:305–309

117. Heilbrun MP, Roberts TS, Apuzzo ML, Wells TH Jr, Sabshin JK. Preliminary experience with Brown-Roberts-Wells (BRW) computerized tomography stereotaxic guidance system. J Neurosurg 1983;59:217–222

118. Bakay RAE. History of functional neurosurgery. In: Winn HR, ed. Youmans Neurological Surgery. Philadelphia: Saunders; 2004:2653–2669

Rationale for Movement Disorder Surgery

Cameron C. McIntyre, Christopher R. Butson, Benjamin L. Walter, and Jerrold L. Vitek

Surgical interventions for movement disorders have been practiced for decades, beginning with early studies that used lesions to eliminate activity in localized brain regions. Later, deep brain stimulation (DBS) grew out of observations during such surgery. Surgeons using stimulating/recording electrodes for target confirmation during ablative surgery found that stimulation of the brain had effects similar to lesioning, specifically that high frequency stimulation (> 100 Hz) of the motor thalamus produced tremor arrest.[1] These early studies eventually proved that functional neurosurgery for movement disorders can alleviate symptoms and improve the quality of life for disabling diseases such as Parkinson disease (PD), essential tremor (ET), and dystonia in appropriately selected patients. Although these surgeries were initially based on empirical observations, the advancement of scientific understanding and medical technology has allowed for an evolution from empirically to rationally based surgical strategies. Current surgical approaches incorporate magnetic resonance imaging (MRI)-based stereotactically and neurophysiologically guided targeting where the selection of the target(s) is based on pathophysiological understanding of the disorder.

Of the three major movement disorders for which surgical efficacy has been demonstrated (PD, ET, and dystonia), each has significant differences in the underlying pathophysiology. The cardinal symptoms of PD include resting tremor, rigidity, bradykinesia, and akinesia, as well as postural and gait disturbances.[2,3] The pathological hallmark of PD is the degeneration of dopaminergic cells within the substantia nigra with deposition of cytoplasmic eosinophilic inclusions (Lewy bodies) and subsequent dopamine depletion of the striatum. Clinical manifestations of PD occur when nigrostriatal dopamine loss reaches ~60%.[4] Dopamine denervation of the striatum triggers a cascade of events within the basal ganglia that impairs its ability to appropriately interact with the rest of the nervous system. Medical treatment of PD with levodopa is not the panacea it was initially thought to be due to the late complications of levodopa-induced dyskinesias and increased motor fluctuations. Even with molecular and genetically based therapies on the horizon aimed at slowing the progression of PD, there is and will be for the foreseeable future a large population of patients significantly burdened by this neurodegenerative disease.

Approximately 4% of the population > 40 years of age exhibit symptoms of ET.[5,6] Most ET patients have mild symptoms that can be controlled with medication. However, a significant number of patients are refractory to medication, have significant disability, and are unable to perform simple activities of daily living or maintain employment. Although the neurophysiological origin of tremor remains debated within the scientific community, there remains a sustained need to address the limitations of current pharmacological approaches to the treatment of ET.

Dystonia is characterized by sustained muscle contractions, leading to twisting, repetitive movements, and abnormal postures. It can be focal, involving a single body region, segmental, involving two or more adjacent regions, or generalized, involving both legs plus at least one other region. Dystonia can be a symptom of destructive disease processes and in such cases is termed secondary dystonia. Dystonia with no obvious pathology is called primary dystonia. Some of these patients have now been found to have an inherited gene mutation, and there are now over 14 gene loci identified in association with dystonia. DYT1 dystonia, the most common of these, typically starts focally with one limb in early childhood and slowly generalizes to involve other body regions. Other genetic loci responsible for primary generalized dystonia include DYT2, 4, 6, 7, and 13.[7]

Reports of neuropathological examination of patients with suspected primary generalized dystonia are limited, and standard MRI scans have been reported as normal. Until recently no neuropathological changes have been reported in the brains of DYT1 patients.[8] However, a recent study found perinuclear inclusion bodies that stain positive for ubiquitin, torsinA, and lamin A/C in the pedunculopontine nucleus, cuneiform nucleus, and griseum centrale mesencephal.[9] Clinicopathological studies in patients with secondary dystonia indicate that the most common site in which a lesion can be identified is in the striatum, or pallidum.[10] Thalamic lesions, although less common, have also been observed in patients with dystonia.[11] Dystonia is a particularly disabling condition, and although many patients with focal dystonias involving small muscle groups may respond to botulinum toxin, others with more diffuse involvement or involvement of larger muscle groups have limited success with traditional medical therapies.

PD, ET, and dystonia each represent especially debilitating diseases that affect significant numbers of patients who do not adequately respond to pharmacological interventions. In turn, functional neurosurgery has been employed in each disease state with substantial degrees of success. The combination of basic science understanding, advancing medical technology, and clinical acceptance has allowed the development of successful surgical practices and clinical centers. Currently there are two forms of surgical intervention for movement disorders that are used most commonly (ablation and DBS), and three general anatomical targets [thalamus, subthalamic nucleus (STN), and globus pallidus (GP)] to which these approaches are applied. Thalamic DBS for intractable tremor has virtually replaced ablative lesions of the thalamus.[12] Similarly, DBS of the STN or internal segment of the globus pallidus (GPi) has largely replaced pallidotomy in the treatment of the cardinal motor features of PD (resting tremor, rigidity, bradykinesia).[13] In addition, multiple pilot studies have begun to examine the utility of DBS for dystonia,[14,15] epilepsy,[16] and obsessive–compulsive disorder (OCD).[17] As data from larger controlled trials become available, neurologists and neurosurgeons will be able to tailor the therapy for their patient based on the patient's disease characteristics (i.e., appropriate choice of target site and mode of treatment, ablation, or stimulation). Furthermore, we will be able to better predict the degree of clinical benefit and risk of adverse side effects based on characteristics of the patient's disease, age, and other clinical variables.

■ Anatomy and Physiology of the Basal Ganglia and Thalamus

The basal ganglia (BG) are located in the basal telencephalon and consist of four interconnected nuclei: the striatum, GP, substantia nigra, and STN (**Fig. 2.1**). The thalamus is a large, oval-shaped structure that constitutes the dorsal portion of the diencephalon and acts as the gateway to the cortex. All sensory pathways (except olfaction) relay in the thalamus en route to the cerebral cortex as well as many of the anatomical circuits of the cerebellum, BG, and limbic structures.

The striatum is the main input structure of the BG; the GPi and the substantia nigra pars reticulata (SNr) are the output nuclei.[18] Glutamatergic projections from virtually all cortical areas, as well as dopaminergic inputs from the substantia nigra pars compacta (SNc), converge onto spiny projection neurons in the striatum. Striatal output typically consists of low-frequency activity (~10 Hz), which is transmitted to the output nuclei (GPi and SNr) via either a direct or an indirect pathway.[18–20] In the direct pathway, one subpopulation of spiny neurons projects directly to the output nuclei (GPi and SNr) of the BG. A separate subpopulation of striatal neurons follows an indirect pathway, first projecting to the external segment of the globus pallidus (GPe), which projects to the STN, which in turn sends projections to the GPi and SNr. The subpopulations of spiny neurons that give rise to the direct and indirect pathways are characterized by their selective expression of neuropeptide and dopamine receptor subtypes.[21] Although all striatal spiny neurons use gamma-amino butyric acid (GABA) as their main neurotransmitter, the subpopulation that gives rise to the direct pathway preferentially express the D1 subtype of the dopamine receptor (primarily excitatory), and the subpopulation that gives rise to the indirect pathway preferentially express the D2 subtype of the dopamine receptor (primarily inhibitory).[20] In turn, dopaminergic inputs from the SNc can explicitly modulate the transmission of neural activity through the direct and indirect pathways (**Fig. 2.1**).

The GPe, GPi, and SNr are each composed primarily of projection neurons that typically exhibit a consistent high-frequency (~60 Hz) firing pattern and use GABA as their main neurotransmitter. The inhibitory GPe output is transmitted to the GPi and STN. The STN is composed primarily of projection neurons that typically exhibit a consistent midfrequency (~40 Hz) firing pattern and use glutamate as their main neurotransmitter. Excitatory STN output makes a feedback loop with GPe and also projects to GPi and SNr. In addition, the STN receives direct excitatory cortical inputs that can modulate its firing rate and pattern. The direct and indirect pathways both project to the GPi and SNr, which sends inhibitory projections to the thalamus (**Fig. 2.1**).

By virtue of the neurotransmitters and baseline activity of neurons in the BG network, activation of the direct or indirect pathways can produce functionally opposite effects on thalamic output.[20] Corticostriatal neurons, thalamocortical neurons, and neurons of the STN are excitatory, utilizing glutamate as a neurotransmitter. All other neurons in the BG network are inhibitory, using GABA as their main neurotransmitter. Under resting conditions, the activity of the output neurons of the striatum is low compared with that of tonically active neurons in the GPe and STN. Activation of the corticostriatal pathway leads to increased firing of striatal neurons. Increased activity of striatal neurons in the direct pathway (striatum ⇢ GPi/SNr) leads to inhibition of the output nuclei (GPi and SNr). A reduction in tonic activity of the neurons in GPi/SNr leads to a reduction in the inhibition of neurons in the thalamus and increased thalamocortical output. In contrast, activation of the indirect pathway (striatum ⇢ GPe ⇢ STN ⇢ GPi/SNr), leads to the opposite functional effect on the thalamus. Increased activity of the striatal output neurons inhibits the tonically active neurons in the GPe. Inhibition of the neurons in GPe disinhibits neurons in the STN. Increased activity of the excitatory neurons of the STN leads to increased firing of neurons in GPi and SNr. An increase in the tonic activity of the neurons in GPi and SNr leads to an increase in the inhibition of neurons in the thalamus and a reduction in thalamocortical output (**Fig. 2.1**).

The thalamus is composed of nuclei most commonly classified into four groups (anterior, medial, ventrolateral, and posterior) based on the anatomical divisions created by the internal medullary lamina. The ventrolateral thalamus constitutes nearly all the nuclei intimately involved in sensorimotor function. The motor thalamus can be further subdivided into distinct relays for BG and cerebellar afferents. These channels in turn gain access to different functional regions of the cerebral cortex.[22] Anatomical tracing studies in nonhuman primates show that pallidal

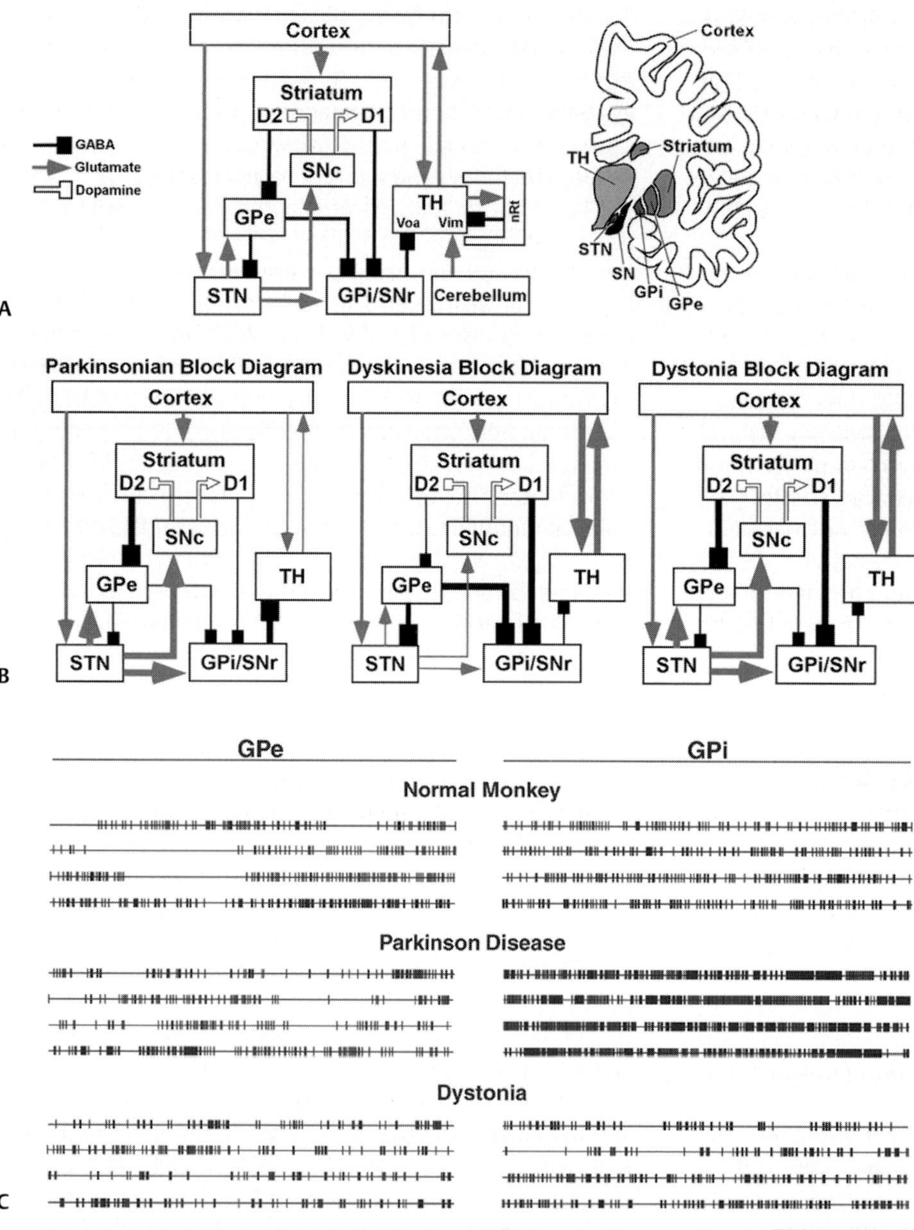

Fig. 2.1 Basal–ganglia–thalamo–cortical network. **(A)** Simplified circuit diagram of the basal ganglia. Relative thickness of the lines indicates degree of activation, arrows represent excitatory synapses, squares represent inhibitory synapses, and line color indicates neurotransmitter [white, dopamine; gray, glutamate; black, gamma-amino butyric acid (GABA)]. Cortical information that reaches the striatum is conveyed to the basal ganglia output structures [internal segment of the globus pallidus (GPi) and the substantia nigra pars reticulata (SNr)] via two pathways, a direct inhibitory projection from the striatum to the GPi/SNr, and an indirect network that involves an inhibitory projection from the striatum to the external segment of the globus pallidus (GPe), an inhibitory projection from the GPe to the subthalamic nucleus (STN), an inhibitory projection from the GPe to the GPi/SNr, and an excitatory projection from the STN to the GPi/SNr. The information is then transmitted back to the cerebral cortex via a relay in the thalamus. **(B)** In Parkinson disease, the dopaminergic cell loss of the substantia nigra pars compacta (SNc) causes a cascade of alterations affecting all the other components of the circuit. The final result is the increased activity of the GABAergic output nuclei GPi/SNr, which causes increased inhibition of the motor thalamus. By contrast, hyperkinetic disorders such as dystonia result in increased inhibition of GPi/SNr, resulting in decreased inhibition of thalamus and overactivity of thalamic projections to cortex. **(C)** Examples of rasters of spontaneous neuronal activity in a normal monkey (top), a patient with Parkinson disease (PD) (middle), and a patient with dystonia (bottom). These illustrate the firing rates in GPi are reduced in dystonia and increased in PD.[93,94] In both PD and dystonia there are abnormal, irregular grouped discharges in GPi, whereas in normal primates GPi has a more tonic regular firing pattern.[93] (Sources: Alexander GE, Crutcher MD, DeLong MR. "Basal ganglia–thalamocortical circuits: parallel substrates for motor, oculomotor, "prefrontal" and "limbic" functions." In: Uylings HBM, Van Eden CG, De Bruin JPC, Corner MA, Feenstra MGP, eds. Progress in Brain Research. New York: Elsevier Science Publishers; 1990 and Smith Y, Bevan MD, Shink E, Bolam JP. Microcircuitry of the direct and indirect pathways of the basal ganglia. Neuroscience 1998;86:353–387.)

and cerebellar receiving areas in the thalamus are largely segregated. GPi projects to the anterior part of the ventrolateral thalamus (human–Voa/Vop; monkey–VLo), which predominantly projects to the supplementary motor cortex. The cerebellum predominantly projects to the posterior part of the ventrolateral thalamus (human–Vim/Voi; monkey–VPLo), which then projects to the motor cortex (area 4) and arcuate premotor area.[23,24]

The majority of neurons within the various thalamic nuclei are thalamocortical projection neurons that use glutamate as their primary neurotransmitter. These neurons typically exhibit a relatively low frequency tonic firing pattern (~20 Hz). However, thalamic neurons transition from a tonic firing pattern to a low-frequency burst firing pattern (~4 to 8 Hz interburst interval) dependent on the behavioral state, which determines the synaptic input conditions.[25,26] Another major component of the thalamic network consists of a thin sheet of inhibitory neurons, known as the reticular nucleus (nRt). The nRt forms the anterior lateral and a portion of the dorsal surfaces of the thalamus. Reticular neurons provide widespread inhibitory input to cells in the entire thalamus. In addition, thalamocortical projection neurons provide direct inputs to reticular thalamic neurons, generating tightly linked feedback loops. In turn, the interaction of the thalamocortical and reticular neurons provides an additional degree of information processing within both motor and nonmotor circuits of the thalamocortical system[27] (**Fig. 2.1**).

The rate-based block diagram of the BG–thalamocortical network is a highly simplified representation. The feedback interaction between the STN and GPe,[28,29] direct cortical inputs to the STN,[30] and the interaction of additional nuclei such as the pedunculopontine nucleus[31] and reticular thalamus[20] complicate our understanding of this network. In addition, this model does not take into account the pattern and/or synchrony of neural activity in each of the interacting nuclei. Although the rate-based model does not capture all of the important details pertinent to this understanding of the pathophysiological basis underlying the development of hypokinetic and hyperkinetic movement disorders, it has provided a great deal of scientific and clinical insight that has led to testable hypotheses and the development of alternate models that take these new observations into account.

■ Pathophysiological Basis of Movement Disorders

Our understanding of the pathophysiological basis of hypo- and hyperkinetic movement disorders has increased significantly over the last decade. The physiology of the normal brain relative to hyper- and hypokinetic disease states is summarized in **Fig. 2.1**, which highlights the neuronal activity changes that take place in the BG and thalamus in these disease states. Sensorimotor, associative, oculomo-

tor, and limbic circuits originate in specific cortical areas, pass through distinct portions of the BG and thalamus, and project back to their cortical area of origin. These circuits are anatomically and functionally segregated throughout the BG–thalamo–cortical network, and disruption of the motor circuit is of primary interest in analysis of movement disorders. Both neuronal firing rates and patterns of activity within the BG network are now considered important in the genesis of movement disorders. In addition, the contribution of altered receptive fields and changes in synchrony are just now being appreciated. These scientific advances are providing a rationale for the selection of anatomical targets for ablative or DBS movement disorder surgery.

The pathophysiological basis underlying the development of PD has been developed from electrophysiological studies in animal models of PD as well as from humans with idiopathic PD undergoing functional neurosurgical procedures. The loss of dopamine from the SNc in PD is proposed to lead to differential changes in neuronal activity of striatal cells in the direct and indirect pathway. In the direct pathway, loss of dopamine at striatal excitatory D1 receptors leads to a decrease of inhibitory activity from the striatum to GPi. In the indirect pathway, there is loss of dopamine at inhibitory D2 receptors leading to increased activity of inhibitory striatal neurons projecting to GPe causing a reduction of GPe activity. The decrease in inhibitory output from GPe to STN leads to excessive excitation from the STN to the GPi. Thus there is an increase in inhibitory activity from the GPi to the thalamus and brain stem, via both the direct and the indirect pathways (**Fig. 2.1B**), which has been implicitly implicated as the change in neuronal circuits that underlies the development of the hypokinetic features associated with PD.[32] Changes in mean firing rates of neurons in GPe, GPi, STN, and VLo in the 1-methyl-4-phenyl-1,2,3,6-tetrahydropyridine (MPTP) monkey model of PD, and in GPe and GPi in patients with idiopathic PD, show a decrease in mean discharge rates in GPe and VLo and an increase in mean discharge rates in STN and GPi.[32–35] These changes are consistent with predictions from the rate-based block diagram of PD. Similarly, a loss or lowering of inhibitory input from GPi to the thalamus has been proposed as the basis for the development of the hyperkinetic movements associated with drug-induced dyskinesias and other hyperkinetic disorders (e.g., dystonia and hemiballismus).

Changes in neuronal firing rates alone, however, are not sufficient to explain the pathophysiology of PD or hyperkinetic movement disorders. Lesions within the motor thalamus do not exacerbate or induce parkinsonian motor signs, but instead, are reported to improve or abolish parkinsonian tremor, rigidity, and drug-induced dyskinesias.[36,37] Similarly, lesions in the GPi do not induce hyperkinetic movement disorders, but instead have been reported to abolish drug-induced dyskinesias as well as the involuntary movements associated with dystonia and hemiballismus. These results suggest that a decrease in activity of thalamic neurons cannot by itself account for the development of parkinsonian motor signs, nor can a reduction in the rate of GPi neurons account for the development of drug-induced dyskinesias, dystonia, or hemiballismus.[38,39] These contradictions of the rate model have led to the incorporation of additional hypotheses to explain the pathophysiology of hypokinetic and hyperkinetic movement disorders.

In addition to the changes in neuronal firing rate, movement disorders are also associated with altered patterns of neuronal activity, changes in somatosensory responsiveness, and the degree of synchrony of neurons within the BG and thalamus (**Fig. 2.1**). The physiological basis for the development of PD has been a much debated issue. However, it appears likely that PD motor symptoms arise from a combination of changes in both rate and pattern. Observations of increased bursting and rhythmic oscillatory patterns within the BG and thalamus are common in both parkinsonian monkeys and humans with PD.[19,40] Bursting activity of thalamic neurons in the cerebellar receiving area of the thalamus is strongly correlated with tremor in PD, as well as ET.[41] In addition, oscillatory activity, changes in somatosensory responsiveness, and degree of synchronization of pallidal and STN neurons are considered prominent features of PD pathophysiology.[29]

Pathophysiologically, dystonia can be viewed as either a hypo- or hyperkinetic movement disorder. Dystonia may be a presenting symptom in parkinsonian patients who are not taking antiparkinsonian medications ("off"-dystonia)

or alternatively may appear as a consequence of L-dopa treatment (peak dose dystonia). Electrophysiological recordings of pallidal neurons in patients with idiopathic dystonia demonstrate a decrease in the mean discharge rates of GPi neurons, consistent with predictions based on the "rate" model for hyperkinetic movement disorders.[42–44] However, in addition to decreased mean discharge rates, neuronal activity in the BG of dystonic patients have also demonstrated altered patterns of activity and widened receptive fields.[44] Uncontrolled changes in synchronization of neuronal populations in GPi may also occur and have been suggested to play an important role in the development of dystonia.[45] However, the exact relationship between changes (rate and pattern) in neural activity and the development of dystonia remains unclear.

The clear clinical improvements in movement disorder symptoms after thalamotomy, subthalamotomy, pallidotomy, or DBS are difficult to reconcile based solely on regularization of firing rate because each intervention should result in a different effect on rate. Therefore, given the pathophysiological characteristics of neuronal firing patterns in movement disorders, it has been suggested that the therapeutic effects of the treatment are dictated primarily by effects on the firing pattern. Based on this hypothesis, both ablation and DBS are effective in the treatment of movement disorders because they replace pathological neuronal activity with either no activity (ablation) or a highly regular firing pattern (DBS).[46–48]

Editor's Comments

For most of the last century, the basal ganglia was viewed as a collection of deep brain nuclei interconnected with the thalamus to form the extrapyramidal system, which, when disrupted, produced diseases quite apart from the pyramidal system. It was not until the 1980s when integration of the basal ganglia, thalamus, and cortex began to emerge from the work of Albin, Alexander, Delong, and colleagues.[95,96] The critical finding in this work was that of a network of basal ganglia/thalamocortical circuits that subserved five separate functions, each segregated from the other, and involved projections from specific cortical areas to separate areas within the subcortical structures that projected recurrently in a closed loop manner back to the original cortical areas through specific thalamic relay nuclei.

In large part, our understanding of these loops relates to many factors, including multiple advances in the neurosciences, but is especially indebted to the MPTP monkey model of Parkinson disease, which allowed the opportunity to characterize biochemical, electrophysiological, and behavioral changes in the basal ganglia as they relate to the parkinsonian state.[32] Of the cortico–striato–pallido–thalamocortical loops, the motor loop is that which is most relevant to movement disorders. Widespread involvement of the nonmotor circuits, such as the oculomotor, dorsolateral prefrontal (executive function), associative, and limbic, may explain many of the nonmotor symptoms that characterize Parkinson disease. But it is the motor circuit that helps us understand the cardinal features of

Parkinson disease.[97] Within the motor loop there are the direct (striatum–GPi) and the indirect (striatum–GPe–STN–GPi) projections to the thalamus that have opposite functional effects and are the basis of what has been widely referred to as the Alexander and Delong model of the basal ganglia.

The original model was a wire diagram, very simplistic in its anatomical and physiological construction. The key is that the direct and indirect pathways not only have opposite functions but are driven by different dopaminergic receptors. Thus the most powerful affect of dopamine in normal humans is mediated through the direct pathway. But in Parkinson disease, the dominant effect shifts to the indirect pathway.[32] These alterations were used to explain the various movement disorders and specifically Parkinson disease. In support of the model, there is a tremendous amount of experimental evidence from microelectrode recording, anatomical tracing, and metabolic studies.[32,96,97] Later, there was additional strong support from intraoperative patient recordings, imaging studies with both PET and functional MRI, pharmacological studies, and surgical outcome from lesioning of the basal ganglia, all of which supported the concept of increased basal ganglia inhibition to the thalamus as a major feature of the parkinsonian state in this model.

Despite the tremendous support for this initial model, it obviously could not explain comprehensively all of the functions of the basal ganglia, either normal or abnormal. This led to rounds of criticisms that the model was limited in its usefulness, if not flawed.[98–100] Although these criticisms were being made, the model was, in fact, continuing to undergo evolution. **Fig. 2.1** represents the accumulation of some of these refinements, although incomplete. There is an increased understanding of the microcircuitry developing into an extremely complex interaction among the various nuclei. It is now clear that the GPe does not simply project to STN but has reciprocal innervation from STN and direct projections GPi/SNr.[101] This loop within the loop may help explain some of the oscillatory behavior of the system.

In addition, direct cortical projections from primary motor cortex, supplementary motor cortex, and premotor cortex to both striatum and STN have also been described and may be important in relaying information into the basal ganglia and synchronizing oscillatory activity. Reciprocal corticothalamic projections occur between Vim and motor cortex as well as VL and VA to secondary motor cortex. The model now includes connections to other networks outside of the basal ganglia. Foremost of these are projections to the pedunculopontine nucleus (PPN) and midbrain extrapyramidal area (MEA), which may have significant effects on balance and gait difficulties.[102] Failure to affect these nuclei could explain why these symptoms are not well controlled by STN or GPi lesions or stimulation. Cortical projections may also reach the striatum through the central median and parafasicularis (CM/PF) thalamic complex, which has reciprocal connections and, in addition, receives excitatory input from PPN/MEA. The CM/PF is an old stereotactic target for movement disorders. GPe has inhibitory projections directly to the thalamus nucleus reticularis and PPN/MEA, suggesting a more widespread effect outside the indirect pathway. The newer anatomical circuits allow for a much richer evaluation of the basal ganglia, thalamic, and cortical interactions with now thalamic output through the striatum allowing for further synchronization along oscillatory pathways.

Along with the need for additional anatomical understanding is the need for additional understanding of the electrophysiology. The main concept initially was one of changes in rate. Although this allows adequate descriptions of classic hypokinetic (PD) and hyperkinetic (dystonia) disorders, it was soon clear that rate alone could not explain many of the subtleties of the disorders. There is a need to explain the difference symptomatologies between hemichorea/ballism, dystonia, and levodopa-induced dyskinesias that all share a common final pathophysiological mechanism.[44,45,91] Although related, there are differences that are more than just the degree of symptomatology and that strongly suggest the need for revision of the rate model. Another deficiency of the rate model is explaining lesions that would produce the so-called Marsden and Obeso paradox.[103] Although many others have described this, these authors crystallized the apparent paradox that if Parkinson disease and hypokinetic disorders represent overly inhibited thalamic motor nuclei, then how can thalamotomy improve parkinsonian symptomatology? It should make it worse. Similarly, why does not pallidotomy increase dyskinesias rather than diminish them? Why do not lesions in general produce adverse motor effects? The effects of DBS can be questioned in the same manner.

The answer came very early on through clinical studies that, not only was rate important but also the alteration in the pattern of activity (**Fig. 2.2**). Thus in Parkinson disease there is within STN, GPi, and Vim a greater tendency to discharge in bursts with a high degree of synchronization with neighboring neurons.[97] The projections from GPe to the thalamus as well as GPi to the PPN should amplify the tendency of the neuronal pools to fire synchronously and in an oscillatory fashion along with their widespread connections to other thalamic subnuclei and cortical regions, thus creating a substantial change in the burst and synchronic activity within the basal ganglia–thalamic complex. If, along with the observation that there is an abnormally wide receptive field in both the MPTP parkinsonian model and Parkinson disease, there is then a suggestion that the oscillatory activity could be erroneously interpreted as excessive sensory feedback. Thus the motor cortex would have a diminished picture of the actual velocity, amplitude, and acceleration of movement activities. This in turn could lead to slowing (bradykinesia) or premature arrest of ongoing motor activity (freezing), and the like. The widened receptive fields and irregular activity may laterally inhibit competing normal motor programs.[104]

Because there is indeed a series of somatotopic representations each of which projects to different cortical areas, multiple differences in symptoms could result from varying degrees of disease within the different subpathways. How specific symptoms develop still remains difficult to resolve with the current model. Parkinsonian tremors are treated by using high frequency stimulation in the thalamus, subthalamus, or globus pallidus. Tremor cells are identified in each of these nuclei; yet neurons in the Vim do not receive afferents from the basal ganglia. All of the long loops that include pacemaker oscillatory bursting activity from elements of the basal ganglia have not yet been established. It is difficult to demonstrate the importance of both rate and frequency in a cartoon (**Fig. 2.2**).

Rigidity likewise is quite difficult to explain with its myriad of manifestations. If the manifestation is at a spinal cord level, again long loop aberrations have been invoked for the symptom. The symptoms may be tied together through thalamocortical dysrhythmia, which would be manifest at the cortical level and could produce these positive symptoms of Parkinson disease.[105] Another alternative, however, includes the identification of PPN and MEA circuitry, which may represent important relays between the thalamus and spinal cord. Lesions of the PPN can induce akinesia, and its importance in balance and gait suggest that this is a tempting target for intervention in Parkinson disease. In fact, stimulation studies have suggested excellent responses with DBS in PPN.[106,107]

Another way of evaluating this problem is to look at it from a totally different model system. Here each loop is a neural optimal control system, which includes a model of object behavior and an error distribution system.[108] In this model, the error distribution system would include the dopaminergic neurons that are necessary to tune the model system to have control by the neural optimal control system (cortex). In such a model, Parkinson disease would be considered a disease of the error distribution system. As a consequence, the system incorrectly predicts the state of the motor system in these patients. The controlling system would then treat the incorrect predictions as if the controlled object were perturbed by an unaccounted for external force and in turn tries to adjust for the error in the next step. In an attempt to correct for the perceived rather than the actual patient's position, the control then introduces specific symptoms such as tremor. Thus at the cortical level, the irregular bursting activity may attempt to be controlled and result in an overshoot rather than an equilibrium.

A similar paradigm can explain rigidity where both agonist and antagonists are simultaneously stimulated rather than alternatively stimulated. The levodopa therapy then becomes a method of increasing the gain in the error distribution system, which proves effective only up until the point that the decreased precision and corresponding increase in dosage fail to obtain the same level of improvement. At this level, the patient begins to exhibit medically induced symptoms (i.e., dyskinesias), because of overamplification of error signals caused by large adjustments in the model from the increased gain in the error distribution system. To explain the Marsden and Obeso paradox, the lesion simply decreases the gain in the error distribution system without fixing the error problem, thus treating the symptoms and not the underlying disease. Therefore, in this theory, optimal treatment would avoid destroying the area responsible for the error distribution within the system. Rather, focal treatment to specific areas within the system should be effective. This theoretical approach, although quite interesting, leaves much to be desired in terms of the model's ability for quantification and prediction.

An important recent finding is that there are multiple oscillatory frequency bands in the local field potentials (LFPs) in STN that relate to disease and treatment. The LFPs are pleomorphic, focal, and synchronized current oscillations produced by local neuronal populations. There are low (13 to 20 Hz) and high (20 to 35 Hz) as well as some very high frequency (70 to 300 Hz) rhythms. The movement-and levodopa-dependent 300 Hz frequency may reflect the normal processing in the basal ganglia and provides support of the excitatory mechanism of high-frequency stimulation.[109] The gamma frequency (70 to 100 Hz) may represent synchronous activity in the upper STN.[110] It is the β (8 to 30 Hz) frequency activity that is abnormal in PD. In the off state or within minutes of turning off the DBS, the frequency dominates and inversely correlates with the akinesia.[111–113] In the on state or with high frequency DBS, the higher frequencies in the gamma range return to dominate, but dyskinesias are marked by an increase in low-frequency bands (4 to 10 Hz).[113,114] Understanding how these LFPs are formed could clarify our modeling of the electrophysiology of the basal ganglia.

The mechanism or mechanisms by which DBS modulates neuronal network function remain controversial. Most likely all of the mechanisms discussed in the chapter are activated. If there is a gradient current density, clearly both inhibitory and excitatory effects must occur.[47] The stimulation is from a high-voltage cathode pulse. The polarization block therefore must occur proximal to this lead. However, at a distance somewhat greater, the cathode pulses will preferentially stimulate axons (of passage or from the depolarized neurons) resulting in both orthodromal and antidromal propagation. Unlike the somata, the axons can follow the high frequency firing rates, and this activation of distal neural elements may lead to the reestablishment of appropriate synchronization that is believed to be the key element to the mechanism of DBS stimulation. Stimulation of presynaptic GABAergic terminals could increase inhibition in this area and potentially stimulate some inhibitory interneurons, but this is probably a trivial mechanism.

In addition, imaging is increasingly suggesting more excitatory evidence rather than inhibitory evidence. The combination of the two may be necessary but the excitatory effects are predominant. Thus several studies have shown that DBS in STN has a net effect of increasing firing rates in GPi rather than decreasing them. But as this chapter points out, the model is not only rate but also pattern. The effect of DBS then is one of increased synchronization rather than the irregular burst activity, which appears to be so disruptive to the cortex. One concept is that this is a stochastic resonance and it is the normal signal that had been lost in the noise and is suddenly revealed by this constructive interference paradigm.[71] There is something about going from beta to gamma activity in STN that is important, and the same may be true of other nuclei. Even direct stimulation of the motor cortex may help parkinsonian symptoms.[115]

Lesioning has very different effects on local and distant circuitry and imaging than DBS, but a common effect of both is increased activity in the motor cortex.[116,117] Lesioning may simply be a different means of removing the disruptive rhythms. It would be interesting to know what happens to the LFPs in lesioning. Meanwhile, it is no longer popular to say that DBS acts as a "functional lesion." However, the bottom line is that, as far as we know, both DBS and lesioning produce identical net effects on movement disorder symptoms.

■ Therapeutic Mechanisms of Movement Disorder Surgery

The clinical effects of ablation or DBS have been well documented, but our understanding of their mechanism(s) of action remains unclear. It is obvious that ablation of a given anatomical nucleus eliminates its neuronal output, but it is not obvious how the nervous system accommodates to that change in terms of its overall network activity. Likewise, it is unclear how stimulation, currently thought to activate neuronal output, can have functional consequences similar to ablation. In addition, questions remain regarding the effects of stimulation at the level of both the neurons surrounding the electrode and the network in which they reside. Answering these questions will provide the foundation for understanding the therapeutic mechanisms of these interventions. In addition, knowledge of the mechanisms of action will provide a fundamental step toward furthering the development of movement disorder surgery strategies and technology.

Although DBS is an attractive alternative to ablation for a variety of reasons, ablation remains a viable strategy, especially in underdeveloped countries where economic and personnel/technological infrastructure are limited. Possibly the most important distinction between DBS and ablation is that DBS allows bilateral procedures without the high incidence of side effects associated with ablative procedures. In addition, side effects associated with DBS are reversible. DBS allows for customization of the therapy that the individual patient needs over time via alteration of the stimulation parameters and electrode contacts. Lastly, DBS does not destroy tissue, allowing the opportunity for patients to benefit from emerging restorative therapies. However, programming DBS devices for maximal clinical benefit can be a difficult and time-consuming process that typically requires a highly trained and experienced individual to achieve optimal results. Programming is typically done with no visual reference to the breadth of effect of stimulation on the stimulated structure. Although guidelines exist on stimulation parameter settings that are typically effective,[49–52] it is unfeasible to clinically evaluate each of the thousands of stimulation parameter combinations that are possible. In addition, application of DBS technology to disorders such as epilepsy, dystonia, and OCD is especially problematic because the beneficial effects of stimulation can take weeks to months to manifest and it is unclear what electrode geometries or stimulation paradigms are optimal for these different disorders.

Several anatomical targets currently exist for movement disorder surgical intervention, but the STN is the most commonly targeted site for the treatment of PD and is reported effective for the control of all the cardinal motor signs of PD.[53] The last 2 decades have provided strong scientific evidence that the increased rate and altered pattern of STN neuronal activity play a paramount role in the development of parkinsonian motor signs. Experimental lesions of the STN in MPTP-treated monkeys have been demonstrated to reverse contralateral akinesia, rigidity, and postural tremor but may also induce hemichorea/ballism.[54–58] Interestingly, early pilot clinical trials of subthalamotomy for PD suggest it can be done safely, with beneficial effects comparable to pallidotomy or DBS of the STN or GPi, and a low prevalence of hemichorea.[59–62] Involuntary movements may occur following STN lesions but are generally transient. For those instances in which

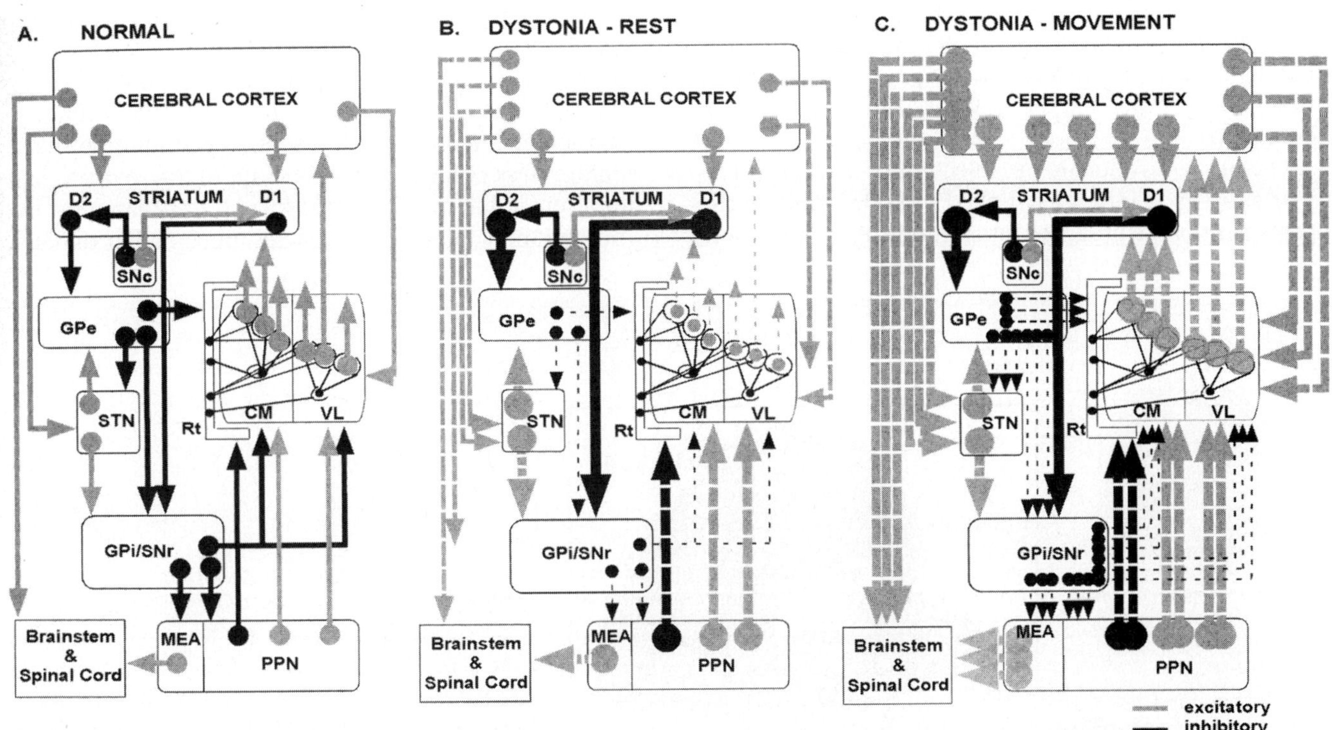

Fig. 2.2 (A–C) Rate and pattern model for primary dystonia. Multiple lines of *different lengths* exiting a nucleus represent *asynchronous* neuronal activity; multiple *broken lines of different lengths* illustrate *altered patterns of asynchronous* neuronal activity; whereas *multiple broken lines of the same length* illustrate *altered patterns of synchronous* activity. The width of the lines depicts the amount of neuronal activity. Consistent with previous reports, thalamic and pallidal activity is reduced at rest. During movement, pallidal activity is further reduced, leading to an increase in thalamic activity and the development of uncontrolled synchrony throughout the subcortical–cortical network. This reduction leads to a disruption in cortical and brain stem output and the disordered movement that occurs in dystonia. This model does not attempt to fully depict the changes in intrathalamic, brain stem, or spinal circuitry. Modification of the present model will occur as new data concerning the neuronal activity changes in thalamus neurons under the foregoing conditions become available. *Abbreviations*: SNc, substantia nigra pars compacta; SNr, substantia nigra pars reticulata; STN, subthalamic nucleus; GPe, globus pallidus pars externa; GPi, globus pallidus pars interna; CM, centromedian; VL, motor thalamus; Rt, reticular nucleus of the thalamus; PPN, pedunculopontine nucleus; MEA, midbrain extrapyramidal area. Dopamine receptor subtypes D1 and D2 . (From: Vitek JL. Pathophysiology of dystonia: a neuronal model. In Mov Disord 2002;17(Suppl 3):S49–S62. Reprinted with permission of Wiley-Liss, Inc., a subsidiary of John Wiley & Sons, Inc.)

involuntary movements are more severe and persistent, pallidotomy has been an effective treatment.

Although the clinical effects of STN DBS and STN lesions are similar, they result in substantially different electrophysiological and metabolic effects on the central nervous system when clinically effective. Analysis of the volumes ablated by STN lesions or stimulated by DBS suggests that these two interventions may affect a similar volume of tissue (**Fig. 2.3**).[62–64] Experimental studies in MPTP monkeys showed that therapeutic STN lesions generated a reduction in pallidal firing, but oscillatory GPi activity persisted.[57] In contrast, therapeutic STN DBS generated a marked increase in GPi firing and overrode low-frequency burst patterns in the pallidum.[46] Functional imaging with positron emission tomography (PET) of human patients with STN lesions showed significant reductions in SNr, GPi, and ventral thalamic metabolic activity,[65,66] whereas PET scans in patients with therapeutic STN DBS showed increased blood flow in STN, pallidum, thalamus, and cortex.[67] Taken together these results suggest that ablation and DBS generate their therapeutic effects via different mechanisms. These observations provide evidence to suggest that the rationale for selection of a surgical target may be different for both the disorder and the surgical strategy (ablation or stimulation).

Developing a rationale for selection of a surgical target or strategy is intimately linked to understanding the mechanisms of the proposed intervention. Presently, there exist four general hypotheses to explain the therapeutic mechanism(s) of DBS: (1) stimulation-induced alterations in the activation of voltage-gated currents that block neural output near the stimulating electrode (depolarization blockade)[68]; (2) indirect inhibition of neuronal output via activation of axon terminals that make synaptic connections with neurons near the stimulating electrode (synaptic inhibition)[69]; (3) synaptic transmission failure of the efferent output of stimulated neurons as a result of transmitter depletion (synaptic depression)[70]; and (4) stimulation-induced disruption of pathological network activity.[46,71]

Depolarization blockade and synaptic inhibition represent two of the earliest hypotheses to explain the similarity between the therapeutic benefit of ablation and stimulation. Single-unit recordings of local cells in the stimulated nucleus support both of these hypotheses.[68,69,72–78] However, the limitation of these hypotheses is that they do not take into account the possible independent activation of the efferent axon of projection neurons. Theoretical and experimental results show that the axon plays the most important role in the activation of neurons surrounding the electrode during extracellular stimulation.[79–83] Additionally, the response of the cell body does not necessarily represent the output of the axon during DBS.[47] Moreover, subthalamic neurons have recently been found to have a unique class of K$^+$ channels (Kv3 type) that reduces spike duration and allows for faster spike trains than most neurons and may tolerate frequencies much higher than used

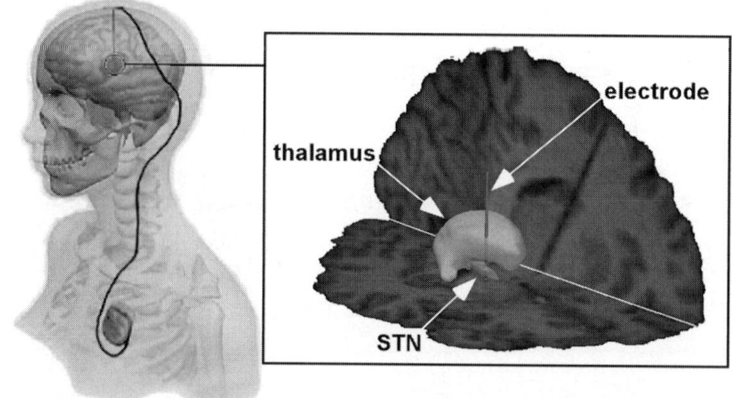

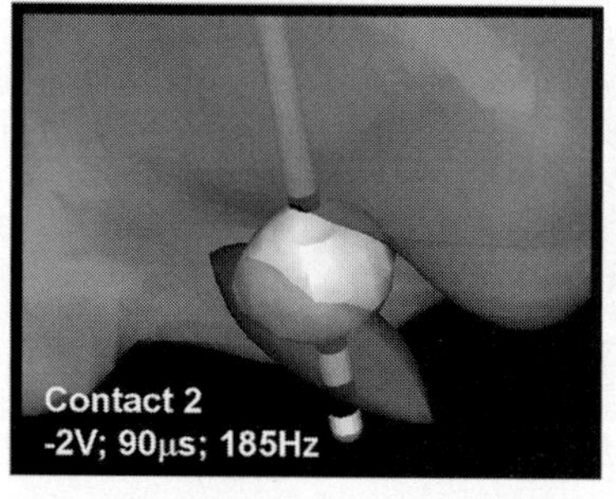

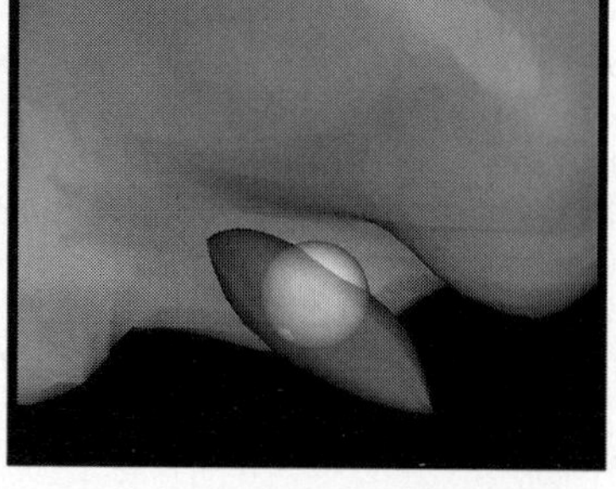

Fig. 2.3 Movement disorder surgical intervention in the subthalamic nucleus (STN). **(A)** The deep brain stimulation (DBS) electrode is implanted in the STN and is connected to the stimulation controller, which is located subcutaneously below the clavicle. The electrode shaft passes through the thalamus, and the four electrode contacts are distributed through the STN. The close-up image on the right shows the thalamus, STN, and electrode coregistered with postoperative anatomical magnetic resonance imaging (MRI). The dark line on the parasagittal MRI slice shows the path of the electrode on the contralateral side of the brain. **(B)** The volume of activation (VOA) under therapeutic stimulation settings (- 2 V, 90 us, 185 Hz) is estimated using a detailed computational model.[64] The VOA encompasses the dorsomedial aspect of the STN along with the zona incerta and fields of Forel. **(C)** STN lesion estimated from postoperative MRI of a Parkinson patient shows a smaller but comparably affected volume.[6]

clinically with DBS.[84] Therefore, although either or both synaptic inhibition and depolarization blockade may occur in the cell body, the functional effect of these phenomena may have limited significance in the therapeutic mechanism(s) of DBS.

If DBS does generate efferent outputs in neurons surrounding the electrode, why do ablation and DBS generate similar therapeutic effects? One possibility is that neurons activated by the stimulus train are unable to sustain high-frequency synaptic action on efferent targets due to depletion of neurotransmitter.[70,85–87] In turn, synaptic depression represents an attractive connection between the functional effects of DBS and ablation. However, several in vivo experimental studies have shown increases in transmitter release and changes in firing of efferent nuclei consistent with activation of neurons around the electrode and subsequent synaptic action on their targets during high-frequency stimulation.[46,88–90] Therefore, although some level of synaptic depression is undoubtedly occurring throughout the stimulated network of neurons, this phenomenon does not appear to be sufficient to block signal transmission between nuclei.

The abnormal motor activity effectively controlled by DBS is most likely generated by altered patterns, increased neuronal synchronization, and/or low frequency rhythmic oscillation of neurons within the BG and thalamus.[19,91,92] It is possible that DBS overrides these altered patterns and low-frequency oscillatory activity and replaces it with tonic high-frequency output, which may be more easily compensated by the remaining elements of the BG–thalamocortical network.[46–48,71]

In summary, several questions remain to be answered before the true mechanisms of movement disorder surgery are explained. Advances in our knowledge of the neural circuitry and the neurophysiological effects of ablation or DBS on the nervous system are necessary for a more detailed understanding. This knowledge will enable definition of the therapeutic mechanisms and provide a more comprehensive rationale for the selection of anatomical target and surgical strategy. In addition, continued scientific advancement in this area may lead to novel target sites, surgical techniques, and medical device designs that will improve the clinical outcomes for patients receiving these therapies in the future.

References

1. Starr PA, Vitek JL, Bakay RA. Ablative surgery and deep brain stimulation for Parkinson's disease. Neurosurgery 1998;43:989–1013

2. Obeso JA, Linazasoro G, Guridi J, Ramos E, Rodriguez-Oroz MC. High frequency stimulation of the subthalamic nucleus and levodopa induced dyskinesias in Parkinson's disease. J Neurol Neurosurg Psychiatry 2000;68:122–123

3. Fahn S. Description of Parkinson's disease as a clinical syndrome. Ann N Y Acad Sci 2003;991:1–14

4. Brooks DJ. The early diagnosis of Parkinson's disease. Ann Neurol 1998;44(3, Suppl 1)S10–S18

5. Louis ED, Fried LP, Fitzpatrick AL, Longstreth WT Jr, Newman AB. Regional and racial differences in the prevalence of physician-diagnosed essential tremor in the United States. Mov Disord 2003;18:1035–1040

6. Dogu O, Sevim S, Camdeviren H, et al. Prevalence of essential tremor: door-to-door neurologic exams in Mersin Province, Turkey. Neurology 2003;61:1804–1806

7. Misbahuddin A, Warner TT. Dystonia: an update on genetics and treatment. Curr Opin Neurol 2001;14:471–475

8. de Carvalho Aguiar PM, Ozelius LJ. Classification and genetics of dystonia. Lancet Neurol 2002;1:316–325

9. McNaught KS, Kapustin A, Jackson T, et al. Brainstem pathology in DYT1 primary torsion dystonia. Ann Neurol 2004;56:540–547

10. Marsden CD, Obeso JA, Zarranz JJ, Lang AE. The anatomical basis of symptomatic hemidystonia. Brain 1985;108:463–483

11. Lee MS, Marsden CD. Movement disorders following lesions of the thalamus or subthalamic region. Mov Disord 1994;9:493–507

12. Benabid AL, Pollak P, Gao D, et al. Chronic electrical stimulation of the ventralis intermedius nucleus of the thalamus as a treatment of movement disorders. J Neurosurg 1996;84:203–214

13. Obeso JA, Olanow CW, Rodriguez-Oroz MC, Krack P, Kumar R, Lang AE. Deep-brain stimulation of the subthalamic nucleus or the pars interna of the globus pallidus in Parkinson's disease. N Engl J Med 2001;345:956–963

14. Coubes P, Roubertie A, Vayssiere N, Hemm S, Echenne B. Treatment of DYT1-generalised dystonia by stimulation of the internal globus pallidus. Lancet 2000;355:2220–2221

15. Yianni J, Bain P, Giladi N, et al. Globus pallidus internus deep brain stimulation for dystonic conditions: a prospective audit. Mov Disord 2003;18:436–442

16. Hodaie M, Wennberg RA, Dostrovsky JO, Lozano AM. Chronic anterior thalamus stimulation for intractable epilepsy. Epilepsia 2002;43:603–608

17. Nuttin BJ, Gabriels LA, Cosyns PR, et al. Long-term electrical capsular stimulation in patients with obsessive-compulsive disorder. Neurosurgery 2003;52:1263–1272 (discussion 1272) (–1264)

18. Alexander GE, Crutcher MD, DeLong MR. Basal ganglia–thalamocortical circuits: parallel substrates for motor, oculomotor, "prefrontal" and "limbic" functions. In: Uylings HBM, Van Eden CG, De Bruin JPC, Corner MA, Feenstra MGP, eds. Progress in Brain Research. New York: Elsevier Science; 1990

19. Bergman H, Feingold A, Nini A, et al. Physiological aspects of information processing in the basal ganglia of normal and parkinsonian primates. Trends Neurosci 1998;21:32–38

20. Smith Y, Bevan MD, Shink E, Bolam JP. Microcircuitry of the direct and indirect pathways of the basal ganglia. Neuroscience 1998;86:353–387

21. Gerfen CR, Engber TM, Mahan LC, et al. D1 and D2 dopamine receptor-regulated gene expression of striatonigral and striatopallidal neurons. Science 1990;250:1429–1432

22. Macchi G, Jones EG. Toward an agreement on terminology of nuclear and subnuclear divisions of the motor thalamus. J Neurosurg 1997;86:670–685

23. Sakai ST, Inase M, Tanji J. Comparison of cerebellothalamic and pallidothalamic projections in the monkey (Macaca fuscata): a double anterograde labeling study. J Comp Neurol 1996;368:215–228

24. Schell GR, Strick PL. The origin of thalamic inputs to the arcuate premotor and supplementary motor areas. J Neurosci 1984;4:539–560

25. Jahnsen H, Llinas R. Electrophysiological properties of guinea-pig thalamic neurones: an in vitro study. J Physiol 1984;349:205–226

26. Jahnsen H, Llinas R. Ionic basis for the electroresponsiveness and oscillatory properties of guinea-pig thalamic neurones in vitro. J Physiol 1984;349:227–247

27. Steriade M. Impact of network activities on neuronal properties in corticothalamic systems. J Neurophysiol 2001;86:1–39

28. Plenz D, Kital ST. A basal ganglia pacemaker formed by the subthalamic nucleus and external globus pallidus. Nature 1999;400:677–682

29. Bevan MD, Magill PJ, Terman D, Bolam JP, Wilson CJ. Move to the rhythm: oscillations in the subthalamic nucleus–external globus pallidus network. Trends Neurosci 2002;25:525–531

30. Nambu A, Tokuno H, Takada M. Functional significance of the cortico–subthalamo–pallidal 'hyperdirect' pathway. Neurosci Res 2002;43:111–117

31. Pahapill PA, Lozano AM. The pedunculopontine nucleus and Parkinson's disease. Brain 2000;123(Pt 9):1767–1783

32. DeLong MR. Primate models of movement disorders of basal ganglia origin. Trends Neurosci 1990;13:281–285

33. Filion M, Tremblay L. Abnormal spontaneous activity of globus pallidus neurons in monkeys with MPTP-induced parkinsonism. Brain Res 1991;547:142–151

34. Bergman H, Wichmann T, Karmon B, DeLong MR. The primate subthalamic nucleus, II: Neuronal activity in the MPTP model of parkinsonism. J Neurophysiol 1994;72:507–520

35. Vitek JL, Bakay RA, Hashimoto T, et al. Microelectrode-guided pallidotomy: technical approach and its application in medically intractable Parkinson's disease. J Neurosurg 1998;88:1027–1043

36. Lim JK, Tasker RR, Scott JW. Quantitative assessment of thalamotomy for Parkinsonism. Confin Neurol 1969;31:11–21

37. Narabayashi H, Yokochi F, Nakajima Y. Levodopa-induced dyskinesia and thalamotomy. J Neurol Neurosurg Psychiatry 1984;47:831–839

38. Laitinen LV, Bergenheim AT, Hariz MI. Ventroposterolateral pallidotomy can abolish all parkinsonian symptoms. Stereotact Funct Neurosurg 1992;58:14–21

39. Vitek JL, Bakay R, DeLong M. Microelectrode-guided pallidotomy for medically intractable Parkinson's disease. Adv Neurol 1997;74:183–198

40. Levy R, Hutchison WD, Lozano AM, Dostrovsky JO. Synchronized neuronal discharge in the basal ganglia of parkinsonian patients is limited to oscillatory activity. J Neurosci 2002;22:2855–2861

41. Lenz FA, Kwan HC, Martin RL, Tasker RR, Dostrovsky JO, Lenz YE. Single unit analysis of the human ventral thalamic nuclear group tremor-related activity in functionally identified cells. Brain 1994;117:531–543

42. Lozano AM, Kumar R, Gross R, et al. Globus pallidus internus pallidotomy for generalized dystonia. Mov Disord 1997;12:865–870

43. Lenz FA, Suarez JI, Metman LV, et al. Pallidal activity during dystonia: somatosensory reorganisation and changes with severity. J Neurol Neurosurg Psychiatry 1998;65:767–770

44. Vitek JL, Chockkan V, Zhang JY, et al. Neuronal activity in the basal ganglia in patients with generalized dystonia and hemiballismus. Ann Neurol 1999;46:22–35

45. Vitek JL. Pathophysiology of dystonia: a neuronal model. Mov Disord 2002;17(Suppl 3):S49–S62

46. Hashimoto T, Elder CM, Okun MS, Patrick SK, Vitek JL. Stimulation of the subthalamic nucleus changes the firing pattern of pallidal neurons. J Neurosci 2003;23:1916–1923

47. McIntyre CC, Grill WM, Sherman DL, Thakor NV. Cellular effects of deep brain stimulation: model-based analysis of activation and inhibition. J Neurophysiol 2004;91:1457–1469

48. Grill WM, Snyder AN, Miocinovic S. Deep brain stimulation creates an informational lesion of the stimulated nucleus. Neuroreport 2004;15:1137–1140

49. Rizzone M, Lanotte M, Bergamasco B, et al. Deep brain stimulation of the subthalamic nucleus in Parkinson's disease: effects of variation in stimulation parameters. J Neurol Neurosurg Psychiatry 2001;71:215–219

50. Moro E, Esselink RJ, Benabid AL, Pollak P. Response to levodopa in parkinsonian patients with bilateral subthalamic nucleus stimulation. Brain 2002;125(Pt 11):2408–2417

51. Volkmann J, Herzog J, Kopper F, Deuschl G. Introduction to the programming of deep brain stimulators. Mov Disord 2002;17(Suppl 3):S181–S187

52. O'Suilleabhain PE, Frawley W, Giller C, Dewey RB Jr. Tremor response to polarity, voltage, pulsewidth and frequency of thalamic stimulation. Neurology 2003;60:786–790

53. Limousin P, Krack P, Pollak P, et al. Electrical stimulation of the subthalamic nucleus in advanced Parkinson's disease. N Engl J Med 1998;339:1105–1111

54. Bergman H, Wichmann T, DeLong MR. Reversal of experimental parkinsonism by lesions of the subthalamic nucleus. Science 1990;249:1436–1438

55. Aziz TZ, Peggs D, Sambrook MA, Crossman AR. Lesion of the subthalamic nucleus for the alleviation of 1-methyl-4-phenyl-1,2,3, 6-tetrahydropyridine (MPTP)-induced parkinsonism in the primate. Mov Disord 1991;6:288–292

56. Aziz TZ, Peggs D, Agarwal E, Sambrook MA, Crossman AR. Subthalamic nucleotomy alleviates parkinsonism in the 1-methyl-4-phenyl-1,2,3,6-tetrahydropyridine (MPTP)-exposed primate. Br J Neurosurg 1992;6:575–582

57. Wichmann T, Bergman H, DeLong MR. The primate subthalamic nucleus, I: Functional properties in intact animals. J Neurophysiol 1994;72:494–506

58. Guridi J, Herrero MT, Luquin MR, et al. Subthalamotomy in parkinsonian monkeys: behavioural and biochemical analysis. Brain 1996;119(Pt 5):1717–1727

59. Alvarez L, Macias R, Guridi J, et al. Dorsal subthalamotomy for Parkinson's disease. Mov Disord 2001;16:72–78

60. Su PC, Tseng HM, Liu HM, Yen RF, Liou HH. Subthalamotomy for advanced Parkinson disease. J Neurosurg 2002;97:598–606

61. Su PC, Tseng HM, Liu HM, Yen RF, Liou HH. Treatment of advanced Parkinson's disease by subthalamotomy: one-year results. Mov Disord 2003;18:531–538

62. Patel NK, Heywood P, O'Sullivan K, McCarter R, Love S, Gill SS. Unilateral subthalamotomy in the treatment of Parkinson's disease. Brain 2003;126(Pt 5):1136–1145

63. McIntyre CC, Mori S, Sherman DL, Thakor NV, Vitek JL. Electric field and stimulating influence generated by deep brain stimulation of the subthalamic nucleus. Clin Neurophysiol 2004;115:589–595

64. Butson CR, Cooper SE, Henderson JM, McIntyre CC. Patient-specific analysis of the volume of tissue activated by deep brain stimulation. Neuroimage 2007;34:661–670

65. Su PC, Tseng HM. Gait freezing and falling related to subthalamic stimulation in patients with a previous pallidotomy. Mov Disord 2001;16:376–377

66. Trost M, Su PC, Barnes A, et al. Evolving metabolic changes during the first postoperative year after subthalamotomy. J Neurosurg 2003;99:872–878

67. Hershey T, Revilla FJ, Wernle AR, et al. Cortical and subcortical blood flow effects of subthalamic nucleus stimulation in PD. Neurology 2003;61:816–821

68. Beurrier C, Bioulac B, Audin J, Hammond C. High-frequency stimulation produces a transient blockade of voltage-gated currents in subthalamic neurons. J Neurophysiol 2001;85:1351–1356

69. Dostrovsky JO, Levy R, Wu JP, Hutchison WD, Tasker RR, Lozano AM. Microstimulation-induced inhibition of neuronal firing in human globus pallidus. J Neurophysiol 2000;84:570–574

70. Urbano FJ, Leznik E, Llinas R. Cortical activation patterns evoked by afferent axons stimuli at different frequencies: an in vitro voltage-sensitive dye imaging study. Thalamus Rel Syst 2002;1:371–378

71. Montgomery EB Jr, Baker KB. Mechanisms of deep brain stimulation and future technical developments. Neurol Res 2000;22:259–266

72. Benazzouz A, Piallat B, Pollak P, Benabid AL. Responses of substantia nigra pars reticulata and globus pallidus complex to high frequency stimulation of the subthalamic nucleus in rats: electrophysiological data. Neurosci Lett 1995;189:77–80

73. Benazzouz A, Gao DM, Ni ZG, Piallat B, Bouali-Benazzouz R, Benabid AL. Effect of high-frequency stimulation of the subthalamic nucleus on the neuronal activities of the substantia nigra pars reticulata and ventrolateral nucleus of the thalamus in the rat. Neuroscience 2000;99:289–295

74. Boraud T, Bezard E, Bioulac B, Gross C. High frequency stimulation of the internal globus pallidus (GPi) simultaneously improves parkinsonian symptoms and reduces the firing frequency of GPi neurons in the MPTP-treated monkey. Neurosci Lett 1996;215:17–20

75. Bikson M, Lian J, Hahn PJ, Stacey WC, Sciortino C, Durand DM. Suppression of epileptiform activity by high frequency sinusoidal fields in rat hippocampal slices. J Physiol 2001;531(Pt 1):181–191

76. Kiss ZH, Mooney DM, Renaud L, Hu B. Neuronal response to local electrical stimulation in rat thalamus: physiological implications for mechanisms of deep brain stimulation. Neuroscience 2002;113:137–143

77. Magarinos-Ascone C, Pazo JH, Macadar O, Buno W. High-frequency stimulation of the subthalamic nucleus silences subthalamic neurons: a possible cellular mechanism in Parkinson's disease. Neuroscience 2002;115:1109–1117

78. Lian J, Bikson M, Sciortino C, Stacey WC, Durand DM. Local suppression of epileptiform activity by electrical stimulation in rat hippocampus in vitro. J Physiol 2003;547(Pt 2):427–434

79. Nowak LG, Bullier J. Axons, but not cell bodies, are activated by electrical stimulation in cortical gray matter, I: Evidence from chronaxie measurements. Exp Brain Res 1998;118:477–488

80. Nowak LG, Bullier J. Axons, but not cell bodies, are activated by electrical stimulation in cortical gray matter, II: Evidence from selective inactivation of cell bodies and axon initial segments. Exp Brain Res 1998;118:489–500

81. Rattay F. The basic mechanism for the electrical stimulation of the nervous system. Neuroscience 1999;89:335–346

82. McIntyre CC, Grill W. Excitation of central nervous system neurons by nonuniform electric fields. Biophys J 1999;76:878–888

83. McIntyre CC, Grill WM. Finite element analysis of the current-density and electric field generated by metal microelectrodes. Ann Biomed Eng 2001;29:227–235

84. Surmeier DJ, Bevan MD. "The little engine that could": voltage-dependent Na(+) channels and the subthalamic nucleus. Neuron 2003;39:5–6

85. Wang LY, Kaczmarek LK. High-frequency firing helps replenish the readily releasable pool of synaptic vesicles. Nature 1998;394:384–388

86. Zucker RS, Regehr WG. Short-term synaptic plasticity. Annu Rev Physiol 2002;64:355–405

87. Shen KZ, Zhu ZT, Munhall A, Johnson SW. Synaptic plasticity in rat subthalamic nucleus induced by high-frequency stimulation. Synapse 2003;50:314–319

88. Windels F, Bruet N, Poupard A, et al. Effects of high frequency stimulation of subthalamic nucleus on extracellular glutamate and GABA in substantia nigra and globus pallidus in the normal rat. Eur J Neurosci 2000;12:4141–4146

89. Windels F, Bruet N, Poupard A, Feuerstein C, Bertrand A, Savasta M. Influence of the frequency parameter on extracellular glutamate and gamma-aminobutyric acid in substantia nigra and globus pallidus during electrical stimulation of subthalamic nucleus in rats. J Neurosci Res 2003;72:259–267

90. Anderson ME, Postupna N, Ruffo M. Effects of high-frequency stimulation in the internal globus pallidus on the activity of thalamic neurons in the awake monkey. J Neurophysiol 2003;89:1150–1160

91. Vitek JL, Giroux M. Physiology of hypokinetic and hyperkinetic movement disorders: model for dyskinesia. Ann Neurol 2000;47(4, Suppl 1)S131–S140

92. Deuschl G, Raethjen J, Lindemann M, Krack P. The pathophysiology of tremor. Muscle Nerve 2001;24:716–735

93. Vitek JL, Zhang J, Evatt M, et al. GPi pallidotomy for dystonia: clinical outcome and neuronal activity. Adv Neurol 1998;78:211–219

94. Starr PA, Turner RS, Rau G, et al. Microelectrode-guided implantation of deep brain stimulators into the globus pallidus internus for dystonia: techniques, electrode locations, and outcomes. Neurosurg Focus 2004;17:E4

95. Albin RL, Young AB, Penney JB. The functional anatomy of basal ganglia disorders. Trends Neurosci 1989;12:366–375

96. Alexander GE, Delong MR, Strick PL. Parallel organization of functionally segregated circuits linking basal ganglia and cortex. Annu Rev Neurosci 1986;9:357–381

97. Wichman T, Delong MR, Vitek JL. Pathophysiological considerations in basal ganglia surgery: role of the basal ganglia in hypokinetic and hyperkinetic movement disorders. Prog Neurol Surg 2000;15:31–57

98. Parent A, Cicchetti F. The current model of basal ganglia organization under scrutiny. Mov Disord 1998;13:199–203

99. Levy R, Hazrati LN, Herrero MT, et al. Re-evaluation of the functional anatomy of the basal ganglia in normal and parkinsonian states. Neuroscience 1997;76:335–343

100. Obeso JA, Guridi J, Rodriguez-Oroz MC, et al. Functional model of the basal ganglia: where are we? Prog Neurol Surg 2000;15:58–77

101. Hazrati LN, Parent A. Projection from the external pallidum to the reticular thalamic nucleus in the squirrel monkey. Brain Res 1991;550:142–146

102. Parent A, Sato F, Wu Y, Gauthier J, Levesque M, Parent M. Organization of the basal ganglia: the importance of axonal collateralization. Trends Neurosci 2000;23(Suppl 10):S20–S27

103. Marsden CD, Obeso JA. The functions of the basal ganglia and the paradox of stereotaxic surgery in Parkinson's disease. Brain 1994;117:877–897

104. Mink JW. The basal ganglia and involuntary movements. Arch Neurol 2003;60:1365–1368

105. Llinas RR, Ribary U, Jeanmonod D. Thalamocortical dysrhythmia: a neurological and neuropsychiatric syndrome characterized by magnetoencephalography. Proc Natl Acad Sci U S A 1999;96:15222–15227

106. Mazzone P, Lozano A, Stanzlione P, et al. Implantation of human pedunclopontine nucleus: safe and clinically relevant target in Parkinson's disease. Neuroreport 2005;16:1877–1881

107. Plaha P, Gill SS. Bilateral deep brain stimulation of the pedunculopontine nucleus for Parkinson's disease. Neuroreport 2005;16:1883–1887

108. Baev KV, Greene KA, Marciano FE, et al. Physiology and pathophysiology of cortico-basal ganglia-thalamocortical loops: theoretical and practical aspects. Prog Neuropsychopharmacol Biol Psychiatry 2002;26:771–804

109. Foffani G, Priori A, Egidi M, et al. 300-Hz subthalamic oscillations in Parkinson's disease. Brain 2003;126:2153–2163

110. Trottenberg T, Fogelson N, Kuhn AA, et al. Subthalamic gamma activity in patients with Parkinson's disease. Exp Neurol 2006;200:56–65

111. Brown P, Williams D. Basal ganglia local field potential activity: character and functional significance in human. Clin Neurophysiol 2005;116:2510–2519

112. Foffani G, Ardolino G, Egidi M, Caputo E, Bossi B, Priori A. Subthalamic oscillatory activities at beta or higher frequency do not change after high-frequency DBS in Parkinson's disease. Brain Res Bull 2006;69:123–130

113. Alonso-Frech F, Zamarbide I, Alegre M, et al. Slow oscillatory activity and levodopa-induced dyskinesias in Parkinson's disease. Brain 2006;129:1748–1757

114. Wingeier B, Tcheng T, Koop MM, Hill BC, Heit G, Bronte-Stewart HM. Intra-operative STN DBS attenuates the prominent beta rhythm in the STN in Parkinson's disease. Exp Neurol 2006;197:244–251

115. Drouot X, Oshino S, Jarraya B, et al. Functional recovery in primate model of Parkinson's disease following motor cortex stimulation. Neuron 2004;44:769–778

116. Ceballos-Baumann AO, Obeso JA, Viteck JL, et al. Restoration of thalamocortical activity after posteroventral pallidotomy for Parkinson's disease. Lancet 1994;344:814

117. Limousin P, Greene J, Pollack P, et al. Changes in cerebral activity pattern due to subthalamic or internal pallidum stimulation in Parkinson's disease. Ann Neurol 1997;42:283–291

3 Setting Up a Movement Disorder Surgery Practice

Brian Harris Kopell, Kenneth Baker, and Nicholas M. Boulis

This chapter addresses practical considerations in starting and building a neurosurgical movement disorder practice. This effort may entail merely adding deep brain stimulation (DBS) to an existing general neurosurgical practice; however, it has traditionally implied the creation of a practice focused on functional neurosurgery, usually in the setting of an academic or large specialty clinic. Because of this association, this chapter addresses both scenarios but focuses on the broader functional neurosurgery practice.

Functional neurosurgery can consist of an intervention to correct aberrant information processing or altered synaptic communication in the nervous system through surgical ablation (anatomical) or electrical stimulation (physiological) to treat neurophysiological abnormalities. The discipline itself remains loosely delineated with no standard syllabus of skills and disease targets. This confusion is reflected in the significant variance in training offered by different fellowships. The core of functional neurosurgery includes the treatment of epilepsy, spasticity, pain, and psychiatric and movement disorders. However, there is a consensus that psychosurgery should be practiced sparingly and with great circumspection, and some contend that epilepsy and pain surgery are entirely independent disciplines. Finally, the emergence of restorative techniques for neuroprotection, axonal regeneration, gene therapy, and cellular grafting promises to further obscure the already imprecise boundaries of this discipline.

It is clear, however, that movement disorders alone will not provide a sufficient caseload to occupy most full-time neurosurgeons. The mix of services offered by functional neurosurgeons must balance the surgeons' interests with the demand in their individual environment. Thus the demand for DBS may motivate generalists in regions lacking the service to add these techniques, whereas young functional neurosurgeons with a specific interest in movement disorders may be forced to practice general neurosurgery as the focused functional practice evolves. Even more than spine or vascular neurosurgery, functional neurosurgery requires an intricate and diverse relationship with a network of referring physicians as well as a variety of integrated teams. The development of the functional practice usually parallels the evolution of these teams. As the application of DBS is expanded to other fields additional teams will be needed. Thus, when DBS is used as an alternative for cingulotomy, subcaudate tractotomy, and capsulotomy in the field of psychosurgery a very different team will be assembled.

Setting up a functional neurosurgical practice poses particular organizational and financial hurdles. This chapter broadly outlines and organizes these challenges. As the technology of functional neurosurgery continues to evolve, some of the specifics discussed in this chapter will cease to be relevant. We anticipate that the technology will become more user friendly, making both acquisition and application easier. However, the hope is that the general principles described will continue to be of use in setting up a practice focusing on movement disorders and functional neurosurgery in general.

■ Capital Expenses

At present, starting a movement disorder practice can require a considerable capital investment. These expenses will include a stereotactic frame, a stereotactic planning software package or planning station, and neurophysiological equipment. Individual surgeons will vary in their utilization of these three core products. Frameless stereotaxis and the integration of these products are trends that may significantly change the nature of the capital expense required to initiate a DBS program. That is, it may become possible to include the cost of such an integrated system into the implanted devices or for hospitals and practices to lease the systems.

Stereotactic Frames

Because presently frame-based stereotaxis remains the gold standard, it is assumed that these devices are essential. Three of the most popular frames will be considered here. Most commercially available frames have similar accuracies and idiosyncrasies.[1] As such, it is important to choose a frame that will have the most robust company support, ease of use, and compatibility with computer planning systems.

The Leksell Stereotactic System (Elekta AB, Stockholm, Sweden, www. electa.com)

Globally, the Leksell Stereotactic System (**Fig. 3.1**) is the most widely used frame. The frame, designed by Lars Leksell in 1949[2] after his period of study with Spiegel and Wycis, is the first stereotactic apparatus based on the

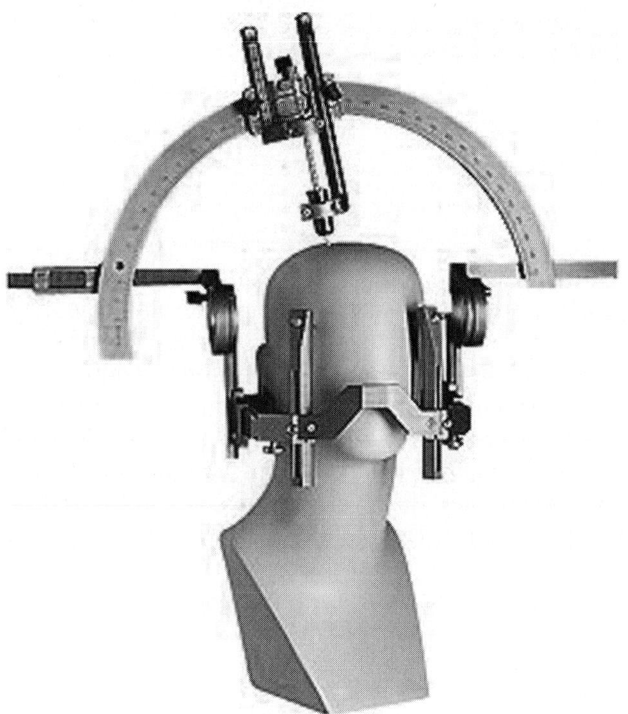

Fig. 3.1 Leksell Stereotactic System (Elekta AB, Stockholm, Sweden, www.electa.com). (See **Color Plate 3.1**.)

arc-centered principle. Leksell's original description of the principle reads as follows:

"Essentially, it consists of a semicircular arc with a movable electrode carrier. The arc is fixed to the patient's head in such a manner that its center corresponds with a selected cerebral target. The electrodes are always directed towards the center and hence the target. Rotation of the arc around the axis rods in association with lateral adjustment of the electrode carrier enables any convenient point of entrance of the electrodes to be chosen independent of the site of the target."[3]

The current model of the Leksell stereotactic headframe (Elekta Instruments, Inc. Norcross, GA, www.eleckta.com), the Model G frame, is nonferromagnetic and compatible with all available imaging techniques, including computed tomography (CT), magnetic resonance imaging and angiography (MRI and MRA), and positron emission tomography (PET). The base ring is rectangular, measuring 190 mm by 210 mm.[4] The x coordinate is set on the arc, whereas y and z coordinates are set on sidepieces attached to the base ring. At the center of the frame $x = 100$ and $y = 100$ and 0,0 in the posterior right corner. The arc attaches to the sidepieces. The x, y, and z coordinates are initially set before sterile draping, and the apparatus needed to adjust these coordinates during the procedure is draped out of the sterile field. Thus, to avoid compromising the sterile field, target adjustments should be done by an individual who is not scrubbed. Frame placement can be easily done on a conscious patient with local anesthesia.

Generally, two people are required for satisfactory placement of the frame. The CT or MRI results can be sent via a network connection to a computerized surgical planning station (SurgiPlan, Elekta). All major planning software packages include settings to register the Leksell frame. A major advantage of the Leksell frame is its long history of proven use in functional neurosurgery as well as stereotactically guided endoscopy, brachytherapy, radiosurgery, and the like. A typical assembly includes the base ring, two front pieces, a collection of MRI-compatible skull fixation pins, and a set of wrenches for pin placement and removal. With some minor variation, the basic set costs $86,000 to $100,000 and includes the Model G headframe, a set of four posts for pin fixation, a titanium pin set, and the arc system.

The Cosman-Roberts-Wells (CRW) Stereotactic Apparatus (Integra Radionics, Burlington, MA, www.radionics.com)

The second most common headframe used in the United States, the CRW Stereotactic Apparatus is another arc-centered system. The CRW frame (**Fig. 3.2**) is the second generation[5] of a stereotactic apparatus first developed by Theodore Roberts, Russell Brown, and Trent Wells in the late 1970s. Most contemporary stereotactic frames use some variation of Brown's vertical triangulation fiducials to convert images to stereotactic space.[6] Like the Leksell frame, it is also a highly versatile, arc-centered system and is compatible with MRI and CT.

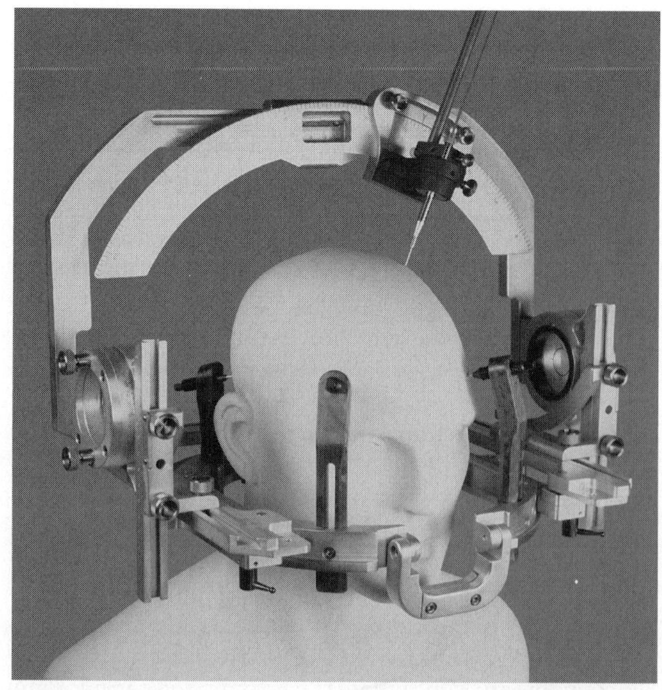

Fig. 3.2 The Cosman-Roberts-Wells (CRW) Stereotactic Apparatus (Integra Radionics, Burlington, MA, www.radionics.com). (See **Color Plate 3.2**.)

The Universal Compact base ring that is affixed to the skull is ovoid and offers a front piece that allows easier airway management. The arc system and targeting sliders are separate from the base ring. Because the head ring is separate from the arc, the CRW system offers a major advantage in sterile draping. The placement of the sterile arc on the head ring in the operating room allows continued sterility and exposure of the anterior-posterior (AP) and lateral (LAT) scales. As a result, target settings and retractor positions can be easily changed with minimal risk of compromising the sterile field. Another advantage is the availability of a phantom base assembly that allows independent verification of target coordinates. All major planning software packages, except SurgiPlan, include settings to register the CRW frame.

A typical assembly includes a head ring, the arc system, a universal CT/MRI localizer, a phantom base assembly, and trunnion reticles. Its estimated cost is $85,000. The functional CRW package includes sidebars for the ears similar to those of the Leskell frame to more easily apply the frame in a rectilinear alignment relative to the skull.

The Riechert/Mundinger (RM) Apparatus

Developed by Fritz Mundinger and Traugott Riechert in 1951,[7] this device is a popular stereotactic system in Europe. The RM frame (**Fig. 3.3**) is a polar coordinate system with the target determined by multiple arcs in lieu of being at the center of an arc. The electrode carrier is offset, and it is desirable to use a phantom (or a computer) to adjust the apparatus. The phantom mechanically simulates the placement of the arc system on the head and the coordinates of the target. Multiple targets require multiple independent calculations and therefore are slower and more complex than on the arc-centered systems discussed earlier.

Using this device, Riechert and Mundinger were the first to execute "open stereotaxy," in which open craniotomy is combined with stereotactic localization. They also used the device in pioneering the use of computers and CT imaging in the targeting of stereotactic procedures. This device can be utilized in a variety of transcranial and transfacial procedures and has also been adapted for radiosurgery. More than 450 of these headframes in over 80 countries are currently in use.[8] However, most planning software packages do not include settings for registration of an RM frame. This system is no longer commercially available.

Frameless Deep Brain Stimulation

Two alternatives to frame-based stereotaxis are currently available. One is the Nexframe system (**Fig. 3.4**). The other is the StarFix system (**Fig. 3.5**). Both allow a frameless solution to DBS and stereotactic lesioning procedures.

Typically, individual CT/MRI compatible fiducials are affixed to the skull prior to surgery. Currently, the only commercially available bone-fixed fiducials for frameless stereotaxis is the Acustar system (z-kat Company, www.z-kat.com). Bone-implanted rather than adhesive fiducials

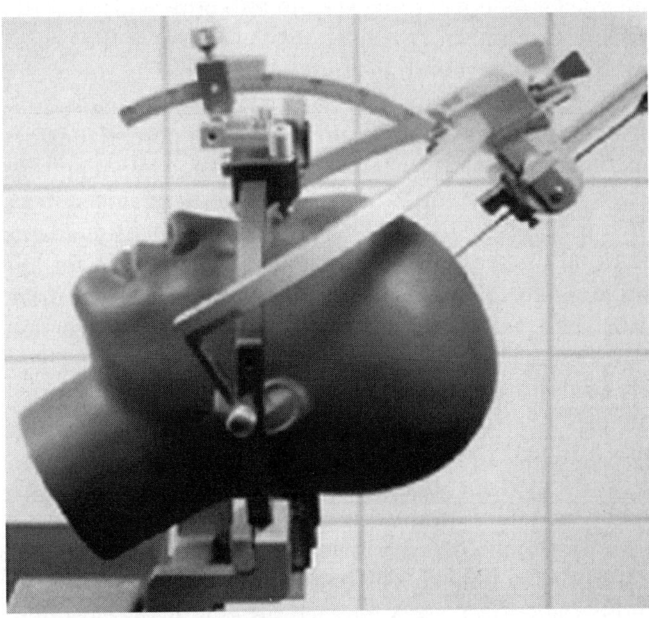

Fig. 3.3 The Riechert-Mundinger Stereotactic frame.

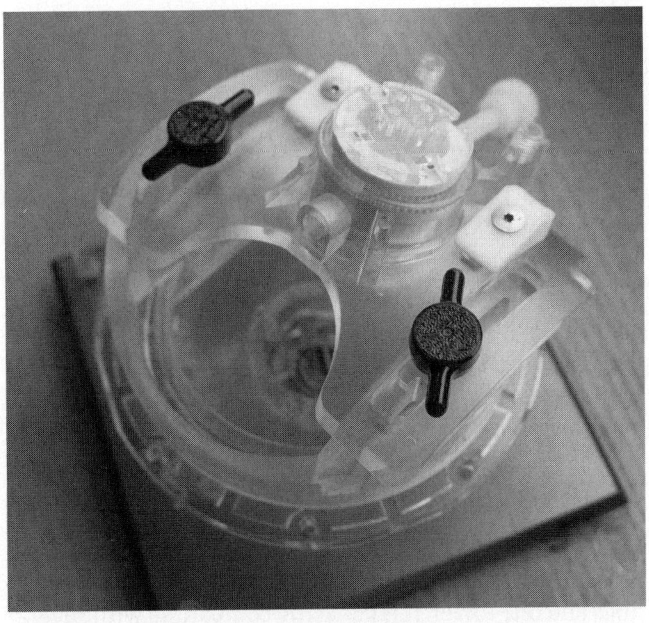

Fig. 3.4 Nexframe Frameless Microelectrode Recording Guidance Assembly (Medtronic, Minneapolis, MN). (See **Color Plate 3.4**.)

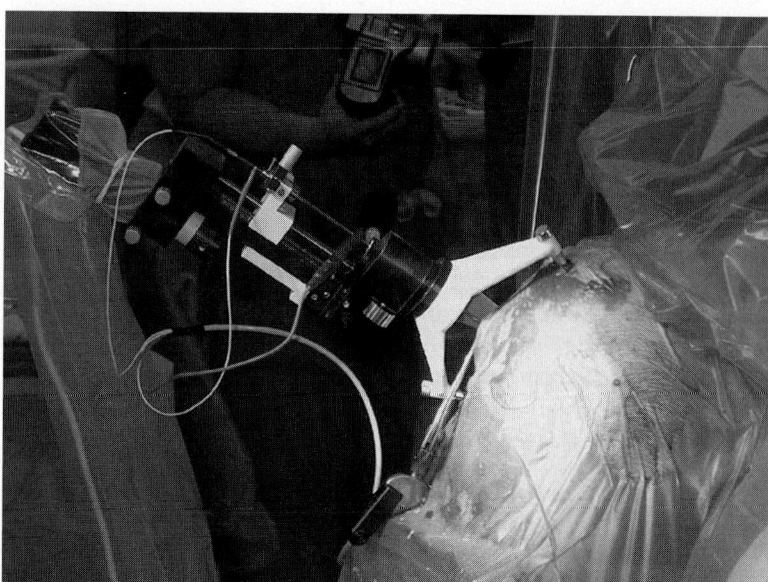

are used to eliminate targeting error due to scalp mobility. Each fiducial is a self-drilling screw assembly, which allows for MRI- and CT-compatible scanning. This process generally involves small stab incisions at each fixation point, done under local anesthesia. This is usually easier for the patient than stereotactic headframe placement. CT and MRI, as well as target planning, can then be done the day before surgery. The fiducials must remain affixed and immobile for the period prior to surgery. Although a study comparing the accuracy of DBS electrode placement utilizing frame and frameless solutions is still ongoing, preliminary data suggest they may be equivalent.[9]

Nexframe Deep Brain Access System

Developed by Image Guided Neurologics (IGN Melbourne, FL, now owned by Medtronic, Neuromodulation [Minneapolis, MN, www.medtronic.com]) this was the first commercially available frameless DBS solution. The Nexframe system includes two burr-hole locking systems for DBS electrode fixation and a tower assembly that allows for targeting in conjunction with a variety of stereotactic planning software packages. A microelectrode recording (MER) guidance assembly that locks in the tower assembly is also available (MicroTargeting from FHC, Inc., Bowdoin, ME, www.fh-co.com).

In this system, only target planning is performed prior to surgery. On the day of surgery, once the tower assembly is fixed to the skull over the burr hole, target trajectory is then established by a swivel/pivot mechanism on the tower itself by active/passive laser guidance. If there is any need to change trajectory, this can be done intraoperatively. The per-use cost of this system is $1800 for two base rings and one tower. It is currently compatible with several stereotactic planning software packages.

The STarFix System

This system offers an approach that is slightly different from that of the Nexframe. Utilizing the STarFix (FHC, Inc., Bowdoin, ME, www.fh-co.com) requires fiducial placement at least 3 days prior to surgery. Target *and* trajectory definition are done using a proprietary software package known as VoXim (IVS Solutions AG, Chemnitz, Germany), although efforts are being made to enable the use of other software packages. This information is sent to FHC, where a STarFix system is custom designed for each patient. During surgery, the STarFix tripod is coupled to the skull via the Acustar bone markers. Note that this system requires the intraoperative application VoXim software as well as a microelectrode recording system also proprietary to FHC. Finally, the trajectory is fixed for the course of the procedure. Any change in trajectory will necessitate the use of a new STarFix system. The advantage of this rigidly constrained system is that it eliminates the potential errors in a "moving-parts" system. There are some initial upfront costs to this system as opposed to the Nexframe system. To utilize this system, the VoXim software, Acustar adapters, and microdrive adapters must be purchased for approximately $90,000. In addition, the FHC microdrive must be used with this system; the motorized version costs $24,000. Each STarFix platform costs $1200. There are several avenues to offset these expenses. The platforms are patient chargeable. Also, placement of fiducials can be billed as placement of cranial tongs.

The added cost of a frameless solution is partially offset by the safety/comfort advantages and time saved in the operating room (because imaging and case planning can be done prior to surgery). Also, although the total cost may be more, the upfront costs for such systems as the Nexframe are essentially nil because each device can be obtained on a per-use basis.

Neuronal Recording Systems

Although the importance of intraoperative physiological mapping with respect to optimizing patient outcome is still debated in some circles,[10–13] it is commonly considered to represent the gold standard approach to DBS surgery. This debate and the utility of MER are discussed at length elsewhere in the book (chapter 8). Although no prospective clinical trials are available to support MER, our group utilizes it for all procedures. Apart from our belief that MER optimizes accurate electrode positioning, it may prove to be important in building a referral base. Patient support groups and the Internet have served to enhance the dissemination of information about DBS. Thus both patients and referring neurologists have often been alerted to the variance in application of these techniques. We make a point to explain our view of the importance of MER to both patients and referring physicians as part of the process of building confidence and credibility.

Electrical noise in the operating room is one of the greatest inconveniences encountered in initiating a movement disorder practice. In general, minimizing the number of electrical devices functioning in the operating suite can eliminate noise. Nonetheless, early in the process of developing a practice an MER system should be tested in the operating room that is to be used for DBS. Some MER systems are more susceptible to noise. Importantly, critical operating room equipment that generates significant noise may need to be replaced. In some cases, architectural issues may require relocation of the planned operating room (personal experience).

The MER equipment constitutes an additional capital investment, currently ranging from $50,000 to $100,000. Although such systems actually consist of numerous components, a typical system can be separated into the microdrive and its accessories, the collection of electronics used to amplify and filter the signal, and an oscilloscope and/or high-quality audio monitor. **Table 3.1** gives a list of some of the more popular commercially available MER systems.

Such systems offer an "all-in-one" package of the various components discussed in this section.

Self-compiled systems, using hardware acquired from various vendors of neurophysiology equipment, can be substantially cheaper than integrated systems. However, this do-it-yourself method requires a high level of expertise for both construction and maintenance. Fortunately, prepackaged MER equipment includes both the recording equipment as well as microdrives with adapters for the Leksell and CRW frames. Slavin recently published a comparative review of the fundamental features of the systems currently available.[14] However, the quality and nuances of any system should be evaluated carefully, and, where possible, it is best to consult others who have used or are using a given system and to observe each system in operation.

Many commercially available MER systems are capable of moving up to five electrodes simultaneously. The movement of each electrode is not independent because these systems rely on a single motor or turn screw to advance and retract the array. If one is considering using more than one simultaneous electrode, we strongly recommend obtaining a commercially available system because custom design and assembly of such a system are complicated and potentially expensive.

The Microdrive

It is important to consider not only the durability of a microdrive in the face of repeated manipulation and sterilization, but also the ease with which its parts can be assembled under sterile conditions. This is particularly important for the guide tubes and cannulae. In addition, the drive and its cables must be as light as possible so as not to induce undesirable torque on the frame system without sacrificing quality. Current drives can be classified as manual, motorized, or hydraulic, with each group having distinct advantages and disadvantages.

Motorized and hydraulic drive types enable the surgical team to control the action of the drive, and hence the microelectrode, from a remote location. In contrast, manual drives require the surgeon to advance or retract the microelectrode by manually rotating a turn screw system. This

Table 3.1 Neuronal Recording Systems

System Name	Guideline–4000*	Stim Pilot	MicroGuide
Manufacturer	FHC, Inc.	Medtronic Functional Diagnostics	Alpha-Omega Engineering
Distributor	FHC, Inc.	Medtronic	Nicolet (US/Asia) /Alpha-Omega (Europe)
Price Range ($US)	$50k–$100k	$60k–$80k	$75k–$100k
Contact	(207) 666–8190	(800) 328–0810	(877) 919–6288
	www.fh-co.com	www.medtronic.com	www.alphaomega-eng.com

*mT Guideline 4000 is in premarket evaluation.

task can be ergonomically awkward and can slow down the process of mapping, which requires an integration of patient examination, evaluation of the recordings, and adjustments to the electrode position.

Motorized drives, which consist of a small electrical motor mounted atop the drive unit, have the advantage of remote control. However, they also carry the potential to introduce substantial artifact or noise into the recording signal as the microelectrode is advanced or retracted. This rather loud noise has the cumulative effect of delaying the procedure. First, amplifiers require a small but finite period of time to recover from such artifact. Second, this noise requires that the user advance and stop in a series of steps to isolate neuronal action potentials. At least one company has attempted to solve this artifact problem by simply "muting" the signal output during electrode movement.

In contrast, hydraulic systems do not generate electrical noise. These systems consist of a slave cylinder placed atop the drive unit. The cylinder is attached to a manual or motorized master cylinder unit by means of hydraulic tubing. This setup has long been preferred in laboratory neurophysiological applications, enabling remote control while keeping the motor, if present, sufficiently distant from the microelectrode so as not to induce artifact. Of greatest importance with respect to efficiency, this setup allows for almost continuous sampling of the trajectory with minimal or no movement-related artifact. The foremost disadvantage to hydraulic systems is the potential for the hydraulic tubing to break or leak, releasing fluid that is potentially nonsterile. Further, hydraulic systems tend to require more maintenance, including the constant need to replenish fluid that has evaporated.

Recording Equipment

The components of the recording equipment are extremely sophisticated and encompass many individual features. The most important of these features is the quality of the signal output. Given their impedance, microelectrodes make superb antennae and quite readily pick up extraneous electrical noise. As such, a good MER system must incorporate both active and passive techniques to shield the signal from noise, as well as subsequent electronics to further filter any pervasive noise. The system should also be simple to operate. Although most systems now include more sophisticated techniques for analyzing the extracellular action potential data, in most cases little more is needed than the raw data signal. Because the human ear is often better at discerning a neuronal action potential and patterns of firing than the eye, a high-quality audio monitor is again warranted.

The microelectrodes themselves are typically tungsten or platinum-iridium metal electrodes with tip exposures of 10 to 20 µm. Platinum-iridium metal electrodes are usually preferred because, in comparison with tungsten electrodes, there is less electrode erosion. Electrode erosion results in impedance changes during microstimulation, degrading recording quality.

One final consideration to be made when exploring commercial MER systems is the potential application of the equipment, particularly the recording components, to non-DBS-related procedures. Many of the systems currently available are suited, though not ideal, for recording evoked potentials and thus may be used for other types of intraoperative and outpatient monitoring.

Stereotactic Targeting Software

Stereotactic software allows the movement disorder surgeon to plan the target and trajectory for a given procedure. A surgical planning software system is not an absolute necessity for a functional practice. Target coordinates for each of the available stereotactic frames can be manually calculated directly from the scanners themselves. However, commercial planning systems can make the process faster and more efficient.

The most prevalent commercial systems are manufactured by Medtronic, Radionics, Elekta, and BrainLab (**Table 3.2**). Each has its own limitations and advantages.[15,16]

Table 3.2 Neuronavigation Systems

System Name	Treon Plus StealthStation: StealthMerge Module Framelink Module	SurgiPlan/ ImageFusion	Leksell SurgiPlan	VectorVision: iVision Module
Manufacturer	Medtronic Surgical Navigation Technology	Radionics	Elekta	BrainLab
Distributor	Medtronic	Radionics	Elekta	BrainLab
Price Range ($US)	$253,500 (Frame and frameless based capabilities) (Compatible with Nexframe)	$100,000–$120,000 (CRW/Leksell frame based only)	$85,000 (Leksell-frame based only)	$250,000 + (Frame and frameless based capabilities) (Compatible with Nexframe)
Contact	(877) 242–9504	(781) 272–1233	(770) 300–9725	(800) 784–7700
	www.stealthstation.com	www.radionics.com	www.elekta.com	www.brainlab.com

Abbreviations: CRW, Cosman-Roberts-Wells.

Some are designed specifically for functional neurosurgery, whereas others allow for tumor and spine stereotaxis. These systems provide features that may improve accuracy like image fusion or corrections for frame misalignments. Further, these systems have features that can save time, including image fusion (allowing MRIs to be done prior to day of surgery), preset indirect targets, and general software navigation protocols that speed the process. The most important considerations when choosing a software package are ease of use, compatibility with frame-based and frameless systems, and company support.

Whether a surgeon is adding movement disorder surgery to a general practice or building a functional neurosurgery practice, the individual's institution may have an existing image-guided system to which the functional software package can be added. Alternatively, it may be best to purchase an entire system for doing various surgeries, or you may consider deferring the higher-cost image-guided platform and purchase a stand-alone functional system. Prices for a complete image-guided surgical system generally vary depending on the number of software modules included, but are typically over $200,000. Stand-alone functional only workstations can be purchased in the $100,000 range.

Editor's Comments

Functional neurosurgeons are not born but created. During residency, stereotactic and functional procedures should be introduced and the concepts grasped. Following graduation, most neurosurgeons interested in focusing on functional neurosurgery should complete a well-structured fellowship program. The time, resources, and intellectual activity going into placement of a DBS lead are far greater than those required for a stereotactic brain biopsy. Although functional and stereotactic fellowships are not yet officially recognized, they do provide sufficient experience and an intensive work experience to allow sufficient expertise to master all the subtleties necessary for a specialized practice in functional and stereotactic neurosurgery. During neurosurgical training, an intimate familiarity with a variety of stereotactic equipment should be developed. In starting a new practice, it is generally this equipment that will be purchased. Nevertheless, it behooves wise neurosurgeons to explore other pieces of equipment because that upon which they were trained may not be optimal for their new venue. At the same time, inadequate temporizing purchases should be avoided.

Our personal preference is for a metal frame. We recognize in a small practice a plastic frame might be of some value,[20] but they simply do not hold up in high-volume practices. Nor do I like externally supported aiming devices (Laitinen Stereoadapter, Sandström Trade and Technology, Inc. Wellard, Ontario, Canada, www.sandstromion.cal.non-invasive-stereoadaptor.com) that are not firmly affixed.[21] I prefer either the Leksell or the functional CRW frame. These are highly versatile, highly durable, and well-established frames with good product support throughout the world. The ear bars are especially useful for aligning the skull and minimizing tilt. Another advantage of the CRW or Leksell system is the ease with which it can integrate with other add-on equipment. I have a great deal of experience with both of these systems, and they are quite useful for routine stereotactic as well as the most advanced stereotactic and functional neurosurgery interventions.

Specialized equipment such as COMPASS (COMPASS International, Inc. Rochester, MN, www.compass.com) provides a unique overall system for multiple stereotactic functions, including functional stereotactic surgery.[22] However, it represents a major commitment of resources that most start-up programs are not willing to commit.

The Riechert/Mundinger (RM) system is simple to use and quite versatile. I have little personal experience with using this device, but it reminds me a great deal of the Brown-Roberts-Wells (BRW) system and the difficulties that arise from a polar system in which movements to multiple targets are much more difficult to calculate. However, it does have a nice phantom, and the few users that I've had interactions with do like the system. The Zamorano-Dujovny frame (F. L. Fischer, Freiberg, Germany, www.flfischer.com) is an arc-centered stereotactic system that is an outgrowth of the RM system.[23] Similarly, the Talairach system has evolved into several new systems (see chapter 91).[24] In Japan, the Sugita apparatus (Mizuho America, Inc., Beverly, MA, www.mizuho.com) has some popularity but no advantages over the systems already discussed.[25]

A great deal of interest has been recently generated by the frameless systems. The initial outline of this book did not contain any information on frameless systems. Unlike the Polaris system (Ohio Medical Instruments, Inc., Cincinnati, OH, www.ohiomed.com), these are specifically designed for functional neurosurgery, and most of the preliminary evaluations have been positive. These are basically plastic systems and for single use. This adds potential cost to these systems, which is already minimally profitable. Frameless units in the short term for low volume programs are quite reasonable. However, a stereotactic frame costing approximately $60,000 to $80,000 amortized over 10 years is $6,000 to $8,000 a year. If you are performing more than 10 cases a year the frame more than pays for itself when compared with the extra cost of the disposable frameless systems ($1800 to $1200 each × 10). Additionally, the extra cost for the disposable frameless platform has to come out of the limited reimbursement under the global cost for the hospitalization. The saving grace for the hospital is that diagnostic MRI studies can be charged to offset the cost of the frameless systems (see Chapter 10).

The next most important piece of equipment is that of image-guided neuronavigation systems. The more multidimensional the images (axial, coronal, sagittal, and special view, i.e., trajectory, probe's eye, look ahead, etc.) and the more the trajectories that can be overlaid and annotated the better. Increasingly, the frame systems are developing their own image-guided platforms. I use both the SurgiPlan (Elekton, Stockholm, Sweden) and the StealthStation (FrameLink Medtronic Navigation, Louisville, CO.) systems. Both of these are excellent systems, but I prefer the ability to image my trajectories and annotate them with FrameLink. The utility of overlaying brain atlases is extremely limited and can be misleading, especially to the novice. Never assume location simply because an overlay would suggest that the location is where you "should be." I use the image data but never fully trust them until they are verified electrophysiologically. Although most of the atlases are somewhat adjustable, they simply do not fully configure the anatomy of the patient. An improved imaging quality in the platforms such as edge enhancement and better tissue contrast is preferred to adjustable atlas overlays. I've also seen far too many poor quality image fusions. As an experiment, I once fused two magnetic resonance images set together, one of which I deliberately invented. It fused and let me proceed as "verified." Wise customers will view each platform before choosing the best possible system for their purposes rather than simply the system on which they were trained.

The equipment for the microelectrode is being integrated with the frame systems. Resist the attempt to simply purchase a single one-step, all-inclusive frame, imaging-guidance platform and microelectrode system simply because of convenience. Many of the early microelectrode systems have been quite substandard in terms of their signal fidelity and audio quality. I have had excellent recordings and service with both the Axon (now manufactured by FHC) and the Alpha-Omega systems (now distributed by FHC). These systems are somewhat archaic with their large cabinets. I have also used the FHC MicroTargeting drive that is satisfactory but has problems with artifact from the motor. FHC's disposable model makes most sense only in very low volume practices. FHC is also supporting the Medtronic Leadpoint MER system. Increasingly, smaller, laptop-type devices are being developed. The multiple electrode arrays have been slow to catch on in the United States but is popular in several locations in Europe (chapter 9). We've had some limited experience with multiple simultaneous electrode recording and we would caution the beginner from stepping into this arena too early because listening to multiple channels can be confusing. FDA-approved commercially constructed microelectrodes are readily available from FHC (MicroTargeting electrodes).

■ Building a Program

Each subdiscipline within functional neurosurgery requires a multidisciplinary approach. Movement disorder surgery epitomizes this characteristic. Appropriate preoperative assessment requires neurological, neuropsychological, and neurosurgical assessment. In the operating room, DBS surgery requires both neurophysiological and stereotactic neurosurgical expertise as well as an anesthesiologist comfortable with the nuances of this operation. Postoperative management requires longitudinal patient relationships that incorporate internal pulse generator (IPG) programming. Lastly, successful care of this patient population requires open communication between physicians, nurses, and clerical staff in each of the areas described. Ideally, the knowledge and expertise of several fields should not only interact but merge in a completely coordinated effort.

The degree to which responsibility is distributed to different individuals will depend on the scale of the practice in question. Our high-volume practice currently involves three neurosurgeons, five neurologists, two neurophysiologists, two neuropsychologists, as well as an ethicist, fellows, nurses, and a variety of other ancillary support staff. This staffing has been organized with the goal of implanting approximately three DBS patients per week. In the early stages of practice development, or if DBS is to be added to a general practice, this level of delegation is not practical. Nonetheless, each of the roles described below must be fulfilled. The greatest challenge to initiating a DBS practice is to provide these various clinical dimensions with the limited resources inherent in an early stage of program building.

The Core Team

In this section, we will attempt to identify the roles and disciplines absolutely necessary to bring a movement disorder patient to surgery. **Fig. 3.6** represents the relationships between these various roles. This sketch will assume that the surgery will take place in a tertiary care, academic medical center. Special considerations for the private practice model are presented in the last sections.

The Movement Disorder Neurologist

The movement disorder neurologist is usually the first member of the team that a DBS candidate sees. Although fellowship training is available in movement disorder neurology, there is no specific board certification process for this subspecialty. DBS patients will either come from within the movement disorder neurologist's own practice or from community neurologists and internists. The next section discusses the referral pool for DBS. As with the neurosurgeon, the movement disorder neurologist should be incorporated into the preoperative, intraoperative, perioperative, and postoperative segments of care.

The movement disorder neurologist should make the ultimate determination of the stage of a candidate's disease progression as well as the diagnosis. At the initial phase of DBS evaluation, it is appropriate to take a fresh look at a patient's diagnosis. The movement disorder neurologist should prevent the implantation of patients with multisystem atrophy or related L-dopa unresponsive conditions. Because these patients are inherently difficult to treat they will often be referred for surgical options. Additionally, the movement disorder neurologist can help to

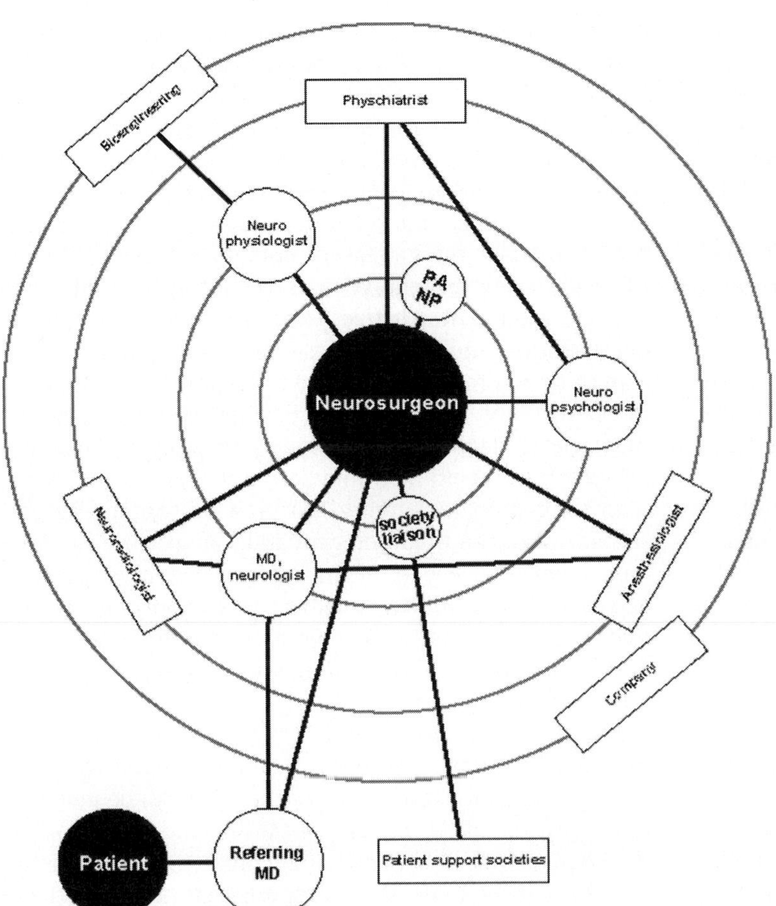

Fig. 3.6 Core relationship between the surgical movement disorder team.

triage patients who have been referred prematurely. This is a delicate task that is addressed in the section on referral base. Premature referrals for DBS surgery can embarrass primary physicians and make them hesitant about further referrals. This issue can best be dealt with through an open line of communication between both the movement disorder surgeon and neurologist and referring physicians.

The most important role of the movement disorder neurologist is to determine whether a patient is medically refractory. The patient's current movement disorder medication profile and history should be evaluated to determine whether further adjustments are justified. If medications can be further optimized, the team neurologist will communicate recommendations to the referring doctor and the neurosurgeon. Importantly, the referring doctor and patient should be given an explicit timeline for initiating these adjustments. We prefer to give patients a delayed surgery date that can be canceled in the event that medical management succeeds. Patients sent back to referring neurologists with recommendations and no timeline will often be lost to follow-up either entirely or for long periods. This approach can be frustrating to both patients and referring doctors. Thus we recommend that the team movement disorder neurologist answer the question, "Is this patient likely to be an acceptable candidate for DBS within the next year?" If so, then remaining medical options should be exhausted in the time preceding a known date for surgery. This ensures that only appropriate, refractory patients come to surgery, which also ensures a good relationship with referring physicians and patients. Direct conversations with referring physicians prior to the initial consultation can avoid time lost on poor candidates.

If a patient is deemed an appropriate candidate by history, medication profile, and disease symptoms, the team neurologist will refer the patient to the surgeon and neuropsychologist. The final task of the team neurologist is to orient the patient to the nature of DBS surgery and appropriate expectations for the individual's response to stimulation. However, an exhaustive discussion of the risks and benefits of surgery and stimulation should be left to the neurosurgeon. In the early stages of setting up a movement disorder practice, some neurosurgeons may choose to solicit direct, nontriaged referrals. Even in this scenario, a movement disorder neurologist should be enlisted to ensure that all possible alternatives to surgery are presented and diagnosis is confirmed.

The movement disorder neurologist can be an essential part of the surgical team. The neurologist can be integral in assessing the correct placement of the DBS electrode by correlating test stimulation parameters with standardized preoperative ratings. The neurologist will also assess neurological side effects. In our practice, the neurologists control neurophysiology and bill for the mapping procedure, including MER, microstimulation, and macrostimulation. Individual functional neurosurgeons in smaller practices may choose to direct mapping with a PhD neurophysiological assistant. This is possible but somewhat awkward and may consequently slow the procedure.

Perioperatively, the team neurologist should be available to assess any changes to symptoms from surgery. We have found that DBS programming through resolving edema in the basal ganglia can be confusing and inefficient. As a result, we delay programming patients until 1 month after surgery. Consequently, medication profiles are generally kept stable from preoperative regimens throughout the surgical hospital stay. This is not always possible because microsubthalamotomy may result in side effects (dyskinesias) after surgery even with doses that were tolerated before surgery. The team neurologist should be integral in guiding medication changes in this period.

Postoperatively, the movement disorder neurologist can assume the point role in programming of the IPGs. Alternatively, the responsibility for programming can be assumed by the neurosurgeon. As with the intraoperative role of the neurologist, this decision should be made by the surgeon as the practice develops. Programming is a billable procedure that can support the costs of maintaining this more intensive role in the longitudinal care of the patient. Nonetheless, neurologists are in the ideal position to do IPG programming because they have the expertise in evaluating movement disorder symptoms and side effects from stimulation and medication. Furthermore, as the stimulation parameters are titrated toward optimal effect, the patient often requires adjustment in medication profiles. Thus the neurologist is uniquely positioned to coordinate medical and electrical therapies. In fact, we instruct our patients that DBS is merely a means to deliver focused electrical current, which itself acts like a new drug in the larger treatment regimen. Once medications and stimulation parameters have reached a therapeutic plateau, the team neurologist will communicate the current regimen with the referring neurologist/internist. The referring doctor should reassume the responsibility for pharmacological therapy and can be trained to make minor adjustments to IPG settings. If any major problems develop or changes need to be made, the relationship between referral doctor and team neurologist will facilitate patient care.

The Neuropsychologist

Although movement disorder surgery can ameliorate the symptoms of Parkinson disease, essential tremor, and dystonia, the operations themselves can affect the patient's cognitive function. Cognitive changes are well documented potential side effects of ablative surgery.[17] Similarly, despite the potential to adjust and even discontinue stimulation, pallidal and subthalamic stimulation can cause permanent changes to the intellectual function.[18] In addition, it is becoming increasingly clear that subthalamic stimulation can induce emotional side effects, including depression and mania. Further, the increased mobility achieved through DBS can cause preoperative manic or impulsive tendencies to become more destructive. Although the risk of cognitive deterioration and stimulation-related emotional lability cannot be rigorously determined preoperatively, the best indicator is the neuropsychological profile of the patient. Any signs of significant executive dysfunction, impulsivity, or dementia should be immediate warnings as to the patient's suitability for surgery. Movement disorder surgeons should make the final determination about surgical candidacy with respect to information on cognitive function and emotional stability. However, it is important to have objective documentation of this status based on reproducible metrics prior to proceeding with surgery. Identifying a specific neuropsychologist with an interest in DBS and Parkinson disease will facilitate this process. In the event that concerns about cognitive and emotional issues develop during stimulation, the neuropsychologist can be involved in the process of objectively measuring and documenting the change. This collaboration becomes indispensable as one seeks to establish DBS programs that minimize these side effects.

Also, because movement disorder surgery deals with chronic debilitating disease, psychopathology can develop in both patients and family members as they attempt to cope both pre- and postoperatively. Anxiety and depression are commonly associated with the disease. Further, the vast improvement in the function of movement disorder patients after surgery can have a significant impact on patients and their support system. The patient's primary caretaker, once heavily depended on for support, may require help dealing with a changed role. The neuropsychologist may help to anticipate these problems, detect them when they occur, and make treatment recommendations.

The Neurophysiologist

Although it is common for a functional neurosurgeon to take an active role in deep brain mapping, it is commonly performed in conjunction with an MD- or PhD-level neurophysiologist with substantial experience in electrophysiology, physiology, or neuroscience. Although experience in the physiology of motor control is useful, the team neurophysiologist should have a working knowledge of the regional anatomy and electrophysiological characteristics of MER in the target site(s) and surrounding structures. Characteristics studied include neuronal waveform, discharge pattern, discharge frequency, changes in activity with sensory stimulation (light touching of skin, palpation of muscle, movement of limbs), and changes in activity with behavior. Optimally, training should consist of a 1-year fellowship in intraoperative MER techniques, covering required knowledge and skills; however, this is not always practical. At a minimum, the neurophysiologist should have a robust understanding of the principles of differential amplification, impedance, and the Nyquist theorem, as well as the safe operations of electronic equipment related to micro- or semi-microelectrode recordings, including amplifiers, filters, and microelectrodes.

Because accurate electrode placement depends on effective mapping, someone in the operating room must be comfortable with the equipment. That individual is responsible for maintaining and trouble shooting the equipment as well as deploying it in the operating room. Technical difficulties with the equipment in the operating room require an experienced, dedicated individual capable of efficient trouble-shooting. This includes searching out and reducing the electrical interference that is present in every operating room. Outside of the operating room, the neurophysiologist ensures that all of the technical equipment is in working order and in good repair. This person also interacts with vendors and bioengineering personnel to enact upgrades and repairs as technology/resources allow. Also, in an academic center, the neurophysiologist will be essential in investigational efforts involving the recorded MER data and functional imaging studies. The degree to which an individual surgeon starting a movement disorder practice takes on this responsibility will again depend on available resources. As more integrated and user-friendly mapping equipment becomes available, this role may be assumed by the neurosurgeon in low-volume practices. However, at the present time, having a team neurophysiologist is critical to most higher volume practices.

The Nurse Practitioner/Physician Assistant

This role is extremely important to the smooth operation of the movement disorder surgery practice. A nurse practitioner/physician assistant (NP/PA) becomes a partner to the functional neurosurgeon in managing this complex and needy patient population. The NP/PA often serves as the main interface between the patient and the neurosurgeon and will likely be more accessible than the busy surgeon. Together with the neurosurgeon, the NP/PA will see the patients preoperatively, establish a rapport, deliver support throughout the operative experience, and see the patient postoperatively. The NP/PA should be the first person on the team that the patient will contact with any question or problems. Thus it is important that the NP/PA is intimately aware of the DBS procedure. This includes indications, the procedure itself, and, importantly, postoperative complications.

If the surgery takes place without resident support, the PA/NP can often serve as first assistant during the head frame or fiducial placement, imaging acquisition, and DBS electrode implantation. In our practice, the neurosurgical NP assists with head frame placement and shepherding the patient through preoperative MRI and CT scanning. The PA/NP then takes the patient to the operating room while stereotactic planning is performed. As discussed earlier, frameless stereotaxis may obfuscate the need for stereotactic planning on the morning of surgery. However, using the frame-based approach, a postframe CT must be obtained even if image fusion is to be utilized. In our practice, the NP has often assisted with comforting the patient throughout the procedure. Many DBS patients will experience transient confusion during the operation. This phenomenon is often attributed to the mild pneumocephalus that occurs during surgery. Although not precisely understood, it occurs more frequently in older patients with more advanced disease. The presence of an individual with whom the patient is well acquainted, who can provide continuous encouragement and orientation, is often critical to completing the case.

In smaller movement disorder practices, particularly ones that are integrated with a broader program of neural augmentation, the neurosurgical PA/NP may play the central role in IPG programming under the guidance of a neurosurgeon. Because this individual may play a similar role in the management of intrathecal pain and spasticity pumps, as well as neural stimulators for pain management, they are often already comfortable with the equipment and basic knowledge necessary for IPG programming. As mentioned earlier, in our practice, IPG programming is largely delegated to the team movement disorder neurologist. In this setting, however, NPs conduct most of the hands-on programming under supervision, whereas the neurologist focuses on patient evaluation, medical management, and troubleshooting. In either scenario, as time passes, the number of patients dependent on the practice will continue to increase given the longitudinal relationship necessary. Thus, in the absence of a skilled PA/NP, the movement disorder neurosurgeon's time will become increasingly occupied with IPG programming, which affects the neurosurgeon's surgical productivity.

Secretary/Patient Liaison

The role of handling appointments and scheduling is common to any medical secretary. However, two features distinguish the demands on a medical secretary in a movement disorder surgery practice. First, navigating the ambiguities and intricacies of reimbursement for DBS remains difficult. More time spent with insurance companies means less time for patient care. Until recently, DBS for subthalamic nucleus stimulation was not approved by the US Food and Drug Administration (FDA). There are future applications of DBS that are still not FDA approved. Examples include DBS for epilepsy, pain, and psychiatric disorders. We expect the demand for these procedures to increase prior to FDA approval. DBS for dystonia is approved by the FDA under the humanitarian device authorization but requires an Investigational Review Board (IRB-) approved protocol. Getting insurance company approval for treatment requires negotiation with labyrinthine systems that are as unique as the different managed care companies they serve. A secretary with some expertise in this area can facilitate this process.

Second, the movement disorder surgery secretary must effectively field the pre- and postoperative outpatient calls. DBS is offered to patients who range from well informed to mildly cognitively impaired. We emphasize that this is a very needy population with whom communication is not always easy. Further, because DBS is elective, a successful practice must cater to the patient. Unlike many of the segments of neurosurgery, patients and families have the liberty to shop for the movement disorder program with which they are most comfortable. Patient access and communication is one of the most critical components to achieving this comfort.

Finally, the movement disorder surgery secretary can serve as a layperson liaison. Patient support groups are often an essential part of the movement disorder surgery experience for the patient. A strong relationship between the practice and these groups, facilitated by the secretary, allows the patients to get the continuing adjunctive support they need and also offers fertile ground for future patients. Finally, for the present, DBS remains novel to the general public. Thus movement disorder surgery practices may be approached by the press with the desire of covering "the story" of these patients and the technology. As will be discussed, such coverage can play an important role in practice building. An articulate secretary knowledgeable in the rudiments of movement disorder surgery can facilitate this process.

The Neurosurgeon

We believe strongly that the movement disorder surgeon must be the team leader. Given that the surgeon must make the ultimate decision concerning who receives surgery and where the electrode will be placed, he or she must command the respect of the team. As such, the surgeon must not only perform the procedure itself but must also be involved in all aspects of care. Depending on the model of the practice and the resources available, the surgeon will need to assume each and every role defined earlier as the circumstances dictate.

In our practice, the neurosurgical preoperative consult focuses on the patient's emotional, cognitive, and medical ability to tolerate surgery. We assess the patient's primary symptoms and expectations in an attempt to determine whether DBS will benefit the patient. Further, we educate patients as to what will be demanded of them on the day of surgery and afterward, as well as the risks of surgery, neural implants, and stimulation itself. Finally, we review

the team neurologist's assessment of whether the patient has exhausted reasonable medical options. Due to the size of our team, we have found that a weekly team meeting is useful to establishing consensus about candidacy as well as pre- and postoperative management.

During procedures, we encourage an open discussion of physiological data (but not in the patient's presence), prior to deciding on new electrode tracts. Nonetheless, disagreements often remain concerning these data. The final decision concerning target adjustments must always be the neurosurgeon's. Thus efficient and accurate interpretation of these data ultimately outweighs the technical demands of movement disorder surgery.

Adjunct Medical Fields

Other medical fields will be essential in the execution of movement disorder surgery. Although not a part of the core team per se, they will have an ongoing relationship with the neurosurgeon.

Anesthesiology

Many of the procedures in movement disorder surgery can present unique challenges for the anesthesiologist. It, therefore, becomes important that the movement disorder neurosurgeon and the anesthesiologist have a particularly strong line of communication. Often, movement disorder patients are older and, because of their disease, more infirm than others in their age group. With few exceptions, the operations are performed awake, with only occasional intravenous (IV) sedation. The lack of general anesthesia takes an element of control away from both the anesthesiologist and the neurosurgeon. Airway issues are of primary concern because the patient is often immobilized in a bulky stereotactic headframe. Pain control and patient comfort often require a delicate balance because sedatives often exacerbate the airway issues and interfere with MER acquisition. The anesthesiologist who is better educated about the mechanics of a given movement disorder procedure will be more able to provide an atmosphere of control in the operating theater. Also the anesthesiologist must have a working knowledge of the impact of various medications on neuronal activity as measured by electrophysiology. This understanding is essential to maintaining patient control, safety, and comfort without negating MER.

Neuroradiology

Image acquisition is central to movement disorder surgery. Excellent anatomical images can help cut down on MER recording passes and ultimately lead to a safer procedure. Further, neural imaging in the presence of implanted stimulators requires an understanding of parameters for safely applying MRI. This imaging plays a critical role in targeting previously implanted patients as well as evaluating complications or DBS failures.

Although MER is currently indispensable, advances in imaging technologies may diminish its future role. Diffusion tensor imaging, connectivity imaging, and advances in functional MRI (fMRI) sequences may ultimately allow the neuroradiologist, together with the neurosurgeon, to define a movement disorder surgery target [fore the patient enters the operating room. Such an endeavor would necessarily result in a shorter operation, thereby conserving resources and providing a safer experience for the patient. Thus the neuroradiologist will play an important role in advancing DBS technique.

Psychiatry

As already mentioned, movement disorder surgery can have significant emotional and psychodynamic consequences. The targets involved in movement disorder surgery can have significant modulatory effects on aspects of mood.[12] Improved patient mobility can render preoperative impulsivity potentially dangerous. As the patient deals with the return of function and the patient's family members deal with changes in their own relationship to the patient, psychiatric assistance may be necessary. Thus it is useful for the movement disorder neurosurgeon to locate a psychiatrist with an interest in DBS who is familiar with these issues and can address them as necessary. This individual plays an expanded role in a functional neurosurgery practice that includes psychosurgery.

Bioengineering

Many academic medical centers have a bioengineering department. Often these facilities will have the expertise for diagnosis and repair of the expensive equipment essential to movement disorder surgery. Importantly, because each operative center has its own unique challenges, this department can help in the modification of standard equipment to optimize resources. As discussed, the team neurophysiologist is the member that must interact with bioengineering most commonly.

Vendors

The movement disorder surgeon should maintain some connections with the vendors of equipment used in movement disorder surgery. These companies often provide training and expertise that can fill gaps in the team's knowledge base. Not only will this keep the surgeon apprised of advances in equipment, it also offers an interface for reciprocal improvement. In addition, vendors of IPGs and electrodes depend on the surgeon's productivity and may help to interface with referring neurologists. This role may include providing support for simple IPG programming in these neurology practices. By maintaining communication with the vendors, neurosurgeons can help to steer research and development in a clinically relevant direction.

Editor's Comments

Unquestionably, the three most important people in building a program are the neurosurgeon, the neurologist, and the nurse practitioner or physician assistant to manage the program. The neurosurgeon and neurologist must be emotionally and scientifically compatible. There is always a tendency for a neurosurgeon to want to proceed with the minimum amount of data and a tendency for a neurologist to want too much data. Compromises by both parties are necessary. In terms of managing patients and determining who should go on to be evaluated as a surgical candidate, the neurologist is clearly the leader. The neurologist manages these patients before and after surgery and has the best handle as to who is a good candidate and who would be a poor candidate based on the patient's disease and psychiatric makeup. The neurosurgeon of course will make the ultimate decision as to whether to proceed with surgery on any particular patient. Many times the neurologist's opinion is colored by factors other than those strictly related to surgery. The neurosurgical evaluation is critical and represents a different aspect of the evaluation; hence this book devotes two chapters (Chapters 4 and 5), one by a neurologist and one by a neurosurgeon, to preoperative evaluation of patients. The neurosurgeon and the neurologist will often have multiple roles in surgery. Sometimes the microelectrode recording will be performed by the neurologist and sometimes by the neurosurgeon. Both should work together in examining and evaluating the electrophysiological and clinical data. A second voice is extremely useful in the operating room; however, it must be remembered that the neurosurgeon is the final arbiter and makes the final decisions. It is the wise neurosurgeon that will take the counsel of the neurologist, though ultimately it is the neurosurgeon's experience and artistry that will finally determine the success of the procedure.

An experienced and compassionate nurse practitioner or physician assistant is necessary to help in all aspects of the pre- and postoperative care of the patient. Frequently, this person's appearance in the operating room is useful for the patient, especially during long, complicated cases. These individuals can also serve to record data and act as a liaison between neurosurgery and neurology. The ancillary members of the team also need to be as expert as possible because there are many characteristics of these patients that require special consideration and evaluation in the performance of the surgery. The smoother the team's performance, the happier will be the patient, the better will be the selection process, and the better will be the ultimate results.

■ The Business of a Movement Disorder Surgery Practice

Once the equipment is procured and the team assembled, the practice faces several challenges. The patients must be found. Once found, the practice must be run in an economically feasible manner for the surgeon, the supporting team members, and the hospital/medical center. The strategies outlined here can address these challenges. **Fig. 3.7** summarizes the various avenues of patient referral sources.

The movement disorder population is a large, relatively untapped patient source. Taking the three top indications for movement disorder surgery, one can get an idea of the numbers of potential cases. Community-based epidemiological studies have found the prevalence of essential tremor to be as high as 3.9% of the population, with estimates as high as 5.5% in patients over 40 years of age.[19] The prevalence of dystonia has been estimated to be 3.4 per 100,000 for generalized and 30 per 100,000 for focal subtypes. Parkinson disease may affect ~650,000 Americans and 1.6 million people worldwide. Based on the incidence of the disease, there are estimates that ~33,000 people worldwide, including 13,000 Americans, could benefit from Activa Parkinson's Control Therapy each year. The total current population of essential tremor/Parkinson disease patients that are surgical candidates in the United States is estimated to be 180,000. Since 1997, more than 14,000 people worldwide have benefited from Activa Therapy for essential tremor and Parkinson disease.[11] Severe spasticity resulting from cerebral palsy, spinal cord injury,

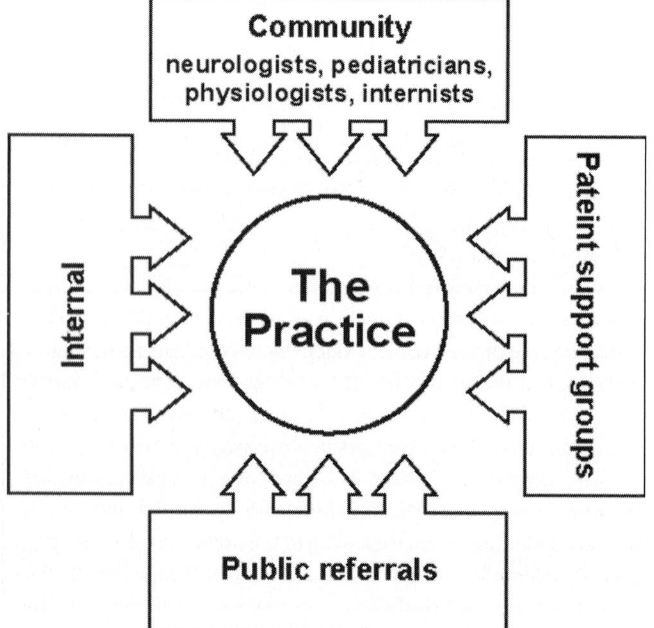

Fig. 3.7 Summary of the various avenues of patient referral sources.

and multiple sclerosis as well as a variety of less common disorders may benefit from surgery. Between 1992 and 2000, ~11,000 intrathecal pumps were implanted for baclofen delivery. Building a successful movement disorder practice depends on finding these patients.

The movement disorder surgeon's relationship with local general neurologists is the most important means of generating referrals. Developing this relationship requires a concerted effort and remains complicated. Because of the novelty of neural augmentation, local hospitals remain interested in hosting movement disorder surgeons to give grand rounds. Similarly, local and state organizations of neurologists may provide venues to reach out to referring neurologists. These presentations serve to build the surgeon's credibility with the local neurological community.

However, in our experience, primary physicians refer their patients predominantly to individuals with whom they have a personal relationship. These relationships must be cultivated by the movement disorder surgeon in the early stages of practice building. As mentioned earlier, device vendors have a shared interest in cultivating these relationships and are often willing to support introductory dinners or meetings. Many referring neurologists lack the knowledge base necessary for effective referrals. The referral process can be a no-win situation for these individuals. Inappropriate referrals result in the patients' expectations being raised and ultimately disappointed. This process undermines the patients' confidence in their primary neurologist. On the other hand, neurologists fear that patients who undergo implantation will be lost to their practice. Thus, whether the patient is appropriate or inappropriate for DBS, many neurologists perceive that their practice will be adversely affected by the referral. This cycle can be overcome by establishing a personal relationship with the primary neurologists. Phone calls should be encouraged to discuss possible referrals. This process educates the neurologists and cuts down on wasted consultations with poor surgical candidates. Further, it provides the primary neurologists with the opportunity to leverage this relationship, enhancing their stature in the eyes of their patients.

Likewise, a personal relationship can address the primary neurologist's fear of losing patients who undergo implantation. Within the context of this relationship, these neurologists can be incorporated into the process of medical adjustment that will occur as IPG programming proceeds. Thus DBS implantation expands rather than limits their role in management. Finally, in some cases, these neurologists can undertake IPG programming as a billable part of their practice. The device vendors provide education and support in this process.

As mentioned earlier, both patients and neurologists can be reached through interfacing with the local media. The appeal of DBS technology persists and makes good public interest subject matter. More importantly, the stark contrast of patients' symptoms before and after DBS, and the ability to recapitulate this contrast by turning off IPGs, creates a story that is easy for the public to understand. The marriage of high technology with manifest human relief continues to attract publicity. This publicity builds credibility with both neurologists and patients. It may also reach patients who are not currently receiving appropriate therapy. It is important to point out, however, that raw publicity is a double-edged sword. The self-referrals that this activity generates will contain many patients that are not appropriate for surgery. The team movement disorder neurologist can be of significant assistance in triaging these individuals.

With the advent of information sharing technologies such as the Internet, patient support groups and disease societies provide a wealth of information for patients regarding treatment for their disease. One aspect of this resource is a list of physicians who provide movement disorder surgery. Getting involved with these patient groups by providing information and speaking at informational sessions can help make the patients aware of a particular practice and its technical expertise in treating movement disorders. These organizations can serve to connect new movement disorder surgeons with the specific organizations active in their practice area. We have paraphrased the descriptions of these organizations that appear on their Web sites below.

National Parkinson Foundation (www.parkinson.org)

The National Parkinson Foundation was founded in 1957 by a Ms. Jeanne Levey. Headquartered in Miami, Florida, the NPF supports researchers; physicians; occupational, physical, and speech therapists; and psychological counseling. It also provides educational and medical information for Parkinson patients, their families, neurologists, and general medical practitioners.

American Parkinson Disease Association Inc. (www.apdaparkinson.org)

The American Parkinson Disease Association Inc. was founded in 1961 to "ease the burden and find a cure" for Parkinson disease. Headquartered in New York, the organization focuses its energies on research, patient support, education, and public awareness of the disease. In 2003–2004, the APDA budget for research was more than $2.5 million and exceeded $2 million for patient support. Each year the APDA scientific advisory board reviews grant requests and submits recommendations for funding researchers whose work shows promise of making scientific breakthroughs or finding improved treatments for Parkinson disease. The APDA national office also coordinates the efforts of 65 chapters, 57 information and referral centers, and 250 affiliated support groups across the nation.

Parkinson's Disease Foundation (www.pdf.org)

Located in New York and Chicago, the PDF is a national not-for-profit organization, a leading presence in the field of Parkinson disease research, education, and public information. The organization has an annual budget of more than $6 million and maintains corresponding relationships with 100,000 Parkinson families and friends.

Rewired for Life Foundation (www.rewiredforlife.org)

Re-Wired for Life Foundation is a nonprofit organization created to promote the understanding of DBS among patients, their families, and medical professionals through dissemination of information, patient support meetings, medical professional meetings, and research development.

International Essential Tremor Foundation (www.essentialtremor.org):

The International Essential Tremor Foundation (IETF) was created in 1988 to provide information, services, and support to individuals and families affected by ET. The organization encourages and promotes research in an effort to determine the causes, the treatment, and, ultimately, the cure for ET. IETF is the only worldwide organization dedicated to meeting the needs of those whose daily lives are challenged by ET.

Dystonia Medical Research Foundation (www.dystoniafoundation.org):

The Dystonia Medical Research Foundation was founded in 1976 by Samuel and Frances Belzberg, of Vancouver, Canada, after their daughter was diagnosed with dystonia. Dedicated to serving the needs of all persons affected with dystonia and their families, the Dystonia Foundation has grown from a small family-based foundation to a membership-driven organization of close to 32,000 persons. The overall membership of the Dystonia Foundation consists of individuals living with all forms dystonia, their friends and families, health care professionals, and researchers. It is multifaceted and broad in its perspective, uniting people on all levels to better serve those living with dystonia.

Huntington's Disease Society of America (www.hdsa.org)

Soon after the legendary folk singer Woody Guthrie lost his battle with Huntington disease (HD), his widow, Marjorie, sought out other families affected by this devastating disease. In 1967, this handful of dedicated volunteers formed the Committee to Combat Huntington's Disease. Today, the Huntington's Disease Society of America (HDSA) continues the mission that Marjorie Guthrie began. HDSA has grown into a national organization consisting of 32 community-based volunteer chapters, two national field directors, and a national office that provides leadership, support, and guidance for HD families through a national network of volunteer-based chapters and affiliates as well as through their newly created Centers of Excellence.

Professional Societies

Another aspect of networking for the neurosurgeon looking to set up a movement disorder practice is the professional society. The professional society allows the movement disorder neurosurgeon a forum to exchange the latest scientific and clinical advancements. Having the latest in information is essential to the movement disorder surgeon, and these societies can be helpful in achieving this goal. Although there are many such societies, we describe the two major groups.

The Movement Disorder Society (www.movementdisorders.org)

The Movement Disorder Society was founded in 1985 on the initiative of Professors Stanley Fahn and C. David Marsden, whose leadership and vision guided the expansion of clinical expertise and research in this field. This is an international multidisciplinary society of clinicians, scientists, and other health care professionals who are interested in Parkinson disease, related neurodegenerative and neurodevelopmental disorders, hyperkinetic movement disorders, and abnormalities in muscle tone and motor control.

American Society for Stereotactic and Functional Neurosurgery (www.assfn.org)

Administered through the Joint Section on Stereotactic and Functional Neurosurgery of the CNS and AANS, this is a neurosurgeon-specific organization that provides a forum for the review of the basic form and function of the human nervous system to improve stereotactic and functional neurosurgical procedures that alleviate human disease and suffering through diagnosis or treatment of the function of the nervous system. As such, movement disorder surgery is a significant focus of the group, which holds biannual meetings.

Essential tremor and focal dystonia present specific challenges with respect to generating referrals. Although referrals from neurologists will form the bulk of Parkinson DBS candidates, many patients with essential tremor and focal dystonia are not in the care of a neurologist. These patients may have symptoms that limit their lifestyle or employment, but they may remain in the care of a generalist who is not aware of modern movement disorder surgery. The Internet, media, and patient support groups may facilitate outreach to these patients.

Reimbursement: Special Considerations

Awareness of the various physician and facility reimbursement scenarios is critical to practice development. There are three reimbursement codes that are relevant to most stereotactic movement disorder operations. The first code is for the frame placement, craniotomy, surgical planning, and implantation of electrodes. The second, is a reimbursement code for intraoperative testing and evaluation. This code may be billed by the neurosurgeon if he or she does this testing but cannot be billed redundantly if a neurologist or other individual is billing for that service. Finally, there is a follow-up and DBS programming code. Of course, this code will be utilized by the member of the movement disorder team that is responsible for this task.

Current professional billing practice in the United States is based on the Resource Based Relative Value System (RBRVS). Each procedure is given a current procedural terminology (CPT) code by a board made up of members from the American Medical Association, the medical insurance industry, and the Centers for Medicare and Medicaid Services (CMS). Each CPT code is assigned a Relative Value Unit (RVU), which takes into account the effort involved in the procedure, the utilization of resources, and the risk of malpractice litigation. Each area of the country has a particular conversion factor (CF); a monetary value that, when multiplied by the RVU, gives the reimbursement for a particular procedure.

In the past, the CPT codes applying to functional neurosurgery underestimate the effort involved in many of the procedures, and many codes have not been updated to account for the evolution of procedures, which have grown more complex and time consuming. In addition, these codes did not take into consideration the cost of expensive implants required for neural augmentation. Recently, however, progress has been made in this arena. The previous CPT code for a bilateral DBS implant, 61862–50, was assigned an RVU of 29. In 2004, code 61862 was deleted and replaced by a new set of CPT codes, which recognized the use of MER. These new codes, 61867 and 61868, represent a RVU of 39.3, and an increase of 35%. In 2004 there are four variations of that reimbursement code depending on the number of electrode arrays (1 or 2) and whether microelectrode mapping was used. Because of this, the reimbursement code for intraoperative testing and evaluation (codes 95961 and 95962) can no longer be billed by the neurosurgeon but can be billed if a neurologist or other individual is performing that service. Implantation of the IPG is billed as 61885 for one electrode array or 61885–50 for two, but Kinetra has a separate 61886 code that is less than bilateral IPG placements. There is also a new set of follow-up and programming codes that may be performed by neurosurgeons on occasion but are most commonly performed by the neurology team (Chapter 13).

Facility reimbursement basically comes in two forms for movement disorder surgery—inpatient and outpatient. Lead implantation is currently only allowed in an inpatient setting. Depending on patient complications and comorbidities, the inpatient implantation of electrodes maps either to DRG001 or to DRG002. Estimated average hospital payments for those DRGs under Medicare are approximately $22,062 and $12,851, respectively. Therefore, it is critical to document the comorbidities of movement disorder patients. Given the demographics of Parkinson disease, many of the patients will qualify for DRG001.

Implantation of the IPGs can be done either within the inpatient admission, and thus be included within the DRGs mentioned previously, or within a separate outpatient admission. In the case of the outpatient admission, the 2004 Medicare reimbursement is approximately $25,217 for a bilateral IPG implantation. This regulatory idiosyncrasy has led to most surgeons electing staged implantation. Nonetheless, because the cost of DBS hardware alone exceeds the DRG002 reimbursement level, hospitals may lose money unless it is staged. Medtronic provides a reimbursement assistant hotline (800–292–2903) and there are helpful Web sites (www.medtronic.com, www.prscoding.com, or www.cms.hhs.gov).

Editor's Comments

We must also remember that medicine, despite its scientific basis and artistry, is also a business and must be run like a business. Begin by assessing the potential climate before starting a practice (**Table 3.3**). Be sure of the support by both the neurosurgery and neurology departments for the functional surgery program and a cooperative intra- and intergroup dynamics. Beware of half-hearted neurology support when their true allegiance is to more and bigger drug studies. Understand the reimbursement strategies and how to optimize them. The revenue generation can be modestly lucrative for the hospital and the physicians, if the appropriate fiduciary responsibilities are taken. In the ever-changing Medicare sphere, one must be very cognizant of where small amounts of benefits may be had. Be sure the billing is done properly (**Table 3.4**). The profitability to the neurosurgeon can be increased by using the appropriate billing codes. These codes changed in 2004 and are listed in **Table 3.5**. The new codes differentiate for single or dual lead placements with or without microelectrode recordings. Microelectrode recordings can now be billed, and there is a small increase in payment. Thus the increased time required for the microelectrode recordings is included in this billing. However, the neurosurgeon can no longer bill separately for microelectrode evaluations (95961 or 95262). Because this is usually done by a neurologist, it can be profitable for neurologists, and they will thus be more readily of assistance in the operating room. I would add fluoroscopy confirmation of the probes to surgery (CPT code 76003). It is not only useful in determining the position of the DBS lead but also in recording position of the microelectrodes throughout the procedure. Thus some of the information that would seem somewhat inconsistent can be corrected by realizing that the microelectrode did not go precisely where directed. The reimbursement for this is relatively small but can be useful when the profitability of the procedure is small.

Table 3.6 demonstrates the numbers generated by a hospital in 2003. Depending on the particular diagnostic code and how the surgery was performed, profitability for a single DBS lead placement and generator to the hospital could vary from plus $8,000 to a negative $10,000. Add to this the bilateral generators and considerable loss can result. Thus performing the surgery in two stages and passing through the equipment cost in an outpatient procedure dramatically increases the profitability to the hospital and makes the hospital's interest in your surgical performances at that facility far more likely than if your surgery is losing money on a consistent basis.

In addition to working with the hospital, work with the community to build a practice. Outreach to the support groups for a variety of neurological diseases in which the functional neurosurgeon may interact is not only useful for developing the practice but is also quite helpful in developing an understanding of what is valuable within this community. Supporting these organizations will ultimately also result in support for your continued practice. A little philanthropy can go a long way in building goodwill. Getting out into the community hospitals is also quite useful in developing a practice. Try to position yourself as the expert in the field by holding seminars and providing grand rounds not only in your hospital but also at local hospitals. Never refuse a chance to present your work. Work with the hospital or institutional marketing department and have them help track your market penetration. Have a Web site that patients can find on the Internet that features your work.

Make a point to meet and socialize with colleagues in the hospital and clinic. A few well-spent minutes in the cafeteria may send referrals your way. Pay attention to where referrals originate. Responding quickly and appropriately to them goes back to the basic principles of availability, affability, and accountability to build good working interactions with your referral base. Never say no to consultations. Be sure your clinic is patient friendly. Make sure the staff is courteous, caring, and professional. Patients want an efficient and professional neurosurgeon who cares about them as a person. Efficiency does not mean cutting short patient questions. Don't keep patients waiting by routinely overbooking. Fully explain cancellations. Most importantly, treat patients as you would like to be treated. Frequent patient complaints can lose a referral base. Patient surveys or even a call to your office by a friend trying to set up an appointment can be an eye opener to identifying problems.

Timely communications are a real asset in building a referral base. Nothing irritates a referring physician more than not hearing from the neurosurgeon, especially if the physician has to deal with the patient in person or on the phone before the follow-up letter arrives. Academic centers are especially poor at getting dictations done quickly or getting letters typed promptly. Two or 3 weeks later the "problems" may result in a lost referral source. A quick phone call, e-mail, or fax helps. It is important to give patients handouts, and it is a good idea to provide educational material to the referral physician, at least the first time a specialty problem is referred and especially if there is a difference of opinion as to optimal treatment. Do not get the reputation of being a "cowboy." Be sure your early cases are ideal candidates. Ultimately, the results of your surgery will be the greatest determinate as to whether continued referrals are made to your practice.

Table 3.3 Assessing the Facilities and Support

What is the size of the market? (Typically functional neurosurgery needs about 1 million people.)

What is the willingness of the hospital/institution to pay for specialized equipment for functional neurosurgery?

Has there been an increase or decrease in neurological procedures in the group or institution, based on previous years?

What are hospital admission volumes for movement disorders?

Is there a movement disorder specialist and a movement disorder clinic in the group or institution? Are they interested in developing a functional surgery program?

Who are your competitors (both functional and nonfunctional neurosurgery)? Which hospital has the biggest market share of the neurosurgery market?

What are competitor hospitals and groups' reputational strengths and weaknesses?

How can you differentiate yourself, based on these strengths and weaknesses?

What are the opportunities for functional neurosurgery procedures, based on the medical dynamics that currently exist?

Is a neuroradiologist available?

What is the availability of computed tomography, magnetic resonance imaging, single-photon emission computed tomography, and positron emission tomography?

Is anesthesia with expertise/interest in neurological patients preferentially assigned to neurosurgery?

Is specialized rehabilitation readily available for movement disorder patients?

What is the availability of physician extenders (i.e., physician assistants, nurse practitioners)?

What is the willingness of the hospital/institution to pay for a dedicated biller/coder, secretary, or physician extender?

Table 3.4 Collection Tips

1. Do not assume billing staff understands functional neurosurgery coding. You are the only one who truly knows what you did in the operating room. Know the current procedural terminology (CPT) and diagnostic codes so you can check overall billings. Understand and use the right modifiers.

2. Dictate documentation that provides a good history and reason for the procedures. Use ICD-9 CM codes to their highest level of specificity. Correlate them with the correct procedure code so staff can clearly understand what diagnosis supports each procedure.

3. Code your visits and procedures quickly so the billing staff can get claims filed in a timely manner. Evaluation and management of codes are important. Speed does matter.

4. Send electronic claims to as many payors as you can, and receive electronic payments from as many payors as you can. This will increase the speed payment and save staff time. Any effective practice management system must edit and verify that all claim form boxes are completed prior to sending claims electronically. An error on the patient's Social Security number or birthday will generate a rejection.

5. Make sure billing staff has a good knowledge base about individual carrier contracts and policies. This makes the staff's follow-up much more effective. They need to know what documentation is required.

6. Dictate appeal letters to carriers as soon as requested. This allows staff to resubmit the claim quickly. Keep a template for common requests. Know how to read Explanation of Benefit forms to respond to denials, incorrect bundling, down coding, and designations of "experimental procedures."

7. Keep abreast of reimbursement rules and regulations. Make sure that CPT books, carrier newsletters, and Medicare resources are up to date, and send staff to as many coding seminars and conferences as possible.

8. Pay attention to accounts receivable. The billing staff needs to be sure to verify appropriate payments. Payers frequently do not pay accurately or according to contracts. Don't allow accounts receivable to pile up. Leave clear parameters on what information you want to review concerning overdue accounts.

Table 3.5 Usual and Customary Billed Charges—Physician Billings

Procedure	CPT Code and Description[1]	2008 Medicare RVUs[2]		2008 Medicare National Average	
		For physician services provided in [4]			
		Physician Office[5]	Facility	Physician Office[5]	Facility
Bone Marker Fiducial Placement[6]	**21499** Unlisted musculoskeletal procedure, head	N/A	0	N/A	Carrier priced[7]
	64999 Unlisted procedure, nervous system	N/A	0	N/A	Carrier priced[7]
Diagnostic Imaging[8] **and Planning**[9]	**70450-26** CT, head or brain without contrast material[10]	1.18	1.18	$41	$41
	70551-26 MRI, brain, without contrast material[10]	2.05	2.05	$71	$71
	76376-26 3D rendering with interpretation and reporting of computed tomography, magnetic resonance imaging, ultrasound or other tomographic modality, not requiring image postprocessing on an independent workstation[10]	0.29	0.29	$10	$10
	76377-26 3D rendering with interpretation and reporting of computed tomography, magnetic resonance imaging, ultrasound or other tomographic modality, requiring image postprocessing on an independent workstation[10]	1.14	1.14	$40	$40
Lead Implantation[11]	**61863** Twist drill, burr hole, craniatomy, or craniectomy with stereotactic implantation of neurostimulator electrode array in subcortical site (e.g., thalamus, globus pallidus, subthalamic nucleus, periventricular, periaqueductal gray) without use of intraoperative microelectrode recording; first array	N/A	38.09	N/A	$1,357
	61864 Each additional array (List separately in addition to primary procedure)	N/A	11.90	N/A	$433
	61867 Twist drill, burr hole, craniotomy, or craniectomy with stereotactic implantation of neurostimulator electrode array in subcortical site (e.g. thalamus, globus pallidus, subthalamic nucleus, periventicular, periaqueductal gray) with use of intraoperative microelectrode recording; first array	N/A	55.51	N/A	$1,965
	61868 Each additional array (List separately in addition to primary procedure.)	N/A	16.82	N/A	$605
Generator Implantation or Replacement[11,12]	**61885 (Soletra)** Insertion or replacement of cranial neurostimulator pulse generator or receiver, direct or inductive coupling; with connection to a single electrode array	N/A	15.15	N/A	$544
	61886 (Kinetra) Insertion or replacement of cranial neurostimulator pulse generator or receiver, direct or inductive coupling; with connection to two or more electrode arrays	N/A	19.14	N/A	$685
	For bilateral stimulation via implantation of two Soletra pulse generators, each connected to a single lead, use 61885-50 plus 61863 and 61864 or 61867 and 61868. For bilateral stimulation via implantation of one Kinetra dual-array pulse generator with connection to two leads, use 61886 plus 61863 and 61864 or 61867 and 61868.				
Intraoperative Stimulation with Microelectrode Recording[13]	**95961-26** Functional cortical and subcortical mapping by stimulation and/or recording of electrodes on brain surface, or depth electrodes, to provoke seizures or identify vital brain structures; initial hour of physician attendance	4.55	4.55	$160	$160
	95962-26 Functional cortical and subcortical mapping by stimulation and/or recording of electrodes on brain surface, or depth electrodes, to provoke seizures or identify vital brain structures; each additional hour of physician attendance (List separately in addition to code for primary procedure)	4.68	4.68	$164	$164

(continued)

Table 3.5 *(continued)*

Procedure	CPT Code and Description[1]	2008 Medicare RVUs[2]		2008 Medicare National Average	
		For physician services provided in [4]			
		Physician Office[5]	Facility	Physician Office[5]	Facility
Revision or Removal of Leads or Generator[11]	**61880** Revision or removal of intracranial neurostimulator electrodes	N/A	13.40	N/A	$480
	61888 Revision or removal of cranial neurostimulator pulse generator or receiver	N/A	10.10	N/A	$361
Analysis and Programming Note: In the office, analysis and programming may be furnished by a physician, practitioner with an "incident to" benefit, or auxiliary personnel under the direct supervision of the physician (or other practitioner), with or without support from a manufacturer's representative. The patient or payor should not be billed for services rendered solely by the manufacturer's representative. Contact your local carrier/payor for interpretation of applicable policies.	**95970** Electronic analysis of implanted neurostimulator pulse generator system (e.g., rate, pulse amplitude and duration, configuration of wave form, battery status, electrode selectability, output modulation, cycling, impedance and patient compliance measurements); simple or complex brain, spinal cord, or peripheral (i.e., cranial nerve, peripheral nerve, autonomic nerve, neuromuscular) neurostimulator pulse generator/transmitter, without reprogramming	1.35	0.61	$50	$21
	95978 Electronic analysis of implanted neurostimulator pulse generator system (e.g., rate, pulse amplitude and duration, battery status, electrode selectability, output modulation, cycling, impedance and patient compliance measurements), complex deep brain neurostimulator pulse generator/transmitter, with initial or subsequent programming, first hour	5.58	4.84	$197	$168
	95979 Each additional 30 minutes after first hour (List separately in addition to code for primary procedure.)	2.52	2.30	$88	$80
Evaluation and Management Note: An office visit can only be billed separately when a full-scale, separately identifiable evaluation and management sevice takes place in addition to analysis and programming. The use of evaluation and management codes may require a -25 modifier and must meet separate coding requirements as well as documentation requirements.	**99211–99215** Office or other outpatient visit	0.54–3.43	0.24–2.71	$20–$109	$8–$94
	99217–99220 Observation care	N/A	1.85–4.06	N/A	$65–$140
	99221–99223 Initial hospital care	N/A	2.45–4.96	N/A	$85–$172
	99354–99355 Prolonged services, office	2.52–2.56	2.38–2.43	$80–$90	$83–$85
	99356–99357 Prolonged service, inpatient	N/A	2.34-2.35	N/A	$82

Data reprinted with the permission of Medtronic, Inc. Copyright 2008.
CPT is a trademark of American Medical Association.

Notes to Table 3.5

[1] Current Procedural Terminology (CPT) is copyright 2007 American Model Association. All rights reserved. No fee schedules, basic units, relative values or related listings are included in CPT. The AMA assumes no liability for the data contained herein. Applicable FARS/DFARS restrictions apply to government use. *(Continued on next page)*

Table 3.6 Comparisons of Deep Brain Stimulation Profitability

	Medicare Reimbursement	Hospital Direct Cost	Contribution Margin	Hospital Total Cost	Net Income/ Loss
Proposed Scenario 1					
Inpatient admission (for insertion of lead) DRG 001 Craniotomy age < 17 with Complications or Comorbidities	27,107	12,779	14,328	19,280	7827
Outpatient Surgery (for insertion of pulse generator)* APC 222 Implantation of Neurological Device	11,877	7766	4111	11,535	342
DBS Procedure Totals	**38,894**	**20,545**	**18,439**	**30,815**	**8169**
Proposed Scenario 2					
Inpatient admission (for insertion of lead) DRG 002 Craniotomy age <17 w/o Complications or Comorbidities	14,301	12,779	1522	19,280	(4979)
Outpatient surgery (for insertion of pulse generator)* APC 222 Implantation of Neurological Device	11,877	7766	4111	11,535	342

(continued)

Notes to Table 3.5 (*continued*):

[2] Federal Register, Volume 72, Number 227, November 2007. The total RVU as shown here is the sum of three components physician work RVU, 2008 transitioned practice expense RVU and malpractice RVU. The work RVU must be modified by the CMS budget neutrality factor in order to calculate Medicare payment.

[3] Medicare national average payment is determined by applying the standard budget neutrality adjustor of 0.8806 to the physician work RVU component, then multiplying the sum of the three component RVUs by the 2008 conversion factor of $34.0682, as published in the Federal Register, Volume 72, Number 227, November 27, 2007. The 2008 Medicare National Average reflects the legislative short-term fix that replaced the 10.1% cut with a 0.5% increase through June 30, 2008. RVUs listed are not adjusted by the budget neutrality factor. Final payment to the physician is also adjusted by the Geographic Practice Cosst Indices (GPCI). Because GPCI varies by area, each physician's specific reimbursement will vary from the national average payment shown. Also note that any applicable coinsurance, deductible and other amounts which are patient obligations are included in the national average payment shown.

[4] The RVUs shown are for the physician's services and payment is made to the physician. However, there are different RVUs and payments depending on the setting in which the physician rendered the service. "Facility" includes physician services rendered in hospitals, ASCs and SNFs. Physician RVus and payments are generally lower in the "Facility" setting because the facility is incurring the cost of some of the supplies and other materials. Physician RVUs and payments are generally higher in the "Office" setting because the physician incurs all costs there.

[5] "N/A" shown in Physician Office setting indicates that Medicare has not developed RVUs in the office setting because the service is typically performed in a facility (e.g., in a hospital). However, if the local carrier determines that it will cover the service in the office, then it is paid using the facility RVUs at the facility rate, per the Federal Register, Volume 72, Number 227, November 27, 2007.

[6] Placement of implanted fiducials should generally be considered integral to lead implantation and should not be coded separately when performed on the same day as the lead implantation by the same physician. Placement of implanted fiducials can be coded separately if performed during a different operative episode on a previous date or by a different physician from the one who performed the lead implantation. Note that medical necessity must be demonstrated and documented for staging the procedure.

[7] This is a *carrier-priced* code. Carriers establish the RVUs and the payment amount, usually on an individual case basis after review of the procedure report.

[8] Preoperative CT and MRI Imaging is separately codable when it represents full-scale diagnostic imaging and the interpretation is documented via a formal imaging report. Intra-operative imaging is a part of surgical navigation and should not be coded separately. Note that although CPT code 61795 exists for computer-assisted surgical navigation, National Correct Coding Initiative (NCCI) edits do not allow this to be coded separately with lead implantation codes 61863 and 61867.

[9] The 3D rendering codes are reported in addition to the code for the base CT or MRI procedure.

[10] This assumes the service is occuring in the hospital facility so the physician is providing the professional interpretation only.

[11] Surgical procedures are subject to a "global period." The global period defines other physician services which are generally considered part of the surgery package. They are not separately coded, billed, or paid when rendered by the physician who performed the surgery for 90 days, treatment of complications unless they require return visit to the operating room, and minor postoperative services such as dressing changes and suture removal.

[12] National Correct Coding Initiative (NCCI) edits do not allow removal of the old device to be coded together with implantation of the new device.

[13] Microelectrode recording is included in codes 61867 – 61868 and cannot be coded separately when performed by the operating surgeon. However, when another physician (e.g., neurologist or neurophysiologist) performs the neuropsychological mapping during the placement of the electrode array, that physician may report codes 95961 – 95962 separately.

Table 3.6 (continued)

DBS Procedure Totals	**26,178**	**20,545**	**5633**	**30,815**	**(4637)**
Current Scenario 3					
Inpatient admission (for insertion of lead) DRG 001 Craniotomy age < 17 with Complications or Comorbidities	27,107	12,779	14,328	19,280	7827
Inpatient Surgery (for insertion of pulse generator)* DRG 012 Degenerative Nervous System Disorder	6464	7766	(1302)	11,535	(5071)
DBS Procedure Totals	**33,571**	**20,545**	**13,026**	**30,815**	**2756**
Current Scenario 4					
Inpatient admission (for insertion of lead) DRG002 Craniotomy age < 17 with Complications of Comorbities	**14,301**	**12,779**	**1522**	**19,280**	**(4979)**
Inpatient Surgery (for insertion of pulse generator)*	6464	7766	(1302)	11,535	(5071)
DRG 012 Degenerative Nervous System Disorder	**20,765**	**20,545**	**220**	**30,815**	**(10,050)**
DBS Procedure Totals					

*There is also potential of $326 for APC 692–Electronic Analysis of Neurostimulator Pulse Generators if done during the visit as well. Numbers in parentheses are negative. Values are set for 2003 and do not reflect the current market, but are meant as examples of the variability that exists with different approaches. You will need to calculate for your particular market.

■ Conclusion

Movement disorder surgery, and functional neurosurgery in general, is still at the frontier of neurosurgical practice. Like all frontiers, there are several significant challenges that must be faced. These include the technical, economic, organizational, and operational aspects of all the diverse elements that are involved in movement disorder surgery. By carefully identifying all of these components one can develop a specific strategy that will allow a successful effort in this venture.

References

1. Maciunas RJ, Galloway RL Jr, Latimer JW. The application accuracy of stereotactic frames. Neurosurgery 1994;35:682–694 (discussion 694–695)
2. Leksell L. A stereotaxic apparatus for intracerebral surgery. Acta Chir Scand 1949;99:229–233
3. Leksell L. Stereotaxis and radiosurgery: an operative system. Springfield, IL: Charles C Thomas, 1971
4. Lunsford DL, Kondziolka D, Leksell D. The Leksell Stereotactic System. Stereotact Funct Neurosurg 1998;26:51–54
5. Cosman E. Development and Technical Features of the Cosman-Roberts-Wells (CRW) Stereotactic System. In: Pell F, Thomas DG (eds.) Handbook of Stereotaxy Using the CRW Apparatus. Baltimore: Williams & Wilkins; 1994: 1–52
6. Brown RA. A stereotactic head frame for use with CT body scanners. Invest Radiol 1979;14:300–304
7. Riechert T. Beschreibung und Anwendung eines Zielgerates für stereotaktische Hirnoperationen. Acta Neurochir (Wien) 1956; (3 Suppl):308–337
8. Mundinger F, Boesecke R. The Riechert/Mundinger apparatus. In: Gildenberg PL, Tasker RR (eds.), Stereotact Funct Neurosurg. New York: McGraw Hill: 1998; 73–78
9. Henderson JM, Holloway KL, Gaede SR, Rosanow JM, Csavoy A. Frameless placement of deep brain stimulation electrodes: an accuracy study. Mov Disord 2004;19(Suppl 9):S302
10. Guridi J, Rodriguez-Oroz MC, Ramos E, et al. Discrepancy between imaging and neurophysiology in deep brain stimulation of medial pallidum and subthalamic nucleus in Parkinson's disease. Neurologia 2002;17:183–192
11. Priori A, Egidi M, Pesenti A, et al. Do intraoperative microrecordings improve subthalamic nucleus targeting in stereotactic neurosurgery for Parkinson's disease? J Neurosurg Sci 2003;47:56–60
12. Hariz MI. Is microelectrode recording necessary in movement disorder? The case against. In: Israel Z, Burchiel KJ, eds. Microelectrode Recording in Movement Disorder Surgery. New York: Thieme; 2004:197–207
13. Sierens DK, Bakay RAE. Is microelectrode technique necessary in movement disorder surgery? The case in favor. In: Israel Z, Burchiel KJ, eds. Microelectrode Recording in Movement Disorder Surgery. New York: Thieme; 2004:186–196
14. Slavin KV. Intra-operative microrecording equipment: comparative analysis of commercially available microrecording systems. Neurol Res 2002;24:544–554
15. Steinmeier R, Rachinger J, Kaus M, et al. Factors influencing the application accuracy of neuronavigation systems. Stereotact Funct Neurosurg 2000;75:188–202
16. Abbasi HR, Hariri S, Martin D, et al. A comparative statistical analysis of neuronavigation systems in a clinical setting. Stud Health Technol Inform 2001;81:11–17
17. Troster AI. Introduction to neurobehavioral issues in the neurosurgical treatment of movement disorders: basic issues, thalamotomy, and nonablative treatments. Brain Cogn 2000;42:173–182

18. Woods SP, Fields JA, Troster AI. Neuropsychological sequelae of subthalamic nucleus deep brain stimulation in Parkinson's disease: a critical review. Neuropsychol Rev 2002;12:111–126

19. Jankovic J. Classification and epidemiology of movement disorders. In: Krauss JK, Grossman RG, eds. Surgery for Parkinson's Disease and Movement Disorders. 2001:21

20. Patil AA. The Patil apparatus. In: Tasker P, Gildenberg P, eds. Textbook of Functional and Stereotactic Neurosurgery. New York: McGraw-Hill; 1998:105–111

21. Hariz MI, Laitinen L. The Laitinen apparatus. In: Tasker P, Gildenberg P, eds. Textbook of Functional and Stereotactic Neurosurgery. New York: McGraw-Hill; 1998:87–94

22. Goerss SJ. The COMPASS system. In: Tasker P, Gildenberg P, eds. Textbook of Functional and Stereotactic Neurosurgery. New York: McGraw-Hill; 1998:151–162

23. Zamorano L, The Zamorano-Dujovny Multipurpose Localizing Unit. Advanced Neurosurgical Navigation. New York: Thieme; 1999: 255–266

24. Benabid A-L, Hoffman D, LeBas J-F, Munari C. The Talairach system. In: Tasker P, Gildenberg P, eds. Textbook of Functional and Stereotactic Neurosurgery. New York: McGraw-Hill; 1998:79–86

25. Sugita K, Mutsuga N. The Sugita apparatus. In: Tasker P, Gildenberg P, eds. Textbook of Functional and Stereotactic Neurosurgery. New York: McGraw-Hill; 1998:131–137

4 Selection of Centers, Diseases, and Patients for Movement Disorder Surgery

Leo Verhagen Metman

Surgery for movement disorders has gained momentum over the last decade, catalyzed by the advent of high-frequency deep brain stimulation (DBS).[1,2] Owing to its reversible nature, DBS is considered a safer method than ablative surgery.[3] Nonetheless, several risks are associated with DBS, some are related to the procedure and hardware, others to the actual stimulation.[4–7] Hardware problems such as lead fracture and migration occur, and hemorrhage and infection can be intraoperative or postoperative problems. Additionally, a variety of cognitive, behavioral, psychiatric, and speech abnormalities have surfaced in the DBS literature.[8–11] Postoperatively, DBS is a costly and time-intensive therapy. Taken together, this list of problems serves as a reminder that DBS, just like ablative surgery, should only be undertaken after carefully weighing risks and benefits for each individual patient.[12] As with any elective surgery, patients and physicians are faced with options that need to be carefully considered as part of a patient selection process that will lead to the best outcome possible. In addition to medical considerations, other factors may play a role in determining whether surgery is the most appropriate treatment option. Nonmedical factors such as economic feasibility and governmental directives are not universal and are therefore not discussed here. Instead, the chapter focuses on a theoretical model which assumes that DBS is the surgical procedure of choice.[13,14] In this case, three "selections" need to be made as discussed in the following sections: (1) the selection of the optimal surgical center, (2) the selection of the appropriate disease amenable to surgical treatment, and (3) the selection of the optimal candidate for surgery.

■ Selection of a Center

The first pivotal component of successful surgery is the selection of a center consisting of a multidisciplinary team that is trained and experienced in the multifaceted management of patients with movement disorders.[6] Only when such an infrastructure is in place can the patient expect to be appropriately diagnosed, evaluated, and treated with the highest chance of a good outcome.[9] The ideal team should consist of several members whose roles in the preoperative, intraoperative, and postoperative periods are briefly discussed here.

Preoperative Period

Movement Disorder Neurologist

A movement disorder neurologist should provide the initial evaluation for any patient that is referred for consideration of a neurosurgical procedure. This key member of the surgical team provides invaluable expertise in diagnostic matters and knowledge of pharmacological as well as surgical treatments for movement disorders. During this visit the neurologist will (1) confirm the diagnosis through a detailed history and physical examination, (2) decide whether pharmacological approaches have been appropriately maximized, (3) determine whether the patient's symptoms can likely benefit from surgical treatment (which may include additional visits to evaluate patients with and without their medications), and (4) determine if the potential benefits outweigh the risks for a particular patient. Following this thorough assessment, the neurologist will provide an opinion to the patient and family and advise them accordingly. Should the neurologist deem surgery appropriate, the patient will be referred to the team's neurosurgeon.

Neurosurgeon

Neurosurgeons will usually rely on the movement disorder neurologist in terms of diagnosis and appropriateness of surgical treatment for an individual patient, but because they are the physicians ultimately responsible at surgery, they play an essential role in patient evaluation prior to surgery as well. They will assess whether patients are sufficiently healthy to undergo brain surgery. Hypertension, coagulopathies, chronic infections, and diabetes mellitus are just some of many comorbidities that do not preclude surgery but need to be dealt with or stabilized together with consulting physicians before neurosurgeons will proceed. During this preoperative visit, an important task for the neurosurgeon is to inform the patient of any possible adverse events. From a patient's perspective, the interaction with the surgeon at this point also provides an opportunity to be fully apprised of the surgeon's (and team's) experience with the procedure.[6] Although some patients may wisely inquire as to how many procedures the surgeon has performed, less assertive individuals may unknowingly contribute to the steepest part of the team's learning curve.

Arguably, surgeons should a priori disclose their record of experience with the procedure proposed.

Psychologist

We consider that the ideal team should have a dedicated movement disorders psychologist/psychiatrist for several reasons.[15] Patients and their families are embarking on a stressful journey and may need mental support from the very start of the evaluation for surgery. In addition, just as patients need to be sufficiently healthy from a physical point of view, they also need to be of sufficient mental health to withstand the rigors of surgery. Thus psychologists will perform a battery of tests to confirm that patients are mentally stable, cognitively intact, and not depressed.[16] They will also be able to assist in the detection of unrealistic expectations or inappropriate motivations for surgery.

Coordinator

Every surgery program needs a central and easily accessible person who can guide patients and their family members through all phases of the surgery process.[17] This role is ideally assumed by a coordinator (physician assistant, nurse practitioner, or other qualified health professional) with responsibilities transcending departmental boundaries. Thus this dedicated coordinator's tasks will include (1) coordinating the visits to individual team members and thereby minimizing inconvenience to patients and family members, (2) providing help with insurance and precertification issues, (3) educating the patient and family members and answering questions that remain after patients have seen the other team members, (4) taking an active role in the patient evaluation process, (5) and most of all, being a constant and visible presence throughout the entire process, providing a familiar personal contact for patients and their loved ones.

Intraoperative Period

Neurosurgeon and Neurologist

During surgery a team approach is crucial for optimizing outcome. Integrated teamwork is especially important when microelectrode recordings are an integral part of the procedure, as many (but not all) centers deem essential.[7,9,18,19] While the neurosurgeon directs the surgical planning and instrumentation, the neurologist/neurophysiologist interprets the recorded signals, examines the patient for motor and sensory responses, and evaluates the effects of macrostimulation to determine the physiological target. Together they decide on the final coordinates for DBS lead placement.

Coordinator

The presence of a trusted ally during a physically and mentally exhausting intervention could make the difference between a cooperative or a belligerent patient. Therefore, in an ideal situation the coordinator should be present in the operating room. The coordinator can also be invaluable as a scribe in the mapping process, and as a communication conduit between the operating room and the patient's family in the waiting room in the case of prolonged procedures.

Postoperative Period

Neurologist and Coordinator

Following the immediate postoperative surgical care, the patient will be returning to the neurologist's office to start the stimulation process. This time-consuming process consists of the initial programming visit and several adjustment visits over the following months.[20-23] Simultaneously, medications may be adjusted downward. Once the patient is on a steady stimulation regimen the neurologist should reevaluate the patient using the same standard assessments as before surgery.[16] Proper determination of the benefit from surgery will aid in patient management and will also provide a "quality control instrument" for the surgical treatment. This formal assessment should be repeated over time to evaluate the long-term results of the procedure. It should be noted that even when the stimulation parameters and the medications are in optimal balance, DBS patients require more frequent attention from the neurologist for a variety of reasons. Initially, fear of the unknown will lead to frequent consultation. Later on, a variety of hardware-related problems can occur, including unexpected outages of the pulse generator due to unsuspected magnetic fields in the patient's environment; discomfort due to the position of the connectors, the extension leads, or the pulse generators; infection, lead erosion, or battery failure. This requires careful and regular monitoring. Importantly, most patients also tend to indefinitely expect or at least hope that as yet untried parameter combinations can further increase the benefit from the stimulation. In addition, stimulation can be so effective that malfunction is perceived as a true emergency.[24] Consequently, a key feature in any stimulation program is that patients can be evaluated in the clinic on short notice. Having only one individual proficient in the management of DBS patients is therefore insufficient, and adequate training of the coordinator and other staff in performing stimulator evaluations and adjustments will enhance the efficiency of the team.

Psychologist

Following surgery, stressors on the patients and their families do not immediately subside and may require intervention by the psychologist. Sometimes unrealistic expectations exceed the outcome and, as a result, disappointment needs to be dealt with. In other instances surgery may have caused cognitive or behavioral changes threatening the status quo and disrupting the family's routines.[25,26] Although such changes are mostly transient, that fact is not known at the time they occur, and the psychologist can offer valuable support during the recuperation. Whether cognitive/behavioral changes did or did not occur, all patients should be routinely evaluated with the same neuropsychological test battery given preoperatively.[16] This will not only establish that they indeed have fully recovered from surgery, but will also serve as a "quality control instrument" from a cognitive perspective for the procedure performed.

■ Selecting Disorders

As with ablative surgery in the past, numerous movement disorders can be and have been surgically addressed with DBS.[13,27] However, DBS is currently only US Food and Drug Administration (FDA)-approved for three indications: Parkinson disease (PD), essential tremor (ET), and dystonia (the latter under the restrictions of a humanitarian device exemption). The collective experience with DBS in other movement disorders is too limited to identify specific patient selection criteria and is therefore not discussed here.

Parkinson Disease

Idiopathic PD is characterized by the presence of two or more cardinal features: rest tremor, rigidity, bradykinesia, and, with advanced disease, impaired postural reflexes. Symptoms initially respond favorably to dopaminergic medication, such as L-dopa. The efficacy of DBS of the globus pallidus internus (GPi) or subthalamic nucleus (STN) has now been demonstrated in several controlled studies.[28–30] PD has many imitators, which is one of the reasons a movement disorders specialist should evaluate potential surgical candidates. Especially early in the disease PD can be difficult to distinguish from parkinsonism caused by a variety of other disorders, such as multiple system atrophy (MSA), progressive supranuclear palsy (PSP), diffuse Lewy body disease, corticobasal ganglionic degeneration, vascular Parkinsonism, normal pressure hydrocephalus, and drug-induced parkinsonism. No data currently exist to support the use of DBS for any of these conditions; their presence therefore needs to be ruled out as part of the selection process.[31] Some of these parkinsonian disorders can be deceivingly responsive to L-dopa, albeit usually for very limited periods of time. Thus, even in specialized movement disorders clinics 10% of cases diagnosed with PD during life may in fact receive a different diagnosis at autopsy. Mostly, however, time is sympathetic to this dilemma and the distinction between PD and other forms of parkinsonism becomes more defined with longer disease duration. This is an argument in favor of an often used rule of thumb that patients should have had PD for at least 5 years before surgery is considered.[16] By that time the diagnosis of idiopathic PD can usually be made beyond reasonable doubt based on the asymmetric onset, the slowly progressive course, the excellent and maintained response to L-dopa, the maintained asymmetry, and the absence of stigmata of the aforementioned other parkinsonian disorders.

Essential Tremor

Classic ET is a monosymptomatic disorder characterized by postural or kinetic tremor (frequency 4 to 12 Hz) involving hands and forearms.[32,33] Rest tremor is absent, except in the most severe cases where the tremor persists even though the patient is seemingly at rest.[34] Head tremor may be an additional or even isolated feature, but only in the absence of abnormal head posturing.[35] Less frequently the tremor is also (but not in isolation) present in the voice, the trunk, the face, and the legs.[36] The remainder of the neurological exam is usually normal, although some patients may have some rigidity or postural instability.[5,36,37] ET is familial in 60% of cases with autosomal dominant transmission with incomplete penetrance. Patients report a beneficial effect from alcohol. With the passage of time, the frequency of ET decreases while the amplitude increases, leading to considerable disability, especially in those with a strong kinetic component.[38] The target of choice for DBS is the ventrointermedius nucleus of the thalamus (Vim), including its anterior border with the ventro-oralis posterior nucleus (Vop),[39] and possibly the subthalamic region.[40] The efficacy of DBS has now been demonstrated in several studies.[14,41,42] The differential diagnosis of ET includes cerebellar and Holmes tremor.[36] Cerebellar tremor is a lower frequency (< 5 Hz) kinetic tremor that is amplified during the last part of the movement trajectory (intention tremor). Depending on the etiology the tremor can be unilateral or bilateral. Common causes are MS, stroke, and trauma. Often the involuntary movement is an inseparable combination of cerebellar tremor and ataxia. The latter may contribute to the incomplete response to DBS (or lesioning) as reported for MS-associated tremor.[43] Holmes tremor (or rubral tremor) is a combination of rest and kinetic tremor (frequency < 4.5 Hz) due to midbrain lesions that involve the cerebellar outflow tract as well as the substantia nigra.[33,36] Case reports suggest that Holmes tremor responds to Vim DBS.[44,45] Another recent report suggests that dual electrodes, one in the cerebellar receiving area (Vim) and one in the pallidal receiving area [Ventro-oralis anterior (Voa) and posterior (Vop)] are a more definitive therapy.[46]

Dystonia

Dystonia is a syndrome of involuntary, patterned, and repetitive contractions of opposing muscles leading to often painful twisting movements and abnormal postures.[47] Primary dystonia is not considered a degenerative disorder but rather one characterized by abnormal physiology at multiple levels along the neuraxis.[48,49] Consistent with this concept, no pathological substrate has been found, making dystonia an attractive target for physiological manipulation with DBS. Several recent case series and a double-blind crossover study have now documented considerable benefit (50 to 90% improvement) of GPi DBS for patients with primary generalized dystonia (PGD).[50–53] The most common (30%) cause of PGD is a single GAG deletion mutation in the DYT1 gene.[54] The commercially available assay for this mutation has provided an opportunity to study this genetically homogeneous subgroup of dystonia patients. Secondary dystonia may be associated with a variety of neurological disorders, trauma, and other insults to the brain. Whether secondary dystonia is generalized or restricted to one side of the body (hemidystonia), the variable underlying etiology makes for a variable outcome of GPi DBS, with reported improvement ranging form 0 to 50%. It has been suggested that secondary dystonia may respond better to thalamic than to pallidal DBS.[51] In a recent case series, on the other hand, dystonia caused by pantothenate-kinase-associated neurodegeneration (PKAN) demonstrated an excellent response to pallidal DBS.[55]

Editor's Comments

This chapter describes how a movement disorder specialist approaches the task of evaluating patients for surgery. Approximately a third of patients that present to a movement disorder center for DBS are not immediate candidates for surgery.[80] The rational for exclusion includes inadequate medical trial, insufficient disability, cognitive and/or psychiatric disorders, incorrect diagnosis, predominantly surgically unresponsive symptoms, and inability to tolerate surgery. The movement disorder neurologist is in the ideal position to initially screen patients so that only the appropriate patients go on to surgery. Surgical intervention for nonidiopathic PD syndromes is generally of little value and frequently results in increased neurological deficits.

Because there is no laboratory test to establish the diagnosis of PD, differentiating PD from MSA or PSP is the biggest challenge in selecting appropriate patients for surgery. MSA is a complex of sporadic neurodegenerative disorders that is usually manifest in the early sixth decade of life and progresses quickly, with a mean survival of approximately 9 years. However, there is some degree of variability in the rate of progression. Symptoms are symmetrical, bradykinetic-rigidity predominant, and may have a modest response to L-dopa. Red flags suggesting MSA include orofacial dystonia, axial dystonia (especially with lateral flexion), an irregular jerk postural tremor, early onset of dysarthria, early onset of gait abnormality, and multiple autonomic dysfunctions such as Raynaud phenomena, emotional instability, orthostatic hypotension, and neurogenic bladder. Classically, three MSA subgroups have been recognized: (1) striatonigral degeneration (SND), where extrapyramidal signs predominate and are therefore most likely confused with PD; (2) Shy-Drager syndrome (SDS), where autonomic failure is predominant; and (3) olivopontocerebellar atrophy (OPCA), where cerebellar signs are predominant. Others will be subtyped by the presence of predominant parkinsonian or cerebellar symptoms.[81] Although a positron emission tomography (PET) scan can be useful in distinguishing MSA from PD, the problem is that there are very few third party payers who will actually reimburse this procedure.

PSP is the most common parkinson-plus neurodegenerative disease. There is early onset of gait disturbance and falls. PD gait disturbance occurs after prolonged duration of symptoms and then in only ~11% of patients. Other common symptoms early in PSP are nonspecific changes in personality, mental and physical slowness, irritability, and social withdrawal, which can sometimes be diagnosed as PD with depression. A minority of the patients actually present with gaze palsy, dysarthria, and dysphagia, and as such the presence of vertical gaze palsy may not always be a useful differential diagnostic tool. The PSP picture can be quite atypical early in the disease, and the addition of time becomes a helpful differential for the diagnosis.[82]

It is extremely uncommon for patients to have idiopathic PD below the age of 21 (juvenile PD). Most parkinsonian symptoms at that age are the result of a multitude of other diseases with the rare exception of a few genetic forms.[83] More difficult to sort out are the manifestations of young-onset PD, which range from age 21 to age 40. These generally represent the lower end of the spectrum for PD and typical Lewy body pathology. Nevertheless, there can be some overlap, and again careful history and neurological examination should sort out most of the unusual cases. Nevertheless, anyone with an onset before the age of 50 should be suspect and a history of the diagnosis for at least 5 years should be present before any surgical intervention is considered.

In addition to the physical examination, no patient should have an evaluation completed until an MRI scan is performed. This will help to identify areas of atrophy that may provide some diagnostic help. In PSP, the patient may have particularly large atrophy of the cortex and midbrain. MSA frequently has marked atrophy of the pons in the olivopontocerebellar form, but not striatonigral degeneration. The presence of strokes may suggest a vascular parkinsonism. However, a mild to moderate degree of periventricular lucency and deep white matter changes are generally not a problem.[84] Severe cerebral atrophy, of course, is not only a technical problem for surgery but also may suggest an impending dementia, if it is not already present. The presence of enlarged ventricles is usually ex vacuo. Their presence on an MRI scan should be a sign that further investigation is necessary. Rarely is shunting effective, although occasionally, if there is true hydrocephalus, shunting may reduce some of the symptomatology. Corticobasal ganglionic degeneration is a degenerative combination of extrapyramidal and cerebral cortical dysfunction. This is a little more insidious than the previously described syndromes and this asymmetric akinetic-rigid syndrome, which is evident early on and can be confused with PD; however, the early onset of cortical sensory loss and apraxia with occasional alien limb phenomena suggests the differentiation from PD. MRI frequently demonstrates asymmetrical cerebral atrophy, especially in the frontal and parietal regions.

In addition to ensuring the proper diagnosis, medical treatment, and suitability for surgery, the movement disorder neurologist can also document the degree of disability with a standardized instrument that ensures the ability to gauge the effectiveness of surgery. These are United Parkinson Disease Rating Scale (UPDRS) and Core Assessment Program for Intracerebral Transplantation-PD (CAPIT-PD) for PD (www.movementdisorders.org & publications). These are very time-consuming and require significant expertise to perform properly. Similarly, the neuropsychologist can provide standardized tests of cognition and psyche. These are the gold standard to evaluate patients and will be performed in centers of excellence.

It is frequently advisable to have the neurosurgeon and neurologist have their clinics on the same day. That way, patients can be exchanged easily back and forth without having to reschedule. In addition, this allows the neurosurgeon the opportunity to see a patient more often in the off state than would otherwise be anticipated. Patients who come in for their off evaluations can frequently be very quickly examined by the neurosurgeon without disrupting the entire day. Certainly, in follow-up visits where the neurosurgeon is simply checking a wound whereas the neurologist will be evaluating medication and stimulation parameters, the one-stop approach satisfies patients. When additional surgery is needed, the ability to immediately contact the neurosurgeon is most useful. By clinical practice, the neurologist will have more clinic days and more clinic time than the neurosurgeon, but keeping the surgical patient appointments on the same day can be advantageous. It is also quite useful to cross train the neurology and neurosurgery physician extender so that there is redundancy in the system and a smooth therapeutic approach can be achieved even in the absence of one or two personnel due to vacations, illness, and so forth.

■ Selecting Patients

Although selecting the appropriate center and the appropriate disease are prerequisites for a successful outcome, the final and most critical selection is that of the appropriate patient. Rigorous predictors of positive and negative outcomes could help identify the "optimal candidates" for surgery, but few have been identified. Surgical studies from which such predictive criteria could be derived are often uncontrolled and have a small sample size, limiting statistical analysis. In addition, the outcome of surgery is critically dependent on the exact location of the lesion or the DBS lead. Separating variability in outcome due to patient characteristics from that related to small variations in location is difficult, especially when the sample is small. Furthermore, most research studies adhere to stringent inclusion and exclusion criteria, and the study sample may therefore not be representative of the patient population referred for surgical evaluation. Finally, on a more philosophical level the question arises whether each patient indeed has to be an optimal candidate for surgery or that on occasion a "good enough" candidate will be acceptable. For instance, an 80-year-old patient with severe tremor interfering with the ability to eat or drink independently may not be an optimal candidate, but eliminating tremor on the patient's dominant side may obviate the need for nursing home placement.

Given all these uncertainties, patient selection will ultimately be a highly individualized process whereby the surgical team draws not only on the available scientific data but also on the experience of its multidisciplinary members.

General Considerations

Before proceeding with elective surgery for any of the disorders described, several general principles apply. The patient should be disabled enough to justify brain surgery.[12,56,57] This implies that pharmacological therapy has been exhausted, as determined by a movement disorder specialist. The latter ensures that, indeed, all appropriate medications have been tried at their optimal doses and in optimal combinations. Related to the foregoing, the target symptoms anticipated to improve with the proposed surgery should indeed be the symptoms causing the most disability. The patient's life expectancy should be taken into account. Thus advanced age or life-threatening comorbidities can potentially disqualify a surgical candidate. There is no absolute cutoff for age, but in general, studies suggest that younger patients do better than older patients.[58,59] The brain magnetic resonance imaging (MRI) should be normal, and the amount of atrophy limited. Regardless of the age, cognition should be intact and the mood stable. Significant impairment in either may lead to uncooperative behavior or uninformative feedback both during surgery and with programming. In addition, preexisting cognitive deficits may be amplified by the surgery, leading to decompensation of a patient who preoperatively was in a delicate neuropsychological balance. Intact cognition is also needed for a patient to understand the risks involved in surgery and the variable degree of improvement after surgery. A cardiac pacemaker is a complicating factor but can coexist with DBS under certain conditions[60]; however, MRI-guided targeting remains contraindicated in such patients and computed tomography (CT) must be used instead. Patients who are critically dependent on electroconvulsive therapy for their depression should not be treated with DBS. Unrealistic expectations may lead to disappointment and depression. Although objective and accurate patient education may seem adequate to prevent unrealistic expectations, it turns out to be insufficient in practice. This has prompted some centers to ask patients for a statement of their expectations in writing or on video prior to surgery, providing a point of reference for future use. Finally, the patient should have a solid support system not only in the perioperative phase but also later on, when multiple clinic visits are required and detailed feedback on the efficacy of different stimulation parameters is essential to maximize the benefit from DBS.

Disease-Specific Considerations

Selection and Evaluation of the Patient with Parkinson Disease

In the late 1980s the development of transplantation programs for PD provided the impetus for the establishment of a "common diagnostic and methodological core evaluation" of participants in surgical trials. In 1992 the Core Assessment Program for Intracerebral Transplantation (CAPIT) was published, followed in 1999 by a sequel applicable to all surgical interventions, the Core Assessment Program for Surgical Interventional Therapies in Parkinson's Disease (CAPSIT-PD).[16,61] Although designed for clinical trials, many of their recommendations apply to clinical practice as well.

Regarding patient selection, the guidelines recommend (1) the presence of two or more of the cardinal features, one of which must be tremor or bradykinesia; (2) the use of published consensus guidelines for MSA, dementia with Lewy bodies, and PSP to exclude patients with atypical parkinsonism; and (3) a disease duration of minimally 5 years. These recommendations are certainly reasonable and should be utilized in clinical practice, as already discussed. Not included in the CAPIT recommendations, neuropsychological selection criteria were first proposed in the CAPSIT-PD guidelines. Thus global intellectual capacity should be assessed with the Mattis Dementia Rating Scale (MDRS), with cutoff scores suggested at 130 or 120; depression should be assessed with the Montgomery and Asberg Depression Rating Scale (MADRS), with cutoff scores of 7 to 19 (mildly depressed); and psychiatric disease should be assessed with the Minnesota Multiphasic Personality Inventory (MMPI).[16] These recommendations are essential for investigational surgical therapies but are also wise guidelines for the selection of patients for DBS in clinical practice. As already commented on, patients with dementia, depression, and psychosis are at risk of critical decompensation throughout the perioperative period and in general have a suboptimal benefit from the procedure. In addition to using these tests to screen out patients unfit for surgery, CAPSIT-PD also proposes a more extensive battery of neuropsychological tests to compare cognition, mood, and behavior before and after surgery, with an emphasis on tests sensitive to frontal lobe dysfunction.[12,16] This, again, is a valuable guideline to be applied in clinical practice because it provides a quality control assessment for the effects of surgery on cognition and behavior for which there is no substitute.[8]

CAPIT/CAPSIT-PD further recommends that patients have an "unequivocal response" to dopaminergic agents, specified as at least 33% improvement in United Parkinson Disease Rating Scale motor subscore (UPDRS-III), following L-dopa or apomorphine challenge.[16,61] This recommendation was made to confirm the diagnosis of idiopathic PD. The pertinence of L-dopa responsiveness has certainly been substantiated in the case of DBS according to several reports. Thus motor improvement with L-dopa preoperatively (as measured by change in UPDRS-III) correlates positively with improvement from stimulation postoperatively and is considered the most valuable predictor of benefit from STN DBS in PD.[62] This correlation holds up when individual symptoms are examined; those symptoms that improve with L-dopa preoperatively are likely to improve with STN DBS.[59] Conversely, residual symptoms in the "on" state (such as on state persistent freezing, dysbalance, and falling) do not improve with surgery.[62] These studies have also examined other preoperative factors predicting a good postoperative outcome. Younger age and shorter disease duration appear to be associated with better overall results.[58,59,62]

CAPIT and CAPSIT guidelines specify the conditions under which the dopaminergic challenge test should be performed. Patients should be first tested in the "defined-off" state, 12 hours after their last dose of medication, and subsequently in the "defined-on" state, ~1 hour after receiving their usual dose of L-dopa. The evaluations should include UPDRS I–IV, Hoehn and Yahr (H&Y) staging, timed tests, and dyskinesia rating.[16,61]

The importance of this type of standardized off–on evaluation goes beyond testing dopaminergic responsiveness and should not be underestimated. At their regular clinic visits most patients are in the on state, and the formal off evaluation may well be the first opportunity for the neurologist to observe the severity and the nature of the individual's parkinsonian symptoms. This will allow the neurologist to decide if the patient's condition in the off state is severe enough to warrant surgery, to identify the most disabling features, and to provide an estimate of the degree of improvement that is to be expected with stimulation. In some cases it may even become clear that the disease has remained asymmetric enough that the procedure can be limited to one hemisphere (Chapter 15).

The CAPIT /CAPSIT-PD guidelines suggest that prior to surgery three core evaluations are performed, over at least a 3-month period.[16,61] This would correct for the day-to-day variability in symptom severity. Except in an occasionally experimental study, this practice is rarely followed because of the burden it poses on patients and staff. Moreover, a recent study suggests that motor, dyskinesia, and timed test scores do not significantly differ from one baseline visit to the next as long as the patient is assessed under standard conditions and by the same rater.[63]

With all these considerations in mind, there are usually two categories of PD patients that proceed to have surgery.

The largest group consists of patients with advanced disease who have L-dopa-associated motor fluctuations and dyskinesias. They still enjoy a good benefit from L-dopa, but the response to each individual dose is short and associated with disabling dyskinesias. They spend a considerable time of the day in the off state. Attempts to increase on time by pharmacological manipulation [using apomorphine, catechol-o-methyltransferase (COMT)-inhibitors, monoamine oxidase (MAO)-B inhibitors] and decrease dyskinesias (using amantadine or liquid L-dopa) have failed in the hands of a movement disorders expert. This group is suitable for DBS because studies have shown reduction of off time, prolongation of on time, and reduction of dyskinesias with both STN and GPI DBS.[28,29]

The smaller group consists of patients with severe tremor.[64] Rest tremor in PD usually responds to L-dopa, but especially in patients with tremor-predominant PD the dose required to substantially diminish disabling tremor can be so high that dose-limiting side effects either occur acutely or are likely to emerge with chronic treatment. In other cases the tremor is truly L-dopa resistant. These types of tremor respond nicely to STN DBS, creating the exception that confirms the rule of L-dopa responsiveness predicting surgical outcome.[65,66] It may therefore occur that patients without significant rigidity, bradykinesia, fluctuations, or dyskinesia are still good candidates for surgery solely due to their severe rest tremor.

Finally, there is an ongoing debate whether STN or GPI is the target of choice in PD.[28,64,67] Although this topic is beyond the scope of this chapter it should be brought up here that most of the scarce literature on patient selection is derived from studies on STN rather than GPI DBS. In the absence of large randomized trials, clinical practice has shifted toward STN DBS based largely on the only undisputed difference that after bilateral STN DBS, dopaminergic medication can be reduced by over 50% on average, whereas there is no such reduction after GPI DBS. In addition STN DBS usually requires a lower current, resulting in longer battery life.[64,68] Recent reports, however, suggest that STN DBS may be associated with more adverse effects than GPI DBS.[28,69] As the differences between these targets become further defined, it is possible that patient characteristics make them more suitable for DBS of STN or GPI.

Selection and Evaluation of the Patient with Tremor

There is no equivalent of L-dopa responsiveness to predict outcome of DBS for ET. However, the type and distribution of the tremor are prognostic factors. Thus postural and distal tremors are usually more completely controlled than kinetic and proximal tremors (Chapter 11). Axial tremors (head, voice) can show significant improvement after unilateral DBS but usually require a bilateral procedure for a more complete response.[70] Bilateral DBS of Vim is not associated with the same adverse effects as bilateral thalamotomy,[14,71] even though mild impairment of speech and

balance can be experienced when higher currents are necessary to suppress tremor.[72,73] A minority of patients may have return of tremor that eventually cannot be fully controlled despite increasing levels of stimulation, similar to the earlier experience with thalamotomy.[5,39,74] It is unclear as to what factors determine which patients are prone to recurrences, but it may be that those with an intention component are especially at risk.[41]

There is no equivalent of the CAPSIT-PD for patients with ET, and no gold standard tremor assessment exists. Most centers employ clinical tremor rating scales quantifying tremor severity in different body parts, and incorporate functional tasks such as writing, drawing a spiral, drinking from a cup, and pouring water from a cup. In addition, quality of life measures and activities of daily living (ADL) measures are used.[70] In advanced ET medications are not very effective and patients do not fluctuate in response to medication as they do in PD. Therefore, in ET patients are not assessed in a defined off and on state. However, for reasons of consistency it is recommended to evaluate patients before and after surgery at the same time of the day, and without their antitremor medications since the night before.

Because of the often dramatic antitremor efficacy in this monosymptomatic disorder, Vim DBS for severe ET can make the difference between independent and dependent lifestyles. This consideration may in rare cases lead to surgery on patients older than 75 or even 80 years of age. In this case a unilateral procedure is preferred, treating the dominant hand. We and others feel that age is not as critical for thalamic DBS as it is for STN DBS.[7] For this reason, we sometimes prefer the Vim to the STN target for elderly individuals with disabling tremor due to PD.

Selection and Evaluation of the Patient with Dystonia

There is no pharmacological test equivalent to L-dopa responsiveness to predict outcome of DBS for dystonia. In addition, GPi DBS for dystonia is a relatively new field, and the few studies published contain insufficient numbers of patients to establish firm prognosticators. However, also in dystonia the type and distribution may turn out to be prognostic factors (Chapter 12).

For generalized dystonia, some studies suggest that DYT1 positive PGD responds better to DBS than DYT1 negative PGD.[53] However, that difference was not confirmed in other recent studies.[50,52] Differences in makeup of the DYT1 groups, which likely represent mixtures of a variety of genetic forms of dystonia, could explain this discrepancy, especially given the small number of patients in each study. Another explanation is that most, but not all, patients with the DYT1 mutation respond to DBS.[75]

Focal or segmental forms of primary dystonia, such as cervical dystonia, are usually treated pharmacologically and with botulinum toxin. Only if these treatments fail and patients are left with disabling symptoms should surgery be considered. Two small studies suggest favorable results.[76,77]

Secondary dystonia, resulting from trauma, stroke, or in association with other neurological disorders, is even more difficult to study in a systematic fashion due to the different etiologies and comorbidities. Usually secondary dystonia exists as part of more complex symptomatology that may include spasticity, paresis, and skeletal deformities, making it difficult to isolate the contribution of the dystonic features to the disability. Not surprisingly, existing reports of DBS in secondary dystonia suggest benefit of smaller proportions than in primary dystonia.[53,78]

No CAPSIT-like core assessment program exists for dystonia. Recently three scales for generalized dystonia were found to have excellent internal consistency and correlation among the raters in a multicenter study[79]: the Global Dystonia Rating Scale (GDRS), the Unified Dystonia Rating Scale, and the most often used scale, the Burke-Fahn-Marsden Scale (BFMS). The latter has a motor subscale based on the exam of the patient and a functional disability subscale based on a questionnaire of ADL. Assessment of cervical dystonia is performed with the Toronto Western Spasmodic Torticollis Scale (TWSTRS). Following DBS the improvement in dystonia is more gradual than that seen in PD or ET. Usually improvement in mobile dystonia starts to occur within hours or days, whereas abnormal postures and functions such as gait take more time to improve.[75] However, in most patients the majority of the eventual benefit is obtained by 3 months, with further improvement continuing for more than 1 year.[50,52] In advanced dystonia patients do not show acute fluctuations in response to medication as they do in PD. Therefore, dystonia patients are not assessed in a defined off and on state. However, for reasons of consistency it is recommendable to evaluate patients before and after surgery at the same time of the day, and without their antidystonia medications since the night before.

■ Future Perspectives

The presented viewpoints are based on the literature but also draw on our own experience in running a movement disorders center and functional neurosurgery service at the Rush University Medical Center. Other centers may use slightly different approaches in the selection and evaluation of surgical candidates depending on their individual setting and resources. Regardless, all surgical teams will recognize the need for evidence-based selection criteria for surgical therapies. The risk:benefit ratio for each surgery needs to be better defined. A larger emphasis needs to be placed on *long-term* efficacy (and adverse events) assessment. Benefits are reported in much more detail, and, thanks to programs such as CAPIT/CAPSIT-PD, in a much more standardized fashion, than adverse events, which are inconsistently classified and almost certainly underreported. Guidelines on how to classify and report adverse events should be developed to improve our ability to compare different targets, procedures, and centers. The search for the optimal target (and subtarget) for each disorder needs to continue through comparative randomized trials. The relationship between lead location/trajectory on the one hand and benefits/adverse events on the other hand needs to be further defined. This would be facilitated by standard, accurate methods for determining postoperative lead placement. Identification of new gene mutations will enable us to better separate different disease entities and thus study the effect of surgery in more homogeneous populations. Finally, as DBS comes of age, new indications for other movement disorders will likely emerge. Although this will be associated with some new disease-specific selection criteria, established surgical teams will be able to utilize their past experiences to refine their surgical techniques, assessment methods, and selection criteria.

References

1. Ashkan K, Wallace B, Bell BA, Benabid AL. Deep brain stimulation of the subthalamic nucleus in Parkinson's disease 1993–2003: where are we 10 years on? Br J Neurosurg 2004;18:19–34
2. Benabid AL. Deep brain stimulation for Parkinson's disease. Curr Opin Neurobiol 2003;13:696–706
3. Pollak P, Fraix V, Krack P, et al. Treatment results: Parkinson's disease. Mov Disord 2002;17(Suppl 3):S75–S83
4. Umemura A, Jaggi JL, Hurtig HI, et al. Deep brain stimulation for movement disorders: morbidity and mortality in 109 patients. J Neurosurg 2003;98:779–784
5. Lyons KE, Pahwa R. Deep brain stimulation and essential tremor. J Clin Neurophysiol 2004;21:2–5
6. Lyons KE, Pahwa R. Deep brain stimulation in Parkinson's disease. Curr Neurol Neurosci Rep 2004;4:290–295
7. Hariz MI. Complications of deep brain stimulation surgery. Mov Disord 2002;17(Suppl 3):S162–S166
8. Anderson KE, Mullins J. Behavioral changes associated with deep brain stimulation surgery for Parkinson's disease. Curr Neurol Neurosci Rep 2003;3:306–313
9. Lozano AM, Mahant N. Deep brain stimulation surgery for Parkinson's disease: mechanisms and consequences. Parkinsonism Relat Disord 2004;10(Suppl 1):S49–S57
10. Piasecki SD, Jefferson JW. Psychiatric complications of deep brain stimulation for Parkinson's disease. J Clin Psychiatry 2004;65:845–849
11. Saint-Cyr JA, Trepanier LL, Kumar R, Lozano AM, Lang AE. Neuropsychological consequences of chronic bilateral stimulation of the subthalamic nucleus in Parkinson's disease. Brain 2000;123(Pt 10):2091–2108
12. Lang AE, Widner H. Deep brain stimulation for Parkinson's disease: patient selection and evaluation. Mov Disord 2002;17(Suppl 3):S94–S101

13. Lozano AM, Hamani C. The future of deep brain stimulation. J Clin Neurophysiol 2004;21:68–69

14. Schuurman PR, Bosch DA, Bossuyt PM, et al. A comparison of continuous thalamic stimulation and thalamotomy for suppression of severe tremor. N Engl J Med 2000;342:461–468

15. Saint-Cyr JA, Trepanier LL. Neuropsychologic assessment of patients for movement disorder surgery. Mov Disord 2000;15:771–783

16. Defer GL, Widner H, Marie RM, Remy P, Levivier M. Core assessment program for surgical interventional therapies in Parkinson's disease (CAPSIT-PD). Mov Disord 1999;14:572–584

17. Young C, Abercrombie M, Beattie A. How a specialist nurse helps patients undergoing deep brain stimulation. Prof Nurse 2003;18:318–321

18. Starr PA, Turner RS, Rau G, et al. Microelectrode-guided implantation of deep brain stimulators into the globus pallidus internus for dystonia: techniques, electrode locations, and outcomes. Neurosurg Focus 2004;17:E4

19. Hariz M, Blomstedt P, Limousin P. The myth of microelectrode recording in ensuring a precise location of the DBS electrode within the sensorimotor part of the subthalamic nucleus. Mov Disord 2004;19:863–864

20. Krack P, Fraix V, Mendes A, Benabid AL, Pollak P. Postoperative management of subthalamic nucleus stimulation for Parkinson's disease. Mov Disord 2002;17(Suppl 3):S188–S197

21. Kumar R. Methods for programming and patient management with deep brain stimulation of the globus pallidus for the treatment of advanced Parkinson's disease and dystonia. Mov Disord 2002;17(Suppl 3):S198–S207

22. Volkmann J, Herzog J, Kopper F, Deuschl G. Introduction to the programming of deep brain stimulators. Mov Disord 2002;17(Suppl 3):S181–S187

23. Dowsey-Limousin P. Postoperative management of Vim DBS for tremor. Mov Disord 2002;17(Suppl 3):S208–S211

24. Hariz MI, Johansson F. Hardware failure in parkinsonian patients with chronic subthalamic nucleus stimulation is a medical emergency. Mov Disord 2001;16:166–168

25. Woods SP, Fields JA, Troster AI. Neuropsychological sequelae of subthalamic nucleus deep brain stimulation in Parkinson's disease: a critical review. Neuropsychol Rev 2002;12:111–126

26. Woods SP, Fields JA, Lyons KE, et al. Neuropsychological and quality of life changes following unilateral thalamic deep brain stimulation in Parkinson's disease: a one-year follow-up. Acta Neurochir (Wien) 2001;143:1273–1277 (discussion 1278)

27. Gross RE. Deep brain stimulation in the treatment of neurological and psychiatric disease. Expert Rev Neurother 2004;4:465–478

28. Anderson VC, Burchiel KJ, Hogarth P, Favre J, Hammerstad JP. Pallidal vs subthalamic nucleus deep brain stimulation in Parkinson disease. Arch Neurol 2005;62:554–560

29. Group D-BSfPsDS. Deep-brain stimulation of the subthalamic nucleus or the pars interna of the globus pallidus in Parkinson's disease. N Engl J Med 2001;345:956–963

30. Esselink RAJ, de Bie RM, de Haan RJ, et al. Unilateral pallidotomy versus bilateral subthalamic nucleus stimulation in PD: a randomized trial. Neurology 2004;62:201–207

31. Chou KL, Forman MS, Trojanowski JQ, Hurtig HI, Baltuch GH. Subthalamic nucleus deep brain stimulation in a patient with L-dopa-responsive multiple system atrophy. Case report. J Neurosurg 2004;100:553–556

32. Jankovic J. Essential tremor: clinical characteristics. Neurology 2000;54(11, Suppl 4)S21–S25

33. Deuschl G, Bain P, Brin M. Consensus statement of the movement disorder society on tremor. Mov Disord 1998;13(Suppl 3):2–23

34. Cohen O, Pullman S, Jurewicz E, Watner D, Louis ED. Rest tremor in patients with essential tremor: prevalence, clinical correlates, and electrophysiologic characteristics. Arch Neurol 2003;60:405–410

35. Deuschl G, Fogel W, Hahne M, et al. Deep-brain stimulation for Parkinson's disease. J Neurol 2002;249(Suppl 3):III/36–39

36. Deuschl G, Volkmann J. Tremors: differential diagnosis, pathophysiology, and therapy. In: Jankovic J, Tolosa E, eds. Parkinson's Disease and Movement Disorders. Philadelphia: Lippincott, Williams & Wilkins; 2002:270–290

37. Hubble JP, Busenbark KL, Pahwa R, Lyons K, Koller WC. Clinical expression of essential tremor: effects of gender and age. Mov Disord 1997;12:969–972

38. Elble RJ. Essential tremor frequency decreases with time. Neurology 2000;55:1547–1551

39. Papavassiliou E, Rau G, Heath S, et al. Thalamic deep brain stimulation for essential tremor: relation of lead location to outcome. Neurosurgery 2004;54:1120–1129 (discussion 1129–1130)

40. Plaha P, Patel NK, Gill SS. Stimulation of the subthalamic region for essential tremor. J Neurosurg 2004;101:48–54

41. Benabid AL, Pollak P, Gao D, et al. Chronic electrical stimulation of the ventralis intermedius nucleus of the thalamus as a treatment of movement disorders. J Neurosurg 1996;84:203–214

42. Limousin P, Speelman JD, Gielen F, Janssens M. Multicentre European study of thalamic stimulation in parkinsonian and essential tremor. J Neurol Neurosurg Psychiatry 1999;66:289–296

43. Wishart HA, Roberts DW, Roth RM, et al. Chronic deep brain stimulation for the treatment of tremor in multiple sclerosis: review and case reports. J Neurol Neurosurg Psychiatry 2003;74:1392–1397

44. Nikkhah G, Prokop T, Hellwig B, Lucking CH, Ostertag CB. Deep brain stimulation of the nucleus ventralis intermedius for Holmes (rubral) tremor and associated dystonia caused by upper brainstem lesions: report of two cases. J Neurosurg 2004;100:1079–1083

45. Romanelli P, Bronte-Stewart H, Courtney T, Heit G. Possible necessity for deep brain stimulation of both the ventralis intermedius and subthalamic nuclei to resolve Holmes tremor: case report. J Neurosurg 2003;99:566–571

46. Foote KD, Okun MS. Ventralis intermedius plus ventralis oralis anterior and posterior deep brain stimulation for posttraumatic Holmes tremor: two leads may be better than one: technical note. Neurosurgery 2005;56(2, Suppl):E445 (discussion E445)

47. Fahn S. Concept and classification of dystonia. Adv Neurol 1988;50:1–8

48. Vitek JL. Pathophysiology of dystonia: a neuronal model. Mov Disord 2002;17(Suppl 3):S49–S62

49. Hallett M. Dystonia: abnormal movements result from loss of inhibition. Adv Neurol 2004;94:1–9

50. Coubes P, Cif L, El Fertit H, et al. Electrical stimulation of the globus pallidus internus in patients with primary generalized dystonia: long-term results. J Neurosurg 2004;101:189–194

51. Krauss JK, Yianni J, Loher TJ, Aziz TZ. Deep brain stimulation for dystonia. J Clin Neurophysiol 2004;21:18–30

52. Vidailhet M, Vercueil L, Houeto JL, et al. Bilateral deep-brain stimulation of the globus pallidus in primary generalized dystonia. N Engl J Med 2005;352:459–467

53. Krause M, Fogel W, Kloss M, Rasche D, Volkmann J, Tronnier V. Pallidal stimulation for dystonia. Neurosurgery 2004;55:1361–1370

54. Ozelius LJ, Hewett JW, Page CE, et al. The early-onset torsion dystonia gene (DYT1) encodes an ATP-binding protein. Nat Genet 1997;17:40–48

55. Castelnau P, Cif L, Valente EM, et al. Pallidal stimulation improves pantothenate kinase-associated neurodegeneration. Ann Neurol 2005;57:738–741

56. Deuschl G, Bain P. Deep brain stimulation for tremor [correction of trauma]: patient selection and evaluation. Mov Disord 2002; 17(Suppl 3):S102–S111

57. Volkmann J, Benecke R. Deep brain stimulation for dystonia: patient selection and evaluation. Mov Disord 2002;17(Suppl 3): S112–S115

58. Russmann H, Ghika J, Villemure JG, et al. Subthalamic nucleus deep brain stimulation in Parkinson disease patients over age 70 years. Neurology 2004;63:1952–1954

59. Charles PD, Van Blercom N, Krack P, et al. Predictors of effective bilateral subthalamic nucleus stimulation for PD. Neurology 2002;59:932–934

60. Capelle HH, Simpson RK Jr, Kronenbuerger M, Michaelsen J, Tronnier V, Krauss JK. Long-term deep brain stimulation in elderly patients with cardiac pacemakers. J Neurosurg 2005;102:53–59

61. Langston JW, Widner H, Goetz CG, et al. Core assessment program for intracerebral transplantations (CAPIT). Mov Disord 1992;7:2–13

62. Welter ML, Houeto JL, Tezenas du Montcel S, et al. Clinical predictive factors of subthalamic stimulation in Parkinson's disease. Brain 2002;125(Pt 3):575–583

63. Metman LV, Myre B, Verwey N, et al. Test-retest reliability of UPDRS-III, dyskinesia scales, and timed motor tests in patients with advanced Parkinson's disease: an argument against multiple baseline assessments. Mov Disord 2004;19:1079–1084

64. Volkmann J. Deep brain stimulation for the treatment of Parkinson's disease. J Clin Neurophysiol 2004;21:6–17

65. Sturman MM, Vaillancourt DE, Metman LV, Bakay RA, Corcos DM. Effects of subthalamic nucleus stimulation and medication on resting and postural tremor in Parkinson's disease. Brain 2004;127 (Pt 9):2131–2143

66. Fraix V, Pollak P, Moro E, et al. Subthalamic nucleus stimulation in tremor dominant parkinsonian patients with previous thalamic surgery. J Neurol Neurosurg Psychiatry 2005;76:246–248

67. Okun MS, Foote KD. Subthalamic nucleus vs globus pallidus interna deep brain stimulation, the rematch: will pallidal deep brain stimulation make a triumphant return? Arch Neurol 2005;62:533–536,

68. Vitek JL. Deep brain stimulation for Parkinson's disease: a critical re-evaluation of STN versus GPi DBS. Stereotact Funct Neurosurg 2002;78:119–131

69. Volkmann J, Allert N, Voges J, Weiss PH, Freund HJ, Sturm V. Safety and efficacy of pallidal or subthalamic nucleus stimulation in advanced PD. Neurology 2001;56:548–551

70. Putzke JD, Uitti RJ, Obwegeser AA, Wszolek ZK, Wharen RE. Bilateral thalamic deep brain stimulation: midline tremor control. J Neurol Neurosurg Psychiatry 2005;76:684–690

71. Pahwa R, Lyons KE, Wilkinson SB, et al. Comparison of thalamotomy to deep brain stimulation of the thalamus in essential tremor. Mov Disord 2001;16:140–143

72. Putzke JD, Wharen RE Jr, Obwegeser AA, et al. Thalamic deep brain stimulation for essential tremor: recommendations for long-term outcome analysis. Can J Neurol Sci 2004;31:333–342

73. Pahwa R, Lyons KL, Wilkinson SB, et al. Bilateral thalamic stimulation for the treatment of essential tremor. Neurology 1999;53:1447–1450

74. Kumar R, Lozano AM, Sime E, Lang AE. Long-term follow-up of thalamic deep brain stimulation for essential and parkinsonian tremor. Neurology 2003;61:1601–1604

75. Vercueil L, Krack P, Pollak P. Results of deep brain stimulation for dystonia: a critical reappraisal. Mov Disord 2002;17(Suppl 3):S89–S93

76. Eltahawy HA, Saint-Cyr J, Poon YY, Moro E, Lang AE, Lozano AM. Pallidal deep brain stimulation in cervical dystonia: clinical outcome in four cases. Can J Neurol Sci 2004;31:328–332

77. Krauss JK. Deep brain stimulation for cervical dystonia. J Neurol Neurosurg Psychiatry 2003;74:1598

78. Eltahawy HA, Saint-Cyr J, Giladi N, Lang AE, Lozano AM. Primary dystonia is more responsive than secondary dystonia to pallidal interventions: outcome after pallidotomy or pallidal deep brain stimulation. Neurosurgery 2004;54:613–619 (discussion 619–621)

79. Comella CL, Leurgans S, Wuu J, Stebbins GT, Chmura T, Group DS. Rating scales for dystonia: a multicenter assessment. Mov Disord 2003;18:303–312

80. Lopiano L, Rizzone M, Bergamasco B, et al. Deep brain stimulation of the subthalamus nucleus in PD: an analysis of the exclusion causes. J Neurol Sci 2002;195:167–170

81. Wenning GK, Geser F, Stampfer-Kountchev M, Tison F. Multiple system atrophy: an update. Mov Disord 2003;18(Suppl 6):S34–S42

82. Osaki Y, Ben-Shlomo Y, Lees AJ, et al. Accuracy of clinical diagnosis of progressive supranuclear palsy. Mov Disord 2004;19:181–189

83. Paviour DC, Surtees RAH, Lees AJ. Diagnostic considerations in juvenile parkinsonism. Mov Disord 2004;19:123–135

84. Desaloms JM, Krauss JK, Lai EC, Jankovic J, Grossman RG. Posteroventral medial pallidotomy for Parkinson's disease: preoperative magnetic resonance imaging features and clinical outcome. J Neurosurg 1998;89:194–199

5 Preparation for Surgery

Ron L. Alterman and Michele Tagliati

The elective nature of movement disorder surgery demands strict patient selection criteria and optimal surgical technique to ensure patient safety. This chapter discusses the preparation for surgery from the neurosurgeon's perspective beginning with the surgical aspects of patient selection and concluding with the various techniques available for anatomical targeting and surgical planning. When appropriate, scientific evidence in support of best practice is presented. Contemporary stereotactic surgeons have at their disposal several techniques that can be used to perform movement disorder surgery. Surgeons must choose an approach that suits their surgical philosophy as well as the strengths of the institution in which they work.

■ Presurgical Evaluation

Surgery should be considered for any patient with Parkinson disease (PD), essential tremor (ET), or primary torsion dystonia who is cognitively intact and disabled by motor symptoms that are poorly responsive to standard medical regimens. Properly diagnosing and treating movement disorders is no simple matter, and it is the wise neurosurgeon who partners with a movement disorder neurologist who will ensure that the patients are properly diagnosed and medically treated before surgical intervention is offered. This topic is well covered in Chapter 4. Nevertheless, the decision to proceed with surgery and the choice of procedure rest with the surgeon, requiring that the surgeon be well acquainted with the more common movement disorders and can screen for potential problem patients.

Parkinson Disease

Selecting PD patients for deep brain stimulation (DBS) or ablative surgery poses a significant challenge for several reasons. First, PD is highly variable in its clinical presentation and progression.[1] Patients suffer from many symptoms, each of which varies in its response to dopaminergic medications and surgery.[2,3] Second, care must be taken to identify patients with atypical parkinsonian syndromes because these disorders may have a limited response to surgery.[4] Finally, cognitive decline, a prominent feature in elderly patients with advancing PD, must be ruled out because it can be worsened by surgical intervention.[5–7] A well-documented history and physical exam are needed to properly screen the candidates.

A clinical diagnosis of idiopathic PD is supported by the presence of at least two of the following four symptoms: resting tremor, rigidity, bradykinesia, and asymmetrical onset.[1] A substantial and sustained response to L-dopa therapy is a key clinical feature confirming the diagnosis and is a strong predictor of the response to subthalamic nucleus (STN) DBS.[3] In general, patients who remain responsive to L-dopa but who suffer with progressive motor fluctuations and L-dopa–induced dyskinesiae are the best candidates for STN DBS surgery.[3,8]

The progression of an individual's disease and the time frame in which L-dopa-resistant symptoms appear must also be considered. Unusual clinical features observed early in the clinical course suggest the possibility of an atypical parkinsonian syndrome.[9] These include (1) prominent postural instability, (2) predominant rigidity or axial symptoms, (3) freezing phenomena (akinesia), (4) hallucinations unrelated to medication, (5) dementia preceding motor symptoms, (6) supranuclear gaze palsy, (7) severe dysautonomia, and (8) early loss of L-dopa response.[9–12] These traits or a history of conditions known to produce parkinsonism (e.g., chronic neuroleptic use, focal brain lesions) strongly suggest a diagnosis of atypical parkinsonism and constitute a relative contraindication to DBS or ablative surgery.

When atypical parkinsonism is suspected on clinical grounds, ^{18}F-fluorodeoxyglucose positron emission tomography (FDG/PET) may be used to determine the proper diagnosis. FDG/PET is the most reliable means of distinguishing idiopathic PD from multiple system atrophy (MSA) or other forms of atypical parkinsonism.[6,13] Idiopathic PD is marked by hypermetabolism of the lentiform nucleus on FDG/PET, whereas MSA is indicated by lentiform hypometabolism.[13] FDG/PET may also serve as a quantitative predictor of the response to pallidotomy, with the degree of hypermetabolism correlating with postoperative motor improvement.[14] The use of metabolic imaging modalities for the evaluation of patients undergoing DBS therapy is currently under investigation.[15,16]

Visual hallucinations unrelated to medication intake may herald the development of Lewy body dementia.[9] Such patients should be excluded from surgical consideration. Patients experiencing medication-induced visual hallucinations may be good surgical candidates, but their surgery should be delayed until they can be stabilized on a medication regimen that does not impair their mental status. We prefer that patients have a clear sensorium for at least 1 month prior to surgery to avoid increased confusion postoperatively.

Dystonia

Dystonia is characterized by sustained, involuntary muscle contractions generating twisting and repetitive movements or abnormal postures.[17] Dystonia may be a primary disorder with no obvious underlying cause or may be secondary, caused by any number of etiologies.[17] With rare exception (e.g., dopa-responsive dystonia), medical therapies yield limited results.[18] Focal dystonias such as spasmodic torticollis or writer's cramp may be treated effectively with local injections of botulinum toxin,[18,19] but this approach is impractical for generalized dystonia, in which many muscles are affected. Multiple reports indicate that DBS can generate profound improvement in patients with primary dystonia, in particular those patients with *DYT1* gene mutation.[20–24] Further study is required to define the optimal clinical indicators for DBS in dystonia.

Essential Tremor

ET is a common movement disorder of the aged, with an estimated prevalence of 0.3 to 5.6% of the general population.[25] This is a monosymptomatic ailment characterized by a 4 to 12 Hz postural tremor that is exacerbated with emotional stress and volitional movement.[26] The hands and arms are predominantly affected. Head tremor occurs in ~40% of cases, voice tremor in 20%.[27] Most patients with ET present with mild, nondisabling tremor.[28] Only 10% or fewer develop severe motor disability that interferes with activities of daily living.[29] In these cases, medical therapies, including β-blockers and barbiturates, yield limited results. Ablation or DBS in the ventrolateral thalamus yields excellent long-term control of ET, especially tremors of the distal extremities.[30–32] Unlike PD, in which tremor is the least disabling feature, control of tremor in ET results in significant improvements in functional capabilities.[30–32]

Editor's Comments

There are important differences between the focus of the neurosurgeon and the neurologist in selecting patients for functional neurosurgery. The neurologist will predominantly consider the appropriateness of the diagnosis and the medical treatment. The neurosurgeon must evaluate the appropriateness of the patient for a surgical procedure but must also overlap with the neurologist in the final screening before surgery. This is especially true for neurosurgeons without the advantage of working in a movement disorder center. Rarely accept the diagnosis without verification by an expert in movement disorders and/or your complete examination.

It all starts with the history. Assume the diagnosis is wrong. It is extremely important that any history which would suggest a different diagnosis be obtained. Although this is certainly possible with a physician extender, the neurosurgeon needs to be involved in this effort to ensure the integrity of the examination diagnosis. Idiopathic PD is a diagnosis of exclusion; therefore, red flags should be noted for patients with a history that includes any of the following: a remitting course, the use of neuroleptic drugs, encephalitis, head injury, stroke, oculogyric crisis, autonomic problems such as hypotension or neurogenic bladder, and rapid progression of disease. Specifically, the history of resting tremor, and a good and sustained response to L-dopa therapy are two of the most critical aspects in defining PD. Tremor is present in ~80% of patients with PD, and its total absence should put up a red flag. Similarly, response to L-dopa is absolutely critical to define idiopathic PD. We do not accept the excuse that the patient is "allergic" to L-dopa because there are multiple agonists that can be used instead. Unfortunately, neither of these is sufficient to exclude other types of diagnoses. The presence of a strong familial tendency in PD suggests that this may not be idiopathic PD, whereas a strong familial history of ET will provide an increased confidence that the ET diagnosis is appropriate. A history of "recreational drug use," or occupational toxic exposure, whether through agriculture or industry, needs to be carefully reviewed. Dopamine blockers (neuroleptics and antiemetics), dopamine depletors (reserpine and tetrabenazine), and dopamine antagonists (metochlopramide, lithium, α-methyl-dopa, and tricyclic antidepressants) can produce parkinsonian features. Some antiepileptics can cause tremor.

The other aspect of the history that is extremely important for the neurosurgeon is what safety factors may be essential to evaluate preoperatively. Certainly, a list of current medications is essential to prescribing accurate postoperative medication. This is the time to be sure the patient is not on medicine that could cause complications at the time of surgery. Because of the heightened necessity for hemostasis, the history and the list of medications should be scrutinized for any factors or drugs that could delay hemostasis. Specifically, how well does the patient heal following injury, whether or not previous surgeries have been performed without difficulty? Also ask about alternative and over-the-counter medicines because these are frequently not volunteered. The latter is especially important given that multiple medications may contain antiplatelet compounds that the patient may be unaware of. These are listed in **Table 5.1**.

Any suggestion of a lack of pulmonary or cardiac reserve needs to be carefully evaluated preoperatively by a specialist. This is especially true in PD where cardiac problems may be difficult to detect. A history of sleep disturbance may also suggest that the patient will not be quiet during sedation. Patients with any other type of electrical stimulation devices are generally acceptable. Of most concern are the cardiac pacemakers, and each manufacturer should be contacted to determine compatibility with DBS.[33,34] Interference between the two pulse generators (IPG) is possible; appropriate sequencing is necessary to avoid problems. In addition, the IPG device may need to be moved to a different location to avoid programming problems. The presence of a shunt would similarly require special consideration for placement of the IPG, as well as the extension lead. The presence of anticoagulation is a relative contraindication for surgery; however, several patients are on anticoagulants that can easily be discontinued

Table 5.1 Medication to Discontinue Two Weeks before Surgery

Aspirin and aspirin-containing products: Alka-Seltzer, Anacin, Ascriptin, Bufferin, Darvon, Compound 65, Ecotrin, Fiorinal, Goody's Powder, Norgesic, Percodan, Soma Compound, Trilisate

Nonsteroidal anti-inflammatory drugs (NSAIDS): Advil, Aleve, Anaprox, Anasaid, Arthrotec, Cataflam, Celebrex, Clinoril, Daypro, Dolobid, Feldene, ibuprofen, Indosin, Lodine, Motrin, Naprosyn, Nurin, Relafen, Tolectin, Toradol, Vioxx, Voltaren

Blood-thinning medications: Aggrenox, Agrylin (anagrelide), Coumadin (warfarin), Plavix (clopidogrel), Persantine (dipyridamole), Pletal (cilostazol), ReoPro (abciximab), Ticlid (ticlopidine), Trental (pertoxifylline), Lovenox

Other medications suspected of blood thinning: valproic acid, Imuran

Vitamins or herbal supplements may affect the ability to clot such as vitamin E, ginger, garlic, ginkgo, and feverfew

Pain medications that may be taken prior to procedures include Tylenol (acetaminophen), Vicodin (Lortab or hydrocodone), and Ultram

for a week with minimal or no risk. In this situation, we have the internist convert the patient from Coumadin (Bristol-Myers Squibb, Princeton, NJ) to heparin, and then we will reverse it just prior to surgery. Postoperatively, we wait from 3 to 7 days before restarting the Coumadin to ensure adequate homeostasis in the immediate postoperative period. Patients must be forewarned that they are at risk while off medication and the presence of a mechanical device their risk of hemorrhage may be increased postoperatively.

The general physical examination should evaluate patients as to how readily they can undergo surgery and magnetic resonance imaging (MRI). The presence of severe spondylosis, contractures, and kyphosis may reduce the ability to perform the imaging procedure; special considerations may be necessary, such as general anesthesia or a frameless technique. On neurological examination, the presence of the pyramidal signs, absent or atypical tremor, early onset of postural instability, neuropathy, myoclonus, focal cortical signs, and any type of ocular difficulties are all red flags. By definition, ET is a monosymptomatic disorder, so the presence of any additional symptomatology should raise a red flag as to the appropriateness of the diagnosis. Dystonia is widely variable in terms of onset, location, and symptom complexes. As a result, its diagnosis and treatment are extremely complex. This is best discussed in Chapter 12.

Any aspects of the history or physical examination that have raised red flags should be discussed with the referring neurologist to ensure that everything has been done to make the correct diagnosis. Misdiagnosis occurs even among the best movement disorder specialists. If there is a good working relationship, questioning the diagnosis should not be an affront but a legitimate concern expressed by a colleague who wishes to reexamine the diagnosis. Such concerns should not be trivialized. Patients with L-dopa-responsive MSA can be easily misdiagnosed as an idiopathic PD, and DBS STN surgery is not effective.[35–37] Patients with other atypical parkinsonisms are also not likely to improve following STN DBS (see Chapter 15).

Although the neurologist may suggest the surgical procedure, the neurosurgeon determines which procedure is best for a particular patient. The hemiparkinson patients do very well with unilateral DBS in the STN or globus pallidus internus (GPi). We have patients in postoperative year 6 who have not needed a second sided surgery. Although in general STN DBS is done for PD, a GPi may be an equally good target (see Chapter 15). The ventralis intermedius nucleus of the thalamus (Vim) is used almost exclusively for ET, but STN can also be used (see Chapter 11). Dystonia is predominantly treated with GPi DBS but can be treated with DBS leads in other sites (see Chapter 12). A GPi DBS works very well opposite a successful pallidotomy. Al-

though concerns have been raised about an STN DBS contralateral to a previous pallidotomy,[38] we have not found this to be a significant problem for the management of L-dopa therapy, gait freezing, or falls. Clearly, bilateral STN DBS placement can be performed following unilateral or bilateral pallidotomy as well as unilateral or bilateral thalamotomy.[71–73]

The discussion with the patient should be very frank, and it is at this point that the neurosurgeon can determine the expectations of the patient and the family. Both are critically important to correct preoperatively. The family needs to be queried as to their expectations. Families often expect their loved one to be "cured." If they are not able to live independently postoperatively, the patient might be placed in the nearest nursing home. A stable support system is essential for patients in the postoperative period. Some patients expect to be cured based on media reports or another patient they have seen with a DBS. If improvement is less than anticipated, patients will be unhappy even in the face of marked improvement. It is frequently advantageous to have patients talk to other patients who have undergone the procedure. There is a general rule that patients will not get better than their best "on" time. This is especially important to tell patients because their anticipation of success may far exceed their symptomatic relief. The patient's age must also be considered. Older patients simply aren't going to see the maximum improvement that occurs in the younger patients.[42] More important than age, however, is cognitive disability. While most patients do not suffer cognitive decline, the potential is always there especially in older patients and patients with less cognitive function preoperatively. Clear dementia or acute psychiatric disorders should be contraindications for surgery. Although gait and postural instability can improve postoperatively, only when these symptoms are minimal in the on stage will improvement be seen.[3,42–44] Therefore, if these symptoms are severe in the on stage, seriously consider not operating upon these patients, especially if they are older with gait difficulty or there is some suggestion of diagnosis other than the idiopathic PD.

Patients must also come to grips with the potential for complications. Patients should be fully informed of the complication risks, and if they are intimidated it is advisable not to proceed with the surgery. Patients and families must understand that complications can occur at any time. Even when the surgery is successful there are potential problems with hardware or infection. A fifth of patients may require some type of DBS revision.[45] They must also understand that their primary doctor postoperatively will be their movement disorder specialist who will manage the medications and the stimulator parameters. Some neurosurgeons do try to manage both, but we have not seen this to be successful. A neurosurgeon can manage the stimulator and the neurologist can manage medications; however, this succeeds only when there is a limited number of patients requiring such interventions. Physician extenders are increasingly called upon to manage these patients, whether they are in neurosurgery, neurology, or both departments.

A few patients will benefit from surgery but will be afraid of the mechanical device and will therefore elect lesioning. In addition, some patients may qualify for surgery, but they may not be candidates for a mechanical device.[45] It must be remembered that DBS is an elective procedure, and there are alternative therapies available. As with any elective surgery, there is always a conflict between being too conservative with the indications and offering the procedure to too few patients that might benefit or being too liberal so as to include some patients that will not benefit from surgery. The procedure offered to the patient should therefore be based on each patient's individual and unique medical, psychological, and social situation.

■ Preoperative Preparation

Routine preoperative blood work includes a complete blood count, prothrombin time test, and electrolyte analysis. A chest X-ray and electrocardiogram are performed when indicated. Patients are instructed to discontinue aspirin and vitamin E for at least 2 weeks prior to surgery because these agents may increase the risk of intracerebral hemorrhage.[46] Antiplatelet agents and warfarin should be discontinued only with the approval of the patient's medical practitioner. We have on two occasions performed DBS surgery on patients with Von Willebrand disease, providing factor VIII at the time of surgery. We have also operated on two young PD patients who were HIV+. In both instances the patients exhibited stable disease states with normal lymphocyte counts and no episodes of opportunistic infection. Neither suffered a surgical complication, and both have responded beautifully to STN DBS.

Patients with hypertension should take their antihypertensive medications on the morning of surgery because elevated blood pressure may increase the risk of perioperative hemorrhage, and withholding Sinemet (carbidopa/L-dopa) (Merck & Co., Inc., Whitehouse Station, NJ) for the surgery often results in rebound hypertension. Although not possible in many institutions, it is our practice to admit PD patients the night before surgery. Withholding dopaminergic medications facilitates microelectrode localization; however, abrupt withdrawal of these medications can result in fever and myolysis similar to that seen in the malignant neuroleptic syndrome.[34] Therefore, we prefer to withdraw the patient's dopaminergic medications in a controlled setting.

■ Surgical Preparation

Stereotactic Head Frames and Frame Application

Several stereotactic head frames are available commercially. See Chapter 3 for a detailed discussion of the advantages and disadvantages of each stereotactic system. Interested parties are directed to additional references,[47,48] which detail the use of the most common stereotactic frames. Most neurosurgeons already have access to a stereotactic frame, which they use for tumor biopsies and difficult ventricular catheterizations. In most instances these frames are serviceable for performing functional neurosurgical procedures; however, we advise having the frame recalibrated by the manufacturer before employing it for this purpose. The accuracy requirements for functional neurosurgical procedures are far greater than those required for brain biopsy, and the performance of frames can degrade over time.

The frame should be selected for its durability, versatility, and ease of use. Most contemporary frames function on the arc-centered principle, which greatly simplifies the targeting process. The frame should allow targeting from both MRI and computed tomography (CT) and should be compatible with the specific independent targeting software that is chosen. The frame should allow the patient to be positioned as comfortably as possible, especially if one plans to use intraoperative microelectrode recording (MER) which can be time consuming. Finally, some form of reticule system should be available so that one may confirm proper intraoperative positioning of the DBS lead or lesioning electrode (**Fig. 5.1**).

We employ the Leksell Model G stereotactic head frame (Elekta Instruments, Atlanta, GA) for all of the foregoing reasons. The Leksell frame is lightweight yet durable, is both MRI and CT compatible, and allows the patient to be positioned comfortably with the head elevated, minimizing cerebrospinal fluid (CSF) egress from precoronal burr holes. In the operating room, the Leksell frame allows targeting adjustments to be made easily and permits fluoroscopic confirmation of the electrode position.

Head Frame Application

Frame application is perhaps the most overlooked step in performing functional neurosurgical procedures. Proper alignment of the frame with the patient's anatomy simplifies targeting adjustments and allows the surgeon to use consistent angles of approach. The ear-bars that are provided with the Leksell frame facilitate frame application by preventing sideward tilt (roll) or axial rotation (yaw) of the frame relative to the patient's head, while permitting the pitch of the frame to be adjusted easily. It is important to use the ear-bar holes that are closest to the frame's base ring because this raises the frame relative to the body, thus

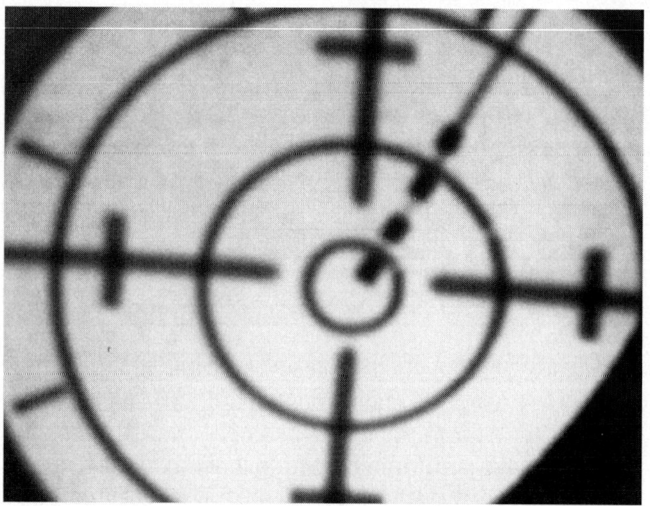

Fig. 5.1 Lateral radiograph with reticules demonstrates proper lead position. An intraoperative fluoroscopic image demonstrates that the distalmost contact of the implanted deep brain stimulation lead is positioned at the target point. The reticule system (i.e., circle and cross-hairs) ensures that pure lateral images are generated and provides a reference from which to judge the lead's position. Serial images can be obtained to control for lead shift during the fixation process. (Source: Hutchison WD, Lang AE, Dostrovsky JO, Lozano AM. Pallidal neuronal activity: implications for models of dystonia. Ann Neurol 2003;53:480–488. Reprinted with permission.)

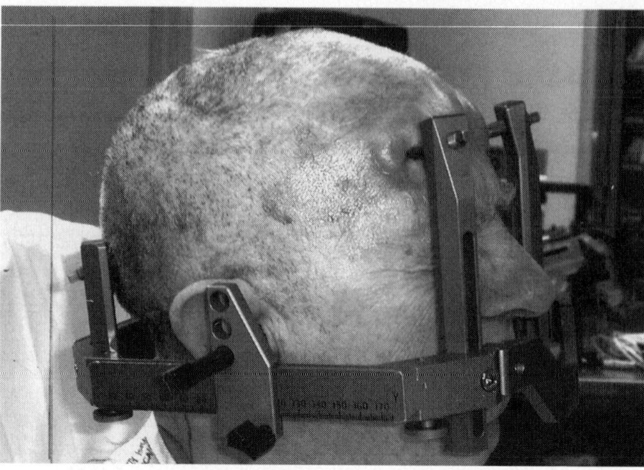

Fig. 5.2 Application of the Leksell frame. Our preferred application of the Leksell frame is demonstrated. The ear bars are employed to prevent sideward tilt (roll) or sagittal rotation (yaw) of the frame relative to the head. The lowest of the three ear bar holes are employed to elevate the frame away from the shoulders, thereby allowing enough space to accommodate the magnetic resonance imaging (MRI) table adapter. The frame is pitched so that the base ring lies roughly parallel to the zygoma, which is used as a proxy for the intercommissural plane. MRI compatible pins are selected of lengths that do not extend far beyond the margins of the vertical posts. The curved front piece is curved downward to minimize the patient's sense of entrapment.

providing enough clearance between the head and shoulders to accommodate the MRI adapter (**Fig. 5.2**).

The frame is pitched so that the base ring lies roughly parallel to the zygoma, which approximates the pitch of the intercommissural (IC) line. So aligned, axial targeting images lie coplanar to the IC plane, the standard meridian for targeting deep brain structures. The length of the fixation pins is selected so that they do not extend beyond the margins of the MRI localizing box so that the frame can fit within the tight confines of the scanner's head coil. Opposing pins should be applied simultaneously to reduce frame rotation.

Once the frame is applied, the patient is transported for imaging. Many frames come equipped with a "reapplication system," which allows the imaging studies to be performed days prior to the surgery and the frame to be reapplied on the day of the procedure. Although this approach can increase operating room efficiency, it requires precise frame reapplication if one is to achieve the desired targeting accuracy. We prefer to perform frame application, imaging, and surgery on the same day, eliminating the possibility of targeting errors due to imprecise reapplication.

Frameless Navigation

Although frameless navigation is used primarily for image-guided craniotomy and tumor biopsy, disposable

platforms, which make "frameless" (or at least miniframe) movement disorder surgery feasible, are now available. Frameless techniques may enhance patient comfort by eliminating the sometimes unpleasant application of the stereotactic head frame. Rigid fixation of the head is obviated because the miniframes are mounted directly to the patient's skull, allowing the patient some head movement during the procedure. Operating room efficiency is also enhanced because the planning images can be obtained days before the surgery without the drawbacks of frame reapplication. Surgical capacity is increased by eliminating the stereotactic head frame, which is expensive to purchase and maintain and can be used just once per day. Preliminary experience suggests that frameless targeting with these platforms can be as accurate as frame-based techniques when skull-mounted fiducial markers and CT/MRI fusion techniques are employed for target determination.[50] More experience is required, however, before we can state with certainty that these systems provide sufficient accuracy to perform functional neurosurgery safely and effectively (see Chapter 10).

Stereotactic Imaging

Three imaging modalities are available for stereotactic targeting: ventriculography, CT, and MRI.

Ventriculography

Air and positive contrast ventriculography were the mainstays of stereotactic targeting prior to the 1970s. Early stereotactic head frames were designed for this imaging modality, and the IC line was selected as the central meridian for stereotactic atlases, both because the anterior and posterior commissures lie close to the majority of therapeutic deep brain targets and because they are visualized reliably on lateral ventriculograms.[51] Though many consider ventriculography the standard for functional neurosurgical targeting, technical complexities, ventricular distortion, and anatomical variability can all result in significant targeting errors.[52] Ventriculography is invasive and can cause significant side effects, including headache, nausea, vomiting, and seizures.[52] Technical advances have enhanced the reliability of stereotactic targeting with both MRI and CT.[53-61] Consequently, these noninvasive imaging techniques, which permit direct targeting of the parenchyma, have supplanted ventriculography as the primary targeting modalities in the current era.

Computed Tomography

The main advantages of CT are its spatial fidelity and the speed with which images can be obtained. Parenchymal targets can be visualized and targeted directly; however, the resolution of many deep brain structures is inferior to that provided by MRI. An additional disadvantage of CT is that images can only be obtained in the axial plane. Although CT is inexpensive, readily available, accurate, and successfully employed by some individuals for functional procedures, we feel that in its present form, CT is best used in conjunction with MRI, utilizing image fusion techniques to take advantage of the complementary strengths of these two modalities.[54,55,58,61]

Magnetic Resonance Imaging

MRI provides high-resolution pictures of the deep brain structures in all three planes of section. Images are obtained quickly and noninvasively, and the imaging technique can be tailored to reveal specific surgical targets. The main disadvantage of MRI is the possibility of targeting inaccuracies secondary to image distortion. Additional drawbacks include the need to sedate patients who are claustrophobic or have significant head tremor and the inability to scan some patients who have previously implanted medical devices. The sources of MRI distortion have been well documented,[62,63] and several papers have been written detailing techniques for overcoming this potential problem.[54-56,58,59,61,64-67] There are two sources of MRI distortion: the scanner and the scanned subject.[62] Scanner-based distortions are caused by heterogeneities in the magnetic field, which can come in a variety of shapes. Heterogeneities tend to be greatest at the periphery of the scanning field[57,62,64] and therefore are more likely to impact the imaging of the stereotactic fiducials rather than the brain itself. This is significant because aberrations of the scanned position of the stereotactic fiducials will yield inaccurate coordinates for the intended target.

Scanner-based image distortions are best controlled via regular shimming of the magnet and calibration of the scanner.[62] Mathematical corrections for gradient field heterogeneities have been described.[65-67] Targeting phantoms may be used periodically to check the accuracy of a specific frame employed with a specific scanner. Though these measures provide valuable controls for scanner-based targeting inaccuracies, none of these interventions control for magnetic susceptibility artifact, the main source of scanned subject-based image distortion.[62,68,69]

When structures of differing magnetic susceptibilities lie adjacent to one another, the apparent border between them may be shifted on the final images.[52] Here again, the stereotactic fiducial markers come into play. The MRI localizer box, which is attached to the stereotactic frame during scanning, contains columns of a substance (typically copper sulfate solution) that is visible on MRI. These fluid columns are encased in plastic, which in turn is surrounded by air, and lie at the periphery of the scanned field. The differences in magnetic susceptibility between the copper sulfate and the surrounding air and plastic may result in small shifts in the apparent location of a fiducial. These shifts may be imperceptible to the human eye but can result in significant targeting errors. For example, Carter et al[70] reported targeting errors of greater than 4 mm when employing a gel-filled localizer that were corrected when they switched to a localizer containing copper sulfate.

Overcoming Magnetic Resonance Imaging Distortion

Several techniques have been developed to overcome the problem of MRI distortion.[54-56,58,59,64-69] Walton et al[59] employed a targeting phantom to demonstrate that targeting accuracy with the Leksell frame degrades for targets located toward the periphery of the targeting field. The stereotactic axis along which targeting is the least accurate is dependent upon the orientation of the targeting images. When using axial images, targeting along the y-axis is the least accurate; however, when using sagittal or coronal images, targeting is least accurate along the z-axis. Interestingly, they also demonstrated that targeting accuracy could be enhanced by eliminating the "third panel" of fiducials (i.e., the anterior plate for axial images or the superior plate for coronal images).[59] Overall, they found that targeting accuracy was inferior when using coronal or sagittal images, a finding that is corroborated by Piovan et al.[71]

The type of MRI employed for targeting can also influence targeting accuracy. Walton et al[59] demonstrated that three-dimensional acquisition techniques are less prone to spatial distortion than are two-dimensional techniques.

Taren et al[68] suggest that fast spin echo/inversion recovery (FSE/IR) is the MRI technique most resistant to magnetic susceptibility artifact. Based on this report and the fact that FSE/IR generates beautiful images of the deep brain structures (**Fig. 5.3**), we have adopted this technique as our sole imaging modality for stereotactic targeting (**Table 5.2**).

Computerized image fusion may also be employed to overcome MRI distortion. Independent workstations such as those sold by Medtronic, Inc. (Minneapolis, MN), BrainLAB, Inc., or Elekta Instruments (Atlanta, GA) employ mathematical paradigms to "fit" the patient's MRI to the stereotactic CT, which is obtained on the morning of surgery. Several authors have demonstrated that CT/MRI fusion techniques can enhance anatomical targeting accuracy.[54,55,58,61,64] These techniques are especially useful when performing stereotactic radiosurgery, procedures in which physiological target refinement is not an option; however, they are not yet so reliable as to eliminate the need for physiological refinement of functional neurosurgical targets and we find that the modest accuracy enhancements do not justify the cost and time of performing both scans.

Table 5.2 Scanning Parameters for Axial Fast Spin Echo Inversion Recovery Images

Excitation time (Te)	120 µsec
Relaxation time (Tr)	10,000 sec
Inversion time (Ti)	2200 sec
Bandwidth	20.83
Field of view (FOV)	24
Slice thickness	3 mm
Slice spacing	0 mm
Frequency	192 Hz
Phase	160
Number of excitations	1
Frequency direction	Anteroposterior
Autocontrol frequency	Water
Flow compensation direction	Slice direction

The scanning parameters that the authors employ for stereotactic targeting are given. Thirty axial images are generated in 6 to 9 minutes. Inverting the raw images generates images similar to those demonstrated in **Fig. 5.3**.

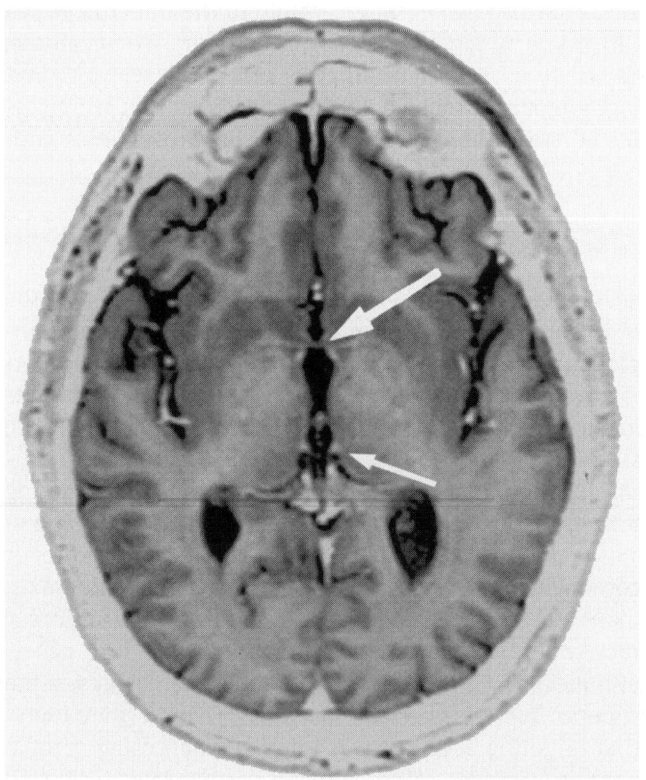

Fig. 5.3 Axial fast spin echo inversion recovery magnetic resonance imaging. The raw image was generated with the scanning parameters given in **Table 5.2**. Inverting the raw image generates the presented image. Both the anterior (*large arrow*) and posterior (*small arrow*) commissures are visualized.

Techniques for Target Selection

The choice of stereotactic imaging technique must complement the surgeon's technique for target selection. In this regard one has three options: direct, indirect, or both. Direct targeting relies on visualization of the surgical target for coordinate determination. Toward this end, coronal and axial T2-weighted images have proven most successful for imaging the STN,[72–75] whereas Spoiled GRASS MRI (SPGR,) FSE/IR, and T2- weighted images will adequately visualize the globus pallidus.[76] Most MRI pulse sequences will image the thalamus as a whole; however, none will demonstrate the subnuclei sufficiently well enough for direct targeting.

Indirect targeting methods rely on the visualization of the commissures and the known relationship of these structures to commonly described surgical targets. Although most MRI pulse sequences will readily visualize the commissures, we employ axial FSE/IR MRI for anatomical targeting for several reasons: (1) these images are acquired rapidly (6 to 9 min); (2) the deep gray matter is well visualized, permitting one to combine both direct and indirect targeting methods; (3) this one technique can be used for indirect targeting of all three primary surgical targets (Vim, GPi, and STN); and (4) FSE/IR is reported to be most resistant to magnetic susceptibility artifact,[68] minimizing the risk of targeting errors due to fiducial shift.

This technique has served the authors well through the performance of 110 pallidotomies and more than 300 DBS lead implants. Previously, Alterman et al[52] demonstrated that the introduction of axial FSE/IR images coincided with a reduction in the number of microelectrode recording tracts required to localize the sensorimotor GPi, sug-

Table 5.3 Indirect Targeting of Deep Brain Targets

	Subthalamic Nucleus (STN)	Globus Pallidus Pars	Nucleus Ventralis Intermedius (Vim)
Mediolateral coordinate	10–12 mm lateral of midline	19–22 mm lateral of midline	12–14 mm lateral of midline (lower extremity) 14–16 mm lateral of midline (upper extremity)
Anteroposterior coordinate	0–4 mm posterior to MCP	2–3 mm anterior to MCP	5–6 mm anterior to PC
Ventrodorsal coordinate	6 mm inferior to MCP	4 mm inferior to MCP	0–2 mm superior to PC
Anteroposterior angle	70 degrees above horizontal	60 degrees above horizontal	60 degrees above horizontal
Mediolateral angle	10–15 degrees lateral of vertical	0–5 degrees lateral of vertical	10–15 degrees lateral of vertical

The calculations employed by the authors to perform indirect targeting of the three primary sites for movement disorder surgery are given. The coordinates for the anterior and posterior commissures are derived directly. The coordinates for the Vim nucleus are calculated relative to the position of the posterior commissure (PC). The coordinates for the GPi and STN are calculated relative to the midcommissural point (MCP), which is derived by calculating the arithmetic mean of the respective coordinates for the commissures.

gesting more accurate image-derived coordinates. The authors recently completed an analysis of over 180 consecutive STN DBS lead implants and again found that, when employing axial FSE/IR images for initial targeting, the final target could be localized with one or two MER trajectories in more than 80% of the procedures, and this in spite of the fact that the STN is not directly visualized with FSE/IR MRI (unpublished results). Although the STN may be visualized and targeted directly on T2-weighted coronal images, stereotactic targeting may be imprecise in the coronal plane.[56,71] Zonenshayn et al[77] compared the accuracy of the coordinates derived from the direct and indirect methods to the final coordinates derived for the STN with MER. They concluded that their "composite" target, which represented a compromise of multiple techniques, yielded the most accurate starting point for STN localization. However, Figure 5.2 of their paper demonstrates that the indirect method based on axial FSE/IR images was superior to direct targeting of the STN on coronal T2-weighted images and closely approximated the overall accuracy generated by their "composite" method. Given our similar experiences and the time required to generate the T2-weighted images, we have continued to employ the indirect method solely to target for DBS implantation.

Our preferred scanning sequence is given in **Table 5.2**. The axial MRI dataset is transferred via hospital network to an independent workstation that is equipped with ste-

reotactic targeting software (@target, BrainLAB, Munich, Germany). Following fiducial registration, the stereotactic coordinates for the commissures are derived. The coordinates for the midcommissural point (MCP) are then calculated by averaging the respective coordinates of the commissures. The target coordinates are calculated relative to the MCP or the posterior commissure as shown in **Table 5.3**.

Computer-Assisted Targeting

Whether performing frame-based or frameless navigation techniques, computer assistance facilitates targeting, reduces human error, and allows one to fine tune the surgical trajectory. Frame-based targeting software is available from commercial entities, including Medtronic, Radionics (Burlington, MA), Elekta, COMPASS International (Rochester, MN), and BrainLAB. All will interface with most commercially available frames. These systems can establish the safest trajectories to the surgical target, avoiding sulci, large cortical veins, and the lateral ventricles. Many of these systems are also equipped with digitized versions of human stereotactic atlases, which can be digitally fit to the patient's anatomy. To date, there is no hard evidence that such techniques enhance targeting accuracy as compared with the techniques already described; however, they may prove helpful to some.

Editor's Comments

There are many factors that limit the accuracy of image-guided stereotaxis. First and foremost is the application accuracy of the frame-based system itself.[78] There is always an application error even with frameless systems. Most commercially available frames are sufficiently accurate for functional neurosurgical procedures. Nevertheless, they can become distorted with time and use. We identify a specific frame for functional stereotactic procedures and keep it sequestered from general stereotactic work. In addition, it should be recalibrated by the manufacturer on a 6-month or yearly basis de-

pending on the degree of use. The application of the frame itself can cause problems because rotation, yaw, or pitch in any direction may prevent imaging the IC in a single slice and may require computer algorithms or image reconstructions for accurate targeting. Even if the IC is observed on an image, accuracy cannot be assured due to yaw. It is really not the IC but the intercommercial plane that we are interested in defining.

The imaging also creates errors. MRI distortions are in the range of 1 to 5 mm. They are caused by multiple factors, including chemical shifts, magnetic field inhomogeneity, and ferromagnetic elements within the field.[62,63] Even T1 magnetization-prepared rapid gradient echo (MPRAGE) sequences that are specifically designed to minimize distortion cause errors estimated to be between 0.5 and 2 mm.[79] Regular shimming of the MRI scanner can minimize the degree of distortion, and use of frequent phantom testing[57] can determine the direction and magnitude of the errors. Despite attempts to make the frames minimally ferromagnetic, there will always be some distortion. In addition, the fiduciaries, whether they are for a frame or frameless system, will introduce some degree of distortion. Any metal in the patient such as amalgams from dental work, metal plates from reconstructive surgery, aneurysm clips, or contralateral DBS systems will all be sources for distortion. Special precautions need to be taken when a previous DBS lead or an electrical stimulator of any sort is present. These are discussed in greater detail in Chapter 14.

Selecting the appropriate sequences can help eliminate some but not all the distortion. The neuroradiologist can be of great help in optimizing the sequences. Every scanner has certain advantages and disadvantages. By optimizing your scanner's parameters, the best possible preoperative imaging can be obtained. For targeting STN, coronal T2-weighted fast spin echo (TR = 2500, TE = 110) are frequently used. For GPi, targeting is frequently on an axial inversion recovery–fast spin echo sequence (TR = 3000, TE = 40, TI = 200). Representative sequences that we have used with various scanners are illustrated in **Table 5.4**. We have had the best imaging with the Philip MR. True inversion recovery–fast spin echo sequences are not possible on the Siemens scanner.

Fusion of MRI and CT has been reported to be a way of improving the spatial integrity and distortion of the MRI scan.[54,80] However, this has not been proven and there is one report suggesting accuracy is not improved.[81] Because much of the inhomogeneities are nonlinear, a linear fusion does not solve the problems. We prefer using a combination of MR T1 three-dimensional and T2 imaging to identify the target. The T2 gives better imaging of the target such as STN,[75,82–86] and the three-planar reconstructions give minimal image degradation. The use of zero inner space (contiguous) slices is necessary to create a three-dimensional acquisition and use computer software for three-planar reconstructions, which are considered to be superior to two-dimensional MRI acquisitions. Optimally, the slice thickness will be as thin as possible to be able to target as accurately as possible. However, this sets up a problem with signal degradation, which becomes greater as the slice thickness decreases.[62,87] Because of the difficulty in seeing the target and recognizing précise boundaries, we and others frequently use a combination of imaging techniques and blend the coordinates together to give the best approximation of target.[77,83–86] Combining both direct and indirect targeting gives a far better feel for the target location and the best initial targeting coordinates. The use of an internal fiduciary such as the red nucleus may actually be a better means of identifying STN than either direct or indirect targeting techniques.[88,89]

The indirect target coordinates given in **Table 5.3** are typical of those used in most neurosurgical practices. Others will correct for the width of the third ventricle. This correction moves the target 11 mm laterally from the ventricle wall for Vim, 18 mm from the third ventricle wall for GPi, and 9 mm from the third ventricular wall for STN. Some have questioned whether the targets are different for DBS and lesioning.[90,91] Direct imaging has advantages that rapid straightforward calculations can be performed. The problem is that there are anatomical variations among individuals and any error in frame placement will produce inaccuracies. Direct targeting has the benefit

Table 5.4 Parameters Used for Preoperative Magnetic Resonance Imaging

Magnetic Resonance Protocol	Siemens Symphony	General Electric Horizon	Philips Gyroscan
T-2-weighted FSE			
TR (msec)	2500	3000	5000
TEeff (msec)	110	87	100
Matrix	252 × 256	384 × 256	256 × 512
NEX	4	4	5
Slice thickness (mm)	2.0	2.0	2.0
Interleaved imaging	0	0	0
Time (min:sec)	12:04	10:48	13:20
Volumetric gradient echo			
Type of acquisition	MPRAGE	SPGR	SPGR
TR (msec)	15	36	33
TE (msec)	7.0	8.0	11
Matrix	512 × 512	256 × 256	256 × 512
Flip angle (°)	30	35	35
NEX	1.0	0.75	2.0
Slice thickness	1.5	1.5	1.0
Imaging time (min:sec)	9:26	11:00	12:00

Abbreviations: NEX, number of excitations; MPRAGE, magnetization—prepared rapid acquisition gradient echo; SPGR, spoiled gradient recalled acquisition; TEeff, effective echo time.

of allowing observation of the target but the target boundaries are somewhat difficult to interpret, which leads to imperfect targeting. Systematic errors in the phase encoding (direction) can result in errors greater than those in indirect techniques. In the future, 3T imaging will allow better direct STN and Vim targeting.

Although on a theoretical basis direct targeting should be more accurate, in fact this has not proven to be the case, and in some ways it is less accurate.[83–89] It should always be remembered that the CT or MRI scans are partial volumes represented in two dimensions. There is a mathematical summary of the density within that volume. Therefore, boundaries will be somewhat indistinct and will be represented with a degree of uncertainty. In addition, whenever there is a chemical shift such as between cerebrospinal fluid and brain or between gray matter and white, there will be some degree of distortion. This will add to the uncertainty as to the distinct border locations. Any patient movement will further degrade the images. The images, no matter how good or how accurate, are historical. Any shifts in the frame, any shifts in the internal structures, any distortion in the probe or systematic error in the head stage will produce errors that will need to be corrected electrophysiologically. In the future, high-quality intraoperative MRI may allow for real-time direct targeting as is being done for brain tumors.

■ Conclusion

The patient is now fully prepared for surgery. If one has paid attention to detail, then the physiological confirmation/ refinement of the target and placement of the therapeutic lesion or DBS lead(s) should proceed smoothly and with few complications.

References

1. Paulson HL, Stern MB. Clinical manifestations of Parkinson's disease. In: Watts RL, Koller WC, eds. Movement Disorders: Neurologic Principles and Practice. New York: McGraw-Hill; 1997:183–199
2. Poewe W, Granata R. Pharmacological treatment of Parkinson's disease. In: Watts RL, Koller WC, eds. Movement Disorders: Neurologic Principles and Practice. New York: McGraw-Hill; 1997:201–219
3. Charles PD, Van Blercom N, Krack P, et al. Predictors of effective bilateral subthalamic nucleus stimulation for PD. Neurology 2002;59:932–934
4. Alterman RL, Kelly PJ. Contemporary pallidotomy for treatment of other parkinsonian syndromes. In: Krauss J, Grossman R, eds. Movement Disorder Surgery. Philadelphia: WB Saunders; 1998:267–272
5. Saint-Cyr JA, Trepanier LL, Kumar R, Lozano AM, Lang AE. Neuropsychological consequences of chronic bilateral stimulation of the subthalamic nucleus in Parkinson's disease. Brain 2000;123:2091–2108
6. Alterman RL, Kelly P, Sterio D, et al. Selection criteria for unilateral posteroventral pallidotomy. Acta Neurochir Suppl (Wien) 1997;68:18–23
7. Fields JA, Trôster A. Cognitive outcomes after deep brain stimulation for Parkinson's disease: a review of initial studies and recommendations for future research. Brain Cogn 2000;42:268–293
8. Krack P, Batir A, Van Blercom N, et al. Five-year follow-up of bilateral stimulation of the subthalamic nucleus in advanced Parkinson's disease. N Engl J Med 2003;349:1925–1934
9. Poewe W, Wenning G. The differential diagnosis of Parkinson's disease. Eur J Neurol 2002;9(Suppl 3):23–30
10. Litvan I, Agid Y, Calne D, et al. Clinical research criteria for the diagnosis of progressive supranuclear palsy (Steele-Richardson-Olszewski syndrome): report of the NINDS-SPSP international workshop. Neurology 1996;47:1–9
11. Jankovic J, Rajput AH, McDermott MP, Perl DP. The evolution of diagnosis in early Parkinson disease. Parkinson Study Group. Arch Neurol 2000;57:369–372
12. Litvan I, Booth V, Wenning GK, et al. Retrospective application of a set of clinical diagnostic criteria for the diagnosis of multiple system atrophy. J Neural Transm 1998;105:217–227
13. Antonini A, Kazumata K, Feigin A, et al. Differential diagnosis of parkinsonism with [18F] fluorodeoxyglucose and PET. Mov Disord 1998;13:268–274
14. Kazumata K, Antonini A, Dhawan V, et al. Preoperative indicators of clinical outcome following stereotaxic pallidotomy. Neurology 1997;49:1083–1090
15. Fukuda M, Mentis MJ, Ma Y, et al. Networks mediating the clinical effects of pallidal brain stimulation for Parkinson's disease: a PET study of resting state glucose metabolism. Brain 2001;124:1601–1608
16. Antonini A, Landi A, Benti R, et al. Functional neuroimaging (PET and SPECT) in the selection and assessment of patients with Parkinson's disease undergoing deep brain stimulation. J Neurosurg Sci 2003;47:40–46
17. Fahn S, Marsden CD, Calne DB. Classification and investigation in dystonia. In: Marsden CD, Fahn S, eds. Movement Disorders 2. London: Buttersworth; 1987:332–358
18. Jankovic J. Dystonia: medical therapy and botulinum toxin. Adv Neurol 2004;94:275–286
19. Bentivoglio AR, Albanese A. Botulinum toxin in motor disorders. Curr Opin Neurol 1999;12:47–56
20. Krauss JK. Deep brain stimulation for dystonia in adults: overview and developments. Stereotact Funct Neurosurg 2002;78:168–182
21. Cif L, Fertit H, Vayssier N, et al. Treatment of dystonic syndromes by chronic electrical stimulation of the internal globus pallidus. J Neurosurg Sci 2003;47:52–55
22. Ford B. Pallidotomy in generalized dystonia. Adv Neurol 2004;94:287–299
23. Lozano AM, Abosch A. Pallidal stimulation for dystonia. Adv Neurol 2004;94:301–308
24. Krauss JK, Yianni J, Loher TJ, Aziz TZ. Deep brain stimulation for dystonia. J Clin Neurophysiol 2004;21:18–30

25. Koller WC, Busenbark KL. Essential tremor. In: Watts RL, Koller WC, eds. Movement Disorders: Neurologic Principles and Practice. New York: McGraw-Hill; 1997:365–385

26. Bain P, Brin M, Deuschl G, et al. Criteria for the diagnosis of essential tremor. Neurology 2000;54(Suppl 4):S7

27. Lou JS, Jankovic J. Essential tremor: clinical correlates in 350 patients. Neurology 1991;41:234–238

28. Koller W, Biary N, Cone S. Disability in essential tremor: effect of treatment. Neurology 1986;36:1001–1004

29. Deuschl G, Bain P. Deep brain stimulation for tremor: patient selection and evaluation. Mov Disord 2002;17(Suppl 3):S102–S111

30. Koller WC, Lyons KE, Wilkinson SB, Troster AI, Pahwa R. Long-term safety and efficacy of unilateral deep brain stimulation of the thalamus in essential tremor. Mov Disord 2001;16:464–468

31. Kumar R, Lozano AM, Sime E, Lang AE. Long-term follow-up of thalamic deep brain stimulation for essential and parkinsonian tremor. Neurology 2003;61:1601–1604

32. Sydow O, Thobois S, Alesch F, Speelman JD. Mulitcentre European study of thalamic stimulation in essential tremor: a six year follow-up. J Neurol Neurosurg Psychiatry 2003;74:1387–1391

33. Senatus PB, McClelland S III, Ferris AD, et al. Implantation of bilateral deep brain stimulators in patients with Parkinson disease and preexisting cardiac pacemakers: report of two cases. J Neurosurg 2004;101:1073–1077

34. Capelle HH, Simpson RK Jr, Kronenbuerger M, Michaelsen J, Tronnier V, Krauss JK. Long-term deep brain stimulation in elderly patients with cardiac pacemakers. J Neurosurg 2005;102: 53–59

35. Chou KL, Forman MS, Trojanowski JQ, Hurtig HI, Baltuch GH. Subthalamic nucleus deep brain stimulation in a patient with levodopa-responsive multiple system atrophy: case report. J Neurosurg 2004;100:553–556

36. Lezcano E, Gomez-Esterban JC, Zarranz JJ, et al. Parkinson's disease-like presentation of multiple system atrophy with poor response to STN stimulation: a clinicopathological case report. Mov Disord 2004;19:973–977

37. Tarsy D, Apetauerova D, Ryan P, Norregaard T. Adverse effects of subthalamic nucleus DBS in a patient with multiple system atrophy. Neurology 2003;61:247–249

38. Merello M. Subthalamic stimulation contralateral to a previous pallidotomy. Mov Disord 1999;14:890

39. Goto S, Yamada K, Ushio Y. Subthalamic nucleus stimulation in a parkinsonian patient with previous bilateral thalamotomy. J Neurol Neurosurg Psychiatry 2004;75:164–165

40. Kleiner-Fisman G, Fisman DN, Zamir O, et al. Subthalamic nucleus deep brain stimulation for Parkinson's disease after successful pallidotomy: clinical and electrophysiological observations. Mov Disord 2004;19:1209–1214

41. Mogilner AY, Sterio D, Razai AR, Zonenshayn M, Kelly PJ, Beric A. Subthalamic nucleus stimulation in patients with a prior pallidotomy. J Neurosurg 2002;96:660–665

42. Russmann H, Ghika J, Villemure JG, et al. Subthalamic nucleus deep brain stimulation in Parkinson disease patients over age 70 years. Neurology 2004;63:1952–1954

43. Welter ML, Houeto JL, Tezenas du Montcel S, et al. Clinical predictive factors of subthalamic in Parkinson's disease. Brain 2002;125:575–583

44. Jaggi JL, Umemura A, Hurtig HI, et al. Bilateral stimulation of the subthalamic nucleus in Parkinson's disease: surgical efficacy and prediction of outcome. Stereotact Funct Neurosurg 2004;82: 104–114

45. Okun MS, Vitek JL. Lesion therapy for Parkinson's disease and other movement disorders: update and controversies. Mov Disord 2004;19:375–389

46. Chang LK, Whitaker DC. The impact of herbal medicines on dermatologic surgery. Dermatol Surg 2001;27:759–763

47. Keyser DL, Rodnitzky RL. Neuroleptic malignant syndrome in Parkinson's disease after withdrawal or alteration of dopaminergic therapy. Arch Intern Med 1991;151:794–796

48. Schulder M, ed. Handbook of Stereotactic and Functional Neurosurgery. New York: Marcel Dekker; 2003

49. Gildenberg PL, Tasker RR, eds. Textbook of Stereotactic and Functional Neurosurgery. New York: McGraw-Hill; 1998

50. Henderson JM, Holloway KL, Gaede SE, Rosanow JM, Csavoy A. Frameless placement of deep brain stimulation electrodes: an accuracy study. Mov Disord 2004;19(Suppl 9):S302

51. Talairach J. Proceedings VI Congreso Latin-Americano de Neurocirugia, Montevideo; 1955:865–925

52. Alterman RL, Kelly PJ. Magnetic resonance image guidance for Parkinson's disease surgery. In: Germano I, ed. Surgery for Movement Disorders. Park Ridge, IL: American Association for Neurological Surgeons; 1998:195–205

53. Kondziolka D, Dempsey PK, Lunsford LD, et al. A comparison between magnetic resonance imaging and computed tomography for stereotactic coordinate determination. Neurosurgery 1992;30:402–406

54. Alexander E III, Kooy HM, van Herk M, et al. Magnetic resonance image–directed stereotactic neurosurgery: use of image fusion with computerized tomography to enhance spatial accuracy. J Neurosurg 1995;83:271–276

55. Cohen DS, Lustgarten JH, Miller E, Khandji AG, Goodman RR. Effects of coregistration of MR to CT images on MR stereotactic accuracy. J Neurosurg 1995;82:772–779

56. Walton L, Hampshire A, Forster DM, Kemeny AA. Stereotactic localization using magnetic resonance imaging. Stereotact Funct Neurosurg 1995;64(Suppl 1):155–163

57. Walton L, Hampshire A, Forster DM, Kemeny AA. A phantom study to assess the accuracy of stereotactic localization using T1-weighted magnetic resonance imaging with the Leksell stereotactic system. Neurosurgery 1996;38:170–176

58. Maurer CR Jr, Aboutanos GB, Dawant BM, et al. Effect of geometric distortion correction in MR on image registration accuracy. J Comput Assist Tomogr 1996;20:666–679

59. Walton L, Hampshire A, Forster DM, Kemeny AA. Stereotactic localization with magnetic resonance imaging: a phantom study to compare the accuracy obtained with two-dimensional and three-dimensional data acquisitions. Neurosurgery 1997;41:131–137

60. Schuurman PR, de Bie RM, Majoie CB, Speelman JD, Bosch DA. A prospective comparison between three-dimensional magnetic resonance imaging and ventriculography for target-coordinate determination in frame-based functional stereotactic neurosurgery. J Neurosurg 1999;91:911–914

61. Yu C, Apuzzo ML, Zee CS, Petrovich Z. A phantom study of the geometric accuracy of computed tomographic and magnetic resonance imaging stereotactic localization with the Leksell stereotactic system. Neurosurgery 2001;48:1092–1098

62. Sumanaweera TS, Adler JR Jr, Napel S, Glover GH. Characterization of spatial distortion in magnetic resonance imaging and its implications for stereotactic surgery. Neurosurgery 1994;35:696–703

63. Burchiel KJ, Nguyen TT, Coombs BD, Szumoski J. MRI distortion and stereotactic neurosurgery using the Cosman-Roberts-Wells and Leksell frames. Stereotact Funct Neurosurg 1996;66:123–136

64. Yu C, Petrovich Z, Apuzzo ML, Luxton G. An image fusion study of the geometric accuracy of magnetic resonance imaging with the Leksell frame. J Appl Clin Med Phys 2001;2:42–50

65. Schad L, Lott S, Schmitt F, Sturm V, Lorenz WJ. Correction of spatial distortion in MR imaging: a prerequisite for accurate stereotaxy. J Comput Assist Tomogr 1987;11:499–505

66. Sumanaweera TS, Glover GH, Hemler PF, et al. MR geometric distortion correction for improved frame-based stereotaxic target localization accuracy. Magn Reson Med 1995;34:106–113

67. Langlois S, Desvignes M, Constans JM, Revenu M. MRI geometric distortion: a simple approach to correcting the effects of non-linear gradient fields. J Magn Reson Imaging 1999;9:821–831

68. Taren JA, Ross DA, Gebarski SS. Stereotactic localization using fast spin-echo imaging in functional disorders. Acta Neurochir (Wien) 1993;58:59–60

69. Dean D, Kamath J, Duerk JL, Ganz E. Validation of object-induced MR distortion correction for frameless stereotactic neurosurgery. IEEE Trans Med Imaging 1998;17:810–816

70. Carter DA, Parsai EI, Ayyangar KM. Accuracy of magnetic resonance imaging stereotactic coordinates with the Cosman-Roberts-Wells frame. Stereotact Funct Neurosurg 1999;72:35–46

71. Piovan E, Zampieri PG, Alessandrini F, et al. Quality assessment of magnetic resonance stereotactic localization for Gamma Knife radiosurgery. Stereotact Funct Neurosurg 1995;64(Suppl 1):228–232

72. Pollo C, Meuli R, Maeder P, Vingerhoets F, Ghika J, Villemure JG. Subthalamic nucleus deep brain stimulation for Parkinson's disease: magnetic resonance imaging targeting using visible anatomical landmarks. Stereotact Funct Neurosurg 2003;80:76–81

73. Hariz MI, Krack P, Melvill R, et al. A quick and universal method for stereotactic visualization of the subthalamic nucleus before and after implantation of deep brain stimulation electrodes. Stereotact Funct Neurosurg 2003;80:96–101

74. Landi A, Grimaldi M, Antonini A, Parolin M, Zincone A. MRI Indirect stereotactic targeting for deep brain stimulation for Parkinson's disease. J Neurosurg Sci 2003;47:26–32

75. Bejjani BP, Dormont D, Pidoux B, et al. Bilateral subthalamic stimulation for Parkinson's disease by using three-dimensional stereotactic magnetic resonance imaging and electrophysiological guidance. J Neurosurg 2000;92:615–625

76. Starr PA. Placement of deep brain stimulators into the subthalamic nucleus or globus pallidus internus: technical approach. Stereotact Funct Neurosurg 2002;79:118–145

77. Zonenshayn M, Rezai AR, Mogilner AY, Beric A, Sterio D, Kelly PJ. Comparison of anatomic and neurophysiological methods for subthalamic nucleus targeting. neurosurgery 2000;47:282–292

78. Maciunas RJ, Galloway RL, Latimer JW. The application accuracy of stereotactic frames. Neurosurgery 1994;35:682–695

79. diPierro CG, Francel PC, Jackson TR, et al. Optimizing accuracy in magnetic resonance imaging-guided stereotaxis: a technique with validation based on the anterior commissure-posterior commissure line. J Neurosurg 1999;90:94–100

80. Scott R, Gregory R, Hines N, et al. Neuropsychological, neurological, functional outcome following pallidotomy for Parkinson's disease: a consecutive series of eight simultaneous and twelve unilateral procedures. Brain 1998;121:659–675

81. Carlson JD, Iacono RP. Electrophysiological versus image-based targeting in the posteroventral pallidotomy. Comput Aided Surg 1999;4:93–100

82. Starr PA, Vitek JL, DeLong M, et al. Magnetic resonance imaging-based stereotactic localization of the globus pallidus and subthalamic nucleus. Neurosurgery 1999;44:303–313 (discussion 313–314)

83. Slavin KV, Anderson GJ, Burchiel KJ. Comparison of three techniques for calculation of target coordinates in functional stereotactic procedures. Stereotact Funct Neurosurg 1999;72:192–195

84. Benabid AL, Benazzouz A, Gao D, et al. Chronic electrical stimulation of the ventralis intermedius nucleus of the thalamus and of other nuclei as a treatment for Parkinson's disease. Tech Neurosurg 1999;5:5–30

85. Voges J, Volkmann J, Allert N, et al. Bilateral high-frequency stimulation in the subthalamic nucleus for the treatment of Parkinson disease: correlation of therapeutic effect with anatomical electrode position. J Neurosurg 2002;96:269–279

86. Starr PA, Christine CW, Theodopoulos PV, et al. Implantation of deep brain stimulators into the subthalamic nucleus: technical approach and magnetic resonance imaging - verified lead locations. J Neurosurg 2002;97:370–387

87. Vlaaringerbroek M, dem Boer J. Magnetic resonance imaging. Berlin: Springer-Verlag; 1996:107–113

88. Andrade-Souza YM, Schwalb JM, Hamani C, et al. Comparison of three methods of targeting the subthalamic nucleus for chronic stimulation in Parkinson's disease. Neurosurgery 2005;56(2, Suppl):360–368

89. Andrade-Souza YM, Schwalb JM, Hamani C, Hoque T, Saint-Cyr J, Lozano AM. Comparison of 2-dimensional magnetic resonance imaging and 3-planar reconstruction methods for targeting the subthalamic nucleus in Parkinson's disease. Surg Neurol 2005;63:357–362 (discussion 362–363)

90. Bejjani B, Damier P, Arnulf I, et al. Pallidal stimulation for Parkinson's disease: two targets? Neurology 1997;49:1564–1569

91. Kiss ZH, Wilkinson M, Krcek J, et al. Is the target for thalamic deep brain stimulation the same as for thalamotomy? Mov Disord 2003;18:1169–1175

6 Anesthesia for Movement Disorder Surgery

Robert E. Gross, Klaus Mewes, and Ghaleb Ghani

Surgical treatment of Parkinson disease (PD) and other movement disorders has been performed with local anesthesia since shortly after the advent of stereotactic functional neurosurgery.[1] Electrophysiological mapping, testing the effects of a radio frequency (RF) lesion, and electrical stimulation testing, both prior to an RF lesion and as part of implantation of a deep brain stimulator (DBS) lead, are all facilitated by having an awake and responsive patient. However, increasing experience and technology and expanding indications are driving a small but increasing number of centers to perform surgery under general anesthesia. The important role of the anesthetist in intraoperative monitoring of local anesthetic procedures is thus expanding to more difficult monitoring of the anesthetized patient, often in more difficult settings such as the intraoperative magnetic resonance imaging (MRI) or the radiology suite.

This chapter reviews anesthetic procedures for surgery on a difficult, often elderly but occasionally pediatric, patient population, before, during, and after the operating room. We also address the use of electrophysiological mapping techniques under general anesthesia. Specific considerations relating to the most common indications for functional stereotactic movement disorder surgery—PD, essential tremor (ET), and dystonia—are highlighted.

■ Preoperative Evaluation

There are unique challenges in treating patients undergoing movement disorder surgery. PD and ET patients are often elderly, which can predispose them to cardiac, respiratory, and other age-related complications. In addition, these patients are usually on several medications related to their movement disorder and other health issues, and such polypharmacy may lead to important drug interactions affecting surgery.[2] Older patients may also have differences in pharmacodynamics and pharmacokinetics affecting many drugs, including those used for anesthesia and sedation (e.g., benzodiazepines).[2,3] It is therefore extremely important that each patient undergo a careful preoperative screening to identify potential risk factors for surgery and drug interactions (**Table 6.1**).

Parkinson Disease

Cardiovascular risks are common in this patient population. Hypertension must be well treated prior to surgery because of the risk of hemorrhage.[4,5] There should be a low threshold to obtain a thallium stress test prior to surgery because ischemic disease may go unnoticed in PD patients who are limited in their mobility. PD patients also commonly suffer from orthostatic hypotension, contributed to by use of L-dopa and dopamine agonists, as well as other autonomic disturbances.[2,3,6] In addition, they can be hypovolemic, malnourished, and debilitated. Respiratory dysfunction is well known in PD.[2] This includes an obstructive ventilatory pattern, dysfunction of upper airway musculature, rigidity, bradykinesia, and dystonia of respiratory muscles.[7] Disturbances of posture and muscle tone can cause atelectasis, restrictive lung disease, and loss in lung volume. These problems are only exacerbated by withdrawal from antiparkinsonian medications. PD patients with significant respiratory issues are predisposed to aspiration in the postoperative period. Cognitive issues affect many PD patients; although frank dementia excludes patients from surgery, nondemented patients may have decreased mental stamina or excessive anxiety that may be indications to perform surgery under general anesthesia.[8]

Essential Tremor

Patients with ET are generally in better physical health than those with PD. However, lifestyle issues related to the disability may lead to poor health. General issues related to older age pertain to this group (we have operated on several patients > 75 years of age with ET), including decline in cognitive function. Possible medication interactions should be noted: most patients will be on a β-adrenergic antagonist such as propanolol, and possibly mysoline, predisposing them to hypotension and bradycardia during surgery.

Dystonia

In general, dystonic patients are younger than most PD and ET patients, and many patients with idiopathic torsion dystonia will be pediatric.[9,10] Severe dystonia can lead to extreme weight loss, malnutrition, and debilitation, with attendant anesthetic risks. Cervicoaxial involvement may

Table 6.1 Preoperative Concomitant Conditions in Patients Undergoing Movement Disorder Surgery

	Parkinson Disease	Dystonia	Essential Tremor
Cardiovascular	Hypertension		Hypertension
	Orthostatic hypotension		
	Coronary artery disease (unrecognized)		Coronary artery disease (unrecognized)
	Cardiac arrythmias		Cardiac arrythmias (medication-related)
	Hypovolemia	Hypovolemia	
	Autonomic dysfunction		
Respiratory	Laryngeal dysfunction	Laryngeal dystonia	
	Restrictive lung disease from rigidity, bradykinesia, dystonia	Aspiration pneumonia	
	Atelectasis		
	Aspiration pneumonia		
Head and neck	Pharyngeal dysfunction	Spasmodic dysphonia	Head tremor
	Dysphagia	Dysphagia	Voice tremor
Gastrointestinal	Poor nutrition	Poor nutrition	
	Weight loss	Weight loss	
	Constipation	Parenteral feeding tube	
Central nervous system (aside from primary disease symptoms)	Depression	Myelopathy	Depression
	Confusion		
	Hallucinations		
Speech impairment			
Medications	Phenothiazines (worsened EPS; malignant syndrome)	Anticholinergics Benzodiazepines	Beta-blockers (bradycardia)
	Droperidol and butyrophenone derivatives (worsened EPS; malignant syndrome)	Baclofen	
	Metoclopramide (worsened EPS; malignant syndrome)		
	Perchlorperazine (worsened EPS; malignant syndrome)		
	MAO inhibitors type A ("cheese effect")		
	Selegiline and meperidine (hyperthermia, etc.)		
	Levodopa and halothane (cardiac arrhythmia)		
	Opioids, including remifentanil (rigidity)		
	Alfentanil (dystonia)		
	Propofol (dystonia; antiparkinsonian effect)		

Source: Mason LJ, Cojocaru TT, Cole DJ. Surgical intervention and anesthetic management of the patient with Parkinson's disease. Int Anesthesiol Clin 1996;34:133–150.
Abbreviations: EPS, extrapyramidal symptoms; MAO, monoamine oxidase inhibitors.

cause respiratory difficulties and, with longstanding disease, spondylosis, kyphoscoliosis, and myelopathy. Careful attention must be directed at determining whether the severity of the dystonia, especially in the cervical and thoracic regions, makes the patient a poor risk for undergoing surgery under local anesthesia. It is not uncommon to operate on these patients under conscious sedation or general anesthesia (see later discussion).

Medication Interactions

Parkinson Disease

It is well known that drugs with dopamine antagonist actions can exacerbate PD and even precipitate "malignant syndrome."[11] These drugs include phenothiazines, butyrophenone derivatives (e.g., droperidol), and other gastrointestinal drugs, including metoclopramide (Reglan, Baxter Healthcare Corp., Deerfield, IL) and prochlorperazine (Compazine, GlaxoSmithKline, Middlesex, England). Monoamine oxidase inhibitors (MAOIs) have multiple potential drug interactions. The commonly used type B MAOIs (e.g., selegiline), do not precipitate tyramine crisis (the "cheese effect") like type A MAOIs, but rigidity, hyperpyrexia, sweating, and agitation have been reported following meperidine in patients on selegiline; this combination should therefore be avoided.[12] Meperidine (Demerol [Sanofi–Aventis, Bridgewater, NJ]) and other opiates may worsen rigidity in both healthy and PD patients. Alfentanil has been reported to cause an acute dystonic reaction in an undertreated PD patient.[2] This problem has not been encountered with the use of remifentanil,[13] although at high doses it can cause rigidity in any patient.[14] PD patients are particularly sensitive to central nervous system (CNS) depressants; thus hypnotics and narcotics should be used judiciously.[15]

Anesthetics can interact with parkinsonian medications. Halothane can lead to dysrhythmias in patients on L-dopa by sensitizing the heart to catecholamines.[3] Propofol is generally well tolerated during surgery[8,16] but can be unpredictable in PD.[17] It can be antiparkinsonian or prodyskinetic or both, which may interfere with surgical treatment if clinical response to stimulation or an RF lesion is to be evaluated in the responsive patient.[18,19]

Essential Tremor

The main drug interaction to be concerned with in patients with ET is related to their use of propanolol, which is a central β-blocker, and care should be taken with the use of other antihypertensives.

Dystonia

Propofol (Diprivan, B. Braun Melsungen AG, Melsungen, Germany) has been reported to precipitate either or both dystonic and myoclonic reactions in healthy patients emerging

from anesthesia.[19,20] Although isolated patients with dystonia have experienced exacerbation of symptoms with propofol,[21] we and others have used propofol in dystonic patients with minimal adverse effects (see **Table 6.2**). Medication interactions should be scrutinized because many patients are on anticholinergics and benzodiazepines, and possibly dopamine antagonists or baclofen. Anticholinergic drugs can predispose to urinary retention, mouth dryness, constipation, and tachycardia. Centrally acting anticholinergics used in anesthetic practice can have additive effects.[2]

■ Peri- and Intraoperative Anesthetic Approaches

Choosing the Anesthetic Approach

Most centers use extensive intraoperative electrophysiological mapping and/or clinical testing of benefits and adverse reactions to electrical stimulation when implanting a DBS or creating an RF lesion. These approaches require an awake, responsive, and reliable patient, most critically at the time of stimulation testing or RF lesion production. For this reason the majority of procedures are done with local anesthetic only, or with some degree of conscious sedation with a rapidly reversible agent such as remifentanil (often with midazolam)[13,16] or low infusion of intravenous propofol because of its rapid onset and emergence.[8,22] However, patients may not tolerate a lengthy awake surgical procedure in the setting of (1) advanced age, (2) mild dementia, (3) pain, (4) adverse health conditions or respiratory difficulties related to the "off medication" state,[8] (5) severe torsion dystonia or choreoathetosis with resultant risk of pulling out of the frame,[9,10,22] or (6) pediatric age.[9,10,22,23] Such patients are operated on under deep sedation, possibly with reversal of the sedation for intraoperative testing at intervals,[23,24] or under general anesthesia throughout (**Table 6.2**). The latter has been facilitated by the advent of DBS, where the position of the lead can be checked prior to removal of the stereotactic frame, and in the worst case, the lead can be repositioned. In contrast, surgeons are less comfortable creating a permanent lesion without having a responsive patient to test during the process.

Stereotactic Frame Placement

Irrespective of the type of anesthesia the patient is to undergo, a careful evaluation of the airway according to the American Society of Anesthesiology (ASA) Guidelines[25] is important to predict the ease of mask ventilation and endotracheal intubation. If general anesthesia is planned, or if the patient has a high-risk airway that may create a higher risk for respiratory compromise intraoperatively (e.g., history of sleep apnea) then a frame with an intubation ring should be used to allow greater airway access, and the frame is positioned with the anesthesia mask in place to ensure the ability to ventilate the patient with the mask before securing the airway.

In most cases, local anesthesia with mild sedation suffices for placement of the stereotactic frame. We routinely use a cocktail of 1% lidocaine, 0.5% bupivacaine, and 1:10 bicarbonate (to decrease the discomfort of the injection in part related to its acidity), infiltrated directly into the pin sites; however, a ring block approach can also be employed. Midazolam and fentanyl are administered prior to local injections. This approach is well tolerated by the vast majority of patients. It is important to anticipate the need for sedation during the imaging or the procedure itself, with possible airway issues, and apply the frame with this in mind. If general anesthesia is to be induced, it can be done either prior to frame placement or in the operating room after imaging. The former helps to achieve a motionless magnetic resonance imaging (MRI) scan.

There is increasing use of frameless DBS placement, which actually involves use of a miniframe and fiducials that, rather than being attached to the frame, are implanted into the patient's skull up to 1 week prior to the actual surgery.[26] The fiducials are implanted with local anesthetic with or without light sedation. If the scan is to be obtained with deeper sedation, the patient may be intubated or have a laryngeal mask (LMA) inserted, which is certainly easier in the absence of the stereotactic frame.

Magnetic Resonance Imaging and Computed Tomographic Scanning

A high-quality MRI scan can be obtained in the vast majority of cases with minimal sedation. PD patients, when scanned on the morning of surgery, are scanned in the off medication state, which eliminates dyskinesia. Because tremor from any etiology disappears with sleep, a small dose of midazolam is usually all that is required, and only very rarely have we needed to use deeper sedation to counter tremor. However, patients with more extreme hyperkinetic movement disorders (e.g., severe generalized dystonia, cervical dystonia, choreoathetosis) or with excessive anxiety will often require deeper sedation with propofol or remifentanil, and intubation or insertion of a laryngeal mask. Although a high-quality MRI scan is always important, it is critical when the procedure is performed with only anatomical control and no electrophysiological mapping or intraoperative stimulation testing.[27–29] Centers that perform surgery in this way generally obtain the MRI scan with the patient under general anesthesia to eliminate any movement artifact and obtain the highest-quality scan.

When imaging the patient under general anesthesia, we prefer to use an LMA rather than endotracheal intubation. The patient does not require muscle relaxants and can be

allowed to ventilate spontaneously in the scanner with monitoring. This avoids the need to bring the ventilator into the MRI chamber.

Surgery under Local Anesthesia

Monitoring

Standard electrocardiography (ECG), pulse oximetry, and blood pressure monitoring are instituted. The pulse oximeter, blood pressure cuff, and intravenous (IV) line, if possible, should be on the side contralateral to the side that is to be tested during the surgery. Rest tremor can interfere with pulse oximetry and give the appearance of fibrillations on ECG. Systolic blood pressure is kept below 150 mm Hg with hydralazine or labetolol, although the latter is contraindicated in the setting of bradycardia, especially in ET patients taking propanolol. We do not typically use arterial monitoring of blood pressure. Oxygen is given via nasal cannula in all patients under local, with or without conscious sedation. We routinely monitor end-tidal CO_2 concentration in all patients because there is a risk of air embolism during the opening (see later discussion). The patient is offered the option of having a catheter inserted in the bladder; some men find it difficult to use a urinal in the supine position. Fluids are monitored and it is important to keep the patient well hydrated throughout the procedure, especially given hypovolemia and hypotension issues with these patients.

Positioning and Draping

The head and neck should be positioned with some degree of flexion at the lower cervical spine and extension at the atlanto-occipital junction. This allows the patient's airway to remain patent and makes it possible for the anesthesiologist to instrument the airway should it become necessary (e.g., in case of airway obstruction, seizures with airway compromise, or neurological deterioration).

PD patients can have moderate to severe kyphosis and, in the extreme, camptocormia,[30] making positioning a challenge. Depending on the stereotactic frame, bars can protrude into the patient's shoulders and need to be carefully padded; this issue needs to be considered during the initial frame application. Severe kyphoscoliosis in PD and dystonia patients can lead to spondylotic decrease in spinal canal diameter and increasing the risk for spinal cord compression, so positioning of the neck in the operating room (OR) must be performed with extreme care.

Extra padding is utilized on our OR table because of the lengthiness of the procedure in an awake patient. We use a mechanical OR bed to avoid interference with the electrophysiological mapping, although given current shielding of the equipment this may not be necessary. In contrast to some, we use only sequential compression stockings in patients under general anesthesia.

Table 6.2 Implantation of Deep Brain Stimulators for Movement Disorders under General Anesthesia

Authors	Anesthesia Type, Indication	N	Anesthesia	Surgical Technique	Findings	Outcome
Parkinson Disease						
Maltete et al[14]	General Severe anxiety, painful dystonia, respiratory difficulties in "off" state, loss of consciousness	15	Propofol 0.8–2 µg/mL concentration in plasma; sedation scale 3–4	Microelectrode mapping of STN; no stimulation mapping	Characteristic STN microrecording; implanted central track 29 of 30 sides	64% decrease in UPDRS motor off score*; stimulation intensity significantly greater for right side not left
	Local	15	Local ± conscious sedation	Microelectrode mapping of STN and stimulation mapping	Implanted central track 25 of 30 sides based on stimulation testing	73% decrease in UPDRS motor off score
	Age- and stage-matched control group		Patel et al[39]	General	19	General NOS
Anatomical targeting of STN without microelectrode or stimulation mapping; confirmation of targeting by stereotactic postop MRI	Repositioned in 1/19 patients; 91.5% within 1 mm medial/lateral and 100% within 1 mm anterior/posterior of intended target	Not provided	Dystonia	Krause et al[16]	General	8
General NOS	Microelectrode mapping of GPi; visual-evoked potential for optic tract; high-frequency, high-intensity stimulation for internal capsule; stereotactic postop MRI	Slower GPi firing rates with long pauses	35.1–55.6% improvement in BFMDRS motor scores	Local	9	Local ± conscious sedation
Microelectrode mapping of GPi and stimulation mapping of optic tract (phosphenes) and internal capsule for paresthesia and dystonia	GPi firing rates and pattern similar to Parkinson patients under local anesthesia	Coubes et al[15,37]	General Young age, poor health, severe dystonia	31	Standard general anesthesia	Anatomical targeting of GPi with no microelectrode mapping or stimulation; immediate stereotactic postop MRI
Postop MRI showed accuracy of DBS position < 1.015 mm^2; surgical treatment time: 1.5 h/electrode	65–79% improvement in BFMDRS		Young age, poor health, severe dystonia			
		Yianni et al[52]	General	25	General NOS	Impedance monitoring with radiofrequency electrode
	45.8% improvement in total BFMDRS	Hutchison et al[30,31]	General	3	Propofol	Microelectrode mapping of GPi and stimulation

GPi firing rate 31 Hz with long pauses; decreased incidence of responses to limb driving	Not provided	Local	7	Local ± conscious sedation with low-dose propofol	Microelectrode mapping of GPi and stimulation	GPi firing rate 77 Hz (~74 Hz found in Parkinson patients) without long pauses; suppression of GPi firing with low-dose propofol in one patient
Keegan et al[41]	General	1	Isofluorane in 50% N$_2$O and O$_2$; 0.4 to 0.7% during mapping	Microelectrode mapping of thalamus; no stimulation mapping	No evidence that anesthesia hindered microelectrode and evoked activity in thalamus	Dystonia improved (Hallevorden-Spatz disease) 2 years postop
Airway obstruction due to excitement	Ghika et al[32]	General	1	General propofol anesthesia	Microelectrode mapping of ventral oral nucleus of thalamus	Could record seemingly normal activity despite burst suppression on EEG
50% decrease in unified dystonia rating scale	Severity	Tremor	Plaha et al[38]	General	4	General anesthesia
Anatomical targeting of subthalamic region (zona incerta) without microelectrode or stimulation mapping; confirmation of targeting by stereotactic postop MRI		80.1% improvement in Fahn-Tolosa-Marin Tremor Rating Scale				

* Statistically significant.

Abbreviations: BFMDRS, Burke-Fahn-Marsden Dystonia Rating Scale; DBS, deep brain stimulator; EEG, electroencephalography; GPi, globus pallidus internus; NOS, not otherwise specified; STN, subthalamic nucleus; MRI, magnetic resonance imaging; UPDRS, Unified Parkinson's Disease Rating Scale.

The drapes are arranged in such a fashion as to allow the anesthesiologist to maintain verbal and eye contact with the patient throughout the case. This is especially important in some PD patients with severe hypophonia and in dystonia patients with spasmodic dysphonia, who have great difficulty in communicating during the procedure under local anesthesia.

The Opening

The skin opening, burr holes, and dural opening can all be done with local anesthesia alone. However, the anxiety and subjective experiences during the burr hole procedure prompt many centers to perform this stage with conscious sedation (low-dose propofol or remifentanil[13]). Short-acting agents are recommended to minimize carryover into the mapping phase. We tend to avoid propofol for conscious sedation in patients with PD because of its antiparkinsonian effect.[18] Although propofol has been found to temporarily induce dystonia in healthy patients as discussed earlier, we do not avoid its use in patients with dystonia who require conscious sedation.

Electrophysiological Mapping and Stimulation Mapping

Electrophysiological mapping and electrical stimulation are best performed with an alert and responsive patient; most centers therefore perform this stage of the procedure under local anesthesia with minimal sedation, letting short-acting agents, if used previously, wear off after the burr holes are made. However, surgery can be performed with conscious sedation with little impact on electrophysiological mapping results and electrical stimulation testing.[8,22,31,32] An important question, however, is how deep can sedation be without interfering with the mapping and stimulation phase of the surgery. Until recently, there was insufficient clinical experience with these situations to even examine these questions.

Surgery under Deep Sedation or General Anesthesia

The goal of microelectrode mapping is to precisely identify the target structure and its borders. For the globus pallidus internus (GPi) and subthalamic nucleus (STN), the sensorimotor region is characterized. For the ventral intermediate (Vim) nucleus in tremor cases, the passive movement-activated cells in Vim and cells with cutaneous sensory receptive fields in the ventral caudal (Vc) thalamic nucleus must be identified. Thus, to accomplish adequate microelectrode mapping, identifiable units must be found, distinctions between adjacent nuclei must be made (e.g., internal and external segments of GP), and movement-related changes in firing rates should be observed. Recent reports demonstrate that these goals can be met, at least in part, with various degrees of anesthesia (**Table 6.2**).

Intubation with the Stereotactic Frame in Place and Airway Control

Anesthesia can be induced prior to the placement of the frame. However, if general anesthesia is to be induced with the stereotactic frame in place, then conventional rigid laryngoscopy will not be easy. Our technique of choice is asleep fiberoptic endotracheal intubation, using the apneic technique through an intubating airway or through an LMA utilizing the Aintree Intubation Catheter (Cook Critical Care, Bloomington, IN). Another option is using an LMA for the entire procedure; the Flexible LMA is our first choice. If one is concerned about gastric distention, especially with controlled ventilation, the ProSeal LMA (LMA North America, San Diego, CA) can be used. When the LMA is used, we prefer to have the patient breathe spontaneously or with assisted ventilation, although some do not hesitate to give the patient some muscle relaxants and control the patient's ventilation.

Microelectrode Mapping under Deep Sedation or General Anesthesia

The effects of anesthetic agents are not homogeneous across different regions of the CNS. For example, brainstem and thalamic evoked potentials can be performed in a patient despite lack of conscious awareness during intravenous or inhalational anesthesia due to the selective effects of anesthetics on the frontal cortex and auditory cortex with preservation of brainstem and thalamic afferent pathways.[33–37] There is a generalized suppression of background activity leaving reactive capabilities facilitated at deep levels, and amplitude of evoked potentials is actually augmented in a dose-related manner.[33] In our experience, this dissociation between neocortical and lower cortical/brain stem effects of intravenous and inhalational agents renders the use of the Bispectral Index (BIS) (Aspect Medical Systems, Natick, MA) for monitoring anesthetic depth[37] somewhat irrelevant for determining whether electrophysiological mapping can be performed.

It is uncertain to what extent general anesthesia affects single-unit recording. In fact, single-unit recordings are routinely obtained in animals under general anesthesia.[38,39] In patients, successful recordings have been made from Vim under propofol narcosis.[31,32] However, there may be differences in characteristics of neuronal activity as a function of anesthetic depth. Compared with dystonia patients mapped under local anesthesia, the firing rates in GPi were substantially decreased, and long pauses were present in dystonia patients mapped with deep sedation or general IV anesthesia (propofol) (**Fig. 6.1**).[10,22] Moreover, although limb driving was obtained under propofol, fewer arm-responsive units were observed.[22] These findings are consistent with enhancement of gamma-aminobutyric acid (GABA)ergic striatal and globus pallidus externus (GPe) afferents to GPi by propofol.[40] We examined GPi firing rates and patterns in the monkey under inhalational general anesthesia and similarly found decreased firing rates and increased pauses in GPi, which

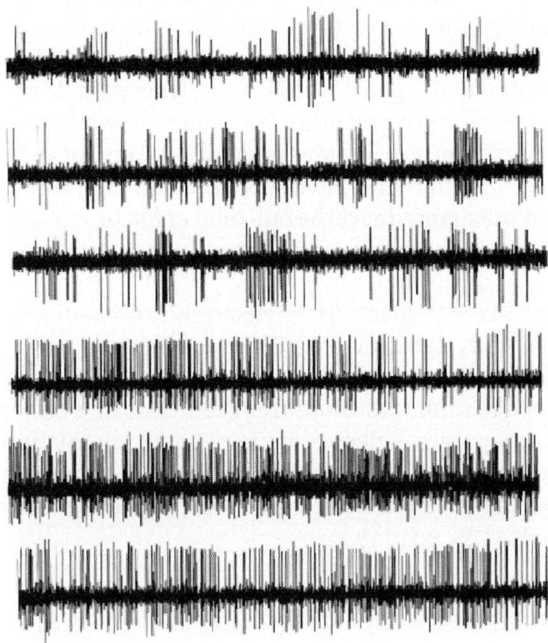

Fig. 6.1 Neuronal recordings of globus pallidus internus (GPi) neurons showing characteristic discharge patterns found in a generalized dystonic patient under propofol anesthesia (top three), and the same patient and region of the GPi recorded in a subsequent procedure with only mild sedation present (bottom three). Three different examples are shown, each of 2-second duration. Reprinted with permission from Hutchinson et al. Pallidal neuronal activity: implications for models of dystonia. Ann Neurol 2003;53:480–488.

substantially blurred the distinction between the external and internal pallidal segment (GPe and GPi) in the 1-methyl-4-phenyl-1,2,3,6-tetrahydropyridine (MPTP)-treated model of PD.[39]

There have been no similar comparative data reported for STN. Maltete et al[8] noted "characteristic" STN recordings in 15 patients recorded under general anesthesia, but the physiology of the recorded neurons was not characterized further. In several nonparkinsonian cases performed under general anesthesia with either propofol or sevoflurane, we were able to adequately map the STN (**Fig. 6.2**). The number of recorded units was similar to those typically found in the STN in PD patients under local anesthesia, and we were able to detect the characteristic increase in activity as the microelectrode entered STN. A sampling of the physiological characteristics of the units, however, did indicate some differences (**Table 6.3**). Under either sevoflurane or propofol, the mean firing rates were somewhat lower, and dispersion, an index of "burstiness," was higher, similar to observations made under anesthesia in the pallidum. Root mean square (RMS), an indicator of the power or signal content of the recorded units, was lower under anesthesia, reflecting a slightly greater difficulty in detecting unit activity. Whether these differences were related to pathophysiology or anesthesia awaits further analysis. In each of the cases we monitored anesthesia depth by BIS monitoring and found no relationship with our ability to detect units, consistent with this parameter as being indicative of anesthetic effects on the neocortex, not the subcortical structures, as discussed earlier.

It is therefore possible to perform microelectrode mapping, even under general anesthesia with propofol or

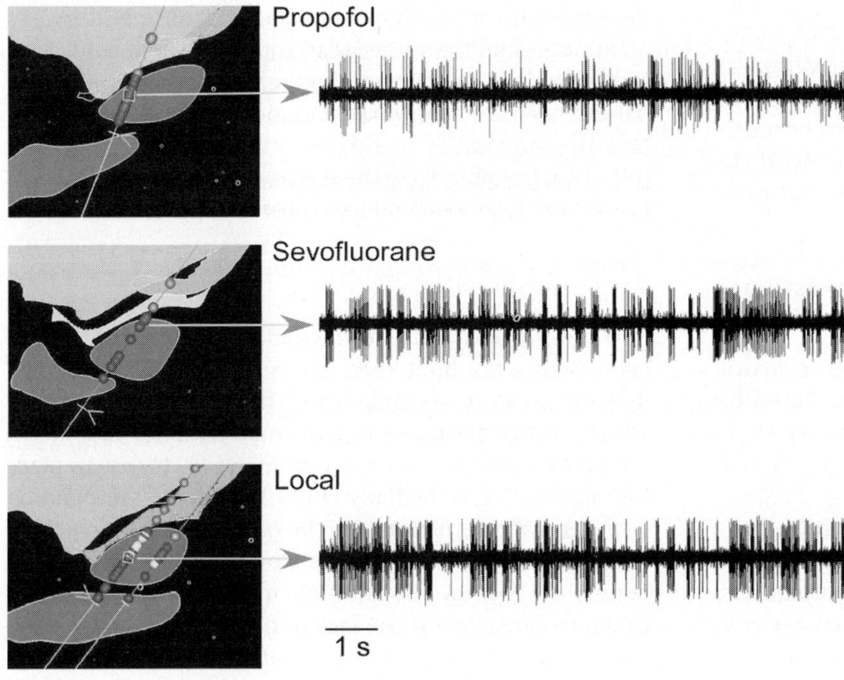

Fig. 6.2 Sagittal maps through three-dimensional surface models of microelectrode tracks performed during mapping of the subthalamic nucleus (STN) under propofol (top), sevoflurane (center), and local anesthesia (bottom). The locations of single units detected are noted by spheres along each track and were found in the thalamus, STN, and substantia nigra (from top down). A representative 10-second sample of the recorded units is shown for each (right).

Table 6.3 Effects of Anesthesia Type on Intraoperative Neuro-physiology

Anesthesia	Physiological Parameter		
	Mean Frequency	Dispersion	Root Mean Square
Local	35.4 ± 12.2	66.4 ± 43.0	1012 ± 343
Propofol	22.7 ± 7.5	92.9 ± 53.7	314 ± 57
Sevofluorane	24.5 ± 0.3	110.2 ± 68.7	276 ± 72

sevofluorane, although the results may be hampered to some degree.[22] Nevertheless, several centers that routinely performing DBS under general anesthesia do not perform microelectrode mapping in the operating room. In these centers, there is greater reliance on anatomical MRI-based confirmation of targeting.[27,29]

Electrical Stimulation under Deep Sedation and General Anesthesia

A pivotal aspect of mapping in movement disorder cases is electrical stimulation to observe clinical benefits and adverse effects. This aspect of mapping is more greatly interfered with under deep sedation because (1) the patient cannot report subjective effects (e.g., paresthesias, visual phosphenes) associated with stimulation spread to structures around the target nucleus (e.g., optic tract, medial lemniscus, internal capsule), and (2) evaluation of clinical benefits is hampered by antiparkinsonian effects of anesthesia (e.g., suppression of tremor and rigidity).[18] Moreover, the patient is incapable of performing voluntary movements to evaluate bradykinesia. However, it is still possible to examine the optic track with flash visual evoked potentials in patients undergoing GPi DBS under general anesthesia.[10,16,22] Internal capsular activation at higher intensities of stimulation has also been observed under general anesthesia.[10] Nevertheless, several centers routinely performing DBS implantation under general anesthesia do not conduct any form of stimulation testing in the operating room.[27–29,41]

Outcome from Deep Brain Stimulator Implantation Under General Anesthesia

There are no prospective, randomized, blinded comparisons of movement disorder surgery, in particular DBS implantation, without and with general anesthesia, so no conclusions can be drawn as to the relative merits of each technique. In a retrospective analysis comparing 15 PD patients that had bilateral STN DBS implantations under general anesthesia and 15 operated with only local anesthesia, Maltete et al[8] found that the general anesthesia patients, despite displaying characteristic STN neuronal activity, had evidence of slightly decreased clinical benefits and re-

quired mildly higher stimulation intensities. This may have been related to the observation that only one of 30 sides were implanted in a trajectory other than the central track when operated under general anesthesia, whereas a different track, based on the results of intraoperative stimulation, was used in five of 30 sides under local. This suggests that the inability to refine the target based on monitoring testing may adversely affect the outcome of the procedure. In those centers that routinely use general anesthesia without any form of intraoperative physiology or testing,[27–29] the location of the implanted DBS electrode is immediately ascertained with stereotactic MRI, repositioning as necessary (which has been rare). Although outcomes from these centers appear similar to those from centers using either or both intraoperative electrophysiology and stimulation testing (currently the gold standard) (**Table 6.2**), definitive answers to the question must await prospective and controlled trials.

Intraoperative Seizures

Occasionally patients undergoing movement disorder surgery will encounter seizures.[4,5,42] Although a cortical hematoma can certainly cause a seizure, we have also encountered them in the absence of any bleeding complication, likely related to pneumocephalus. They typically begin with focal motor manifestations but more often than not generalize. We typically administer midazolam, and the events are usually self-limited. If not, thiopental is administered. Once the seizure is broken we administer IV fosphenytoin (Cerebyx, Parke-Davis, Morris Plains, NJ). The patient's clinical status is then evaluated to search for other focal signs which, if present, lead to termination of the procedure and emergent CT scanning. However, patients who have not received too much sedation from anticonvulsant medications will usually arouse within 5 to 10 minutes and the surgery can continue. Obviously, if the seizure(s) lead to concern about airway compromise, the patient needs to be intubated. Under these circumstances, inserting an LMA is an easy way to secure the airway. If this is not possible, then the stereotactic frame is removed, the airway is secured, and the procedure is terminated.

Air Embolism

Burr holes placed close to the midline can expose venous lakes within the bone that, because they are noncollapsible, may lead to air embolism. This may be exacerbated when functional surgery is performed with the patient in a semisitting position. For this reason, we (1) try not to place the burr hole too medially, and (2) perform the opening with the patient recumbent (the patient can sit up later if desired, after all bleeding, if encountered, is halted with bone wax). We do not routinely monitor with precordial Doppler. However, in the face of declining vital signs and decreasing end-tidal CO_2 the possibility of air embolism is entertained, and the head level is lowered, the wound irrigated, and the bone rewaxed.

Airway Obstruction

In awake patients, airway compromise is occasionally encountered. Usually this is related to poor positioning of the head and neck and can be dealt with easily by repositioning. If more ominous respiratory failure occurs, the airway must be secured. Hopefully, patients at risk for airway obstruction have been identified beforehand, and the frame has been positioned to allow for airway access. Means to secure the airway in patients in the stereotactic frame were

discussed earlier. In rare instances, however, the frame must be removed to secure the airway, and the procedure must be aborted.

Neurological Deterioration

The possibility of a seizure can be entertained and treated as already described, but in the presence of focal deficits or declining consciousness, the procedure is aborted, the airway is secured, and the patient is scanned. Pneumocephalus can account for mild depression in level of consciousness or confusion; when clinically significant it is treated with 100% O_2 by nonrebreathing facemask.

Editor's Comments

Although most functional neurosurgical procedures are performed under local anesthesia, the participation of an experienced anesthesiologist will help the efficiency, comfort, and safety of the patient. Likewise, having an inexperienced anesthesiologist risks just the opposite. Movement disorder patients require special treatment, and they should not be medicated as a general surgery patient of the same age. This is especially true with PD patients who may be medicated with polypharmacy and frequently have hypovolemia, respiratory dysfunction, problems with swallowing, and overall limited mental and physical reserves. A clear understanding of these issues by the neuroanesthesia service is essential to appropriate patient management.

We prefer having the anesthesia team involved from the initiation of the surgical procedure (Chapter 7). This begins with the application of the frame. IV sedation can be extremely helpful with smoothing out the process. The anesthesia team's expertise is extremely useful when evaluating the airway and when titrating sedation to ensure that adequate images can be obtained. In the rare patient with severe cervical lordosis or respiratory compromise, the patient may need endotracheal intubation. We prefer not to use LMA given that gastric reflux is always a potential problem, and it does not always prevent respiratory movement artifacts within the MRI scan. We prefer not to use midazolam because it can have unpredictable sedative effects that cannot be reversed. Propofol can be used in small amounts, but we avoid it in elderly patients with low initial blood pressure or history of dysautonomia because it can produce mark hypotension.

Our preference is for dexmedetomidine (DEX) (Precedex, Abbott Laboratories, North Chicago, IL), which is an α 2-adrenoreceptor agonist that produces dose-dependent sedation, anxiolysis, and analgesia without respiratory depression.[43] The α 2-adrenoreceptors in the brain are concentrated predominantly in the pons and the medulla. These areas include the sympathetic nervous system such as the locus ceruleus, which is a major site of noradrenergic innervation of the CNS. The sedation produced by this α 2-adrenoreceptor agonist, unlike that produced by traditional sedatives, such as benzodiazepines and propofol, does not depend primarily on the activation of the GABA system. DEX has a significant analgesic effect and consistently reduces the requirement for opioids. The cardiovascular effects are complex, but the summary effect is that of a modest reduction in blood pressure and a modest reduction in heart rate. Nevertheless, care must be used in the loading dose to prevent initial hypertension and subsequent hypotension. Patients in whom heart block is evident are relatively contraindicated because arrhythmias or cardiac arrest may be produced. This risk may be increased if β-blockers are used. Additional beneficial effects include control of shivering, reduced anxiety, and minimal affects on ventilation.

Although it is a safe and effective adjuvant to neurosurgery, there is a learning curve to properly bolus and titrate DEX to produce a cooperative sedative state without inducing hypotension or bradycardia. In a randomized, double-blind study of sedated patients undergoing awake carotid endarterectomy, DEX produced less fluctuation in level of sedation, greater comfort, and lower postoperative hypertension compared with the control group (midazolam/fentanyl/propofol management).[44] DEX supplemented with fentanyl is useful for sedation and pain control during placement of the stereotactic frame and for MRI sedation to prevent motion artifacts.

We generally prefer to use DEX as a sole agent for the awake portion of the stereotactic procedure. We infuse DEX at a rate of 0.2 to 1.0 μg/kg/h during surgical stimulation (i.e., scalp incision and burr hole placement) as well as at closure. And we discontinue or place it at an extremely low maintenance infusion dose (0.1 to 0.3 μg/kg/h) for intraoperative recording and electrophysiological testing. It appears to produce minimal effect on electrophysiological recording for electroencephalography (EEG)[45] or evoked potentials.[46] We have used DEX in over 80 DBS patients with minimal effect on microelectrode recordings as long as the patient is awake. There is a mild decrease in tremor but with stress or stopping the DEX it readily returns.

As part of the procedure, tight antihypertensive control is required. DEX is also helpful in reducing the need for antihypertensive drugs. Because of the importance we place on maintaining blood pressure control with a mean of ~90, arterial lines are frequently placed for blood pressure monitoring purposes. Should additional medication be needed, labetolol and hydralazine are the antihypertensives of choice, depending on the cardiac rate. In the setting of marked bradycardia, nitroglycerin may be necessary. Rarely is nitroprusside or nicardipine required.

Although fewer than 1 in 100 PD patients may require intubation, general anesthesia is frequently necessary in patients who have dystonia due to the uncontrolled movements that may cause injury to the patients or caregivers. In some cases, IV general sedation can be performed with propofol or DEX but in most cases the use will be insufficient and evaluation ahead of time by the neurosurgeon and the neuroanesthesiologist should give a clear plan as to whether to try deep IV sedation or general inhalation anesthesia. Care must be exercised when using nitrous oxide because, despite attempts at keeping the CSF space sealed, pneumocephalus can occur at any time during the procedure.

General anesthesia of course has its difficulties in diminishing the electrophysiological activity that can be obtained. General anesthesia will alter the characteristics of the microelectrode recordings, rendering identification of the anatomical regions difficult. In some cases, no useful electrophysiological stimulation data can be obtained in defining the optic tracts, medial lemniscus, or internal capsule. Because in dystonia most of the stimulation effect is looking for adverse effects, these patients are at greater risks for potential postoperative problems.

If the patient has a seizure at the time of surgery, it is usually over before any medication can be delivered, and we avoid giving medication to "stop" the seizure. We do not give Dilantin (Pfizer Inc., New York, NY) or Cerebyx (Parke-Davis) after the seizure is over because they are sedating, and the seizure is almost always a single event. Waiting 15 to 30 minutes to resume the procedure is merited, but if there is any doubt about the patient's ability to continue, the procedure must be terminated. An isolated postoperative seizure is usually not treated but if there are any potential risk factors, a short course of anticonvulsant medication is given.

An emergent intubation should be an extremely rare event but one that the neuroanesthesiologist must always be prepared to perform. However, it is a rare situation that the surgery must be discontinued due to neurological deterioration. Several factors can cause decreased responsiveness and confusion, including withdrawal of medication, hypertension, seizures, air embolism, brain edema, hemorrhage, airway obstruction, and oversedation. Pneumocephalus has the potential to induce a seizure, confusion, or loss of consciousness. Air embolism may have a different presentation in the awake patient, with coughing, tachypnea, and hypoxia.[47] Early recognition and immediate treatment can resolve the problems as quickly as they arise. In evaluating the patient, both the neuroanesthesiologist and the neurologist can be extremely useful. On rare occasions, we have elected to intubate a patient to facilitate expeditious conclusion of the procedure. Immediate postoperative CT or MRI studies are essential.

◼ Postoperative Anesthetic Issues

Following local anesthetic, the postoperative period is relatively straightforward, and the patient is observed in the postanesthesia care unit (PACU) for a standard period. Following general anesthesia, emergence can be delayed in patients with PD. Given the respiratory issues in these patients, careful observation in the PACU is critical. In PD patients, and patients with dystonia, we occasionally encounter laryngospasm, which may require reintubation.

We always obtain postoperative imaging (usually MRI) to evaluate for a hematoma before discharging the patient to the floor; we do not routinely observe in the intensive care unit unless there has been a complication. If the patient has been anesthetized for the surgery then we generally perform the imaging under general anesthesia. Following the imaging, antiparkinsonian medications are started. It sometimes takes awhile for the patient to attain an "on-medication" state after the extended period without medications. Conversely, temporary lesion effects often mitigate parkinsonian signs, and occasionally patients are even dyskinetic. We continue preoperative medication dosages, even after STN DBS, unless the patient has excessive dyskinesia. Patients are allowed to self-administer their own medications, usually with the assistance of family members, because their regimens are never in step with the usual medications rounds by the nursing staff.

◼ Anesthetic Complications

Patients with PD, dystonia, and ET are predisposed to complications from any surgical and anesthetic experience.[2,3] With careful screening, preoperative optimization, and aggressive intraoperative treatment of fluid status, despite the incidence of cardiovascular and respiratory risk factors in this patient population, the serious intraoperative complication rate is relatively low. However, arterial hypertension (59.4%) and hypotension (7.9%), bradycardia (18.0%) and tachycardia (6.2%), and dyspnea or airway obstruction (5.4%) or both were noted relatively frequently.[42] As mentioned, laryngospasm in patients with PD and generalized dystonia might be encountered.

◼ Conclusion

Anesthesia is critical to the successful and uncomplicated completion of any surgical procedure and always presents particular concerns in specialized surgical procedures. Although many functional neurosurgical procedures for movement disorders can appear relatively routine and unchallenging when performed under local anesthesia, careful preparation and vigilant monitoring in this chronic neurodegenerative patient population will prevent most complications. New challenges include the expansion of the procedures to include more difficult patients, with severe hyperkinetic movement disorders (e.g., dystonia, choreoathetosis, Tourette syndrome) or other contraindications to surgery under local anesthesia, and therefore an increasing number of surgeries are being performed under general anesthesia. This relatively uncharted ground presents unresolved issues, including whether and how to perform intraoperative physiological monitoring in the anesthetized patient, as well as how best to administer anesthesia during perioperative and intraoperative MRI scanning.

References

1. Bertrand CM. Surgery of involuntary movements, particularly stereotactic surgery: reminiscences. Neurosurgery 2004;55:698–703 (discussion 703–694)
2. Nicholson G, Pereira AC, Hall GM. Parkinson's disease and anaesthesia. Br J Anaesth 2002;89:904–916
3. Mason LJ, Cojocaru TT, Cole DJ. Surgical intervention and anesthetic management of the patient with Parkinson's disease. Int Anesthesiol Clin 1996;34:133–150
4. Alkhani A, Lozano AM. Pallidotomy for Parkinson disease: a review of contemporary literature. J Neurosurg 2001;94:43–49
5. Beric A, Kelly PJ, Rezai A, et al. Complications of deep brain stimulation surgery. Stereotact Funct Neurosurg 2001;77:73–78
6. Gross M, Bannister R, Godwin-Austen R. Orthostatic hypotension in Parkinson's disease. Lancet 1972;1:174–176
7. Vincken WG, Gauthier SG, Dollfuss RE, Hanson RE, Darauay CM, Cosio MG. Involvement of upper-airway muscles in extrapyramidal disorders: a cause of airflow limitation. N Engl J Med 1984;311:438–442
8. Maltete D, Navarro S, Welter ML, et al. Subthalamic stimulation in Parkinson disease: with or without anesthesia? Arch Neurol 2004;61:390–392
9. Coubes P, Cif L, El Fertit H, et al. Electrical stimulation of the globus pallidus internus in patients with primary generalized dystonia: long-term results. J Neurosurg 2004;101:189–194
10. Krause M, Fogel W, Kloss M, Rasche D, Volkmann J, Tronnier V. Pallidal stimulation for dystonia. Neurosurgery 2004;55:1361–1370
11. Ikebe S, Harada T, Hashimoto T, et al. Prevention and treatment of malignant syndrome in Parkinson's disease: a consensus statement of the malignant syndrome research group. Parkinsonism Relat Disord 2003;9(Suppl 1):S47–S49
12. Pfeiffer RF. Antiparkinsonian agents: drug interactions of clinical significance. Drug Saf 1996;14:343–354
13. Gray H, Wilson S, Sidebottom P. Parkinson's disease and anaesthesia. Br J Anaesth 2003;90:524–525
14. Glass PS, Gan TJ, Howell S. A review of the pharmacokinetics and pharmacodynamics of remifentanil. Anesth Analg 1999;89(4, Suppl) S7–S14
15. Hyman SA, Rogers WD, Smith DW, Maciunas RJ, Allen GS, Berman ML. Perioperative management for transplant of autologous adrenal medulla to the brain for parkinsonism. Anesthesiology 1988;69:618–622
16. Fukuda M, Kameyama S, Kawaguchi T, Yamashita S, Tanaka R. Stereotaxy during intravenous anesthesia with propofol. No Shinkei Geka 1998;26:709–715
17. Fabregas N, Rapado J, Gambus PL, et al. Modeling of the sedative and airway obstruction effects of propofol in patients with Parkinson disease undergoing stereotactic surgery. Anesthesiology 2002;97:1378–1386
18. Anderson BJ, Marks PV, Futter ME. Propofol–contrasting effects in movement disorders. Br J Neurosurg 1994;8:387–388
19. Krauss JK, Akeyson EW, Giam P, Jankovic J. Propofol-induced dyskinesias in Parkinson's disease. Anesth Analg 1996;83:420–422
20. Bragonier R, Bartle D, Langton-Hewer S. Acute dystonia in a 14-yr-old following propofol and fentanyl anaesthesia. Br J Anaesth 2000;84:828–829
21. Zabani I, Vaghadia H. Refractory dystonia during propofol anaesthesia in a patient with torticollis-dystonia disorder. Can J Anaesth 1996;43:1062–1064
22. Hutchison WD, Lang AE, Dostrovsky JO, Lozano AM. Pallidal neuronal activity: implications for models of dystonia. Ann Neurol 2003;53:480–488
23. Lozano AM, Kumar R, Gross RE, et al. Globus pallidus internus pallidotomy for generalized dystonia. Mov Disord 1997;12:865–870
24. Ondo WG, Desaloms JM, Jankovic J, Grossman RG. Pallidotomy for generalized dystonia. Mov Disord 1998;13:693–698
25. American Society of Anesthesiologists Task Force on Management of the Difficult Airway. Practice guidelines for management of the difficult airway: an update report by the American Society of Anesthesiologists Task Force on Management of the Difficult Airway. Anesthesiology 2003;98:1269–1277
26. Henderson JM. Frameless localization for functional neurosurgical procedures: a preliminary accuracy study. Stereotact Funct Neurosurg 2004;82:135–141
27. Coubes P, Vayssiere N, El Fertit H, et al. Deep brain stimulation for dystonia. Surgical technique. Stereotact Funct Neurosurg 2002;78:183–191
28. Plaha P, Patel NK, Gill SS. Stimulation of the subthalamic region for essential tremor. J Neurosurg 2004;101:48–54
29. Patel NK, Heywood P, O'Sullivan K, Love S, Gill SS. MRI-directed subthalamic nucleus surgery for Parkinson's disease. Stereotact Funct Neurosurg 2002;78:132–145
30. Slawek J, Derejko M, Lass P. Camptocormia as a form of dystonia in Parkinson's disease. Eur J Neurol 2003;10:107–108
31. Keegan MT, Flick RP, Matsumoto JY, Davis DH, Lanier WL. Anesthetic management for two-stage computer-assisted, stereotactic thalamotomy in a child with Hallervorden-Spatz Disease. J Neurosurg Anesthesiol 2000;12:107–111
32. Ghika J, Villemure JG, Miklossy J, et al. Postanoxic generalized dystonia improved by bilateral Voa thalamic deep brain stimulation. Neurology 2002;58:311–313
33. Osawa M, Shingu K, Murakawa M, et al. Effects of sevofluorane on central nervous system electrical activity in cats. Anesth Analg 1994;79:52–57
34. Jessop J, Jones JG. Evaluation of the actions of general anaesthetics in the human brain. Gen Pharmacol 1992;23:927–935
35. Kochs E, Schulte am Esch J. Evoked potentials and intravenous anesthetics. Klin Wochenschr 1988;66(Suppl 14):1–10
36. Klostermann F, Funk T, Vesper J, Siedenberg R, Curio G. Propofol narcosis dissociates human intrathalamic and cortical high-frequency (> 400 Hz) SEP components. Neuroreport 2000;11:2607–2610

37. Heinke W, Kenntner R, Gunter TC, Sammler D, Olthoff D, Koelsch S. Sequential effects of increasing propofol sedation on frontal and temporal cortices as indexed by auditory event-related potentials. Anesthesiology 2004;100:617–625

38. Yamamoto T, Hassler R, Huber C, Wagner A, Sasaki K. Electrophysiologic studies on the pallido- and cerebellothalamic projections in squirrel monkeys (*Saimiri sciureus*). Exp Brain Res 1983;51:77–87

39. Mewes K, Zhang J, Vitek JL, DeLong MR, Baron M. Effects of inhalational anesthetics on neuronal discharge patterns and mapping procedures in the primate pallidum. Paper presented at: Society for Neuroscience, October 23–28, 1999, Miami Beach, FL

40. Peduto VA, Concas A, Santoro G, Biggio G, Gessa GL. Biochemical and electrophysiologic evidence that propofol enhances GABAergic transmission in the rat brain. Anesthesiology 1991;75:1000–1009

41. Yianni J, Bain P, Giladi N, et al. Globus pallidus internus deep brain stimulation for dystonic conditions: a prospective audit. Mov Disord 2003;18:436–442

42. Santos P, Valero R, Arguis MJ, et al. Preoperative adverse events during stereotactic microelectrode-guided deep brain surgery in Parkinson's disease. Rev Esp Anestesiol Reanim 2004;51:523–530

43. Bekker A, Sturaitis M. Dexmedetomidine for neurosurgical surgery. Neurosurgery 2005;57:1–10

44. Bekker AY, Basile J, Gold M, et al. Dexmedetomidine for awake carotid endarterectomy: efficacy, hemodynamic profile, and side effects. J Neurosurg Anesthesiol 2004;16:126–135

45. Ard J, Doyle W, Bekker A. Awake craniotomy with dexmedetomidine in pediatric patients. J Neurosurg Anesthesiol 2003;15:263–266

46. Thornton C, Lucas MA, Newton DE, Dore CJ, Jones RM. Effects of dexmedetomidine on isoflurane requirements in healthy volunteers, II: Auditory and somatosensory evoked potentials. Br J Anaesth 1999;83:381–386

47. Deogaonkar A, Avitsian R, Henderson JM, Schubert A. Venous air embolism during deep brain stimulation. Stereotact Funct Neurosurg 2005;83:32–35

7 Stereotactic Surgery with Microelectrode Recordings

Diane Sierens, Scott Kutz, Julie G. Pilitsis, and Roy A. E. Bakay

Stereotactic surgery was developed to access and manipulate deep structures within the brain while minimizing trauma to the surrounding structures. The precision with which the target is reached is essential to accomplish this goal. We have found that use of both indirect and direct magnetic resonance imaging (MRI) targeting methods followed by electrophysiological confirmation with microelectrode recordings (MERs) yields precise results.[1-3] Direct targeting is based on the use of radiological images that allow direct visualization of the target.[2-13] However, MRI scans are not always of sufficient quality to visualize the target because nuclear boundaries are indistinct. Use of higher field strength 3 Tesla (tesla 3T) may improve the reliability of this technique.[14,15] Indirect targeting can be the primary targeting method but more often it is complementary. Indirect targeting is based upon identification of the anterior and posterior commissures (AC and PC, respectively) and then using standard distances from the midcommisural point (MCP) of a line connecting them to approximate the location of a desired target. The distance between AC and PC may vary significantly between individuals, which limits the accuracy of this technique.[16,17] However, direct targeting is not as accurate as initially believed, and indirect methods may be more accurate even when the target can be seen.[18-24] MRI is highly susceptible to image distortion. Although the degree of error can be estimated by phantom studies, individual patient correction may be attempted by MRI fusion with computed tomography (CT). Image fusion does not eliminate errors.[25] Regardless of the targeting method, errors are introduced (see Chapters 5 and 8 for nuances). This chapter describes the use of MER to definitively localize the stereotactic target intraoperatively by electrophysiological means.

The microelectrode had been invaluable in allowing the precise identification of neural structures in the immediate vicinity of the electrode tip.[1-3,26] In 1961, Albe-Fessard et al[27] provided the first report of electrode recordings obtained from humans during stereotactic surgery. During that decade, the technique was incorporated by many others to define the borders of anatomical structures and targets during stereotactic procedures.[28-30] Currently, the science of MER has advanced to the point where it is considered a routine technique in stereotactic and functional neurosurgery. Bertrand, Jasper, and coworkers[31-33] were probably the first to record single units in the human thalamus. Many groups have described MER activity of the human thalamus and consider it a routine technique for thalamotomy or thalamic deep brain stimulation (DBS).[1,34-41] Multiple functional neurosurgical centers that perform pallidotomy and pallidal DBS routinely use MER.[2,42-67] The first case report of subthalamic nucleus (STN) DBS was published in 1994 by Benabid et al, who described a unique approach to the use of MER for optimizing lead placement.[68] Although quality results can be obtained by experts with other electrophysiological techniques (see Chapter 8), the majority of investigators experienced in performing STN DBS surgery today use MER as the definitive targeting method.[3,7,69-78] Reports of sustained improvements based upon long-term follow-up of greater than 1 year after bilateral DBS for movement disorders are predominantly from centers that use MER guidance.[79-83] Thus, although there is no scientific proof of the utility of MER, it is the preferred method of most functional neurosurgeons.

■ Operative Techniques and Patient Positioning

The success of the operation is often dependent on the close communication between the stereotactic neurosurgeon, the anesthesiologist, and the movement disorders neurologist. Other personnel would ideally include a neurophysiologist and a physician extender specializing in movement disorders. Before surgery, all medical and psychiatric problems must be resolved (see Chapter 4). Antiparkinsonian medications are withheld 12 hours prior to surgery to obtain an "off" state for evaluation at surgery. Most patients are uncomfortable with the thought of prolonged periods in the off state, but they must be encouraged not to take their antiparkinsonian medications to avoid drug-induced dyskinesias, which could interfere with stereotactic frame placement, proper imaging, and MER. Furthermore, improvements in clinical symptoms intraoperatively are useful to confirm accurate lead placement. This improvement is masked by antiparkinsonian medication. It also alters the firing rates, which lessens the value of MER. In patients with Parkinson disease (PD), apomorphine significantly decreased the overall firing rates of globus pallidus internus (GPi) neurons, but there was no change in the overall firing rate of neurons in the STN.[84] We allow patients to take medications unrelated to their movement disorder with a sip of water on the morning of surgery.

Typically, the patient is admitted to the hospital the morning of the procedure. An intravenous infusion line is inserted in the patient's arm ipsilateral to the side of surgery, or the first side if bilateral. This allows for unimpeded movement of the contralateral extremity during intraoperative neurological examination. A short half-life drug such as propofol, remifentanyl, or dexmedetomidine may be used for frame placement and image acquisition. We use predominantly the Leksell series G (Elekta, Atlanta, GA; www.elekta.com/healthcare international stereotactic neurosurgery.php). Proper alignment of the frame with the patient's anatomy simplifies targeting adjustments, allows consistent angles of approach, and decreases error that can be introduced by correcting for malposition. Although there are algorithms and computer imaging software that can correct imperfect alignment, each manipulation adds to the potential for inaccuracy. The ear-bars that are provided with either the Leksell or the Cosman-Roberts-Wells (CRW)-fn frame (Integra Radionics, Burlington, MA; www.radionics. com) prevent sideward tilt (roll) or axial rotation (yaw) of the frame relative to the patient's head while permitting the pitch of the frame (anteroposterior axis) to be set so that the base ring lies roughly parallel to the AC–PC plane (**Fig. 5.2**). For the axial MRI to lie coplanar with the AC–PC, the frame needs to be parallel to a line from the inferior orbital rim to the external auditory canal. Foam pads or strips to the ear-bars can decrease the patient discomfort but must not distort the alignment. Use the ear-bar holes that are closest to the frame's base ring and adjust the ear-bar base to center the patient in the frame. The fixation pins should not extend beyond the margins of the vertical posts so that the frame will fit within the confines of the scanner's head coil. Opposing pins should be applied simultaneously to reduce the frame rotation; once engaged the ear-bars should be removed for patient comfort. The pins must be tightened enough to prevent slippage but not overtightened so as to distort the frame. When finished, the frame should be pulled on and any slippage or presence of pain suggests the need for further tightening. If the patient has kyphosis, the table adaptor will limit neck extension. Aligning the head more anteriorly in the frame and placing a pillow under the buttocks should correct this problem. Rarely, because of airway obstruction, endotracheal intubation is needed. The final and most important check is to have the MRI alignment beam symmetrically superimposed on both the lateral and the anterior fiducial channels of the localizer. MRI sequences and target coordinates are discussed in Chapter 5.

It is preferable to perform surgery with minimal sedation. However, this may be difficult in children or adults with severe dystonia and therefore can require a general anesthetic (Chapter 6). Starr et al[61] reported a case in which propofol was used as the anesthetic agent for a child with dystonia during MER. The pallidal discharges were depressed greatly. Krauss et al[65] confirmed this finding. A better choice to avoid effects on spontaneous neuronal discharge is a mixture of ketamine and remifentanyl. We have

also had success with dexmedetomidine. The stereotactic head frame typically renders the airway difficult to access for the duration of the procedure so that if general anesthesia is to be used it should be started before frame placement.[85,86] Furthermore, the effects of any sedation given for the frame placement, image acquisition, or burr hole placement must be resolved prior to MER for which an awake, alert patient is essential for optimal recordings.[1–3]

Perioperative antibiotics, antibiotic-containing irrigation solutions and careful attention to sterile technique appear to be instrumental in maintaining a low infection rate. Hood et al[87] performed 365 consecutive intracranial stereotactic procedures over a 6-year period with only three postoperative infections. Similar to other meta-analyses of antibiotic prophylaxis for prosthetics, a systematic review of antibiotic prophylaxis for surgical introduction of ventricular shunts clearly demonstrated the utility of systemic antibiotics in preventing shunt infections.[88] In light of this, we use perioperative cephalosporin or vancomycin if the patient is allergic to penicillin. The use of prophylactic anticonvulsants is controversial and has not been studied in DBS to date. Although Shrivastava et al[89] give patients a loading dose of phenytoin, we and others[90] do not because seizures are rare and allergic reactions are common. We do not use corticosteroids. Intracranial hemorrhage is a well known and potentially devastating complication of stereotactic surgery. Careful control of perioperative blood pressure is important and may reduce the occurrence of this complication.[91] Because hypotensive patients can become hypertensive in surgery, continuous blood pressure monitoring and the use of intravenous antihypertensive medications should be encouraged to keep systolic blood pressure less than 140 mm Hg or a mean arterial pressure below 90 mm Hg or both. An arterial line may be necessary. Also avoid all antiplatelet agents such as aspirin, nonsteroidal anti-inflammatory drugs, antiplatelet agents, or herbal supplements such as ginkgo, garlic, and ginger for at least 2 weeks prior to surgery. Anticoagulants require special preparation (see Chapter 5).

Before starting surgery, the patient is positioned in a semisitting position with the side of initial surgery toward the anesthesiologist to allow the neurologist access to the contralateral side of the body during MER and test stimulation. Be aware that uncomfortable rigidity, akinesia, and off dystonia may become an issue intraoperatively after draping. Every effort to interact with the patient to provide optimal padding and neck positioning will pay off several hours into the case. It is important to attach the stereotactic head frame to the Mayfield headrest in a neutral neck position. Be sure that the Mayfield controls are readily available to adjust during the case as needed for patient comfort. The patient's head is shaved according to the desire of the patient. Aziz et al[92] do not shave the patient's head, but they wash the hair with aqueous and then alcoholic chlorhexidine. We prefer to shave the entire head and drape so the patient's face and eyes are visible on the nonsterile side of the drape. It is especially useful to mark the location of any hardware and thereby avoid damage to it during delayed second sides, reoperations, or in patients with other devices such as shunts. The eyes are only covered briefly during draping to minimize the patient's sense of entrapment. Two sterile towels are folded into quarters that loop in the front and wrap around the base of the frame before placing the rings of the arc axes, and the operative area is covered with a 25 to 30 cm wide Ioban 2 (3M Health Care, St. Paul, MN; www.3m.com). The towels will keep the Ioban from adhering to the eyebrows or ears and protect the surgeon from potential contamination when placing the rings. We then use a clear plastic drape, either the Elekta stereotactic drape (www.ensproducts.elekta.com) for the Leksell, the Apuzzo stereotactic drape for the CRW (Integra Radionics; www.radionics.com/products/stereotaxy/), or the Ortho Bar drape (Kimberly-Clark Roswell, GA, http:// nacrm.kcmkt.com/ourbrands/ healthcare.asp) as a universal drape. The drape is then attached to an ether screen bar that can be angled as needed. A C-arm should be draped separately using sterile technique for intraoperative fluoroscopy. Many centers incorporate the drape with an overhead C-arm, but we prefer it to be independent and below the table to maximize mobility for aligning the fluoroscopic beam and ease of access to work above the frame.

Infiltrating the incision line and reinfiltrating the four pin sites with 1% lidocaine and 1:100,000 epinephrine mixed with 0.5% marcaine in equal concentrations provides the patient with 6 to 8 hours of comfort. Some rapidly reversible sedation is frequently useful at the start of the procedure. We use a coronal incision 1 to 2 cm posterior to the proposed entry site to remove any tension on the suture line at closure. We take care to separate the pericranium so it can be used in the closure. After local infiltration, a large posterior and lateral subgaleal pocket is created with blunt dissection below the galea and above the temporalis fascia for the excess lead at the end of the case. Prior surgery or scars will require innovation and flexibility in the incision design.

It is prudent to place the patient in a slight Trendelenburg position during the burr hole opening to reduce the possibility of air embolus. The team should realize that a venous air embolism will present differently in an awake patient and look for coughing, tachypnea, and hypoxemia.[93] Prior to making a burr hole, surgical planning software and image fusion provides the technology to simulate the electrode's trajectory and avoid blood vessels, sulci, eloquent structures, and, when possible, the ventricular cavity (**Fig. 7.1**). Surgical planning on the StealthStation using FrameLink (Medtronic Navigation, Louisville, CO; www. archive.stealthstation.com/physician/neuro/library/).jsp

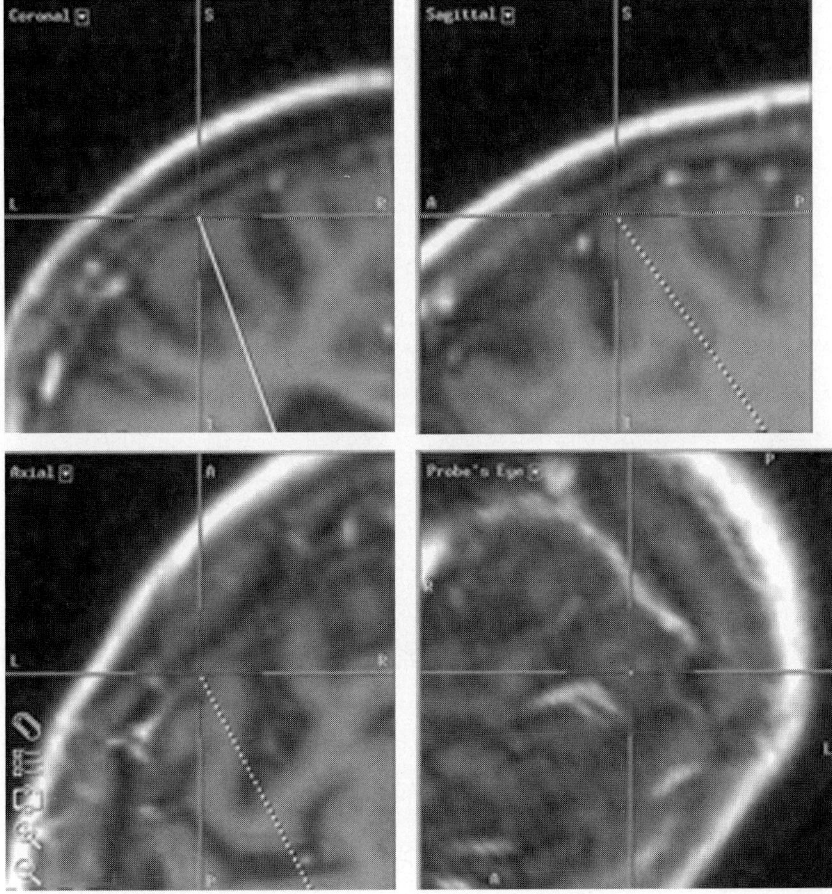

Fig. 7.1 Surgical planning on the StealthStation using Framelink (Medtronic Navigation, Louisville, CO) allows multiplanar imaging of the planned trajectory(s) with routine axial, coronal, and sagittal planes in relation to the anterior–posterior commissure (AC–PC) plane and specific trajectory planes. Additional images, including magnetic resonance imaging (MRI) or computed tomography (CT) but not X-ray or ventriculography, can be fused by a best-fit technique, but it is not a true three-dimensional fusion. A Schaltenbrand and Wahren deformable atlas can be overlaid onto the brain image, but rarely is the fit good enough to use for surgical planning. Volumetric MRI with contrast allows a high degree of resolution in the reformatted images (orthogonal to AC–PC) and visualization of vessels as demonstrated in this photograph. A tract with an entry point that avoids the large superficial veins is planned. The section along the trajectory is indicated by the center of the crosshairs at the location that is being indicated in each plane. The probe's eye view is perpendicular to the trajectory and allows the best view of the anatomical relationships along each slice.

allows multiplanar imaging of the planned trajectory(s) with frame coordinates, and angles for the arc and ring are quickly and accurately calculated so adjustments can be made rapidly to maximize the safety of the tracts. To help prevent hemorrhagic complications, we give gadolinium prior to the three-dimensional T1-weighted MRI scan to enhance the vasculature and avoid superficial veins or sulci near the entry point. The burr hole should be placed anterior to the coronal suture. Inadvertent coagulation of a large draining vein anterior to the coronal suture will be more likely to be asymptomatic,[91] but venous infarctions have been reported[94] so it is best to plan a trajectory to avoid all visible vessels. Additionally, avoiding passage through sensitive cortex may minimize the incidence of postoperative epilepsy.[90]

For STN, we plan the entry site slightly lateral to the eventual target (0 to 8 degrees). Otherwise we try to maintain a strict parasagittal approach. This allows the entire MER trajectory with the collected physiological data to be plotted on a single sagittal slice from a brain atlas and analyzed for target localization. At the same time, the slightly

more lateral approach avoids penetration of the medial caudate and medial thalamus, damage of which is believed to be associated with possible cognitive impairment. Others prefer to place the burr hole 3 to 4 cm lateral to the midline and plan their trajectory of the probe to avoid penetration of the ventricular ependyma, which can deflect the MER or DBS lead.[7,95] Typically this will result in a trajectory 50 to 60 degrees from the AC–PC line in the sagittal plane and a coronal angle 10 to 30 degrees from midline depending on ventricular size. This renders any rectilinear atlases useless. By restricting the coronal offset to 0 to 8 degrees the error is less than 1 mm through the target and will miss most ventricular walls. This is not always possible. In older patients where the shift after decompression of the ventricle can be significant, we will frequently use a more lateral approach to avoid the ventricles. If there is not a lot of atrophy, we do not have a problem going through the ventricle if need be, but realize that there can be deflections off of the ventricular wall. Fluoroscopic and anteroposterior (AP) radiographic imaging is most helpful in these cases (**Fig. 7.2**).

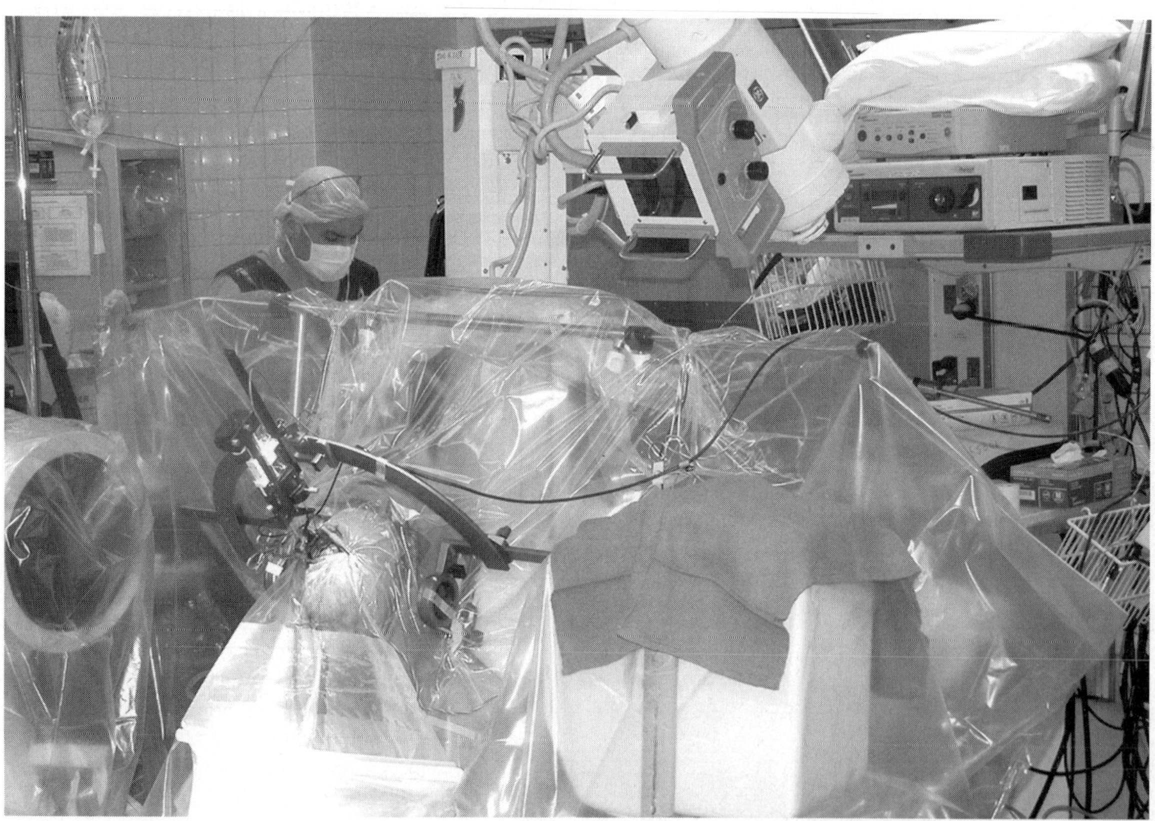

Fig. 7.2 This photograph of the operating suite demonstrates a typical setup for electrophysiology and intraoperative radiography during neurosurgery for deep brain implantation in the treatment of movement disorders. A clear plastic barrier separates the patient from the operative field with complete sterility behind the barrier and yet allows the surgeon to view direct interactions between the patient and movement disorders neurologist. Intraoperative fluoroscopy is set up in anticipation of confirmation of both microelectrode and deep brain stimulation (DBS) tracts. Fluoroscopic equipment is covered with a separate plastic drape allowing complete mobility during the procedure while at the same time not impeding access to the headstage. A portable X-ray machine is brought in only after there is a lead in place to allow anteroposterior skull X-rays to help determine the distance between the implanted lead and the electrode or second DBS lead.

A 14 mm burr hole is made and the diploe and inner cortical bone are undermined with a high-speed drill to form a cone that will maximize the microelectrode trajectories without striking dura or the bony edges of the burr hole. To secure the lead, we use the Stimloc from Medtronic Inc. The burr hole edge needs to be slightly enlarged from 14 to 15 mm to accommodate the Stimloc base and clip. When bilateral placements are planned, we drill the second side first but do not open the dura. If an unexpected dural vein is encountered, the hole can be expanded away from the vein to avoid opening the dura in that position. If that is not reasonable, a new hole is created. The dura below the Stimloc should then be free of venous structures. It is important to remove all visible dura to optimize probe exploration without deflection. The dura is cut in a cruciate manner and cauterized to expose the entire underlying cortex. Continuous irrigation is used to minimize cerebrospinal fluid (CSF) loss and pneumocephalus. Immediately after opening the dura widely, the pia-arachnoid is opened at the entry point to ensure smooth passage of the probe. The burr hole is filled with fibrin glue (Evicel; Johnson and Johnson Gateway, Somerville, NJ; www.Evicel.com) to reduce CSF loss and dampen pulsation artifacts during MER. If there is an unexpected cortical vein, we free it from the pia-arachnoid and push it aside before applying the fibrin glue to keep it out of the primary trajectory and avoid injury. If this is not possible or we still have concerns later in the case, we will remove the fibrin glue and visualize subsequent entries into the cortex before resealing the CSF space with fibrin glue. Now is a good time to stop all anesthetic agents except for blood pressure control.

The Stimloc base is centered and attached to the skull with the groove for the lead pointing posterior and slightly laterally. A fractured screw can be replaced by a screw from a skull fixation tray rather than opening another Stimloc kit. Avoid putting screws into the coronal suture. At this point the risk of air embolism is small, and it is important to elevate the patient's head to a semireclining position with knees bent for patient comfort. This also helps to avoid leakage of CSF and decreases the mechanical load of the micropositioner on the frame. Two observers should independently check all calculations and settings to avoid errors. Remember the "Left" or "Right" on the Leksell arc refers to the side the calibrations are on relative to the patient and not the side of surgery. We always use the left side to avoid confusion. Again, be sure not to overtighten the arc or distortion of 1 to 2 mm can occur. Also be careful to read the direction of the numbering. Failure to do so can result in approaching from the opposite side or recording from GPi rather than STN. All probes used must be carefully inspected for slight bends before each case. It is prudent to have a special case to store the guide tubes to prevent mishandling during the sterilization process. We replace all probes every 6 months to ensure rectilinear approaches.

By this time, there are a tremendous number of points where errors can be introduced (i.e., malposition of the frame requiring corrections for pitch, yaw or roll, overtightening of the pins causing distortion of the frame, measurement limitations, inaccuracies of the frame, distortion from the MRI field, slice thickness, targeting errors, mechanical loading effects on the frame from positioning or headstage, brain shift from CSF loss, or decompression of the ventricles, etc.). The errors may effectively cancel each other out or they may be additive. The net effect is that the theoretical accuracy of stereotactic systems is rarely achieved, and significant inaccuracies can occur.[96] There is then a need to correct for those errors before the lead is placed.

Microelectrode Recording

MER is a neurophysiological technique that detects and amplifies the activity of individual neurons[97] and that performs the following tasks:

1. Identifies the structural borders
2. Identifies eloquent structures
3. Identifies the sensorimotor territory
4. Localizes somatotopic arrangement
5. Outlines the three-dimensional shape of the targeted nuclei

We record single-unit action potentials with tungsten or platinum-iridium-tipped microelectrodes with an impedance of 0.1 to 1 Mohm at 1000 Hz FHC, Brunswick, ME; www.fh-co.com/microelectrodes.html. Typically microelectrode recordings begin 20–30 mm above the proposed target. The depth of recording is determined by the length of the guide tube. Longer routes record more information about the approach but also could result in greater deviations. The amplitude, frequency, and pattern of action potentials are recorded. Due to the extreme fragility of the microelectrode, it must not be touched; when not in use it should be withdrawn into the guide tube. The electrode is advanced in a precisely controlled manner with a micropositioner system. Several systems are commercially available such as Guideline System 4000 Clinical Micropositioner (FHC, www.fh-co.com; FHC Micro-Drive, FHC, Brunswick, ME; www.fh-co.com/microtargeting.html); Nexdrive, Medtronic (www.medtronic.com), Stereoplan with NeuroMap (Integra Radionics, Burlington, MA; www.radionics.com) and Microguide microelectrode recording system manufactured by Alpha-Omega Instruments, Nazareth Illit, Israel, MicroGuide (www.alphaomega-eng.com).[2,98,99] They all provide signal amplification, filtering, visual displays, audio monitoring, impedance monitoring, and stimulation. The Axon micropositioner has an X-Y stage that permits precise movement in the anteroposterior and mediolateral directions. The FHC, Nexdrive, and MicroGuide have five channels separated by

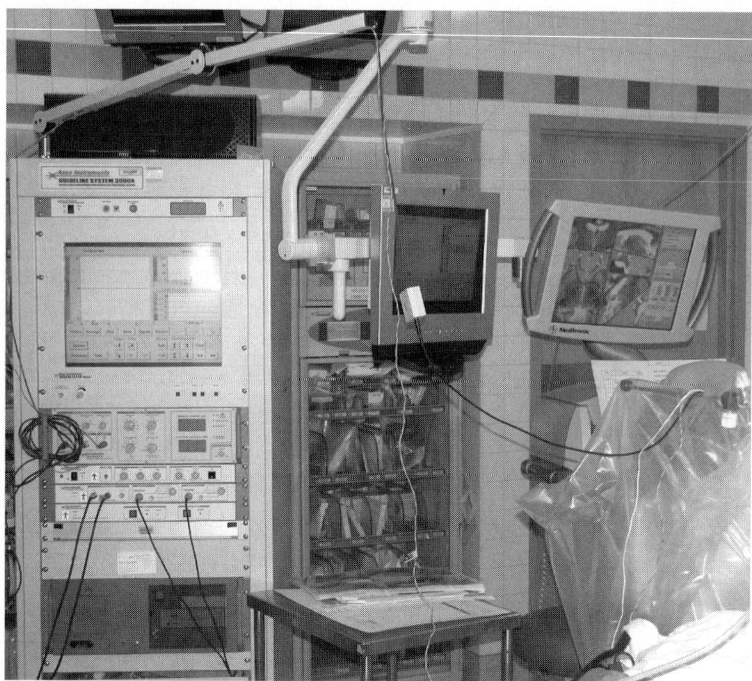

Fig. 7.3 On the left, the intraoperative microelectrode recordings (MERs) are processed and the data stored in an Axon Guideline 3000A (Frederick Haer Co., (FHC), Brunswick, ME). All data and spike sorted imaging can be viewed simultaneously. On the right, this information can also be shared with the StealthStation Treon (Medtronic Navigation, Louisville, CO). Sophisticated trajectory planning can be made on the StealthStation. The data can be annotated along with trajectory to allow electrophysiology data and anatomical data to be compared. Unfortunately, there is no way to link the anatomical database with electrophysiology at this time. The data can be stored for later review.

2 mm, and depending on the orientation and 3 mm offset, allow for 49 separate tracks. Nexdrive now has grids to reach anywhere in a 1 cm × 1 cm area. The recording system must distinguish single-unit action potentials from background neural activity and extraneous electrical noise. Fluorescent lights, heaters, operating room (OR) table motors, and all electrical devices (bipolar, Bovie, etc.) are turned off or unplugged. All OR monitoring equipment that contacts the patient should be battery powered to minimize potential interference with electrophysiological recordings. Electrical noise can range from 1 mV to > 1 V if the patient is not properly grounded.[98] The microelectrode guide tube is an excellent ground. High (> 200 Hz), low pass (< 2 Hz), and adaptive noise filters are used, and there is almost never a need for a notch filter (60 Hz). The neurophysiologist and/or neurologist and neurosurgeon interpret the signal once it is optimized. This is done by examining both visual and auditory amplifications of the local neural electrical output. Due to the rapid appearance of spikes across the screen, the ear can distinguish small changes in the neural signal better than the eye. A good auditory amplifier and trained ear are essential for properly interpreting MER. Headphones are not necessary. There is only one opportunity to correctly evaluate a tract. The microdrive is essential to slowly transverse the tract. Moving too quickly through an area will miss boundaries and opportunities to interrogate cells.

We use the Axon Instruments Guideline System 3000A (distributed by FHC, Brunswick, ME) (**Fig. 7.3**) and are testing multiple MER systems (**Fig. 7.4**). There are several systems available for multiple simultaneous MERs (i.e., Alpha Omega Microguide system, Medtronic StimPilot, and FHC microtargeting drive system). The multiple MER systems

appear to allow greater amounts of data to be more efficiently obtained. This has been our experience with either two, three, or five microelectrodes. Whether single or multiple MERs are used, the number of tracts needs to

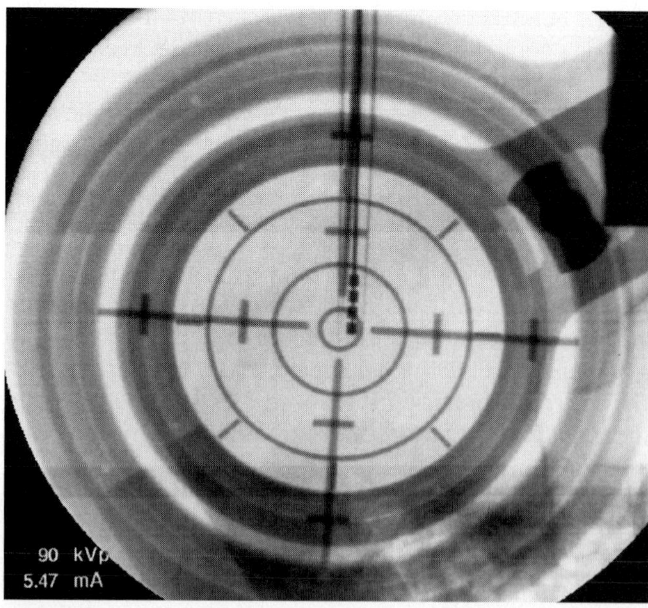

Fig. 7.4 Intraoperative fluoroscopy of a five microelectrode recording (MER) approach to the subthalamic nucleus is shown. The nucleus has been mapped and the medial microelectrode had the longest and most active tract. This electrode has been removed and the deep brain stimulation lead inserted in its place. The guide cannulae of the other four microelectrodes act to "fix" the brain in place to help maintain spatial accuracy and prevent "brain shift" before lead placement.

Table 7.1 Sources of Noise during Microelectrode Recording

ROOM	Headstage
	ELECTRODE
Fluorescent lights	Too high impedance
Bovie	Too low impedance
Bipolar	Damaged or bent tip
Metal to metal contact on the frame	Poor contact
Electrocardiogram	
PATIENT	GROUND
	Improper location
Cerebrospinal fluid pulse artifact	Poor contact
Headstage movement	
Patient speaking or coughing	CABLE
	Wire damaged or broken
	Failed shielding
	Crossed wires

be sufficient to ensure the optimal target. This decision is based on experience and the art of functional neurosurgery. There is the strong but unproven belief that the fewer the tracts the safer the procedure. The rate of symptomatic hemorrhages between single and multiple MERs is similar, with an incidence of 1 to 3% (see Chapter 8). For DBS this low rate is expected. Furthermore, many centers using five simultaneous MERs have few complications and excellent efficacy.[82] It is not likely that results will vary based only on the number of microelectrode penetrations. We primarily use multiple single MER tracts but are increasingly testing multiple (simultaneous) MER and prefer three tracts to obtain maximum information with minimal trauma.

We and others[98] routinely perform microstimulation to "condition" the microelectrode to enhance its recording performance. Sometimes the sterilization process can leave a layer of oxidative by-products on the electrode, which interferes with MER. A short burst of current (25 to 40 µA, 500 µs, and 300 Hz) "cleans" the electrode tip. Frequent impedance checks to keep it in the 0.3 to 0.6 Mohm range are performed throughout a tract, and the cleaning process may need to be repeated. The patient must be completely awake during recording because stupor will dramatically suppress the electrical activity. During the recording of single units, the microdriver is paused and the contralateral body is manipulated to trigger firing of neurons that respond to either active, passive, or tremor movements called sensorimotor responses. In all structures, we search for kinesthetic responses to passive movements about joints or voluntary movements. In the thalamus, we also search for responses to light touch, deep pressure, and hot/cold stimuli. At the end of the pallidal tract, if visual responses are expected due to proximity to the optic tract, a bright light (fiberoptic cable works best) is flashed back and forth into the eyes. Just as important in plotting the map are the quiet areas. These can be used to clearly define nuclei even when the individual unit activity is unclear or not present due to poor recordings or general anesthesia. Also very useful is the

recognition of cellular background or neural noise (the primary function of semimicroelectrodes). The increased activity that occurs when a nucleus is entered and lost when exited is similarly helpful in defining boundaries parallel to the quiet areas. Increased background can be heard and seen. Thus, even if no action potentials are recorded for a good length of time, as long as the background is active the nuclear boundary has not been crossed, nor should a lamina be suspected as long as the volume setting is unchanged.

There are many possible artifacts that can occur (**Table 7.1**). Mechanical artifacts are common and frequently misinterpreted by the inexperienced examiner (**Fig. 7.5**). A little blood on the MER or guide tubes is meaningless but unexpected electrical silence should raise the suspicion of hemorrhage, and careful clinical evaluation is mandated. Isolation of individual neurons is optimal but not essential for interrogation of sensorimotor responses. Passive and active joint movements should be sought in a systematic fashion. Assessment of the movement-related neuronal activity provides important information in isolating the motor territory. Movements should be vigorous and any increase or decrease in firing rates should be confirmed by reexamination at a later time. Always doubt any positive results and try to prove them wrong. Fast firing rhythmic neurons and bursting cells can present a problem for interrogation. Rhythmic movements of the joints may result in false-positive conclusions of kinesthetic response, and irregular movements of the joints may be needed to bring about a correct conclusion.

Intraoperative Testing

During MER, data are gathered and the physiological information is annotated on the corresponding stereotactic atlases.[100,101] Maps such as the Schaltenbrand and Wahren atlas were not prepared using brains of patients with severe movement disorders and may not represent the true anatomical mapping in this group of patients, but it is the

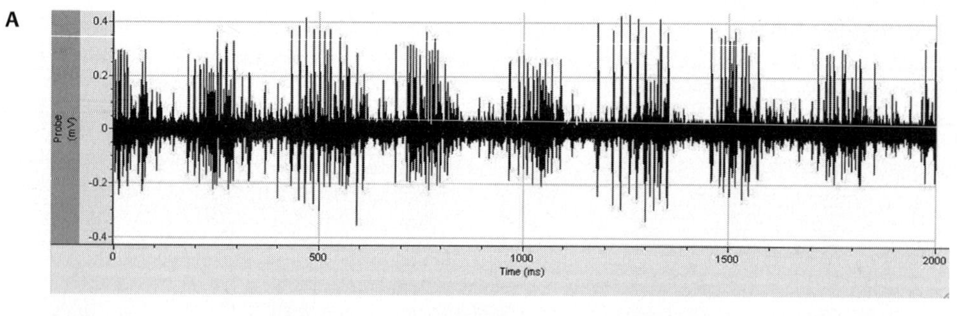

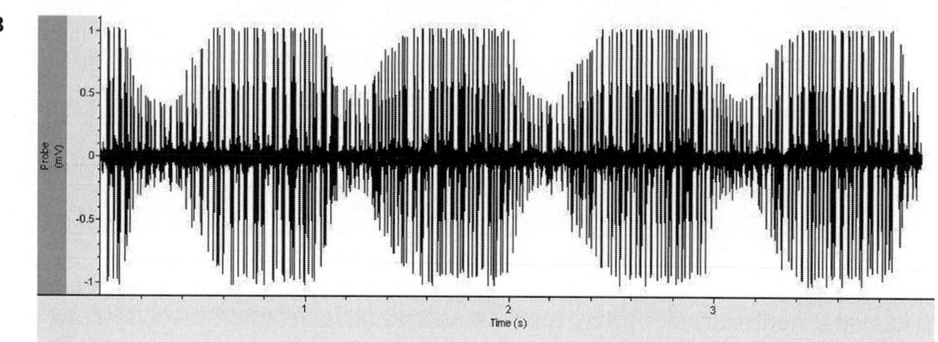

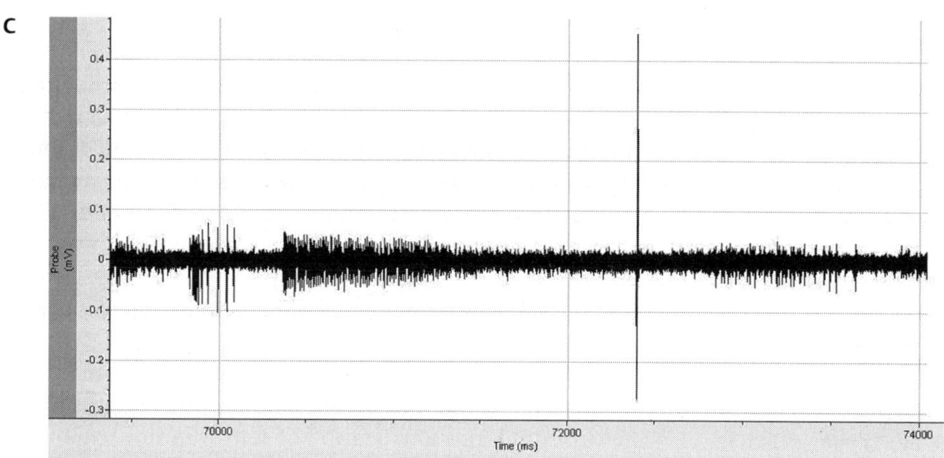

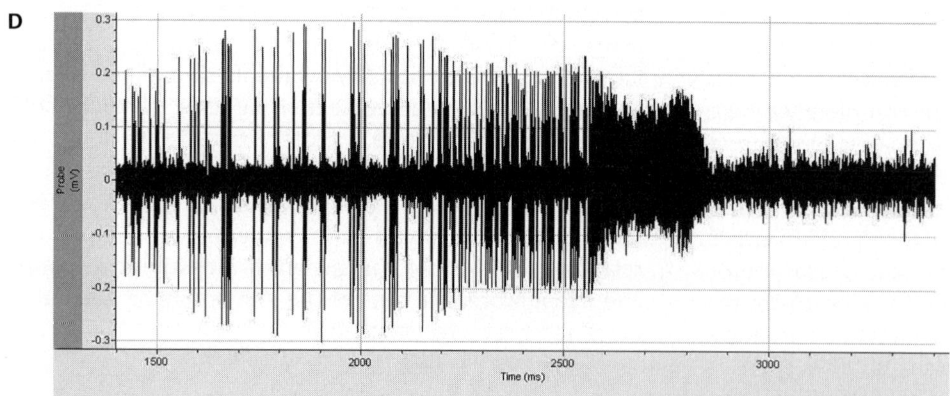

Fig. 7.5 Several unusual electrophysiological tracings are demonstrated in this figure: **(A)** Mechanical artifact is demonstrated in this electrophysiological tracing. The intermittent increase in activity represents an artificial increase in the action potential height of a poorly isolated cell in relation to mechanical effects of tremor on the frame. **(B)** Pulse artifact is demonstrated with a rate that will parallel the electrocardiographic tracing. **(C)** Insertional activity is demonstrated in the striatum. The initial activity from inserting the microelectrode initiates action potentials, which gradually fade. In addition, there is fiber activity seen as a very large action potential. If this were to be placed on a longer time scale, one would see that the wave form of the fiber is inverted. **(D)** Mechanical injury potential with loss of membrane integrity and rupture of the cell leading to aberrant action potentials followed by silence.

best map available to date.[102] Precise mapping of any target nucleus often requires multiple trajectories to complete the electrophysiological map and determine the best fit. Just because the frame is set at 11 or 20 mm from midline does not mean the map will fit on the atlas at 11 mm or 20 mm. The individual variability must be form fitted so the MER and the atlas align reasonably well. Thus the anatomical 20 mm location may fit best at 21.5 mm by the electrophysiology. At the conclusion of each track, we perform microstimulation with the same microelectrode starting at 5 µA and increasing up to 100 µA (biphasic pulses) to elicit responses. Localization of the optimal target is followed either by the insertion of a radio frequency (RF) probe and generation of a lesion or by insertion of the DBS lead. Macrostimulation is then performed to physiologically confirm the anatomical target prior to lesioning or stimulator placement. Intraoperative stimulation tests for efficacy and confirms lack of side effects to an acceptable threshold. Intraoperative neurological examination may demonstrate functional improvement of the patient during MER, lesion generation, or lead placement, which is a good indicator of the ultimate clinical outcome. We will describe the typical neurophysiological characteristics of the thalamus, GPi, and STN.

Thalamic Microelectrode Recordings

Using the sagittal diagrams of the human brain from the Schaltenbrand and Bailey atlas,[101] the anatomy of the thalamus can be defined (see Chapter 11) with the ventralis intermedius nucleus (Vim) being the target (**Fig. 11.5**). This is a small (2 mm wide) subnucleus. The target is the hand area at the Vim and ventralis oralis posterior (Vop) border (~6 mm anterior to the PC, 10 to 10.5 lateral to the third ventricular wall, and in the AC–PC plane). This is an ill-defined

target on MRI (Fig. 11.6). The optimal angle is 60 degrees from the AC–PC to parallel the Vim and Vop subnuclear borders. Notice that the ventralis caudalis (Vc) nucleus constitutes the relay for sensory or tactile stimuli transmitted in the medial lemniscus.[26] Interestingly, neurons in the dorsal portion of the Vc and central and dorsal nuclear subdivisions that lie more superiorly in the thalamus do not respond to any known stimuli. Caudal Vc (ventracaudalis parcocellularis externus, Vcpe) is identified when high-amplitude evoked responses are obtained when the contralateral body is lightly touched. Low threshold (5 to 10 µA) microstimulation resulting in a precise paresthesia will help to confirm the location, as opposed to the medial lemniscus, which produces widespread paresthesia (hemiparesthesia or whole limb). Just anterior to the Vc is what has been described as the "shell" nucleus (ventrocaudalis anterior externus, Vcae), which responds best to deep pressure.[1] The Vc nucleus serves as a "navigational landmark," and MER movements are based on this information (**Table 7.2**).

The somatotopic organization of the thalamus has been well described with the lower-limb sensory neurons lying more laterally (14 to 16 mm) than hand (14 to 12 mm), or mouth (12 to 10 mm), and more medially no kinesthetic cells can be recorded.[1,38] We prefer to target the Vc and by advancing through the Vim (26 ± 4 Hz) identify both in the first pass (**Fig. 11.4**). Bursting cells synchronous to tremor are a significant feature of the Vim. Immediately anterior to the Vim is the Vop (18 ± 3 Hz), which represents the pallidothalamic relay.[26] "Tremor" cells can also occur in Vop but are infrequent. Another potential difference between the two is the kinethetic (movement sensing) response: Vim cells respond primarily to passive movement and Vop cells respond primarily to active movement of contralateral joints (voluntary cells). Our second pass is 2 to 4 mm anterior to the first to identify Vim/Vop and determine the bottom of

Table 7.2 Findings and General Rules for Possible Corrections for Suboptimal Vim Deep Brain Stimulation Trajectories*

	Anterior	Posterior	Medial	Lateral
Caudate	Present	Possibly absent	Possibly absent	Present
Anterior thalamus	Longer	Shorter	Longer	Shorter
Vop/Vim	Same or longer; few SM or tremor cells	Shorter; few to no SM or tremor cells	Shorter; many SM and tremor cells	Longer; many SM and tremor cells
Vc	Absent	Early entry; responds to sensory arm	Early entry; responds to sensory face	Late or no entry; responds to sensory leg
End of tract	Zona incerta	Stop after in Vc	Medial lemniscus	Zona incerta
Corrections	Move 2–3 mm posterior to identify Vc and adjust accordingly	Move 3–4 mm anterior to be at the Vop/Vim boundary	Move 2–4 mm anterior and 1–2 mm lateral to be at the Vop/Vim boundary	Move 2–4 mm anterior and 2 mm medial to be at the Vop/Vim boundary

* The trajectory is designed to find the Vc (crossing mid to lower Vim) at the level of the sensorimotor hand area in the initial tract and move 3 to 4 mm anterior for deep brain stimulation lead placement at the Vop/Vim border. The approach is rectilinear at 60 degrees, and targeting errors are ~2 mm. Findings are compared with the ideal tract. Vc medially is more anterior. Different angles, nonrectilinear approach, or greater targeting errors could produce different findings and require different corrections.

Abbreviations: SM, sensorimotor response; Vc, ventralis caudatus; Vim, ventralis intermedias; Vop, ventralis oralis posterior.

the thalamus. If we have a dual MER setup, we target 4 mm apart in AP (2 and 6 mm anterior to PC) with the anterior MER at target.

Certain pitfalls should be kept in mind when one is exploring the thalamus. The posterior ventromedial nucleus (Vmpo) has been shown in the monkey to receive direct inputs from spinal cord lamina I nociceptive and thermoreceptive neurons.[103] This ventral nucleus is located at the inferoposterior rim of the Vc, and neurons may respond to warm, cold, or noxious stimuli. The Vmpo nucleus overlaps with the Hassler parvocellular Vc (Vcpc) nucleus.[104] Interrogation and stimulation of this area can confuse less experienced investigators because the somatotopy is not the same as the Vc. Another pitfall is that quiet areas in the body of the thalamus may exist due to previous brain lesions, trauma, or infarcts. These lesions may disrupt the homuncular arrangement.[26] The bottom of the thalamus is usually clear with loss of background activity and only infrequent neurons recorded in the zona incerta (Zi) or fibers of the medial lemniscus. The key to success is to find the appropriate somatotropic area of the Vc and put the lead 3 to 4 mm anterior to it. Microstimulation (60 to 100 µA, 500 µs, and 300 Hz) can frequently but not reliably decrease tremor, so primarily we look for side effects. If positive, the MER is < 2 mm from the Vc or capsule, and a move is necessary. If negative, it is not informative. Additional details can be found in Chapter 11.

Globus Pallidus Internus Microelectrode Recording

Using the sagittal diagrams of the human brain ~20 mm from the midline based on the Schaltenbrand and Bailey atlas,[101] the anatomy of the GPi can be defined (**Fig. 7.6**). It is a lens-shaped nucleus ~500 mm³ (**Fig. 7.7**). The optimal angle is 45 degrees from the AC–PC. The initial trajectory is the ~3 mm anterior to the MCP, 17.5 mm lateral from the third ventricular wall (the equivalent of lateral 20), and 4 to 6 mm below the AC–PC plane.[2,6] A typical first microelectrode trajectory courses through the striatum (putamen), the globus pallidus externus (GPe), and finally the GPi. Ventrally beyond the GPi, the electrode crosses the pallidofugal axons (ansa lenticularis) and enters the optic tract. Because of the importance of finding the optic tract, adjustments are made to directly target the lateral edge of it on the first tract even if it is 19 or 18 mm lateral on coronal T1 images to assure this trajectory identifies this landmark (**Fig. 7.8**). The striatum shows a tonically active slow rate of firing, ranging from < 1 to 6 Hz. It frequently exhibits insertional activity that quickly fades, leaving only faint noise of background activity. Passage through the lateral medullary lamina, the background activity is quiet with rare border cells or fibers. Border cells fire regularly at 30 to 40 Hz, do not have receptive fields, and do not respond to movements.[2] When

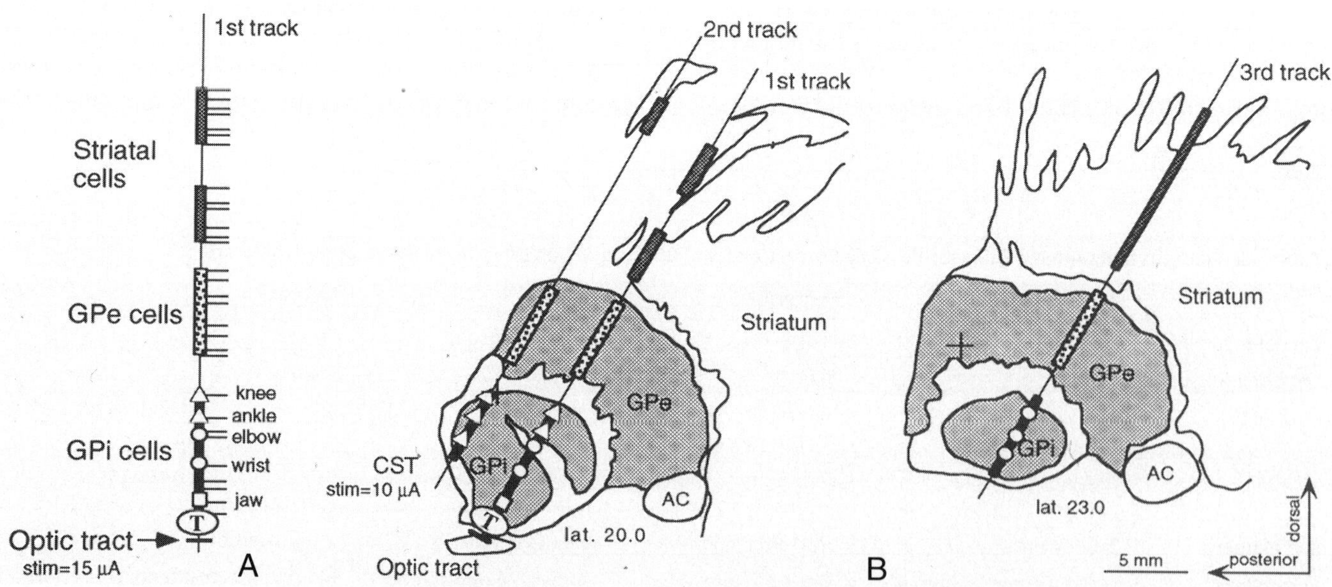

Fig. 7.6 Microelectrode mapping from a case of globus pallidus internus (GPi) is demonstrated. **(A)** The first track is directed toward the optic tract. Detailed findings are represented on the left. Nuclei, lamina, kinesthetic cells. and optic tract are recorded. **(B)** The microelectrode reconstructions are superimposed on sagittal drawings of the Schaltenbrand and Bailey atlas. The open rectangle segment represents putamen, the gray-shaded segments represent external pallidal activity (GPe), and the black-shaded segments, internal pallidal activity (GPi). Light-evoked action potential discharges (LED) were recorded 1 mm below the exit from the GPi at the end of track 1. We would place the deep brain stimulation lead 1 mm lateral and 0.5 mm anterior to track 1 to get further away from the corticospinal tract. The lead would terminate at the ventral border of the GPi. CST, corticospinal tracts. Adapted from Starr et al with permission.[3]

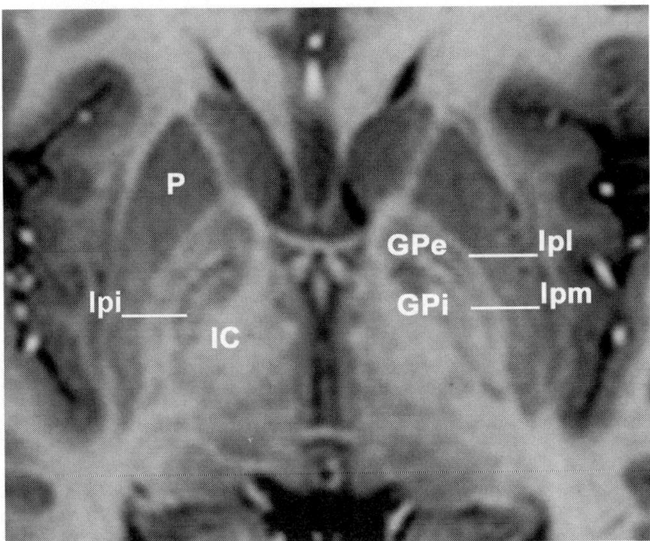

Fig. 7.7 Magnetic resonance imaging demonstrates an axial section in the anterior–posterior commissural plane. The globus pallidus is well demonstrated. Between the putamen (P) and the globus pallidus externa (GPe) is the lateral medullary lamina (lpl or Hassler's lamina pallidi lateralis) and between the GPe and globus pallidi interna (GPi) is the medial medullary lamina (lpm or Hassler's lamina pallidi medialis). Medial and posterior to the GPi is the internal capsule (IC). On the patient's right side in addition to the two laminae surrounding GPe, an additional lamina within the GPi, the accessory medullary lamina (lpi or Hassler's lamina pallidi incompleta) is present. Hassler used lpi to divide GPi into pme and pmi, but that only serves to unnecessarily confuse the nomenclature.

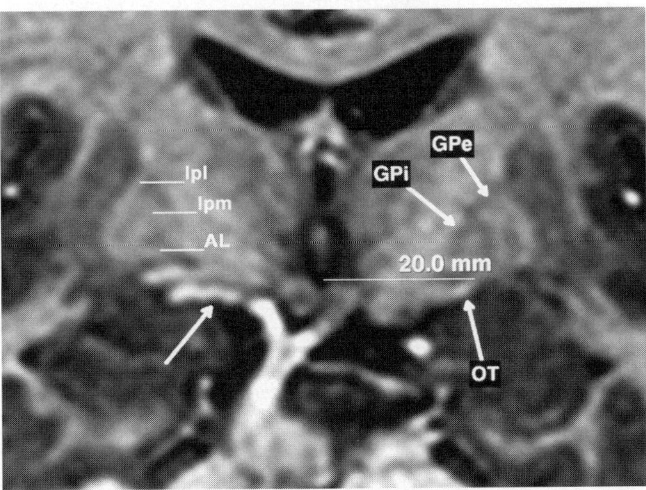

Fig. 7.8 Coronal magnetic resonance imaging at the level of the mammillary bodies demonstrating the globus pallidus externus (GPe) and internus (GPi) with the lateral (lpl) and medial (lpm) medullary lamina surrounding the GPe and the ansa lenticularis (AL) at the base of GPi. The optic tract (OT) is seen well on both sides allowing direct targeting. The patient's right side demonstrates a blood vessel (unmarked arrow), which can frequently accompany the optic tract in the ambient cistern and must be avoided. If the optic tract is not encountered within 1 to 2 mm of the anticipated location, it is not pursued deeper when a vessel is in the area.

entering the GPe, the background increases due to neural activity. Both the rate and the firing pattern will vary in GPe and GPi with the disease process and state of alertness.[2] Two types of GPe neurons are identifiable (**Fig. 7.9**). Most GPe neurons "sputter" with irregular pausing patterns with a firing rate of 50 ± 21 Hz. Rates may be slower with hyperkinetic disorders. About 10 to 20% of GPe neurons fire at low frequency (18 ± 12 Hz) with high-frequency, short duration bursts. Kinesthetic responses are not generally observed in the trajectories used for this approach, because they reside in the posterior putamen. As the electrode leaves the GPe, the medial medullary lamina is crossed, which is a 1 to 3 mm wide band of fibers characterized by the absence of somatodendritic action potentials and no neural background activity (electrical silence except for background noise). If too lateral, this lamina is 4 to 6 mm thick. This is a key finding and will assist separating the GPe from the GPi even under general anesthesia. The accessory medullary lamina partially divides the GPi into inner and outer subdivisions. Again, this will assist in determining laterality. A short GPi and large accessory medullary lamina should not be confused for the internal medullary lamina and a too lateral plane. A posterior move will make the lateralization clear. At the periphery of the GPi in any of the lamina, border cells frequently occur. Border cells are believed to be aberrantly located neurons of the nucleus basalis of Meynert.[2,105] A very large number of these cells at the end of a tract suggest far anterior location in the basal forebrain.

In PD, GPi neurons fire faster than GPe neurons at 82 ± 24 Hz with a less irregular discharge pattern and shorter pauses. Vitek et al[2] report that other patterns may be present such as high-frequency bursts or activity with little pauses between the bursts, creating a "chugging" sound, or lower frequency bursts in the range of 4 to 6 Hz in patients with PD. The 4 to 6 Hz pattern may or may not be associated with overt tremor. The optimal target within the globus pallidus has been a subject of debate.[106–111] The target most commonly used today is the posteroventral GPi.[108] The same target is used for dystonia but the rates of firing of GPe and GPi are similar, and careful attention to boundaries is essential.[112] Additional details on dystonia can be found in Chapter 12. The sensorimotor area resides in the most posterior and lateral region of the GPi. The sensorimotor territory is bounded by the ambient cistern and the optic tract ventrally and the internal capsule at the posterior and medial borders. The manipulation of the individual joints of the contralateral body will localize the sensorimotor territory of the GPi (**Fig. 7.10**). Approximately 25% of neurons in the posteroventral portion of the GPi respond to kinesthetic movements, and many will respond to multiple joints. The GPi is somatotopically organized with the lower extremity represented more medial and dorsal than the upper extremity.[2,60,113–115] This is the inverse of Vim but similar to STN. The jaw represen-

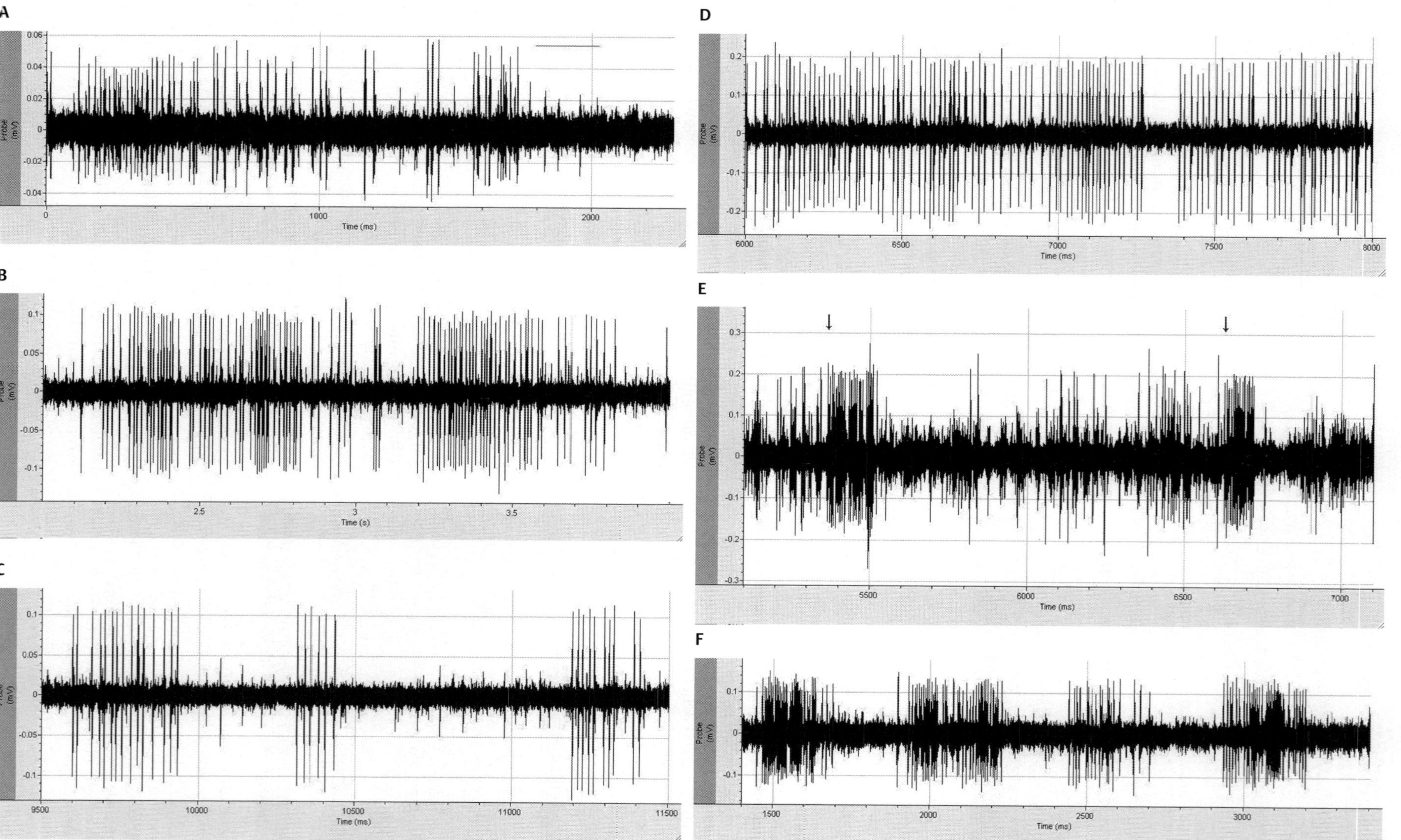

Fig. 7.9 Electrophysiological recordings on the way toward demarcation of the sensorimotor area of the globus pallidus internus (GPi) are illustrated: **(A)** Insertional activity is demonstrated from recordings in the putamen. **(B)** A high-frequency firing pattern with irregular and intermittent pausing is characteristic of the most common type of globus pallidus externus (GPe) cells. **(C)** Less common is the regular bursting activity seen in this GPe cell. **(D)** A typical GPi high-frequency neuron has very few and very short pauses. **(E)** A GPi cell responds to flexion at the elbow (*arrows*). This is a poorly isolated cell and there are mechanical artifacts, but the response pattern can still be seen. **(F)** Rhythmic activity in the GPi is uncommon.

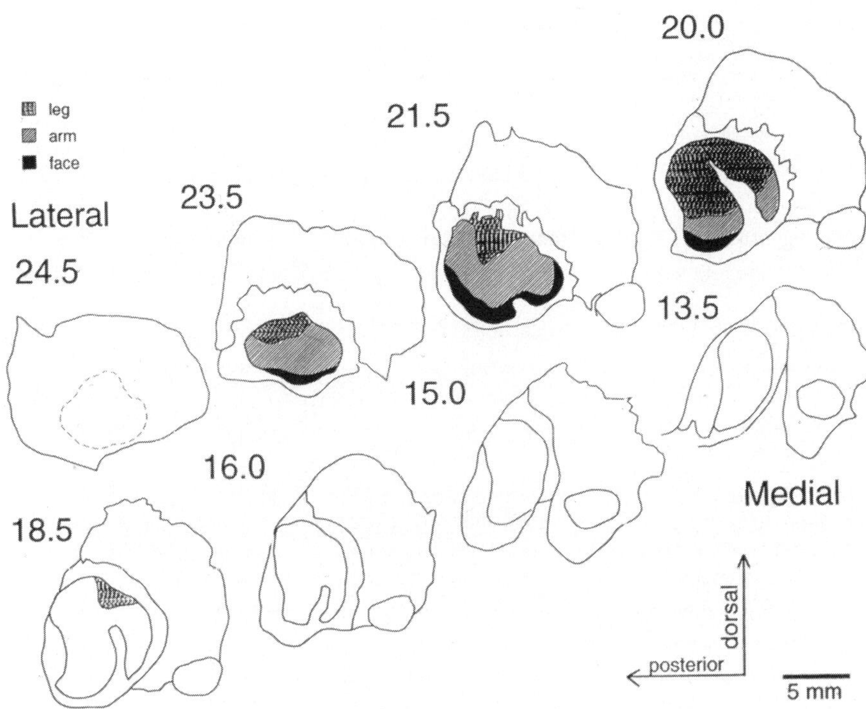

Fig. 7.10 This drawing represents a composite of the sensorimotor responsive areas in the globus pallidus internus (GPi) from 10 patients, with different body areas demonstrated in different shades. The leg kinesthetic area is demonstrated predominantly dorsally and medially, whereas the arm is more evident laterally and ventrally. Far less common are responses to the face, which are usually very ventral. A track with a predominance of leg responsive cells would be medial, whereas a track with a predominance of arm cells would be lateral. There are cells that will respond to multiple joints, including some that respond to both upper and lower extremities. These are predominantly near the border between the two and are ignored in this diagram. Note a very short segment of the GPi with only the upper extremity could occur in an anterior tract at 20.0, 21.5, or 23.0 mm lateral, and a posterior tract is needed for lateralization. The anterior medial areas (associative) lack responsive cells. The anterior commissure is anterior and the internal capsule is posterior except at 24, where the putamen surrounds the GPe. Nucleus basalis is anterior and ventral. (Adapted from Vitek et al[2] with permission.)

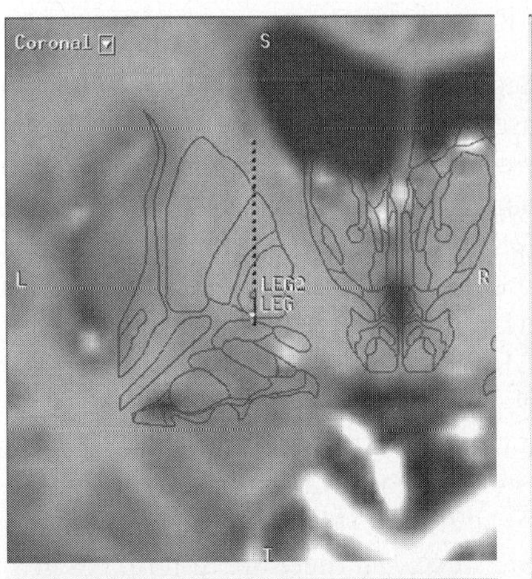

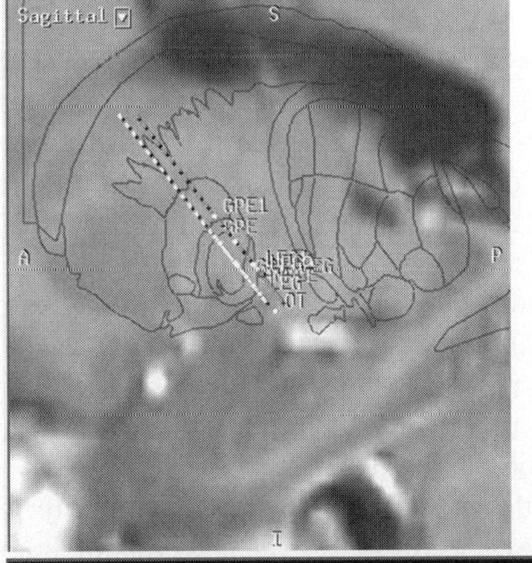

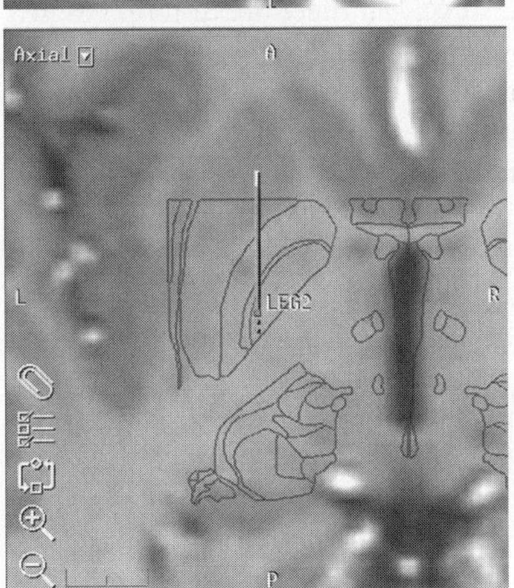

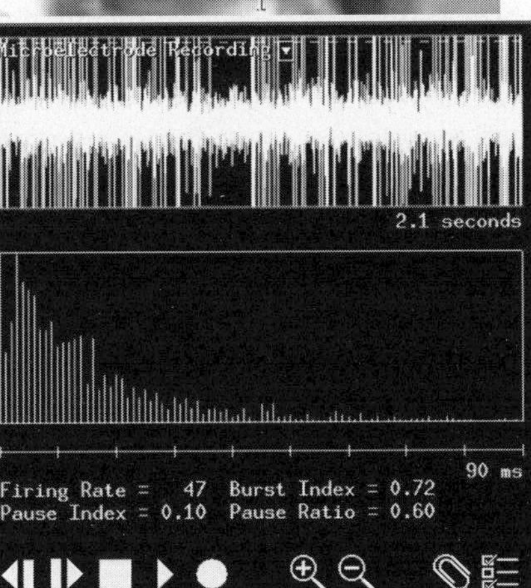

Fig. 7.11 This is an image from the StealthStation (Medtronic Navigation, Louisville, CO) during intraoperative tracings for globus pallidus internus (GPi) deep brain stimulation (DBS). Coronal, axial, sagittal, and electrophysiological recording views are demonstrated in four separate panels. Details can be lost in the transformation of reformatted images. Therefore, we prefer to calculate the initial coordinates from the volumetric axial images using an independent console software in the magnetic resonance suite to maximize the anatomical details and adjust them if the *x* and/or *y* planes are not aligned perpendicular or parallel, respectively, to the anterior–posterior commissure (AC–PC). The computer-calculated coordinates also act as a confirmation of the console calculations. A standardized Schaltenbrand atlas is overlaid and stretched for the best possible fit with this patient's anatomy. The previous tract is shown with annotations to the optic tract (OT) on the sagittal view. Note that the dense concentration of kinesthetic cells makes individual cell identification difficult (see sagittal view). The recording on the right is from a GPi leg2 cell (leg responsive cell in tract #2). This tract will eventually identify the corticospinal tract.

Table 7.3 Findings and General Rules for Possible Corrections for Suboptimal Globus Pallidus Internus Deep Brain Stimulation Trajectories*

	Anterior	Posterior	Medial	Lateral
Putamen	Short length	Short or absent	Absent	Long length
GPe	Enter slightly lower	Enter slightly higher	Enter higher	Enter lower
GPi	Enter lower SM = primarily upper extremities; may have lamina	Enter higher Short length SM = primarily lower extremities	Enter higher SM = primarily lower extremities or none	Enter lower Short length SM = primarily upper extremities
Ratio GPe/GPi	Equal or greater than 1	Greater than 1	Equal or less than 1	Greater than 1
End of tract	Ambient cistern or basal forebrain	Internal capsule	Internal capsule	Ambient cistern
Macrostimulation effect, if any	None	Corticospinal	Corticospinal	None
Corrections	Move posterior 2–4 mm to increase GPi and find OT; an additional lateral tract needed for confirmation	Move anterior 2–4 mm to increase GPi and find OT; an additional lateral tract needed for confirmation	Move lateral 2 mm to obtain SM responses and find OT; an additional posterior tract needed for confirmation	Move medial 2 mm to increase GPi and find OT; an additional posterior tract needed for confirmation

* The initial target is a tract through the GPi to the optic tract at about lateral 20. This assumes a 45 degree angle and rectilinear approach to the GPi with an error of ~3 mm. Findings are compared with an ideal tract. The GPi laterally is more posterior. We eventually want to end up at approximately lateral 21. Different angles, nonlinear approaches, or greater errors could give different findings and require different corrections. *Abbreviations*: AP, anteroposterior; M-L, medial-lateral; GPi, globus pallidus internus; GPe, globus pallidus externus; OT, optic tract; SM, sensorimotor response.

tation is found more ventrally. With adequate sampling (4–6 kinestetic cells), the GPi somatotopy can be trusted in helping determine laterality.

The optic tract can be identified electrophysiologically ventral to the GPi by darkening the room and flashing a light in the patient's eyes and listening for high-frequency modulation of the background audio signal coincident with the light stimulus. Microstimulation (5 to 20 µA, 500 µs, and 300 Hz) of the optic tract produces brief speckles or flashes of light of various colors in the contralateral visual field (focal scintillating scotomata) in ~80% of patients. By using contrast MRI, we avoid causing hemorrhages in the ambient cistern (**Fig. 7.11**). We and others[116] ultimately want to be at the equivalent of lateral 21.5 rather than 20 lateral or ~4 mm from the pallidal capsular borders. A second tract 3 to 4 mm posterior is needed to define the posterior border and corticospinal tract. The internal capsule can be identified by observing stimulation-induced (5 to 60 µA, 500 µs, and 300 Hz) movement of the contralateral tongue, face, or limbs. The somatotopy of the corticospinal system suggests stimulation of the tongue or face is medial to the appropriate target, whereas hand responses suggest a position too anterior. Both the optic and corticospinal tracts are landmarks for MER moves (**Table 7.3**). A final lateral tract should complete the mapping, but if uncertainty exists do additional tracts. Microstimulation (60 to 100 µA, 500 µs, and 300 Hz) does not reliably decrease rigidity so primarily we look for side effects. Even with MER, the nucleus is large, and using relative heights and not completely mapping GPi can result in lesion all over the GPi.[55]

Subthalamic Nucleus Microelectrode Recording

Using the sagittal diagrams of the human brain ~12 mm from the midline based on the Schaltenbrand and Bailey atlas,[101] the anatomy of the STN can be defined (**Fig. 7.12**). This is an almond-shaped nucleus with a volume reported from 125 mm^3 to 238 mm^3.[7,117] The optimal approach is 60 degrees from the AC–PC. The target is 3 mm posterior to the MCP, 11 to 12 mm lateral from the midline, and 4 mm below the AC–PC plane. Direct visualization can be performed on T2 or inversion recovery (IR) coronal (**Fig. 7.13**) or axial images (**Fig 7.14**), but the accuracy is questionable.[19,21,22] We and others[19,20,72] use indirect localization based on the red nucleus as an internal landmark (**Fig. 7.14**) but others find the relationship inconsistent.[118] If there are differences in x, y, or z calculations between indirect and direct targeting, we modified them slightly in the direction of the direct imaging. The STN dimensions are ~4 to 6 mm dorsoventral, 6 to 8 mm mediolateral, and 11 to 13 mm anteroposterior.[7,70,119] Detailed studies in primates demonstrate that the STN is obliquely oriented along the three anatomical axes, with its own axis being 20 degrees oblique to the horizontal plane, 35 degrees oblique to the sagittal plane, and 55 degrees oblique to the frontal plane.[120] These oblique orientations make it somewhat difficult to target.[7] Thus a slight lateral to medial approach results in a longer tract through the STN.

We start 30 mm from the target and record the striatum (caudate) with its insertional activity at < 1 to 6 Hz or if too lateral enter the capsule with occasional fiber

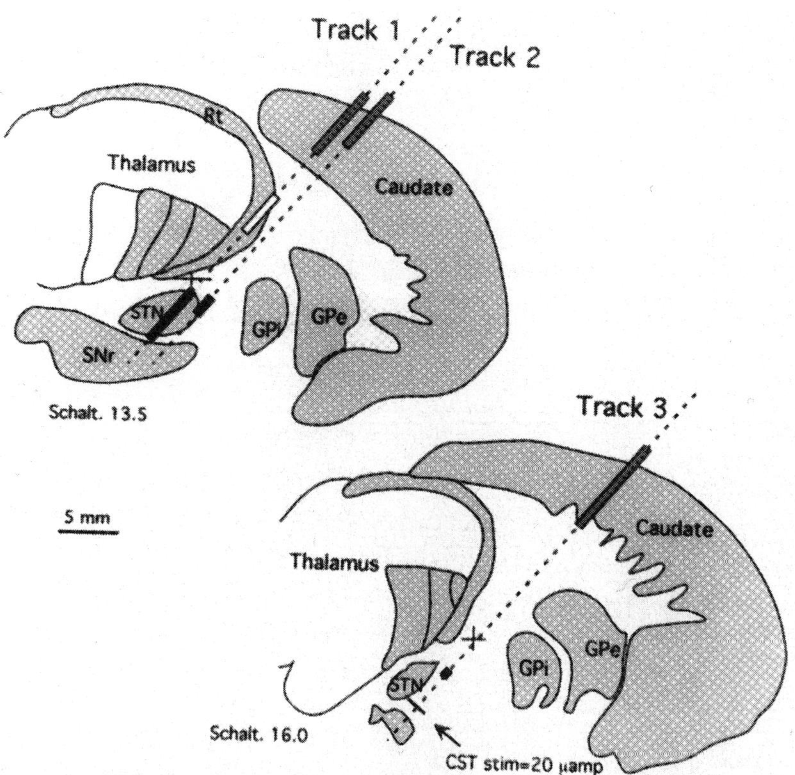

Fig. 7.12 Our method of microelectrode mapping of subthalamic nucleus and surrounding structures before placement of a deep brain stimulation (DBS) lead. Microelectrode track reconstructions are superimposed on parasagittal Schaltenbrand and Bailey brain atlas drawings. Segments of the track reconstructions are shaded to indicate striatal cells (*gray-shaded segment*), dorsal thalamic cells (*open segment*), or subthalamic nucleus (STN) cells (*black segment*). Note tracts 1 and 2 could not fit more laterally because there would be no STN in tract 3; nor could they fit more medially because tract 3 would be much longer. We would place the lead 1 mm medial to tract 1 given that there is no STN in tract 3, which is parallel to tract 1. The lead would terminate at the ventral border of the STN. The microstimulation threshold for corticospinal tract activation (CST stim) was determined at the end of track 3 (frequency = 300 Hz, pulse width = 200 μs). The + is the midcommissural point. (Adapted from Starr et al[3] with permission.)

activity. A typical trajectory passes through the anterior thalamus, followed by the relatively electrically quiet Zi and fields of Forel (H1 and H2), then the STN, and finally the substantia nigra pars reticulata (SNr).[3,19] Depending on the anteroposterior and lateral approach angles, the most anterior and dorsal portions of the trajectory may be silent if passing through the white matter of the internal capsule. Alternatively, if the trajectory is more medial or posterior, the anterior thalamic nuclei are penetrated. Typically, the reticular nucleus or the anterior thalamic nuclei (nucleus

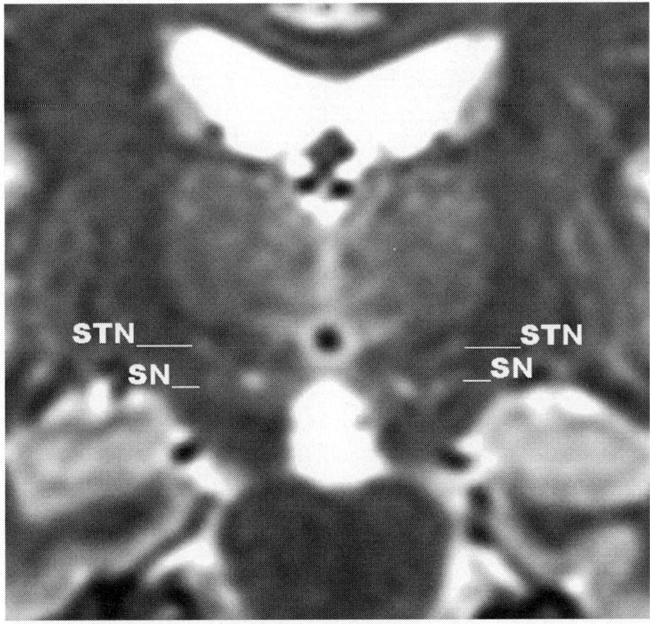

Fig. 7.13 Magnetic resonance coronal inversion recovery–Turbo spin echo (IR-TSE) image demonstrates very nicely the subthalamic nucleus (hyperintensity) at the top of the substantia nigra (SN). The SN is easily identifiable as a "mustache" below and medial to the STN.

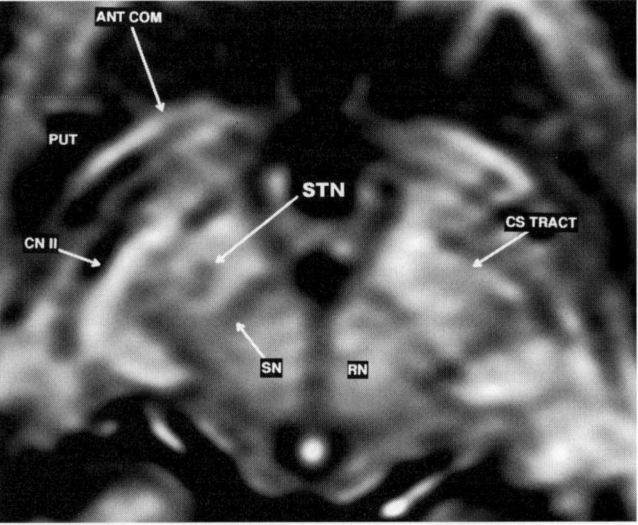

Fig. 7.14 Magnetic resonance axial IR-TSE image at the brain stem level that demonstrates both the subthalamic nucleus (STN) and the substantia nigra pars reticulata (SN). Rarely can images such as this be used for direct targeting; they are not always available nor is it always clear where the optimal STN target is located. The STN on the patient's right (*arrow*) is clear but incomplete. That on the left is unclear if the shadow is the STN or partial volume effect. In slices at higher levels, the STN and SNr become almost indistinct. RN is the red nucleus.

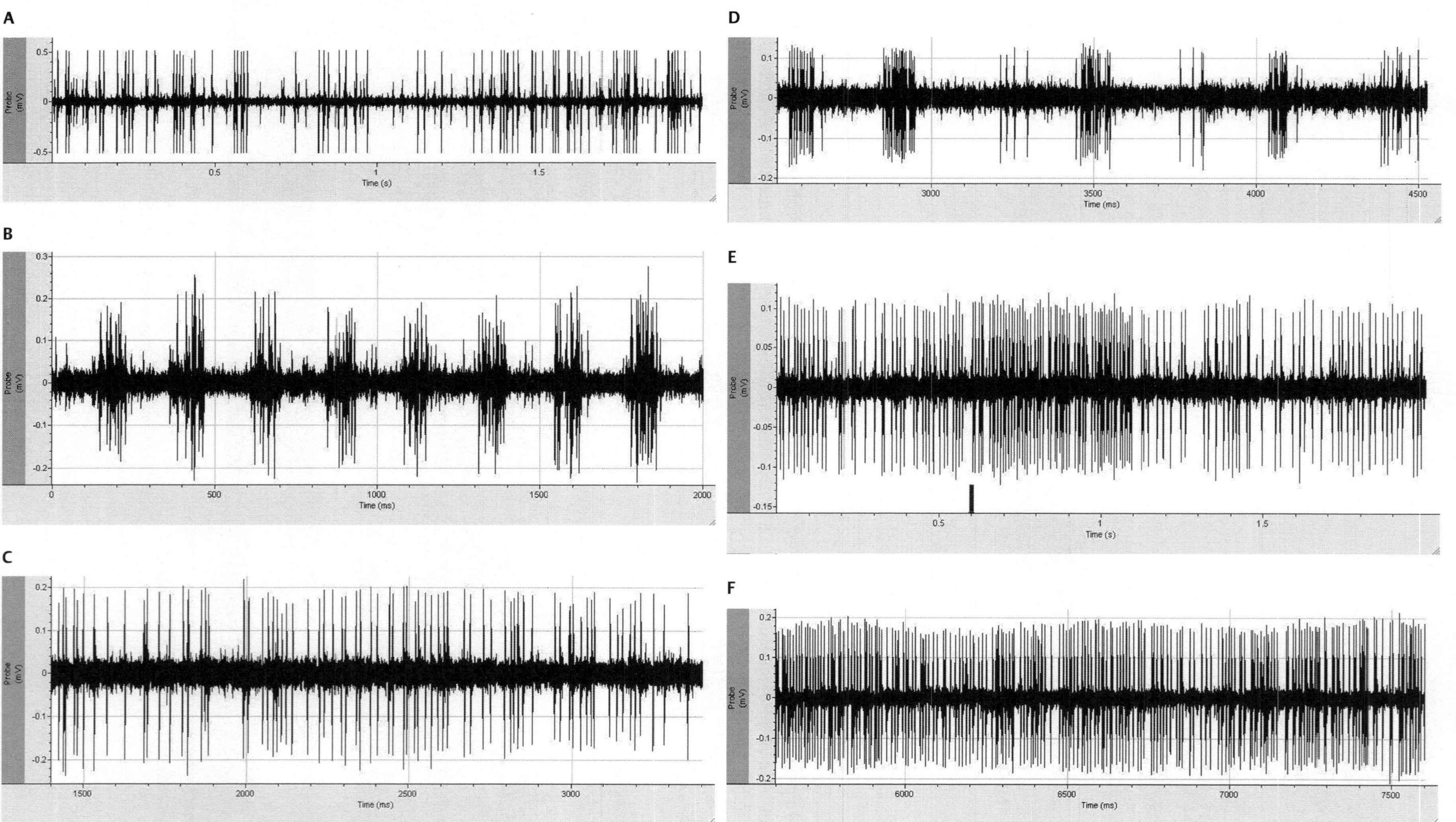

Fig. 7.15 This series of electrophysiological recordings demonstrates findings from a case of subthalamic nucleus (STN) deep brain stimulation (DBS). **(A)** A nonbursting thalamic cell is recorded. The anterior thalamus is usually low density and low amplitude. If a series of high amplitude cells in high density is encountered the tract may be posterior in the ventro-oralis posterior (Vop) nucleus. **(B)** A bursting thalamic cell is recorded whose firing pattern is un-related to tremor. **(C)** Typical STN recordings are demonstrated. Although not well isolated, it can be seen that there is a high-frequency cell with short pauses. Recording multiple units is typical of the densely packed STN. **(D)** An unusual STN cell with tremor-related activity. **(E)** A kinesthetic STN cell that responds to wrist flexion with increased activity (starting at the 6 second mark). **(F)** A typical substantia nigra pars reticulata cell is shown with high-frequency regular firing rates.

lateropolaris and nucleus ventralis oralis anterior) are encountered (**Fig. 7.15**). Cells in this region exhibit a low density and slow firing interposed with rapid bursts of activity called "bursting" cells (~15 Hz). Another cell type encountered exhibits nonbursting irregularly firing activity.[70] The ventral cells are more tonic and faster (28 Hz). A relatively quiet region is encountered as the electrode enters the thalamic fasciculus (H1 field of Forel), which contains very few cells. The Zi is a thin strip of gray matter below this fiber tract. The Zi may have an occasional large-amplitude tonic neuron, or less frequently, bursting neurons (25 to 45 Hz). Ventral to the Zi is another relatively quiet region containing the lenticular fasciculus (H2 fields of Forel), which carries pallidofugal fibers. There is no reliable landmark prior to STN (**Table 7.4**).

As the background noise increases, this indicates a region of increased cell density of the STN. The separation of the thalamus and STN is wider anteriorly and shorter posteriorly. The STN neurons exhibit irregular firing patterns with rates of 30 to 50 Hz. Occasionally (< 10%), regular bursting pattern in the 4 to 6 Hz synchronous with tremor are observed. The STN has somatic motor, limbic, associative, and oculomotor territories.[120] Multiple groups have demonstrated the somatotopic organization of the STN (**Fig. 7.16**) indicating that the leg territory is medial to the arm territory.[3,121–123] Because the overlap is so great, the somatotopy is not very reliable. A clinical pearl during STN MER in patients with a previous pallidotomy is that the activity in the STN appears to be decreased. When the patient is fully anesthetized, MERs in STN are lower voltage and have decreased neural background, and kinesthetic cells cannot be identified. Minimizing sedation may help but this can still lead to poorer targeting and less improvement when the patient is operated upon asleep as opposed to awake.[124]

While some groups look primarily at the length of the STN, others find the length alone does not correlate with optimal clinical results.[125,126] Long tracts of the STN with scant or no kinesthetic cells suggest a too medial tract. The lead should be in the sensorimotor area. We look for long tracts (4 to 6 mm) with multiple kinesthetic cells, preferably with both upper and lower sensorimotor responses and 3 mm from the anterior and lateral borders. Cells in the STN are densely packed, and individual cells may be difficult to isolate. Once STN cells are encountered, the microdriver is paused and the cells assessed for the presence of movement-related responses. Sixty-five percent of movement-related receptive fields were located in the dorsal half of the STN and 96.8% of these were located in the rostral two thirds.[127] Multiple studies suggest that the anterodorsal sector of the STN (especially laterally) or just dorsal within the Zi is the most clinically effective site for stimulation, which correlates with the sensorimotor part.[5,75,102,116,119] MRI resolution does not allow differentiation of the two sites.

As the microelectrode passes through the inferior border of the STN toward the SNr, the discharge pattern changes abruptly as the neuronal background activity is lost. There may be a few slow, low-voltage cells recorded. The SNr is

Table 7.4 Findings and General Rules for Possible Corrections for Suboptimal Subthalamic Nucleus Deep Brain Stimulation Trajectories*

	Anterior	Posterior	Medial	Lateral
Thalamus	Little or no thalamus; bottom of thalamus higher	Long thalamus; possible Vop; bottom of thalamus lower	Long thalamus; bottom of thalamus lower	Short or no thalamus; bottom of thalamus lower
Distance between thalamus and STN	Wider than 3 mm	Wider than 3 mm	Less than 3 mm	Less than 3 mm
STN	Short length; SM cells present	Short length; few SM cells present	Long length; few or no SM cells present (leg)	Long length; or smaller if > 2 mm; SM cells present (arm)
Distance between STN and SNr	Wider than 1mm; if > 2 mm anterior may not find SNr	Wider than 1 mm	Less than 1 mm	Less than 1 mm; or wider if > 2 mm lateral and may not find SNR
Microstimulation effect, if present	None, rarely corticospinal	Paresthesias	Oculomotor	Corticospinal
Corrections	Move 2 mm (4 mm if no STN) posterior to increase STN length; M-L moves may not make a difference or make it worse as will an anterior move	Move 2 mm (4 mm if no STN) anterior to increase STN; M-L moves may not make a difference or make it worse as will a posterior move and may miss posteriorly	Move 2 mm lateral to enter STN higher and record SM cells; AP moves may make no difference and medial will still lack SM cells and may miss posteriorly	Move 2 mm medial to enter STN higher and increase STN length; AP moves will not make a difference and may make it worse as will a lateral move and may miss anteriorly

* The target is a 4 to 6 mm length of STN with SM cells and no adverse effect with stimulation at approximately lateral 12. This assumes a 60 to 70 degree angle and near rectilinear approach to STN with an error of ~2 mm. Findings are compared with an ideal tract. STN laterally is more posterior. Different angles, nonrectilinear approaches, or greater errors could give different finings and require different corrections. *Abbreviations*: AP, anteroposterior; M-L, medial-lateral; SM, sensorimotor responsive; STN, subthalamic nucleus; SNr, substantia nigra pars reticulata; Vop, ventralis oralis posterior.

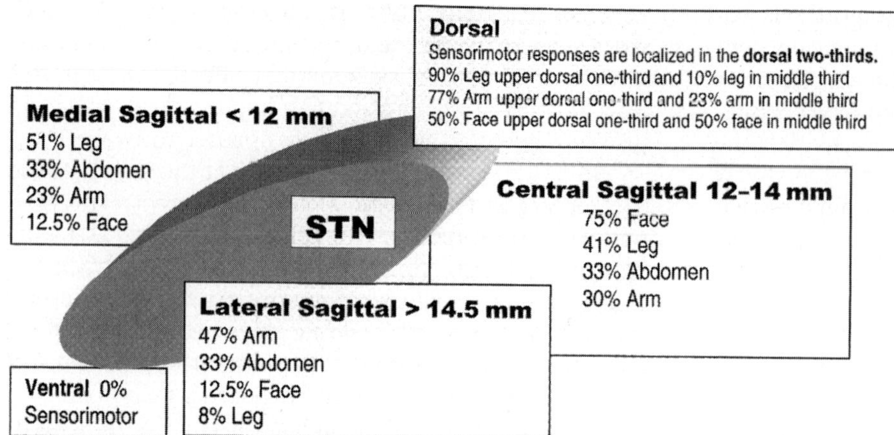

Fig. 7.16 Somatotopic organization of the subthalamic nucleus (STN) with representation of the arm, leg, and face demonstrated in percentages in relation to medial and lateral directions, respectively. Because of the cell density and difficulty isolating cells there are "cells" that will respond to multiple joints, including response to both upper and lower extremities. These occur throughout this diagram. It should be clear that overlap is so great that somatotopic findings are potentially unreliable for localization. (Adapted from Sierens and Bakay with permission.[97])

characterized by a lower density of cells with a regular pattern of firing and higher rates of discharge, ranging from 50 to 70 Hz. MER differentiation between the STN and the SNr can be difficult at times. The keys are the loss of neural background, faster single cell activity, and more tonic activity in the SNr. Distance between the STN and the SNr can be occasionally useful in localization. With a long STN and a short STN to SNr distance (0.5 to 1 mm) the tract is probably medial, whereas a longer separation (2 to 3 mm) or absence suggests a more lateral tract or posterior tract. We only record the first 2 or 3 mm of the SNr to confirm the cell type. Interestingly, intraoperative MER can contribute to the precise localization of STN without demonstrating significantly increased injury at the histopathological level as demonstrated by Counelis et al[128] in a postmortem study. However, a microlesion effect is frequently observed with well-placed STN leads. Microstimulation (60 to 100 µA, 500 µs, and 300 Hz) can decrease rigidity or tremor and may induce dyskinesias, but stimulation effects are not reliable. Primarily, we look for side effects, which, if present, will suggest the need to move the target. Additional details on Benabid's approach can be found in Chapter 9.

Implanting the Lead

After localization of the target is satisfactorily confirmed by MER, a permanent lead may be implanted into the Vim, GPi, or STN. Drills, sharp instruments, and forceps with teeth should not be used around the DBS equipment. We use rubber shodded instruments but care must still be taken not to crush the wire. The DBS lead has an inner stylet but it is still flexible. We use a rigid guide cannula that is placed at the target and allows the DBS lead to be inserted through this cannula. We do not like to drive the DBS lead through tissue because the lead can easily be deflected even over short distances. The DBS lead is a quadripolar electrode, and each contact is made of cylindrical platinum/iridium alloy that is 1.5 mm long and 1.27 mm in diameter. DBS leads can be obtained with contacts spaced 1.5 mm apart, which is typically used for GPi and occasionally Vim (Model 3387, Medtronic, Inc; www.medtronic.com/physician/activa/ downloadable-files/197928_a_005.pdf). Alternatively, contacts spaced 0.5 mm apart are often used for STN or Vim (Model 3389, Medtronic). The proximal portion of the lead consists of four nickel conductor wires insulated with a polytetrafluoroethylene jacket. The contact at the most distal tip is named contact 0 and the most proximal contact is named contact 3. To confirm the position and trajectory of the MER and DBS lead, the use of intraoperative fluoroscopy through the bombsites, or cross-hairs is recommended. Lateral fluoroscopy prior to removal of the microelectrode and after the DBS lead is seated should be compared. When using the frameless system a ring and dot can be made from a standard electrocardiogram (EKG) pad and applied to the temples of the patient to be used as a reference point (see Chapter 10).

For intraoperative DBS bipolar screening, the black (cathode) and red (anode) alligator clips are attached to the DBS lead (most distal is now contact 3) and the other end is connected to a Medtronic model 3625 hand-held pulse generator. Many of the effects are not dissimilar to the programming problem discussed in Chapter 13. Symptomatic relief of tremor and rigidity is evaluated as the current is slowly increased. Vim stimulation (1 to 2 V, 90 µs, and 130 Hz) effectively suppresses PD and essential tremor (ET) (the latter may be less effective acutely). Tremor is less clearly affected by GPi or STN stimulation, and evaluation of rigidity (2 to 3 V, 90 µs, and 130 Hz) is generally a better predictor of efficacy.[129] The "microlesion" effect from placing the lead may partially or completely suppress the patient's symptoms. The voltage threshold for undesirable side effects such as persistent paresthesias, contralateral tonic contractions, ocular phenomena, mydriasis, fear, or dizziness is determined. For Vim the 0 contact is placed at the bottom of the thalamus and stimulated from 0 to 2. Macrostimulation (1 to 3 V, 90 µs, 130 Hz) must confirm effective tremor reduction unless the microlesion of lead placement has abolished the tremor. In that case, we insist on no side effects at voltages below 3 except transient paresthesia (10 to 20 sec). The most commonly observed side effects in Vim are contralateral paresthesias or contralateral contractions, indicating the lead is too posterior or too lateral, respectively.

For GPi, we use a Medtronic 3387 DBS lead and place the 0 contact at the bottom of GPi and stimulate from 1 cathode to 3 anode. Macrostimulation (1 to 3 V, 90 μs, 130 Hz) must confirm effective rigidity reduction unless the microlesion of lead placement has abolished the rigidity.[53] Macrostimulation in PD patients may decrease the tremor but this is not totally reliable.[53,71] In that case, we insist on no side effects at voltage below 4 (we will test up to 10 to be sure we have some effect). The bottom contact is not used, and visual stimulation is not a concern. The only reason to use this contact would be to confirm approximation to the optic tract (0 to 1 at 4 to 10 V, 90 μs, and 130 Hz), but with MER and fluoroscopy to determine depth this is usually unnecessary. There are also ~20 to 30% of patients who will not report visual responses, so a negative finding is not conclusive. Both PD and dystonic patients should have decreased tone with stimulation if not already improved by lead placement. The presence of dyskinesia is felt to be a good sign. The primary purpose of stimulation is to look for adverse effects to determine if the lead needs to be moved. The DBS pallidal target for PD or dystonia is slightly anterior and lateral to the usual pallidotomy target by 1–2 mm to prevent the spread of current to the internal capsule (dysarthria or contractures of face or arm). With higher-intensity stimulation necessary in many patients with dystonia,[61,65] we insist on no adverse effect with stimulation up to 5V. We always like to observe capsular side effect to confirm proper electrical function. If we have a good effect on rigidity from lead placement or stimulation, this is less important, but if not we will go up to 10 V and if necessary 200 μs in an attempt to observe capsular effects. Lack of a good effect on rigidity and no corticospinal effect suggest either a too lateral or a too anterior position. Be sure the Medtronic 3625 has fresh batteries, the proper polarity is set on the programmer, the circuit is not open and there is no short from the alligator clips touching each other or the headstage. Recheck the mapping and reposition the lead only if there is a very good reason to move it. The lead must be moved at least 2 mm or risk returning into the old tract. Fluoroscopy is essential to confirm AP moves and AP skull X-ray for lateral movement.

For STN, we use the Medtronic 3389 DBS lead and place the 0 contact at the bottom of the STN. This places the 1 contact in the dorsal STN and we expect effective stimulation between 0 cathode and 2 anode at 1 to 3 V, 90 μs, and 130 Hz. Macrostimulation must confirm effective rigidity reduction (tremor is less reliable) unless the microlesion of lead placement has abolished the rigidity.[7,77,119,129–132] In that case, we insist on no side effects at voltages below 3 V except transient paresthesia (10 to 20 seconds). Induction of dyskinesias during DBS lead placement generally predicts a good antikinetic effect of chronic STN stimula-

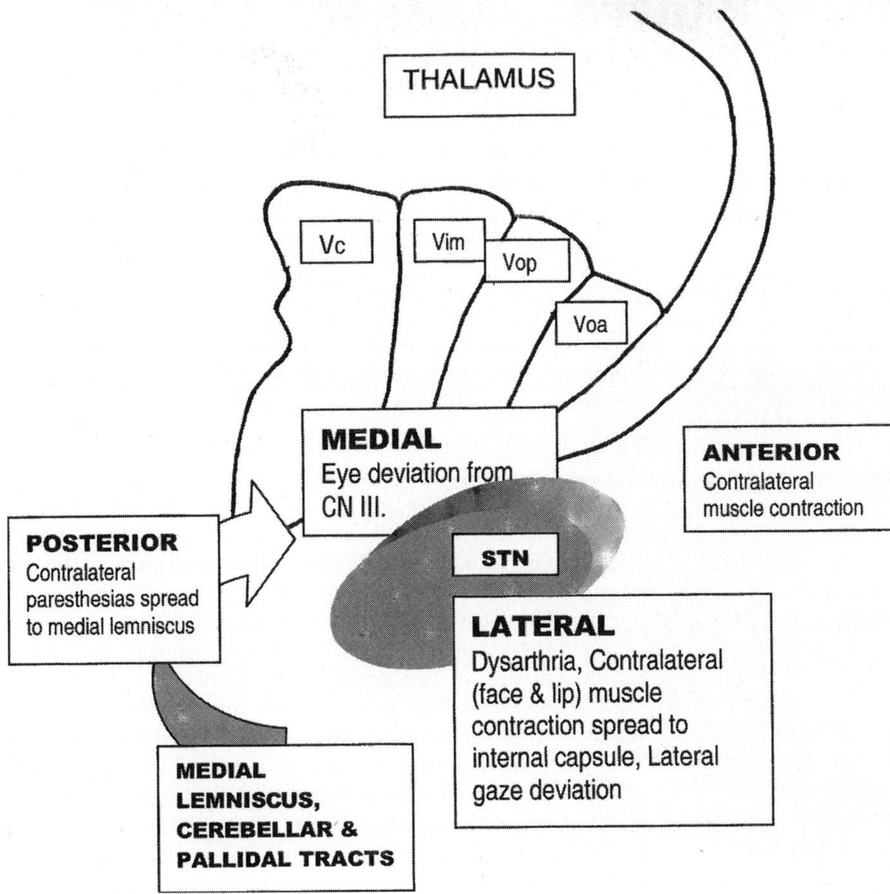

Fig. 7.17 Acute stimulation effects typically seen when stimulating near the border of the subthalamic nucleus (STN) include contralateral muscle contractions and paresthesias. Low voltage stimulation (1–3 V, 90 μs, and 130 Hz) that produces speech or contractures of the face or limb suggests a lead placement too lateral, whereas sustained paresthesias suggest a too posterior position. Conjugate gaze suggests too lateral placement, whereas dysconjugate deviation suggests too medial and inferior location. There can be overlap, so oculomotor symptoms need to be combined with other findings to be reliable (i.e., speech or contractions laterally and nausea or vegetative symptoms medially). Mood changes suggest stimulation of the substantia nigra pars reticulata or lower associative areas of STN but higher leads may be effective without needing to move the lead. Vc, ventralis caudalis; Vim, ventralis intermedius nucleus; Vop, ventralis oralis posterior; Voa, nucleus ventro-oralis anterior. Adapted from Sierens and Bakay[97] with permission.

tion.[74,125,131] Other signs induced by stimulation are side effects such as paresthesias, ocular deviations, tetanic muscular contractions, dysarthria, vegetative symptoms, or visual disturbances.[78] Bejjani et al[7] described possible side effects seen with stimulation at the borders of the STN, which is similar to our findings (**Fig. 7.17**). Difficulties with speech or contractures of the face or limb at less than 3 V suggest a lead placement too lateral, whereas sustained paresthesias suggest a too posterior position, and nausea or vegetative symptoms suggest a too medial lead location. Conjugate gaze suggests too lateral placement, whereas dysconjugate deviation suggests too medial location. However, oculomotor symptoms need to be combined with other findings to be reliable. Mood changes suggest stimulation of the SNr, but higher leads may be effective without needing to move the lead. If the patient can tolerate the side effect, increasing the stimulation to induce a second side effect can help in deciding where to move the lead. We need to observe a side effect to confirm proper electrical function. If we do not have a good effect on rigidity by lead placement or stimulation and there is no electrical problem, the lack of a corticospinal effect suggests too medial a position. Recheck the mapping, consider repositioning the lead by 2 mm in a direction away from the side effects, and confirm the new location with fluoroscopy and AP skull X-ray. The STN is a small target so it is better to have overmapped it than to have to reposition the lead. Again, the lead must be moved at least 2 mm or risk returning to the old tract, and fluoroscopy and AP X-ray are essential to confirm the new location.

Securing the Lead

Once properly in place, great care needs to be taken to ensure that the DBS lead does not move while one is disassembling the headstage and securing the lead. Hardware complications are common and start with cap placement.[133–135] The silicone burr hole fastening device and cap previously supplied by Medtronic in the DBS lead kit can be used to secure the lead, but it is associated with a higher profile on the scalp and frequent vertical lead migrations.[91,133] Intraoperative fluoroscopy is essential to confirm lead location. If movement occurs, we will immediately reposition the lead to the proper position. The Stimloc has a lower profile, reducing the potential for erosion, and has a support clip mechanism, which secures the lead and helps prevent lead migration. The clip can slip, so we mark the exit point on the lead and hold it with a rubber shodded hemostat to prevent any movement during stylet removal and disassembling the headstage. Be sure the lead is secured in the groove on the base ring and cap the Stimloc. A final fluoroscopic image is taken to confirm lead placement. Other neurosurgeons report the use of methylmethacrylate and a straight titanium miniplate and screw fixation.[133,136] However, the former technique increases the difficulty for revision or replacement, and the later technique is associated with a higher risk of lead fracture. The subgaleal pocket made at the start of the case is then used to bury the distal end of the lead posterior and lateral to the incision for the next stage. If extraoperative testing is not being performed, connect the distal DBS lead to the lead cap and boot provided in the DBS lead kit. Placing the lead cap facilitates palpation of the distal end of the lead under the scalp, avoiding the need to later reopen the frontal incision to locate the lead for connection to the extension lead and internal pulse generator (IPG). Vigorous irrigation of the surgical field with antibiotic solution is recommended to help reduce the risk of infection. We also recommend a multilayer scalp closure using the available periosteum to cover the Stimloc base and cap (**Fig.**

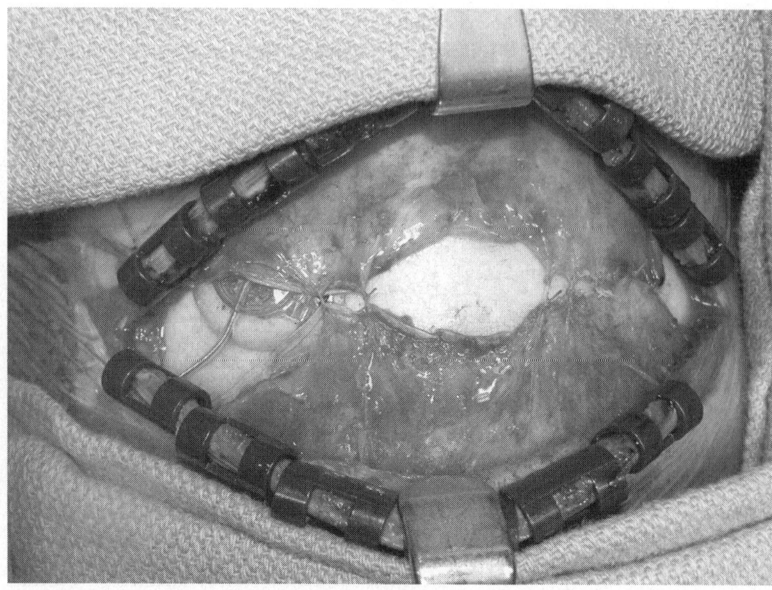

Fig. 7.18 Looking down on the coronal incision, the two Stimloc (Medtronic, Inc., Minneapolis, MN) devices are being covered by the pericranium. The one on the right is completely covered and the one on the left is in the process of being covered. The pericranium posterior is dissected free, and the edges cut toward the center to stretch as far as possible before the lead is placed so no sharp dissection occurs around the lead. The anterior pericranium is dissected free after lead placement to keep it intact as long as possible. In some cases, it is necessary to split the pericranium to maximize coverage.

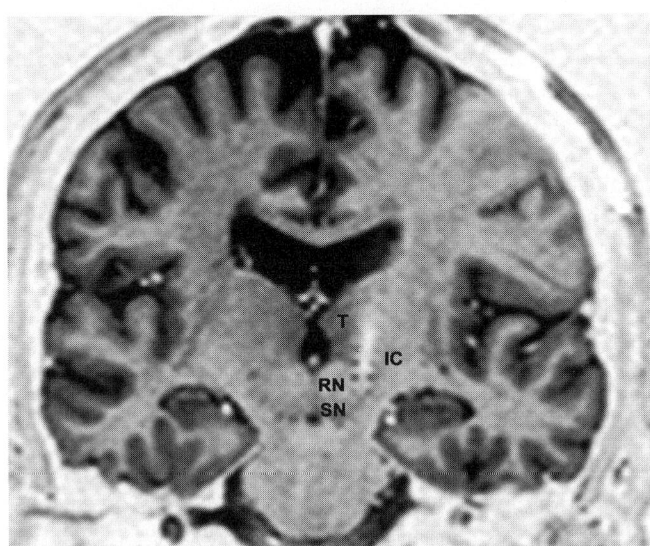

Fig. 7.19 Magnetic resonance inversion recovery–Turbo spin echo (IR-TSE) real image demonstrates the location of the subthalamic nucleus deep brain stimulation (DBS) on the left. The coronal section demonstrates the artifact from the DBS lead is lateral and anterior to the red nucleus and medial to the internal capsule. Overall function was excellent in this patient. *Abbreviations*: RN, red nucleus; IC, internal capsule, T, thalamus; SN, substantia nigra.

7.18). Since using this technique, we have not had an infection at this site in over 200 lead placements. We strongly recommend postoperative MRI prior to IPG placement to confirm lead locations and allow early revision if needed (**Fig. 7.19**). Safety techniques are discussed in Chapter 14. We also fuse the postoperative MRI with the preoperative MRI on the StealthStation to identify the lead location versus the planned location. This will show systematic errors and may suggest better targeting stratagems.

Lesioning

Lesioning is performed with RF (500,000 Hz) thermocoagulation with monopolar electrodes.[137] We use an RFG-3C lesion generator system (Integra Radionics, Burlington, MA). The place of lesioning in the treatment of movement disorders is being reevaluated. Three class I randomized trials compare pallidotomy versus medical therapy,[138] pallidotomy versus GPi DBS,[139] or thalamotomy versus thalamic DBS.[140] Others debate this topic with observational case series and few controls.[39,40,65,77,78,141–144] Most lesioning occurs where DBS is not available, in patients that refuse DBS, before the DBS equipment must be removed, or with radiosurgery for poor surgical candidates (see Chapter 16). There is general agreement that bilateral thalamotomy or pallidotomy is strongly discouraged due to the association with very high complication rates especially speech problems, dysphagia, and cognitive deficits.

Thalamotomy

Once the Vim has been adequately mapped, an RF probe with a 1.1 mm diameter and 2 to 4 mm exposed tip (Integra Radionics Burlington, MA) is inserted.[1] Macrostimulation with the RF probe is similar to DBS but is constant current rather than constant voltage. Minimal acceptable stimulation for speech and motor is > 2 mA at 5 Hz and for sensory > 1 mA at 100 Hz.[1] The RFG-3C lesion generator then performs a test (reversible) lesion of 42°C for 60 seconds and the effects on contralateral tremor, strength, coordination, and speech are noted. In PD, speech problems may preexist, and care must be taken not to exacerbate them. Speech testing needs to be more than simple counting or ABCs. The size of the lesion depends on the size of the electrode tip, temperature, and time. An irreversible lesion is made by heating the electrode tip to 65°C for 60 seconds (longer times do little to expand the size of the lesion). During the heating, the patient is continuously examined and any slight change in exam will terminate the procedure. If it is a false alarm, we will try again. If not, the surgery is ended. After the lesion, the patient is carefully examined; as long as there are no adverse effects the lesioning is repeated at 10 degree increments up to 85°C. A 1.1 × 3 mm RF probe at 65°C for 60 seconds will produce approximately a 2 mm diameter lesion, at 75°C a 3 mm, and at 85°C a 4 mm diameter lesion.[137] The lesion is elliptical, and the length of the lesion will increase inferiorly so the probe needs to be at least 1 to 2 mm from the bottom of the Vim. The patient is reassessed neurologically, and if there is residual tremor the probe is retracted 2 mm dorsally to improve proximal arm tremor or positioned further laterally to improve lower extremity tremor.[1,145–148] Larger lesions are needed for ET compared with PD and even larger ones are needed for kinetic tremor, which increases the risk of complications.

Pallidotomy

Once a sufficient number of microelectrode trajectories have clearly identified the sensorimotor responsive GPi, optic tract, and internal capsule, a Radionics RF electrode with a 1.1 × 3 mm exposed tip replaces the microelectrode.[54] Acceptable macrostimulation for visual is > 2 mA at 300 Hz and for speech and motor > 1 mA at 300 Hz.[2] Vitek et al[2] use a triangular pattern of lesioning with multiple adjacent tracks to match the shape of the posterior GPi. Initially the probe is warmed to 42°C, and the patient is examined for any change in strength, speech, or vision. The probe is then heated to 60°C for 60 seconds with the patient continuously examined. If there are no motor, speech or visual disturbances, the probe is reheated to 75°C at the same site. The probe is then moved 2 mm dorsally and the lesion extended by heating at 75 to 80°C. A second lesion tract is made 3 mm anterior to the first. A third lesion tract

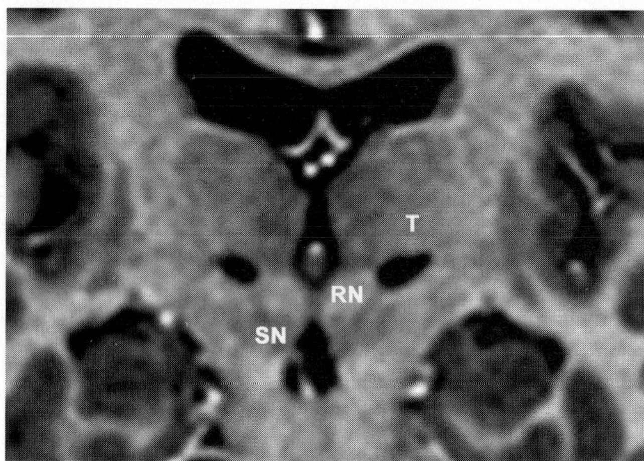

Fig. 7.20 Coronal magnetic resonance imaging demonstrates bilateral subthalamic lesions in the zona incerta and fields of Forel. The lesion is lateral and dorsal to the red nucleus (RN) and ventral to the ventrolateral nucleus of the thalamus (T). Although primarily used to treat Parkinson disease, this type of lesion was also used to treat dystonia. *Abbreviations*: SN, substantial nigra.

may be placed if we do not observe much improvement in the tone of the leg; we perform more medial lesioning carefully with continuous monitoring of strength and speech.

Subthalamotomy

Subthalamotomy or campotomy was used during the 1960s as an alternative to thalamic surgery for the alleviation of tremor and rigidity.[149–151] Well-placed lesions could be very effective, but complications carried a greater risk than thalamotomy, especially ataxia, dysarthria, and cerebellar symptoms (**Fig. 7.20**). Because of the success of STN DBS stimulation and the potential for development of hemiballism as a complication, this technique is primarily of historical interest.[152] However, these white matter areas are being explored with DBS.[153–155] STN lesioning has been described, but results do not appear as good as DBS, and significant complications can occur.[152,156]

Second Side

There are many reasons to operate on just one side. If bilateral surgery is indicated, where it should be performed simultaneously or staged is controversial (see Chapter 15). We tend to stage older and very asymmetric patients. If we plan a bilateral simultaneous case, the patient is informed that the decision to do the second side will be made after the first side is complete. The decision is based on the patient's desire to continue, how the patient is doing clinically, how satisfied we are with the initial placement, and other factors. It is better to be

sure of the correct lead placement before starting the second side and being misled. The burr hole is already prepared and the conversion of the frame to the other side, opening of the dura, and preparation of the headstage should take only a few minutes. Frequently, the neurologist or our nurse will be able to give an update to the family. The procedure is the same, but there is an advantage in that the first lead helps localize the target and almost always fewer tracts are required (**Fig. 7.21**). We perform lateral fluoroscopy and AP skull x-rays for each pass. The distance between the electrode (or lead) and the contralateral lead divided by the length of the contacts and multiplied by the known length of the contacts gives a very accurate distance between the electrode (or lead) and the contralateral lead. This helps confirm that the electrode and lead go where they are directed. In a second side of a staged operation, the location of an effective contralateral lead facilitates target adjustment (**Fig. 7.22**). When performing bilateral STN DBS, Benabid et al[132] note that the positioning of the contralateral STN lead is symmetrical in only ~60% of the cases, emphasizing the importance of assessing the functional location of the target during surgery.

Extraoperative Testing

Some groups previously recommended a trial of in-hospital external stimulation.[39,133] The Medtronic DBS lead kit no longer provides the components for externalizing the lead temporarily for extraoperative testing but they can still be purchased separately. The DBS distal lead is connected to the percutaneous extension wire that is tunneled subcutaneously from the subgaleal pocket to a separate exit site in the skin, usually posterior. A simple nylon suture is used to tighten the skin around the extension lead. A simple dressing is used to keep the lead clean and prevent entanglement until needed. The pin connector on the percutaneous extension wire connects to the twist-lock connector on the screening cable, and the plug end of the screening cable plugs in to the Model 3625 test stimulator. Different lead configurations should be evaluated at various parameter settings of rate, amplitude, and pulse width. Oh et al[133] externalized 96% of their patients for approximately 1 week of trial stimulation, which may have contributed to an erosion rate of 2.5% and an infection rate of 1.5%. In our opinion, externalized leads increase complication risks and add no value except for screening pain patients where the success rate is low and an IPG may not need to be implanted.

Simultaneous or Staged Second Side Lesioning

The patient returns in 5 to 14 days after DBS lead insertion for IPG placement under general anesthesia. The need to separate the procedures in the United States is in part related to reimbursement (see Chapter 3) but is also beneficial in elderly and severely debilitated patients. This does not delay

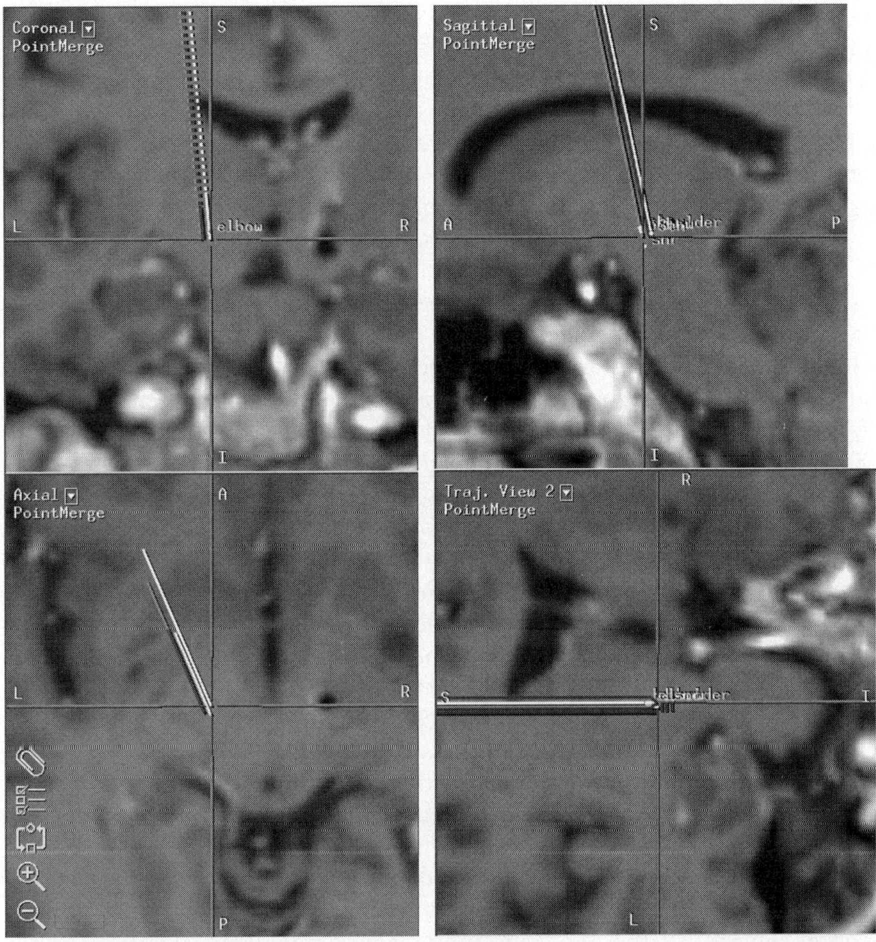

Fig. 7.21 This StealthStation image (Medtronic Navigation, Louisville, CO) demonstrates coronal, axial, sagittal, and trajectory views during subthalamic nucleus (STN) exploration for a staged deep brain stimulation (DBS) lead placement. The previously placed DBS lead is on the right (the patient's right too). Three recording tracts are shown and a few of the recorded STN cells are annotated. The trajectory view is parallel to the off-sagittal plane or, as in this case, the off-coronal plane and hence the distortion of the ventricles. The most medial tract does not enter the ventricle.

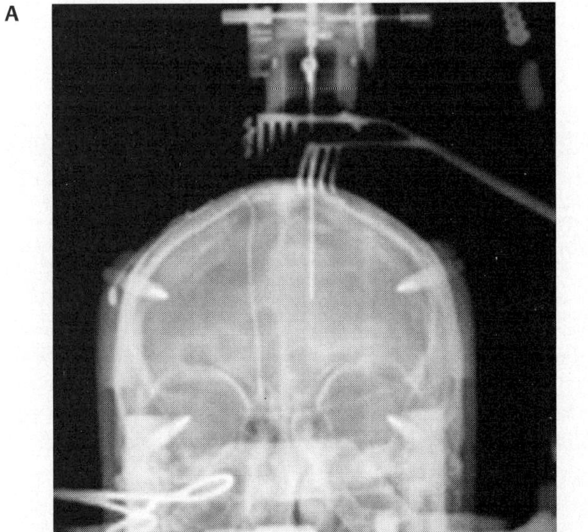

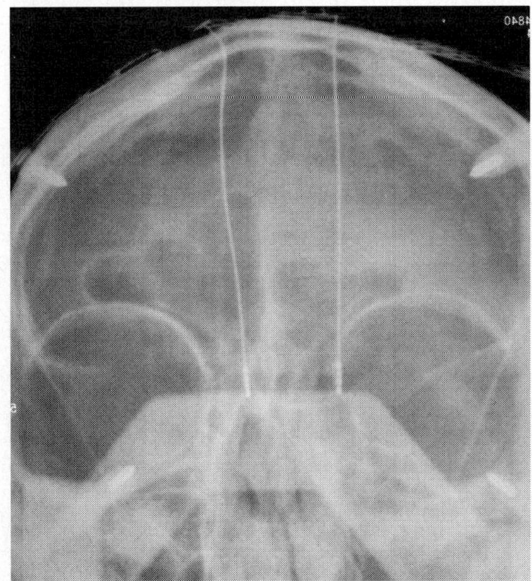

Fig. 7.22 Intraoperative anteroposterior (AP) skull X-rays demonstrate the position of a previously placed lead on the patient's right and probes on the left. **(A)** The bottom of the headstage, a guide tube and microelectrode can be identified on the way to target. This provides excellent confirmation of any movements in the mediolateral direction. **(B)** The second lead has been placed based on the optimal microelectrode recording (MER) site. In **(A)**, the distance between the initial lead and the MER target can be easily calculated. With the second DBS lead, those calculations can confirm that the lead went into the same location. The measured distance between the two leads (16 cm) is divided by the measured height of the contacts (5 cm) multiplied by the known height of the contacts (7.5 mm), and gives reasonable confidence that the two leads are ~24 mm apart. This calculation correlates well with postoperative magnetic resonance imaging measurements.

therapy, which is typically not started until 4 weeks postoperative. We use the bilateral Medtronic Soletra Model 7426 Neurostimulator (Medtronic, Inc., Minneapolis, MN) for each quadripolar lead connection. The Medtronic Kinetra Model 7428 Neurostimulator allows bilateral DBS control with two quadripolar leads connected into one pulse generator. They both contain a silver vanadium oxide battery housed in a titanium case. Vesper et al[157] describe advantages and the special programming features of the Kinetra system (see Chapter 13). It is US Food and Drug Administration (FDA) approved for PD, but the reimbursement is less than that for the bilateral Soletra. It is not frequently used in the United States. The dual-channel Kinetra is more useful for dystonia because power consumption is linear and battery life is longer in the higher voltage range,[65] but it is not FDA approved for use in dystonia to date. It is more than twice as large as the Soletra, and it is not advisable in thin-skinned and small patients. For the Kinetra, both extension leads must be tunneled down on the same side to prevent a loop effect that could be dangerous during MRI studies. In converting from two Soletra to Kinetra, remember to reroute the lead on the contralateral side to prevent this looping effect (www.medtronic.com/physician/activa/downloadablefiles/M220822A_a_003.pdf).

Surgery is performed under general anesthesia with endotracheal intubation. We prep and drape each side separately to allow the head to be turned away from the side of the implant. The subcutaneous pocket for the IPG is made two fingerbreadths below and parallel to the clavicle just above the pectoral fascia. The pocket should be big enough to accommodate the entire IPG and avoid having the skin incision cross over the generator. If the pocket is made too large, formation of a hematoma may occur. Postoperative sterile seromas also occur at the site of the IPG. This should be drained by needle puncture only if the suture line is threatened because it will frequently reaccumulate and can get secondarily infected.[91] It is best just watched.

For connection of the extension lead to the DBS lead, we do not reopen the scalp incision near the burr hole, but palpate for the distal lead temporarily housed in the lead cap and placed in the temporoparietal region as previously described. With the head turned toward the opposite side, a 3 cm horizontal skin incision is made below the parietal boss and posterior to the pinna down to the temporalis fascia (**Fig. 7.23**). Avoid the area where the glasses would rest. This plane is opened inferiorly with blunt dissection, and a closed curved Mayo scissors is passed over the temporalis fascia until the craniocervical fascia is penetrated. Using careful blunt dissection superiorly, the distal DBS lead and temporary connector are withdrawn minimally from this skin incision. The old boot and connector are discarded. A shunt passer or tunneling device provided in the Medtronic lead extension kit may be used to tunnel the lead extension between the scalp and chest incisions. We prefer the standard shunt passer with a plastic sheath because it is firmer and maintains a curvature. There is less potential traumatic damage while one is passing the extension lead inside the plastic sheath. We have had multiple fractures of the plastic Medtronic carrier, especially the Kinetra dual carriers. We use two separate shunt passers to separate the two leads and prevent entanglement (**Fig. 7.24**). It is important to secure the connector to the temporalis fascia to prevent migration. We accomplish this by opening the

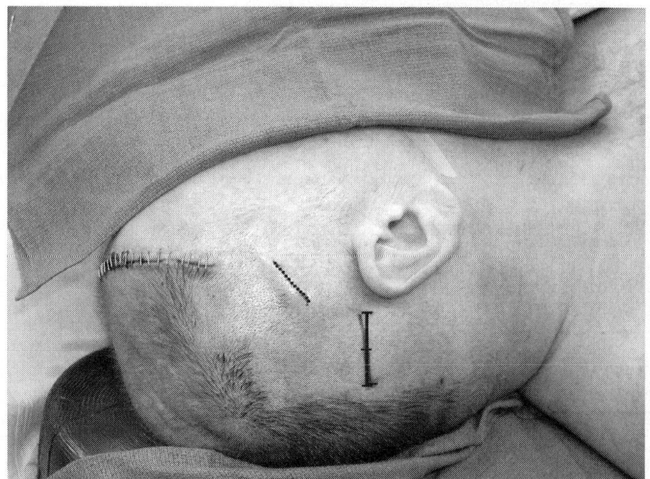

Fig. 7.23 The patient is positioned for the extension lead and internal pulse generator (IPG) placement. The previously placed lead cap is identified (more superior and anterior than usual) and marked. An incision line is marked behind the ear over the temporalis muscle for securing the connector. The old incision is not opened.

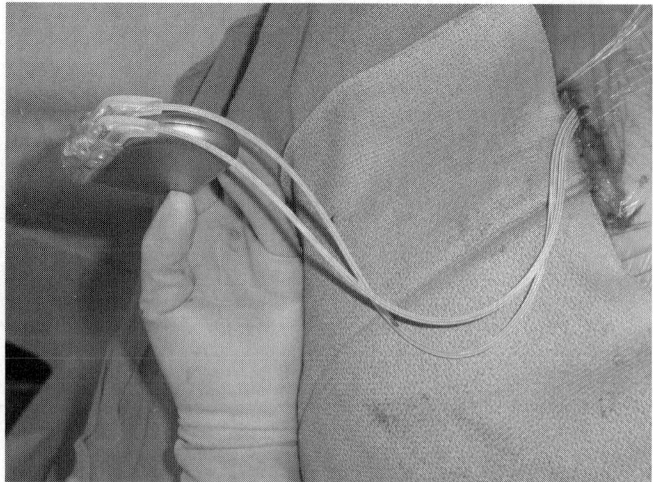

Fig. 7.24 This operative photograph shows the two extension leads connected to the Kinetra (Medtronic, Inc., Minneapolis, MN). Each extension lead is brought through a separate tunnel and attached. The pocket needs to be large for the Kinetra and excess leads, which should be wrapped around it.

temporalis fascia and splitting the muscle longitudinally and perpendicular to the scalp incision as far as possible above and below as exposure allows. The new connector will sit above the scalp incision and below the fascia; a 2–0 silk is used to secure it at the distal end of the connector to the fascia. The fascia is oversown with 2–0 Vicryl (Ethicon, Somerville, NJ) (**Fig. 7.25**). This will take pressure off the skin closure and add a layer of coverage over the extension lead. We bury the two leads for the Kinetra the same way in parallel tunnels below the temporalis fascia. This will require a larger skin incision extended posteriorly. Since using this technique we have not had an infection or erosion of the connector in over a 100 cases. The galea is closed with 2–0 Vicryl and the scalp with stainless steel staples (Proximate Skin Staplers, Johnson and Johnson Gateway; www.jnjgateway.com).

The early bulky lead connector might have contributed to skin erosions and infections.[91] The release of the low-profile connector (Model 7482;(Medtronic, Inc. Minneapolis, MN)) has decreased the occurrence of erosions in this area. Currently, most infections occurred as erosions at the connector site as reported by Oh et al.[133] The multilayer closure and vigorous use of antibiotics before, during, and after surgery has reduced our infection rate to 2% in over 300 cases. Several lead fractures occurred when the connectors were previously placed below the mastoid in the neck.[133] By securing the connector with a nonabsorbable suture to the temporalis fascia, we try to prevent lead fracture and migration. Anchoring the connector helps prevent excessive traction on the lead and slippage through the Stimloc clip mechanism, contributing to possible lead migration or fracture. This is more likely to occur in patients with prominent cervical tremor, dystonia, or dyskinesia. Overtightening the connector screws may cause contact damage and possibly a short circuit. An open circuit can be caused by failure to tighten one or more of the screws. Color coding is a must for the Kinetra but useful in all cases for identification. "White on the right, clear on the left" is a good mnemonic (**Fig. 7.26**).

Lastly, once all connections are secured, the IPG is placed in the subcutaneous pocket with the etched identification side facing outward. The excess extension wire is coiled around and behind the IPG so there are no sharp bends in the wire. Two suture holes are provided in the connector block of the IPG to secure it to the pectoral fascia. Rarely, in children or very thin adults, is there a need to place the IPG in or below the muscle. We avoid the abdomen because there is a high incidence of flipping the IPG so it cannot be interrogated or twisting of the extension lead. To close the dead space, the deep connective tissues are sutured with 2–0 Vicryl, the dermis with 3–0 Vicryl, and the skin approximated with a running subcuticular 4–0 Monocryl (Ethicon) and the skin incision sealed with Dermabond (Ethicon). For the second side, we make sure all instruments used in closure are discarded and there is no contamination of the back table. The patient is then turned toward the opposite direction and reprepped, redraped, and the procedure repeated. The two IPGs need to be at least 22 cm apart to prevent interference and unintended program changes. A similar distance is used if a pacemaker is present. At the end of the case, collect all uncontaminated

A
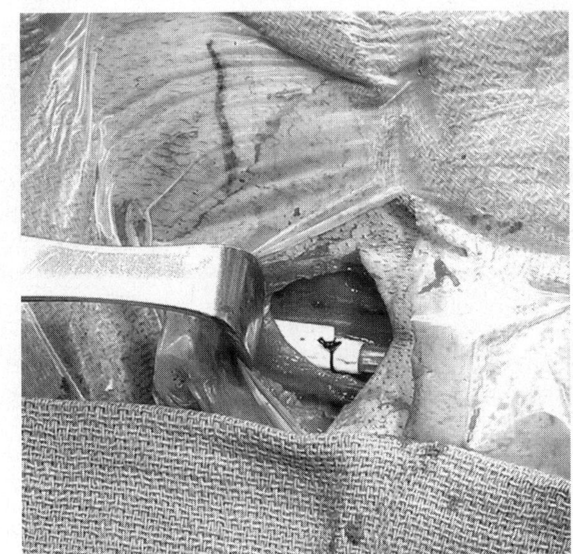

B
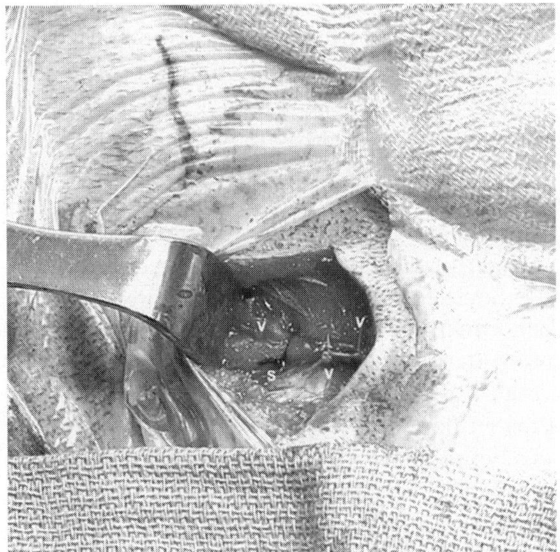

Fig. 7.25 These operative photographs are follow-up images to **Fig. 7.23**. **(A)** The postauricular incision is open and the lead cap has been retrieved and removed. The boot (white) covers the connector of the extension lead which is attached to the DBS lead. **(B)** The connector and extension lead are covered by the temporalis fascia. A silk suture (S) is looped around the extension lead just below the connector and secures it to the fascia. Three Vicryl (V) sutures close the fascia over the top of the connector and extension lead.

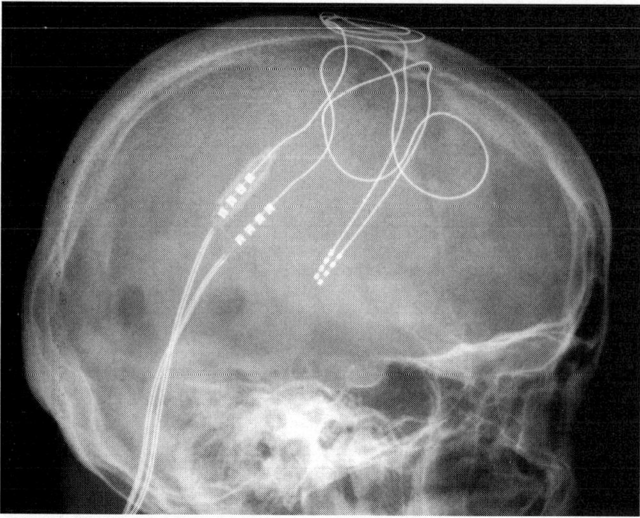

Fig. 7.26 Skull X-ray demonstrates two deep brain stimulation (DBS) leads both coming off the right side connected to a Kinetra (Medtronic, Inc., Minneapolis, MN). The DBS lead wires are obviously so entangled on the skull that there is great difficulty in knowing which connector is which; therefore, using the white (radiographically identifiable) boot on the right side allows right and left connectors to be distinguished. There is frequently a slight space disparity in the extension lead below the connector that is often misread as fractured. These two extension leads were working perfectly well at the time of this X-ray. It would be difficult should there be a short circuit to know which if either of these has become disconnected.

loose parts and sterilize them as recommended by the Medtronic *Physician and Hospital Manual*. They will come in handy in other cases.

For end-of-life (EOL) IPG replacement (battery < 3.0 V and status EOL, if telemetry is still possible), we cover with perioperative and postoperative antibiotics. The procedure is straightforward if care has been taken in placing the original IPG. The procedure is done with local and IV sedation except for children and extremely anxious adults. The IPG is set to off and 0 volts if still programmable. Local anesthetic is kept at a minimum and injected only superficially to avoid the extension lead. After the dermis is opened, we use Bovie electrocautery at low energy (provided there is no fracture) to dissect around the IPG and leads. The ground plate should be far away from the surgical field. Short burst and low power followed by irrigation are used to prevent heat injury to the lead plastic cover. We feel this is a better alternative to sharp dissection and decreases the potential for damage to the lead. After the exchange, the IPG is secured to the pseudocapsule, and the cavity is irrigated with antibiotics and local anesthetic. A three-layer closure is then performed. If there are two IPGs and one is EOL and the other is low (3.0 to 3.3 V and status "Low"), it is better to replace both at the same time than to have to come back in a month.

Special Problems

Reoperation for lead fracture or migration is uncommon with placement of the connector on the skull and securing it to the fascia. When it happens, we target the fractured lead or the cavity as evidence of the prior tract on the MRI and do not feel the need for MER. Failure of the lead to effectively treat the symptoms is far more common, especially in larger centers with many outside referrals.[158] We operate on these and previously removed infected leads as if they were virgin cases. Failure to respond may mean a wrong diagnosis or wrong lead placement or a malfunctioning system. Careful clinical assessment and screening to be sure the diagnosis and primary symptoms to be treated are correct is essential to prevent improper reoperations. Preoperative MRI (assuming the wires are not broken) and X-rays of the entire system are essential for planning. The surgery is as already described, with reopening of the prior operative site unless it was initially chosen improperly. Even if the lead is suboptimally placed, we leave it in place as a landmark and record around it. Removal may create edema that could hinder recordings. The signal artifact of

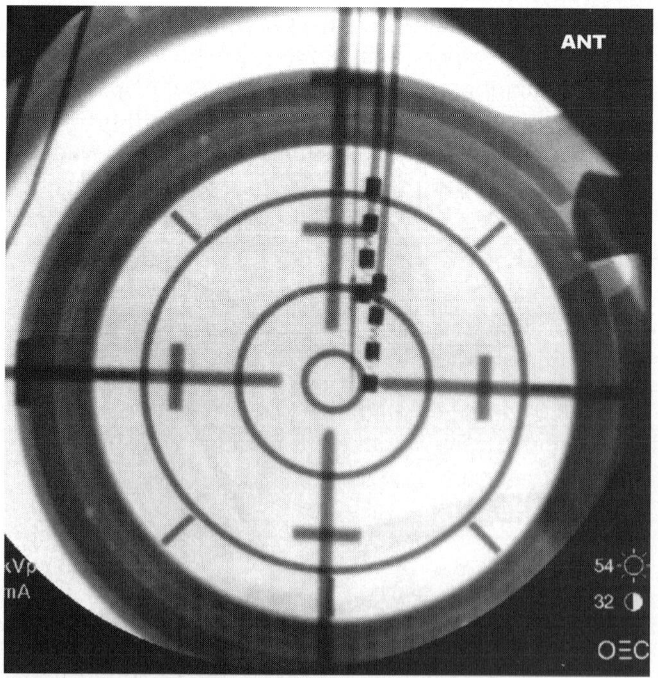

Fig. 7.27 This radiographic image demonstrates two deep brain stimulation leads and a microelectrode. The anterior (ANT) is to the right. The most anterior lead is functioning well but that on the left never functioned and has migrated dorsally. Magnetic resonance imaging suggests it was placed too medially and migrated at closure or shortly thereafter based on history. We elected to explore the subthalamic nucleus with a microelectrode only millimeters ventrally and laterally to the misplaced lead. When the mapping was done a functional lead was inserted and the old lead removed.

the lead on MRI is ~2 to 3 times the actual dimension so we can easily explore > 2 mm from the center of the signal artifact with tracts parallel to the lead. Leaving the old lead in place during placement of the new lead allows intraoperative confirmation of placement and prevents the new lead from going into the old tract (**Fig. 7.27**).

We are very aggressive about treating infections. Any superficial wound erythema is suspect, and local inspection for foreign body is performed. The "stitch infection" is treated with topical and oral antibiotics for 1 week. Re-evaluation in 10 days almost always demonstrates successful treatment. If not, either a second course of treatment or operative exploration is performed. For clear infections with expressible pus, the wound is cultured and the patient admitted for IV triple antibiotics prior to surgery. Gross contamination of the entire system is rare and requires prompt removal of the entire device. Far more commonly there is segmental infection that may be successfully treated. Infections over the burr hole are now rare with low profile caps and three-layer closure of an incision that is not over the burr hole cover. The exception is reoperations where the closure is not as good as primary closures. An elliptical incision is made around the drainage site to remove all the contaminated skin. After generous sharp or mechanical debridement of affected tissue, we use vigorous irrigation with a liter of hydrogen peroxide and then with a liter of normal saline with vancomycin in an attempt to sterilize the area. If infected, we remove the plastic of the Stimloc or burr hole cover after securing the lead to the skull with a titanium miniplate and screw fixation to prevent movement. This requires rongeur or drill opening of the base ring. Once all infected tissue is removed and the area is irrigated, we reglove and close with 2–0 nylon in a horizontal mattress pattern with a new set of sterile instruments. CSF leakage is rare but if present the lead needs to be removed. Long-term (4 to 8 weeks) IV antibiotics selected for the specific organism are necessary. In addition, we like to add rifampin for its synergistic effects in the treatment of foreign body infections.

Infection in combination with erosion over the connector is the most common deep scalp infection. We use the same technique but also remove the connector boot as the most contaminated element and replace it with a new one after the antibiotic irrigation. The new boot connector is applied after changing all gloves and operative equipment. This is then secured with a single Vicryl stitch in a pocket away from the incision line and if possible below the temporalis. It is usually not necessary to remove the extension lead, but if gross contamination extends deep around the extension lead or the extension lead is the eroded element then removal is performed. If this is known or suspected preoperatively, we open the chest incision first, take cultures, and cut the extension lead. Regardless of the approach, we always pull the lead into the infected area after vigorous irrigation as already described to minimize the opportunity for contamination. The extension lead is replaced after the antibiotic course. A

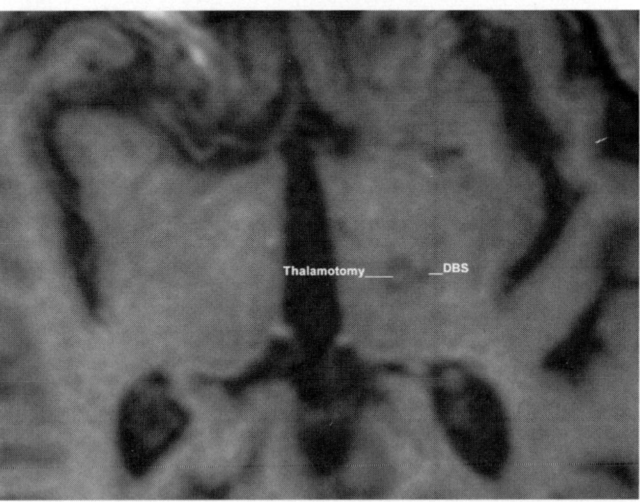

Fig. 7.28 Axial magnetic resonance imaging demonstrates a radio frequency thalamotomy medial to a prior deep brain stimulation lead. The lead was successful in relieving tremor but at high voltage caused corticospinal symptoms. When the erosion at the connector required the DBS removal, a lesion probe was placed medial to the DBS lead and tested. The DBS lead was removed and a radiofrequency lesion produced a thalamotomy (bull's-eye appearance). The result was excellent tremor control.

new lead cap is used to cover the DBS lead and assist in finding the lead on reoperation. The DBS lead is always carefully wiped clean and dried. The DBS lead and lead cap are placed in a new pocket away from the incision line. Occasionally, if the Gram stain is negative from the chest and the organism is highly sensitive, then a new extension lead with a new tunnel can be connected to the DBS lead and the old IPG. Long-term (4 to 8 weeks) IV antibiotics selected for the specific organism are necessary. If the DBS lead has to be removed, some neurosurgeons attempt to lesion through the DBS lead.[159] If the area of the burr hole is sterile, we have performed RF lesioning in a standard fashion with an RF probe at the lead site or adjacent to it (**Fig. 7.28**) at the time of removal.

For infection in the chest, we open the incision at the connector first, culture the connector, and cut the proximal extension lead. This site is vigorously irrigated with antibiotic solution and closed. The IPG and the extension lead are then removed as a separate field. The cavity is vigorously irrigated and chronic IV antibiotics used. If the Gram stains are positive at the connector site, the entire system should be removed. Recurrence on antibiotics or after completion of the course of antibiotics should result in removal of the entire system. Although high rates of antibiotic failure have been reported,[91,133] we have had success in more than 60% of patients. The presence of unusual organisms (i.e., gram-negative bacteria) or infections in diabetic patients are more likely to lead to antibiotic failure. Intracranial infection is very rare and requires removal and specialized antibiotic treatment. Similar to cardiac pacemakers, the best precaution is aggressive antibiotic prophylaxis.[160]

■ Conclusion

Unfortunately, there has not been a randomized, controlled trial comparing the results of microelectrode versus nonmicroelectrode techniques for targeting the STN, but several groups suggest that electrophysiological guidance has modified lead implantation and improved outcomes.[7,19–21,72,161–164] Millimeters matter in an ill-defined target like STN that changes shape throughout life[165] and where atrophy of this nucleus may affect outcome.[166] There is a definite learning curve associated with stereotactic surgery for movement disorders. Multiple centers[2,41,97,134] have reported that the majority of problems occur early in their series. In addition, we are learning more about the basal ganglion and where DBS may be most effective.[167,168] Particularly promising is the pedunculopontine nucleus.[169,170] Due to the advancements in radiographic imaging, neuronavigational software, surgical technique, and the refinement of microelectrode recordings, many patients have experienced dramatic clinical improvements with a relatively low risk of permanent neurological deficit. DBS is increasingly recognized as safe and effective therapy.[167] Future device optimizations and the possibility of customized stimulation delivery will likely further improve outcome. The skills required are easily obtained but the intellectual insights suggest the distinct advantages of fellowship training.

References

1. Bakay RAE, Vitek JL, Delong MR. Thalamotomy for tremor. In: Rengechary SS, Wilkins RR, eds. Neurosurgical Operative Atlas. Vol 2. Park Ridge, IL: American Association of Neurological Surgeons; 1992:299–312

2. Vitek JL, Bakay RA, Hashimoto T, et al. Microelectrode-guided pallidotomy: technical approach and its application in medically intractable Parkinson's disease. J Neurosurg 1998;88:1027–1043

3. Starr PA, Vitek JL, Bakay RAE. Deep brain stimulation for movement disorders. Neurosurg Clin N Am 1998;9:381–402

4. Dormont D, Ricciardi KG, Tande D, et al. Is the subthalamic nucleus hypointense on T2-weighted images? A correlation study using MR imaging and stereotactic atlas data. AJNR Am J Neuroradiol 2004;25:1516–1523

5. Saint-Cyr JA, Hoque T, Pereira LC, et al. Localization of clinically effective stimulating electrodes in the human subthalamic nucleus on magnetic resonance imaging. J Neurosurg 2002;97:1152–1166

6. Starr PA, Vitek JL, DeLong M, Bakay RA. Magnetic resonance imaging-based stereotactic localization of the globus pallidus and subthalamic nucleus. Neurosurgery 1999;44:303–313 (discussion 313–314)

7. Bejjani BP, Dormont D, Pidoux B, et al. Bilateral subthalamic stimulation for Parkinson's disease by using three-dimensional stereotactic magnetic resonance imaging and electrophysiological guidance. J Neurosurg 2000;92:615–625

8. Schlaier J, Schoedel P, Lange M, et al. Reliability of atlas-derived coordinates in deep brain stimulation. Acta Neurochir (Wien) 2005;147:1175–1180 (discussion 1180)

9. Dormont D, Cornu P, Pidoux B, et al. Chronic thalamic stimulation with three-dimensional MR stereotactic guidance. AJNR Am J Neuroradiol 1997;18:1093–1107

10. Kondziolka D, Bonaroti E, Baser S, Brandt F, Kim YS, Lunsford LD. Outcomes after stereotactically guided pallidotomy for advanced Parkinson's disease. J Neurosurg 1999;90:197–202

11. Patil AA, Falloon T, Hahn F, Cheng J, Wang S. Direct identification of ventrointermediate nucleus of the thalamus on magnetic resonance and computed tomography images. Surg Neurol 1999;51:674–678

12. Reich CA, Hudgins PA, Sheppard SK, Starr PA, Bakay RAEA. High-resolution fast spin-echo inversion-recovery sequence for preoperative localization of the internal globus pallidus. AJNR Am J Neuroradiol 2000;21:928–931

13. Vayssiere N, Hemm S, Zanca M, et al. Magnetic resonance imaging stereotactic target localization for deep brain stimulation in dystonic children. J Neurosurg 2000;93:784–790

14. Slavin KV, Thulborn KR, Wess C, Nesesyan H. Direct visualization of the human subthalamic nucleus with 3T MR imaging. AJNR Am J Neuroradiol 2006;27:80–84

15. Mercado R, Madat T, Moore GR, Li D, MacKay A, Honey C. Three-tesla magnetic resonance imaging of the ventrolateral thalamus: a correlative anatomical description. J Neurosurg 2006;105:279–283

16. Van Buren JM, Maccubbin DA. An outline atlas of the human basal ganglia with estimation of anatomical variants. J Neurosurg 1962;19:811–839

17. Brierley JB, Beck E. The significance in human stereotactic brain surgery of individual variation in the diencephalon and globus pallidus. J Neurol Neurosurg Psychiatry 1959;22:287–298

18. Schuurman PR, de Bie RM, Majoie CB, Speelman JD, Bosch DA. A prospective comparison between three-dimensional magnetic resonance imaging and ventriculography for target-coordinate determination in frame-based functional stereotactic neurosurgery. J Neurosurg 1999;91:911–914

19. Zonenshayn M, Rezai AR, Mogilner AY, Beric A, Sterio D, Kelly PJ. Comparison of anatomic and neurophysiological methods for subthalamic nucleus targeting. Neurosurgery 2000;47:282–292 (discussion 292–294)

20. Cuny E, Guehl D, Burbaud P, Gross C, Dousset V, Rougier A. Lack of agreement between direct magnetic resonance imaging and statistical determination of a subthalamic target: the role of electrophysiological guidance. J Neurosurg 2002;97:591–597

21. Rodriguez-Oroz MC, Gorospe A, Guridi J, et al. Bilateral deep brain stem stimulation of the subthalamic nucleus in Parkinson's disease. Neurology 2000;55:S45–S51

22. Andrade-Souza YM, Schwalb JM, Hamani C, et al. Comparison of three methods of targeting the subthalamic nucleus for chronic stimulation in Parkinson's disease. Neurosurgery 2005; 56(2, Suppl) 360–368

23. Richter EO, Hoque T, Halliday W, Lozano AM, Saint-Cyr JA. Determining the position and size of the subthalamic nucleus based on magnetic resonance imaging results in patients with advanced Parkinson's disease. J Neurosurg 2004;100:541–546

24. Menuel C, Garnero L, Bardinet E, Poupon F, Phalippou D, Dormont D. Characterization and correction of distortions in stereotactic magnetic resonance imaging for bilateral subthalamic stimulation in Parkinson disease. J Neurosurg 2005;103:256–266

25. Duffner F, Schiffbauer H, Breit S, Friese S, Freudenstein D. Relevance of image fusion for target point determination in functional neurosurgery. Acta Neurochir (Wien) 2002;144:445–451

26. Tasker R, Hutchison JD, Richardson WD. Microelectrode recording technology. Tech Neurosurg 1999;5:46–64

27. Albe-Fessard D, Arfel G, Guiot G, Hardy J, Hertzog E, Aleonard P. Identification et delimitation precise de certaines structures sous-corticales de l'homme par l'electro-physiolgie. CR Acad Sci (Paris) 1961;243:2412–2414

28. Fukamachi A, Oye C, Narabayashi H. Delineation of the thalamic nuclei with a microelectrode in stereotaxic surgery for parkinsonism and cerebral palsy. J Neurosurg 1973;39:214–225

29. Hardy J, Bertrand C. Electrophysiological exploration of sub-cortical structures with microelectrode during stereotaxic surgery. Confin Neurol 1965;26:201–204

30. Albe-Fessard D, Guiot G, Lamarre Y, Arfel G. Activation of thalamo-cortical projections related to tremorogenic processes. In: Purpura DP, Yahr MD, eds. The Thalamus. New York: Columbia University Press; 1966:237–253.

31. Bertrand G, Jasper H, Wong A, Mathews G. Microelectrode recording during stereotactic surgery. Clin Neurosurg 1969;16:328–356

32. Jasper H, Bertrand G. Thalamic units involved in somatic sensation and voluntary and involuntary movements in man. In: Purpura DP, Yahr MD, eds. The Thalamus. New York: Columbia University Press; 1966:365–390.

33. Bertrand G, Jasper H. Microelectrode recording of unit activity in the human thalamus. Confin Neurol 1965;26:205–208

34. Gaze RM, Gillingham FJ, Kalyanaraman S, Porter RW, Donaldson AA, Donaldson IML. Microelectrode recordings from the human thalamus. Brain 1964;87:691–706

35. Narabayashi H, Ohye C. Importance of microstereoencephalotomy for tremor alleviation. Appl Neurophysiol 1980;43:222–227

36. Kelly PJ, Ahlskog JE, Goerss SJ, Daube JR, Duffy JR, Kall BA. Computer-assisted stereotactic ventralis lateralis thalamotomy with microelectrode recording control in patients with Parkinson's disease. Mayo Clin Proc 1987;62:655–664

37. Tasker RR, Dostrovsky O. What goes on in the motor thalamus? Stereotact Funct Neurosurg 1993;60:121–126

38. Garonzik IM, Hua SE, Ohara S, Lenz FA. Intraoperative microelectrode and semi-microelectrode recording during the physiological localization of the thalamic nucleus ventral intermediate. Mov Disord 2002;17(Suppl 3):S135–S144

39. Benabid AL, Pollak P, Gao D, et al. Chronic electrical stimulation of the ventralis intermedius nucleus of the thalamus as a treatment of movement disorders. J Neurosurg 1996;84:203–214

40. Tasker RR. Deep brain stimulation is preferable to thalamotomy for tremor suppression. Surg Neurol 1998;49:145–153 (discussion 153–154)

41. Linhares MN, Tasker RR. Microelectrode-guided thalamotomy for Parkinson's disease. Neurosurgery 2000;46:390–395 (discussion 395–398)

42. Dogali M, Fazzini E, Kolodny E, et al. Stereotactic ventral pallidotomy for Parkinson's disease. Neurology 1995;45:753–761

43. Baron MS, Vitek JL, Bakay RA, et al. Treatment of advanced Parkinson's disease by posterior GPi pallidotomy: 1-year results of a pilot study. Ann Neurol 1996;40:355–366

44. Kopyov O, Jacques D, Duma C, et al. Microelectrode-guided posteroventral medial radiofrequency pallidotomy for Parkinson's disease. J Neurosurg 1997;87:52–59

45. Lang AE, Lozano AM, Montgomery E, Duff J, Tasker R, Hutchison W. Posteroventral medial pallidotomy in advanced Parkinson's disease. N Engl J Med 1997;337:1036–1042

46. Uitti RJ, Wharen RE, Turk MF, et al. Unilateral pallidotomy for Parkinson's disease: comparison of outcome in younger versus elderly patients. Neurology 1997;49:1072–1077

47. Masterman D, DeSalles A, Baloh RW, et al. Motor, cognitive, and behavioral performance following unilateral ventroposterior pallidotomy for Parkinson disease. Arch Neurol 1998;55:1201–1208

48. Samuel M, Caputo E, Brooks DJ, et al. A study of medial pallidotomy for Parkinson's disease: clinical outcome, MRI location and complications. Brain 1998;121(Pt 1):59–75

49. Lai EC, Jankovic J, Krauss JK, Ondo WG, Grossman RG. Long-term efficacy of posteroventral pallidotomy in the treatment of Parkinson's disease. Neurology 2000;55:1218–1222

50. Favre J, Burchiel KJ, Taha JM, Hammerstad J. Outcome of unilateral and bilateral pallidotomy for Parkinson's disease: patient assessment. Neurosurgery 2000;46:344–353 (discussion 353–355)

51. Van Horn G, Hassenbusch SJ, Zouridakis G, Mullani NA, Wilde MC, Papanicolaou AC. Pallidotomy: a comparison of responders and nonresponders. Neurosurgery 2001;48:263–271 (discussion 271–273)

52. Vitek JL, Giroux M. Physiology of hypokinetic and hyperkinetic movement disorders: model for dyskinesia. Ann Neurol 2000;47(4, Suppl 1)S131–S140

53. Taha JM, Favre J, Baumann TK, Burchiel KJ. Tremor control after pallidotomy in patients with Parkinson's disease: correlation with microrecording findings. J Neurosurg 1997;86:642–647

54. Bakay RAE, Starr PA, Vitek JL, DeLong MR. Posterior ventral pallidotomy: techniques and theoretical considerations. Clin Neurosurg 1997;44:197–210

55. Gross RE, Lombardi WJ, Hutchison WD, et al. Variability in lesion location after microelectrode-guided pallidotomy for Parkinson's disease: anatomical, physiological, and technical factors that determine lesion distribution. J Neurosurg 1999;90:468–477

56. Krauss JK, Desaloms JM, Lai EC, King DE, Jankovic J, Grossman RG. Microelectrode-guided posteroventral pallidotomy for treatment of Parkinson's disease: postoperative magnetic resonance imaging analysis. J Neurosurg 1997;87:358–367

57. Lozano A, Hutchison W, Kiss Z, Tasker R, Davis K, Dostrovsky J. Methods for microelectrode-guided posteroventral pallidotomy. J Neurosurg 1996;84:194–202

58. Tsao K, Wilkinson S, Overman J, Koller WC, Batnitzky S, Gordon MA. Pallidotomy lesion locations: significance of microelectrode refinement. Neurosurgery 1998;43:506–512 (discussion 512–513)

59. Alterman RL, Sterio D, Beric A, Kelly PJ. Microelectrode recording during posteroventral pallidotomy: impact on target selection and complications. Neurosurgery 1999;44:315–321 (discussion 321–323)

60. Guridi J, Gorospe A, Ramos E, Linazasoro G, Rodriguez MC, Obeso JA. Stereotactic targeting of the globus pallidus internus in Parkinson's disease: imaging versus electrophysiological mapping. Neurosurgery 1999;45:278–287 (discussion 287–289)

61. Starr PA, Turner RS, Rau G, et al. Microelectrode-guided implantation of deep brain stimulators into the globus pallidus internus for dystonia: techniques, electrode locations, and outcomes. Neurosurg Focus 2004;17:E4

62. Troster AI, Fields JA, Wilkinson SB, et al. Unilateral pallidal stimulation for Parkinson's disease: neurobehavioral functioning before and 3 months after electrode implantation. Neurology 1997;49:1078–1083

63. Tronnier VM, Fogel W, Kronenbuerger M, Krause M, Steinvorth S. Is the medial globus pallidus a site for stimulation or lesioning in the treatment of Parkinson's disease? Stereotact Funct Neurosurg 1997;69(1–4, Pt 2):62–68

64. Krauss JK, Loher TJ, Pohle T, et al. Pallidal deep brain stimulation in patients with cervical dystonia and severe cervical dyskinesias with cervical myelopathy. J Neurol Neurosurg Psychiatry 2002;72:249–256

65. Krauss JK, Yianni J, Loher TJ, Aziz TZ. Deep brain stimulation for dystonia. J Clin Neurophysiol 2004;21:18–30

66. Starr PA, Vitek JL, DeLong M, Mewes K, Bakay RAE. Pallidotomy: theory and technique. Tech Neurosurg 1999;5:31–45

67. Sierens D, Bakay RAE. Pallidotomy for Parkinson's Disease. In: Tarsy D, Vitek JL, Lozano AM, Eds. Surgical treatment of Parkinson's disease and other movement disorders. Totowa, NJ: Humana Press; 2003:115–128

68. Benabid AL, Pollak P, Gross C, et al. Acute and long-term effects of subthalamic nucleus stimulation in Parkinson's disease. Stereotact Funct Neurosurg 1994;62:76–84

69. Krack P, Benazzouz A, Pollak P, et al. Treatment of tremor in Parkinson's disease by subthalamic nucleus stimulation. Mov Disord 1998;13:907–914

70. Sterio D, Zonenshayn M, Mogilner AY, et al. Neurophysiological refinement of subthalamic nucleus targeting. Neurosurgery 2002;50:58–67 (Discussion 67–69)

71. Rodriguez MC, Guridi OJ, Alvarez L, et al. The subthalamic nucleus and tremor in Parkinson's disease. Mov Disord 1998;13(Suppl 3):111–118

72. Starr PA, Christine CW, Theodosopoulos PV, et al. Implantation of deep brain stimulators into the subthalamic nucleus: technical approach and magnetic resonance imaging-verified lead locations. J Neurosurg 2002;97:370–387

73. Yelnik J, Damier P, Demeret S, et al. Localization of stimulating electrodes in patients with Parkinson disease by using a three-dimensional atlas-magnetic resonance imaging coregistration method. J Neurosurg 2003;99:89–99

74. Benazzouz A, Breit S, Koudsie A, et al. Intraoperative microrecordings of the subthalamic nucleus in Parkinson's disease. Mov Disord 2002;17(Suppl 3):S145–S149

75. Hamel W, Fietzek U, Morsnowski A, et al. Subthalamic nucleus stimulation in Parkinson's disease: correlation of active electrode contacts with intraoperative microrecordings. Stereotact Funct Neurosurg 2003;80:37–42

76. Benabid AL, Koudsie A, Benazzouz A, et al. Subthalamic stimulation for Parkinson's disease. Arch Med Res 2000;31:282–289

77. Limousin P, Krack P, Pollak P, et al. Electrical stimulation of the subthalamic nucleus in advanced Parkinson's disease. N Engl J Med 1998;339:1105–1111

78. Volkmann J. Deep brain stimulation for the treatment of Parkinson's disease. J Clin Neurophysiol 2004;21:6–17

79. Kleiner-Fisman G, Fisman DN, Sime E, Saint-Cyr JA, Lozano AM, Lang AE. Long-term follow up of bilateral deep brain stimulation of the subthalamic nucleus in patients with advanced Parkinson disease. J Neurosurg 2003;99:489–495

80. Rodriguez-Oroz MC, Obeso JA, Lang AE, et al. Bilateral deep brain stimulation in Parkinson's disease: a multicentre study with 4 years follow-up. Brain 2005;128(pt 10):2240–2249

81. Visser-Vandewalle V, van der Linden C, Temel Y, et al. Long-term effects of bilateral subthalamic nucleus stimulation in advanced Parkinson disease: a four year follow-up study. Parkinsonism Relat Disord 2005;11:157–165

82. Krack P, Batir A, Van Blercom N, et al. Five-year follow-up of bilateral stimulation of the subthalamic nucleus in advanced Parkinson's disease. N Engl J Med 2003;349:1925–1934

83. Schupbach WM, Chastan N, Welter ML, et al. Stimulation of the subthalamic nucleus in Parkinson's disease: a 5 year follow-up. J Neurol Neurosurg Psychiatry 2005;76:1640–1644

84. Levy R, Dostrovsky JO, Lang AE, Sime E, Hutchison WD, Lozano AM. Effects of apomorphine on subthalamic nucleus and globus pallidus internus neurons in patients with Parkinson's disease. J Neurophysiol 2001;86:249–260

85. Gray H, Wilson S, Sidebottom P. Parkinson's disease and anaesthesia. Br J Anaesth 2003;90:524 (author reply 524–525)

86. Nicholson G, Pereira AC, Hall GM. Parkinson's disease and anaesthesia. Br J Anaesth 2002;89:904–916

87. Hood TW, Yap JC. A survey of infections in stereotactic surgery. Appl Neurophysiol 1981;44:314–319

88. Ratilal B, Costa J, Sampaio C. Antibiotic prophylaxis for surgical introduction of intracranial ventricular shunts. Cochrane Database Syst Rev 2006;3

89. Shrivastava RK, Germano I. Deep brain stimulation for the treatment of Parkinson's disease. Contemp Neurosurgery 2001;23:1–9

90. Tasker R. Movement disorders. In: Apuzzo MLJ, ed. Brain Surgery: Complication Avoidance and Management. New York: Churchill Livingstone: 1993:1509–1524

91. Umemura A, Jaggi JL, Hurtig HI, et al. Deep brain stimulation for movement disorders: morbidity and mortality in 109 patients. J Neurosurg 2003;98:779–784

92. Aziz TZ, Nandi D, Parkin S, et al. Targeting the subthalamic nucleus. Stereotact Funct Neurosurg 2001;77:87–90

93. Deogaonkar A, Avitsian R, Henderson JM, Schubert A. Venous air embolism during deep brain stimulation surgery in an awake supine patient. Stereotact Funct Neurosurg 2005;83:32–35

94. Binder DK, Rau GM, Starr PA. Risk factors for hemorrhage during microelectrode-guided deep brain stimulator implantation for movement disorders. Neurosurgery 2005;56:722–732

95. Iacopino DG, Conti A, Angileri FF, Tomasello F. Different methods for anatomical targeting. J Neurosurg Sci 2003;47:18–25

96. Maciunas RJ, Galloway RL, Latimer JW. The application accuracy of stereotactic frames. Neurosurgery 1994;35:682–695

97. Sierens D, Bakay RAE. Is microelectrode recording necessary? The case in favor. In: Israel Z, Burchiel KJ, eds. Microelectrode Recording in Movement Disorder Surgery. New York: Thieme; 2004:186–196

98. Shils JL, Tagliati M, Alterman RL. Intraoperative microelectrode recording equipment: what features are necessary? Stereotact Funct Neurosurg 2001;77:101–107

99. Slavin KV, Holsapple J. Microelectrode techniques: equipment, components, and systems. In: Israel Z, Burchiel KJ, eds. Microelectrode Recording in Movement Disorder Surgery. New York: Thieme; 2004:14–27

100. Schaltenbrand G, Hassler RG, Wahren W. Atlas for Stereotaxy of the Human Brain. Stuttgart: Thieme; 1977

101. Schaltenbrand G, Bailey P. Introduction to Stereotaxis with an Atlas of the Human Brain. Stuttgart: Thieme; 1959

102. Littlechild P, Varma TR, Eldridge PR, et al. Variability in position of the subthalamic nucleus targeted by magnetic resonance imaging and microelectrode recordings as compared to atlas co-ordinates. Stereotact Funct Neurosurg 2003;80:82–87

103. Craig AD, Bushnell MC, Zhang ET, Blomquist A. A thalamic nucleus specific for pain and temperature sensation. Nature 1994;372: 770–773, 7695716.

104. Hassler R. The division of pain conduction into systems of pain sensation and pain awareness. In: Weigel K, Janzen R, Herz A, Steichele C, eds. Pain: Basic Principles–Pharmacology–Therapy. London: Churchill Livingstone; 1972:98–112

105. Lozano AM, Hutchison WD. Microelectrode recordings in the pallidum. Mov Disord 2002;17(Suppl 3):S150–S154

106. Krauss JK, Grossman RG. Optimal Target of Pallidotomy: A Controversy. Philadelphia: Lippincott-Raven; 1998:291–296

107. Laitinen L. Optimal Target of Pallidotomy: A Controversy. Philadelphia: Lippincott-Raven; 1998:285–289

108. Bakay RAE, Starr P. Optimal target of pallidotomy: a controversy. In: Krauss JK, Grossman, Jankovic J, eds. Pallidotomy for the Treatment of Parkinson's Disease and Movement Disorders. Philadelphia: Lippincott-Raven; 1998:275–283

109. Hariz MI, Hirabayashi H. Is there a relationship between size and site of the stereotactic lesion and symptomatic results of pallidotomy and thalamotomy? Stereotact Funct Neurosurg 1997;69(1–4, Pt 2):28–45

110. Gross RE, Lombardi WJ, Lang AE, et al. Relationship of lesion location to clinical outcome following microelectrode-guided pallidotomy for Parkinson's disease. Brain 1999;122(Pt 3): 405–416

111. Lombardi WJ, Gross RE, Trepanier LL, et al. Relationship of lesion location to cognitive outcome following microelectrode-guided pallidotomy for Parkinson's disease: support for the existence of cognitive circuits in the human pallidum. Brain 2000;123(Pt 4):746–758

112. Vitek JL, Bakay RA. The role of pallidotomy in Parkinson's disease and dystonia. Curr Opin Neurol 1997;10:332–339

113. Vitek JL, Bakay RA, DeLong MR. Microelectrode-guided pallidotomy for medically intractable Parkinson's disease. Adv Neurol 1997;74:183–198

114. Dogali M, Beric A, Sterio D, et al. Anatomic and physiological considerations in pallidotomy for Parkinson's disease. Stereotact Funct Neurosurg 1994;62(1–4):53–60

115. Taha JM, Favre J, Baumann TK, Burchiel KJ. Characteristics and somatotopic organization of kinesthetic cells in the globus pallidus of patients with Parkinson's disease. J Neurosurg 1996;85: 1005–1012

116. Starr PA. Placement of deep brain stimulators into the subthalamic nucleus or globus pallidus internus: technical approach. Stereotact Funct Neurosurg 2002;79:118–145

117. Henderson JM, Pell M, O'Sullivan DJ, et al. Postmortem analysis of bilateral subthalamic electrode implants in Parkinson's disease. Mov Disord 2002;17:133–137

118. Danish SF, Jaggi JL, Moyer JT, Finkel L, Baltuch GH. Conventional MRI is inadequate to delineate the relationship between the red nucleus and subthalamic nucleus in Parkinson's disease. Stereotact Funct Neurosurg 2006;84:12–18

119. Voges J, Volkmann J, Allert N, et al. Bilateral high-frequency stimulation in the subthalamic nucleus for the treatment of Parkinson disease: correlation of therapeutic effect with anatomical electrode position. J Neurosurg 2002;96:269–279

120. Yelnik J, Percheron G. Subthalamic neurons in primates: a quantitative and comparative analysis. Neuroscience 1979;4:1717–1743

121. Starr PA, Theodosopoulos PV, Turner R. Surgery of the subthalamic nucleus: use of movement-related neuronal activity for surgical navigation. Neurosurgery 2003;53:1146–1149

122. Rodriguez-Oroz MC, Rodriguez M, Guridi J, et al. The subthalamic nucleus in Parkinson's disease: somatotopic organization and physiological characteristics. Brain 2001;124(Pt 9):1777–1790

123. Romanelli P, Heit G, Hill BC, et al. Microelectrode recording revealing a somatotopic body map in the subthalamic nucleus in humans with Parkinson disease. J Neurosurg 2004;100:611–618

124. Maltete D, Navarro S, Welter ML, et al. Subthalamic stimulation in Parkinson disease: with or without anesthesia? Arch Neurol 2004;61:390–392

125. Houeto JL, Welter ML, Bejjani PB, et al. Subthalamic stimulation in Parkinson disease: intraoperative predictive factors. Arch Neurol 2003;60:690–694

126. McClelland S, Kim B, Winfield LM, et al. Microelectrode recording-determined subthalamic nucleus length not predictive of stimulation-induced side effects. Neurosurg Focus 2005;19:E13

127. Abosch A, Hutchison WD, Saint-Cyr JA, Dostrovsky JO, Lozano AM. Movement-related neurons of the subthalamic nucleus in patients with Parkinson disease. J Neurosurg 2002;97:1167–1172

128. Counelis GJ, Simuni T, Forman MS, Jaggi JL, Trojanowski JQ, Baltuch GH. Bilateral subthalamic nucleus deep brain stimulation for advanced PD: correlation of intraoperative MER and postoperative MRI with neuropathological findings. Mov Disord 2003;18:1062–1065

129. Pollak P, Krack P, Fraix V, et al. Intraoperative micro- and macro-stimulation of the subthalamic nucleus in Parkinson's disease. Mov Disord 2002;17(Suppl 3):S155–S161

130. Moro E, Scerrati M, Romito LM, et al. Chronic subthalamic stimulation reduces medication requirements in Parkinson disease. Neurology 1999;53:85–90

131. Benabid AL, Benazzouz A, Limousin P, et al. Dyskinesias and the subthalamic nucleus. Ann Neurol 2000;47(4, Suppl 1)S189–S192

132. Benabid AL, Koudsie A, Benazzouz A, et al. Deep brain stimulation for Parkinson's disease. Adv Neurol 2001;86:405–412

133. Oh MY, Abosch A, Kim SH, Lang AE, Lozano AM. Long-term hardware-related complications of deep brain stimulation. Neurosurgery 2002;50:1268–1274 (discussion 1274–1276)

134. Joint C, Nandi D, Parkin S, Gregory R, Aziz T. Hardware-related problems of deep brain stimulation. Mov Disord 2002;17(Suppl 3): S175–S180

135. Kondziolka D, Whiting D, Germanawala A, Oh M. Hardware-related complications after placement of thalamic deep brain stimulator systems. Stereotact Funct Neurosurg 2002;79:228–233

136. Favre J, Taha JM, Nguyen TT, Gildenberg PL, Burchiel KJ. Pallidotomy: a survey of current practice in North America. Neurosurgery 1996;39:883–890 (discussion 890–892)

137. Cosman ER. Radiofrequency lesions. In: Gildenberg PL, Taker RR, eds. Textbook of Stereotactic and Functional Neurosurgery. New York: McGraw-Hill; 1997:973–986

138. Vitek JL, Bakay RA, Freeman A, et al. Randomized trial of pallidotomy versus medical therapy for Parkinson's disease. Ann Neurol 2003;53:558–569

139. Merello M, Nouzeilles MI, Kuzos G, et al. Unilateral radiofrequency lesion versus electrostimulation of posteroventral pallidum: a prospective randomized comparison. Mov Disord 1999;14:50–56

140. Schuurman PR, Bruins J, Merkus MP, Bosch DA, Speelman JD. A comparison of neuropsychological effects of thalamotomy and thalamic stimulation. Neurology 2002;59:1232–1239

141. Benabid AL, Vercueil L, Benazzouz A, et al. Deep brain stimulation: what does it offer? In: Ariel Gordin, ed. Parkinson's Disease: Advances in Neurology. Philadelphia: Lippincott Williams & Wilkins; 2003:293–302

142. Pahwa R, Lyons KE, Wilkinson SB, et al. Comparison of thalamotomy to deep brain stimulation of the thalamus in essential tremor. Mov Disord 2001;16:140–143

143. Koller WC, Lyons KE, Wilkinson SB, Troster AI, Pahwa R. Long-term safety and efficacy of unilateral deep brain stimulation of the thalamus in essential tremor. Mov Disord 2001;16:464–468

144. Pinter MM, Murg M, Alesch F, Freundl B, Helscher RJ, Binder H. Does deep brain stimulation of the nucleus ventralis intermedius affect postural control and locomotion in Parkinson's disease? Mov Disord 1999;14:958–963

145. Tasker R. Thalamotomy. In: WA F, ed. Stereotactic Neurosurgery: Neurosurgical Clinics of North America. Philadelphia: Saunders; 1990:841–864

146. Akbostanci MC, Slavin KV, Burchiel KJ. Stereotactic ventral intermedial thalamotomy for the treatment of essential tremor: results of a series of 37 patients. Stereotact Funct Neurosurg 1999;72:174–177

147. Fox MW, Ahlskog JE, Kelly PJ. Stereotactic ventrolateralis thalamotomy for medically refractory tremor in post-levodopa era Parkinson's disease patients. J Neurosurg 1991;75:723–730

148. Goodman SH, Wilkinson S, Overman J, et al. Lesion volume and clinical outcome in stereotactic pallidotomy and thalamotomy. Stereotact Funct Neurosurg 1998;71:164–172

149. Andy OJ, Jurko MF. Posterior subthalamic lesions in Parkinson tremor. Surg Forum 1963;14:434–435

150. Mundinger F. Stereotaxic interventions on the zona incerta area for treatment of extrapyramidal motor disturbances and their results. Confin Neurol 1965;26:222–230

151. Spiegel EA, Wycis HT, Szekely EG, Adams DJ, Flanagan M, Baird HW. Campotomy in various extrapyramidal disorders. J Neurosurg 1963;20:871–884

152. Guridi J, Obeso JA. The subthalamic nucleus, hemiballismus and Parkinson's disease: reappraisal of a neurosurgical dogma. Brain 2001;124(Pt 1):5–19

153. Velasco F, Jimenez F, Perez ML, et al. Electrical stimulation of the prelemniscal radiation in the treatment of Parkinson's disease: an old target revised with new techniques. Neurosurgery 2001;49:293–308

154. Plaha P, Ben-Shlomo Y, Patel NK, et al. Stimulation of the caudal zona incerta is superior to stimulation of the subthalamic nucleus in improving contralateral parkinsonism. Brain 2006;129(pt 7):1732–1747

155. Kitagawa M, Murata J, Uesugii H, et al. Two-year follow-up of chronic stimulation of the posterior subthalamic white matter for tremor-dominant Parkinson's disease. Neurosurgery 2005;56:281–289

156. Lopez-Flores G, Miguel-Morales J, Teijeiro-Amador J, et al. Anatomic and neurophysiological methods for the targeting and lesioning of the subthalamic nucleus: Cuban experience and review. Neurosurgery 2003;52:817–830

157. Vesper J, Chabardes S, Fraix V, Sunde N, Ostergaard K, Kinetra Study Group. Dual channel deep brain stimulation system (Kinetra) for Parkinson's disease and essential tremor: a prospective multicentre open label clinical study. J Neurol Neurosurg Psychiatry 2002;73:275–280

158. Okun MS, Tagliati M, Pourfar M, et al. Management of referred deep brain stimulation failures: a retrospective analysis from 2 movement disorders centers. Arch Neurol 2005;62:1250–1255

159. Oh MY, Hodaie M, Kim SH, Alkhani A, Land AE, Lozano AM. Deep brain stimulator electrodes used for lesioning: proof of principle. Neurosurgery 2001;49:363–369

160. Da Costa A, Kirkorian G, Cucherat M, et al. Antibiotic prophylaxis for permanent pacemaker implantation: a meta-analysis. Circulation 1998;97:1796–1801

161. Priori A, Egidi M, Presenti A, et al. Do intraoperative microrecordings improve subthalamic nucleus targeting in stereotactic neurosurgery for Parkinson's disease? J Neurosurg Sci 2003;47:56–60

162. Alterman RL, Shils JL, Gudesblatt M, Tagliati M. Immediate and sustained relief of levodopa-induced dyskinesias after dorsal relocation of a deep brain stimulation lead: case report. Neurosurg Focus 2004;17:E6

163. Papavassiliou E, Rau G, Heath S, et al. Thalamic deep brain stimulation for essential tremor: relation of lead location to outcome. Neurosurgery 2004;54:1120–1129

164. Hamani C, Richter EO, Andrade-Souza Y, Saint-Cyr JA, Lozano AM. Correspondence of microelectrode mapping with magnetic resonance imaging for subthalamic nucleus procedures. Surg Neurol 2005;63:249–253 (discussion 253)

165. den Dunnen WF, Staal MJ. Anatomical alterations of the subthalamic nucleus in relation to age: a postmortem study. Mov Disord 2005;20:893–898

166. Bonneville F, Welter ML, Elie C, et al. Parkinson disease, brain volumes, and subthalamic nucleus stimulation. Neurology 2005;64:1598–1604

167. Goetz CG, Poewe W, Rascol O, Sampaio C. Evidence-based medical review update: pharmacological and surgical treatments of Parkinson's disease: 2001 to 2004. Mov Disord 2005;20:523–539

168. Temel Y, Visser-Vandewalle V. Targets for deep brain stimulation in Parkinson's disease. Expert Opin Ther Targets 2006;10:355–362

169. Mazzone P, Lozano A, Stanzione P, et al. Implantation of human pedunculopontine nucleus: a safe and clinically relevant target in Parkinson's disease. Neuroreport 2005;16:1877–1881

170. Plaha P, Gill SS. Bilateral deep brain stimulation of the pedunculopontine nucleus for Parkinson's disease. Neuroreport 2005;16:1883–1887

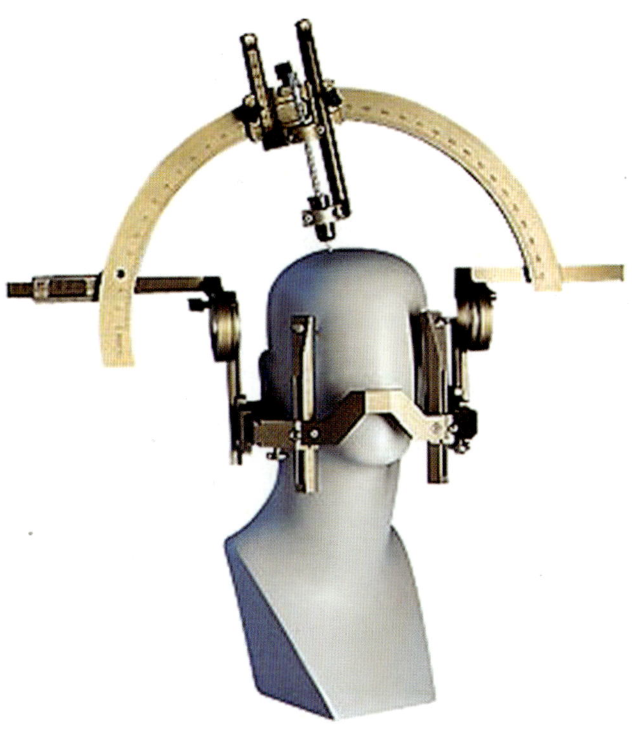

Color Plate 3.1 Leksell Stereotactic System (Elekta AB, Stockholm, Sweden, www.electa.com). (See **Fig. 3.1**, page 26.)

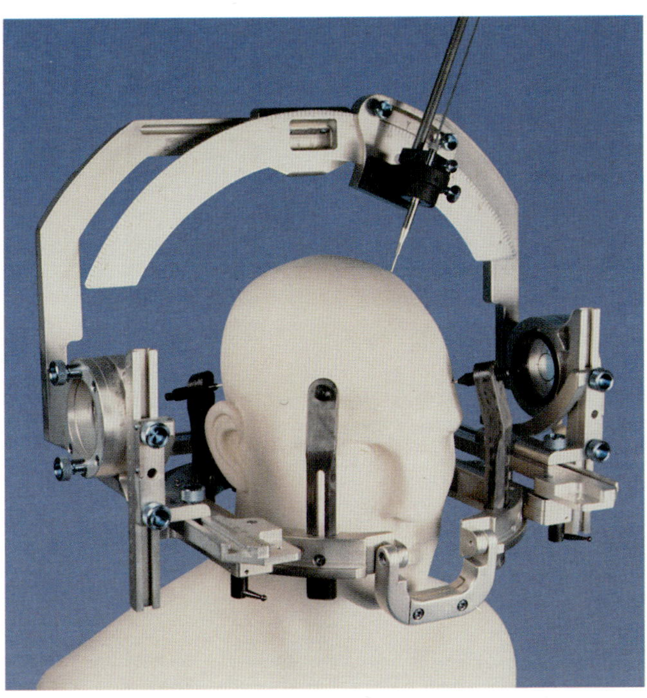

Color Plate 3.2 The Cosman-Roberts-Wells (CRW) Stereotactic Apparatus (Integra Radionics, Burlington, MA, www.radionics.com). (See **Fig. 3.2**, page 26)

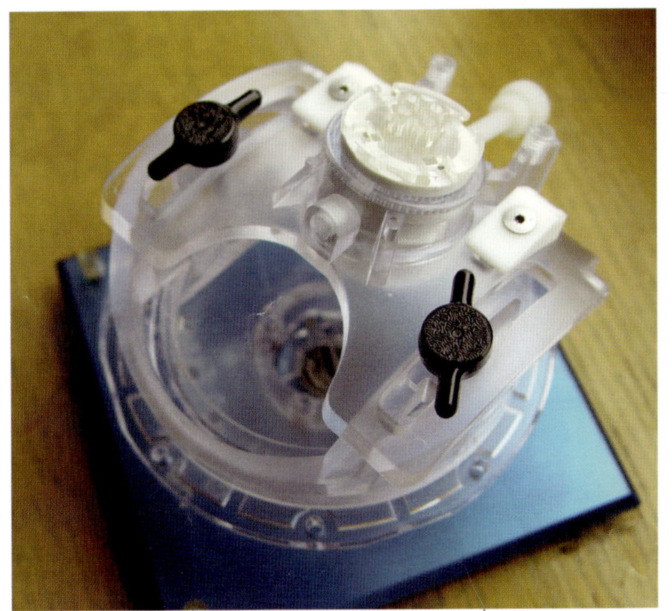

Color Plate 3.4 Nexframe Frameless Microelectrode Recording Guidance Assembly (Medtronic, Minneapolis, MN). (See **Fig. 3.4**, page 27.)

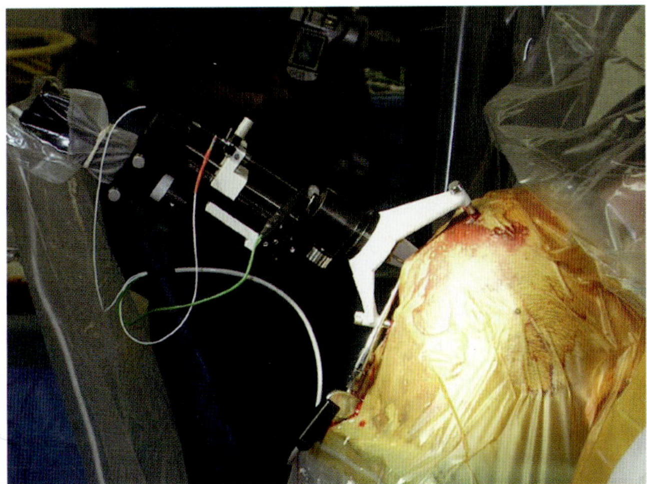

Color Plate 3.5 STarFix tripod (FHC, Inc., Bowdoin, ME, www.fh-co.com) coupled to the skull via the Acustar bone markers (z-kat Company, www.z-kat.com). (See **Fig. 3.5**, page 28.)

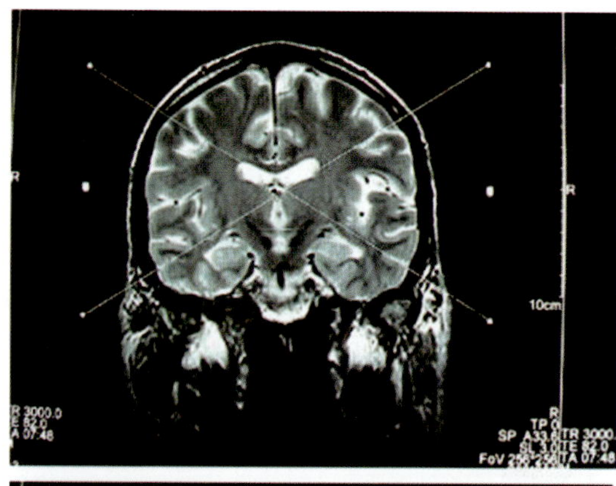
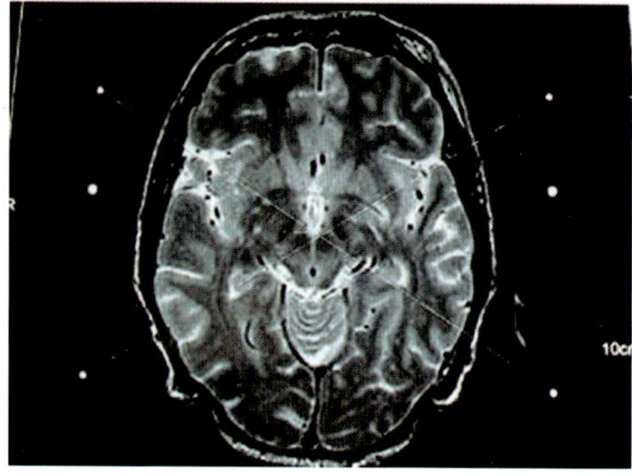

Color Plate 8.2 Axial and coronal stereotactic magnetic resonance imaging showing the subthalamic nucleus. (See **Fig. 8.2**, page 117.)

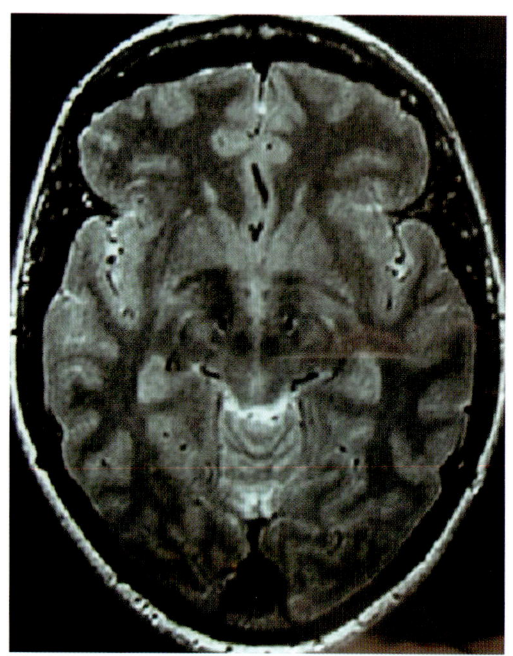

Color Plate 8.5 Stereotactic thin-slice magnetic resonance imaging showing deep brain stimulation leads in the subthalamic nucleus bilaterally. (See **Fig. 8.5**, page 121.)

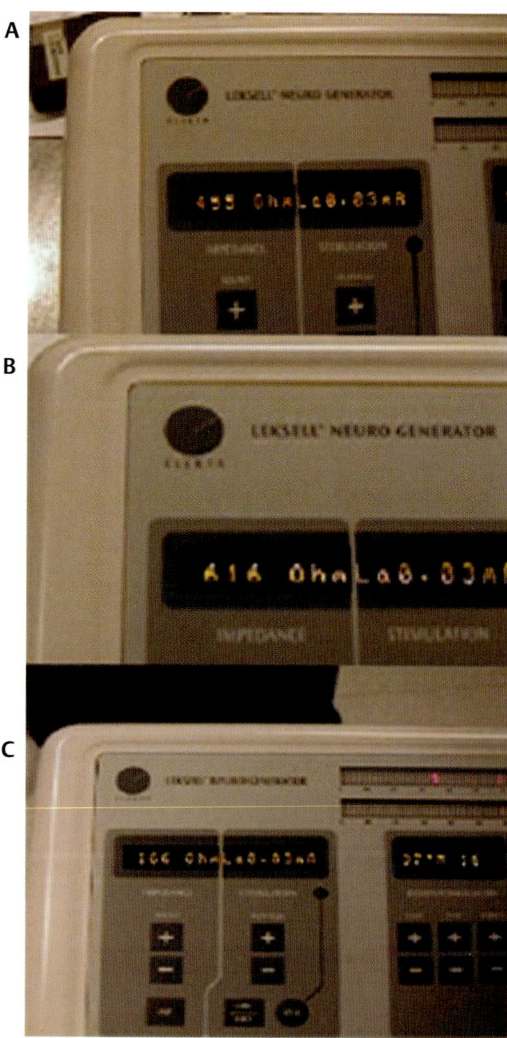

Color Plate 8.3 Impedance values in **(A)** gray matter, **(B)** white matter, and **(C)** cerebrospinal fluid measured with a 2 mm thick radiofrequency electrode. (See **Fig. 8.3**, page 118.)

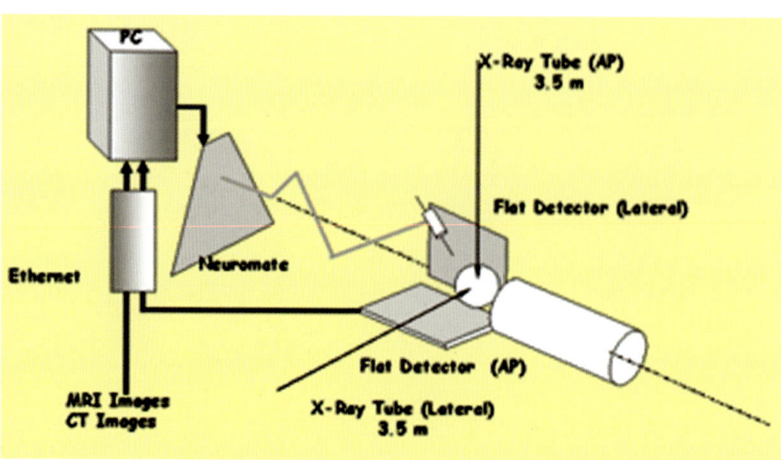

Color Plate 9.1 Flow chart of the NeuroMate robotized stereotactic system. (See **Fig. 9.1**, page 127.)

Color Plate 9.2 General pictures of the NeuroMate robotized arm, the ultrasound guidance system, and the "flight simulator." (See **Fig. 9.2**, page 127.)

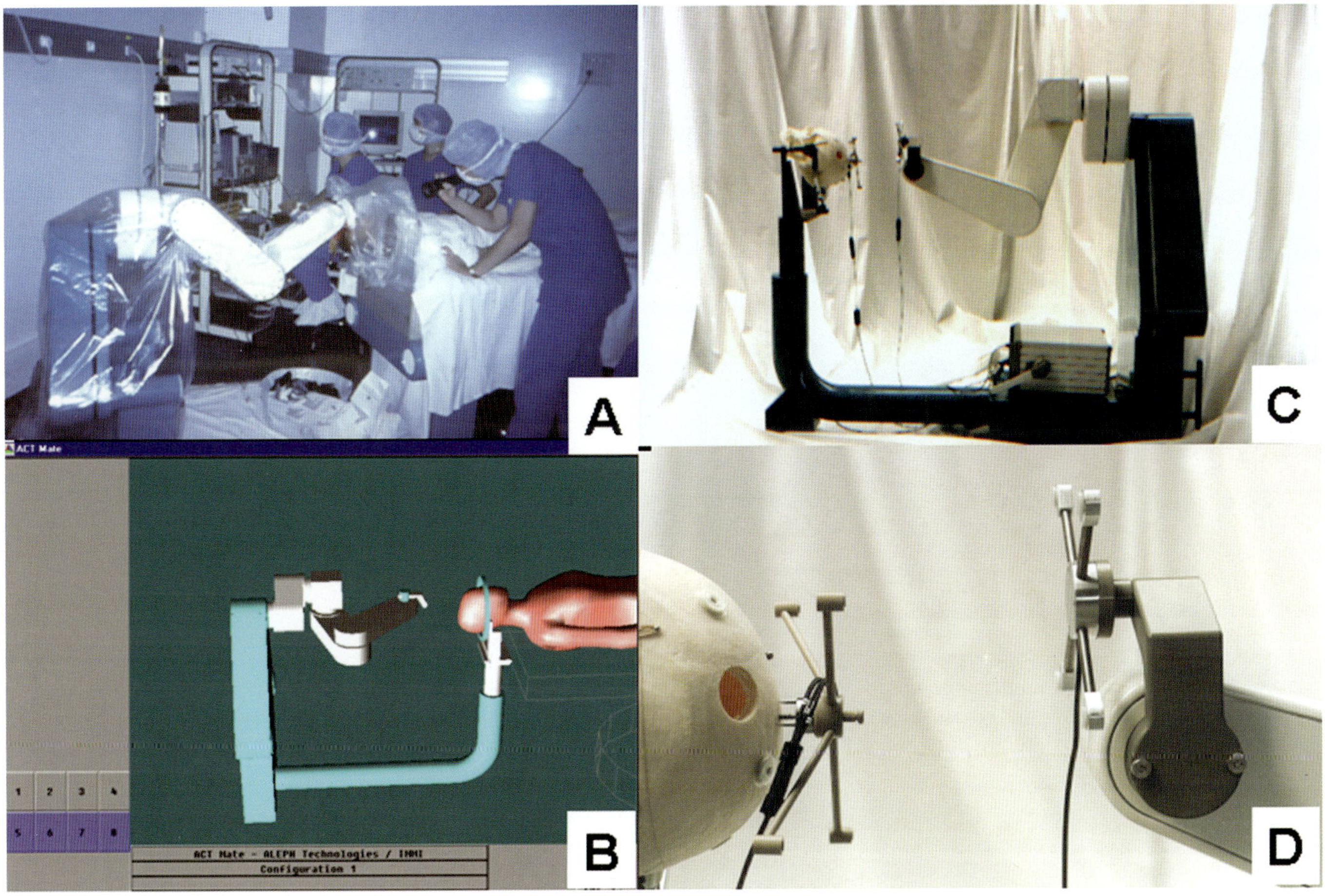

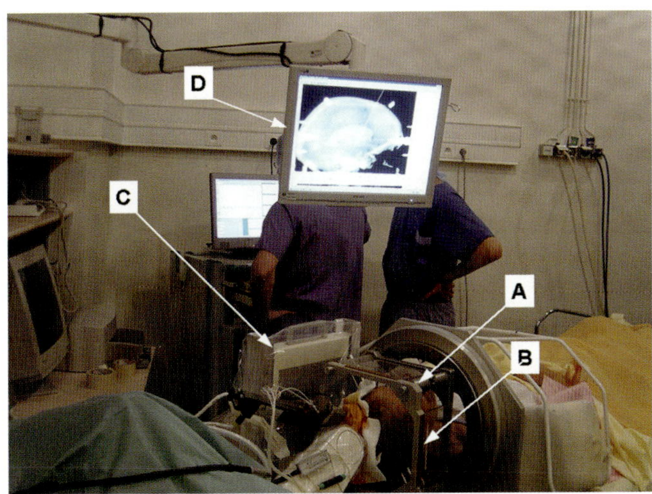

Color Plate 9.3 Stereotactic frame and flat detectors. (**A**) Stereotactic frame mounted on a rotating solid-state stand. (**B**) X-ray Plexiglas localizers mounted on the stereotactic frame. (**C**) Flat angiography digitizers mounted in orthogonal setup with long-distance X-ray generators. (**D**) Display of X-ray images. (See **Fig. 9.3**, page 128.)

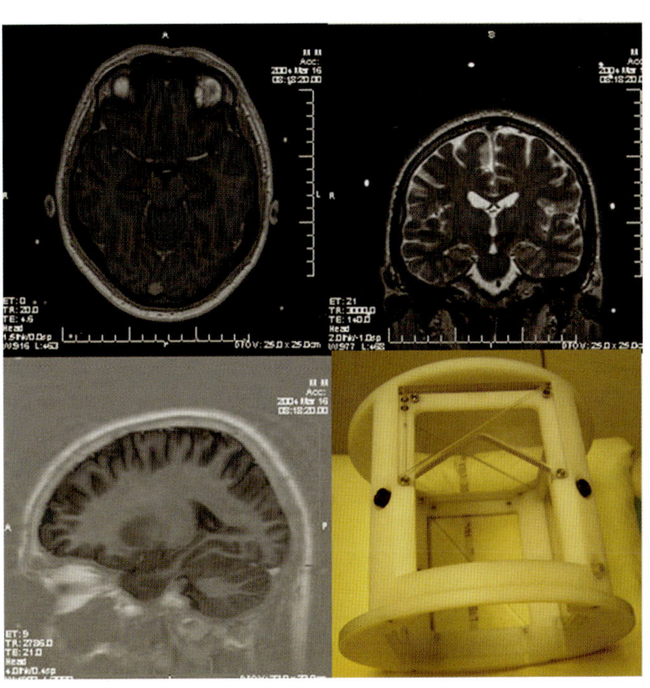

Color Plate 9.6 Stereotactic magnetic resonance imaging (MRI) and MRI localizer head set. (See **Fig. 9.6**, page 131.)

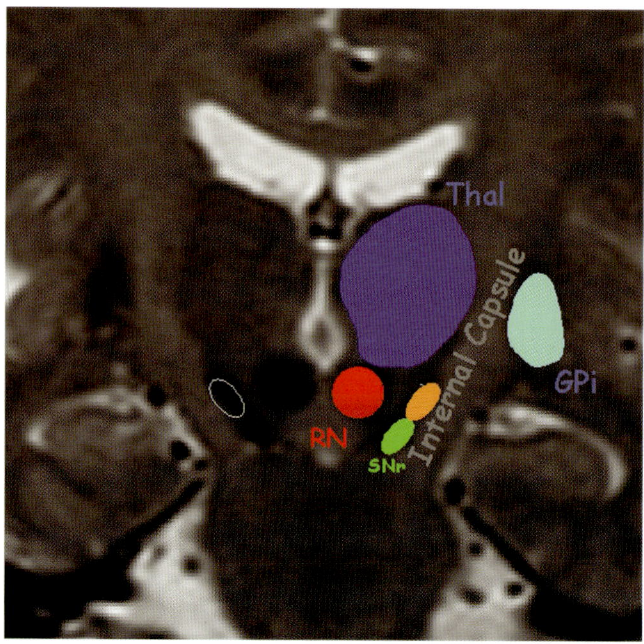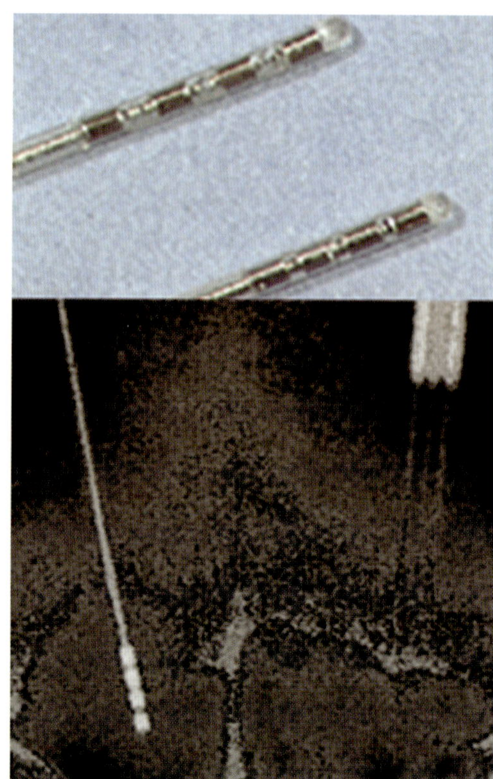

Color Plate 9.7 Magnetic resonance imaging visualization of the movement disorder targets: subthalamic nucleus (STN), thalamus (Thal), and pallidum as well as the red nucleus (NR) and the internal capsule. GPi, globus pallidus internus. (See **Fig. 9.7**, page 132.)

Color Plate 9.8 Chronic deep brain stimulation tetrapolar electrodes and acute recording micro-electrodes in a five-electrode setting. (See **Fig. 9.8**, page 133.)

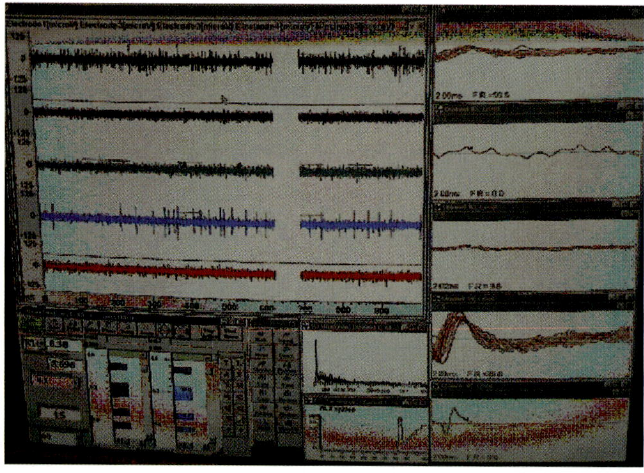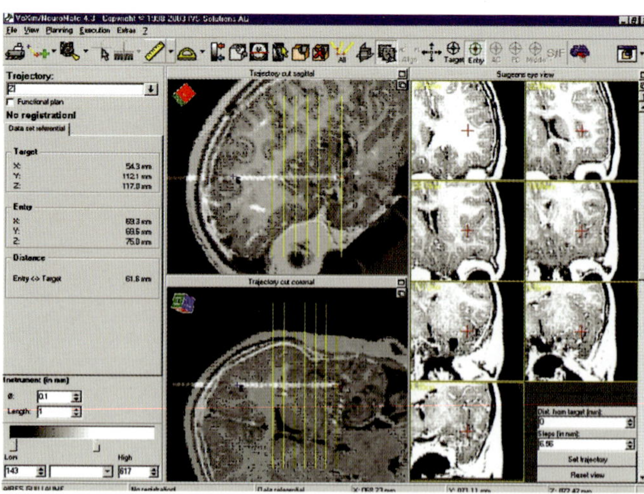

Color Plate 9.9 Five microelectrode simultaneous recording traces. (See **Fig. 9.9**, page 133.)

Color Plate 9.13 Deep brain stimulation planning of stereoelectroencephalography electrodes on the VoXim neuronavigation software (Integrated Visualization Systems, Chemnitz, Germany). (See **Fig. 9.13**, page 137.)

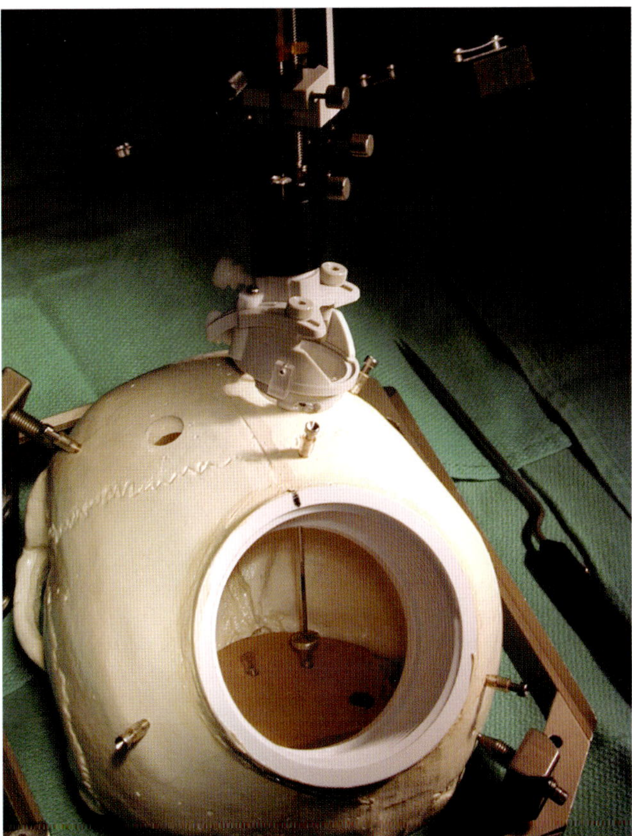

Color Plate 10.1A A plastic skull phantom used for verification of the image-guided navigation system. A localizing probe is being introduced to the expected target point. (See **Fig. 10.1A**, page 141.)

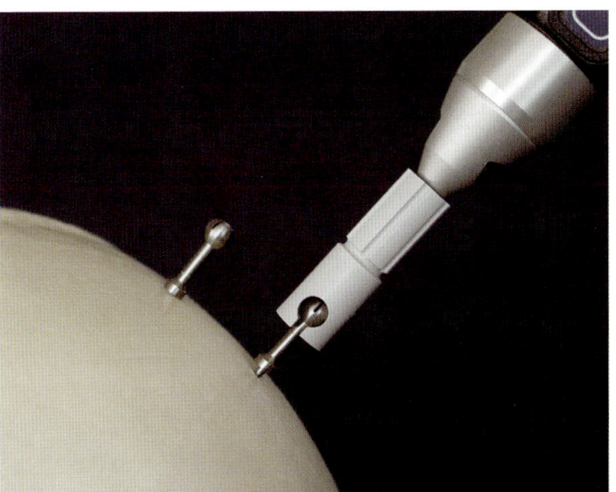

Color Plate 10.2 The one-piece titanium fiducial is pictured with a battery-powered autodriver. (See **Fig. 10.2**, page 142.)

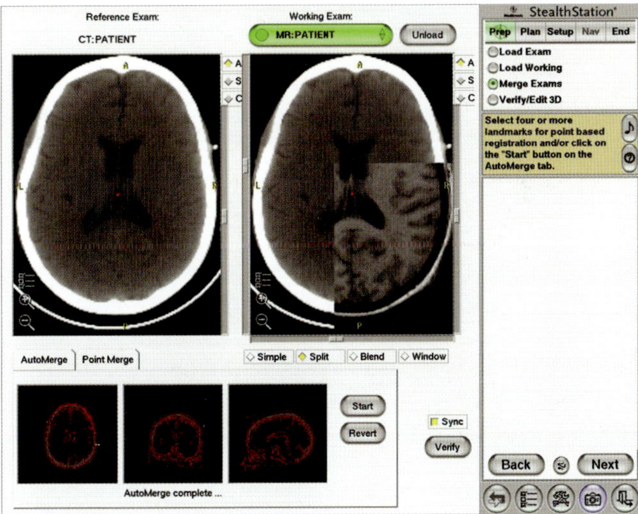

Color Plate 10.5 Note the excellent agreement of the fusion of the magnetic resonance scan done 3 weeks prior to surgery and computed tomography performed the day prior to surgery at the boundaries of the ventricles and in the cerebral sulci. (See **Fig. 10.5**, page 143.)

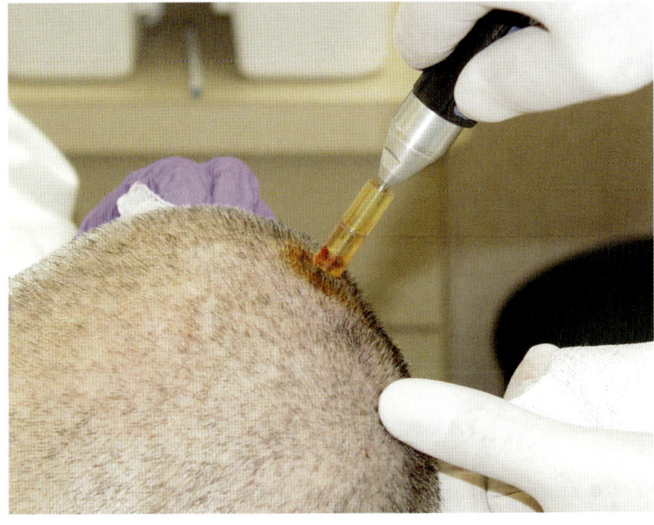

Color Plate 10.3 Placement of a fiducial marker is pictured following sterile preparation, infiltration of local anesthetic, and creation of a small stab incision. (See **Fig. 10.3**, page 142.)

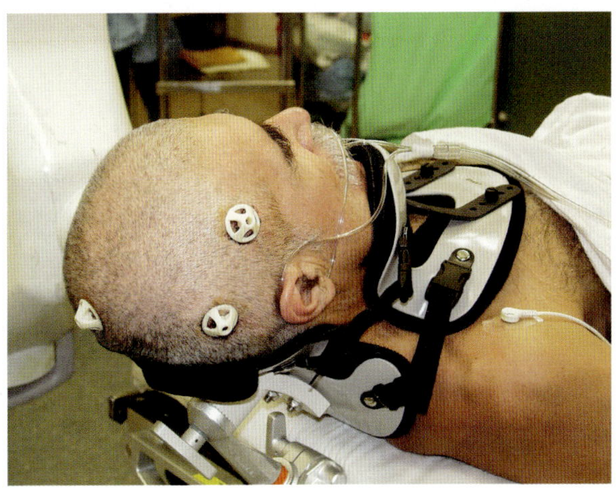

Color Plate 10.6 A patient positioned for deep brain stimulator insertion. A collar attachment helps stabilize the head during the initial localization and drilling steps; this is removed once electrophysiological monitoring begins. (See **Fig. 10.6**, page 143.)

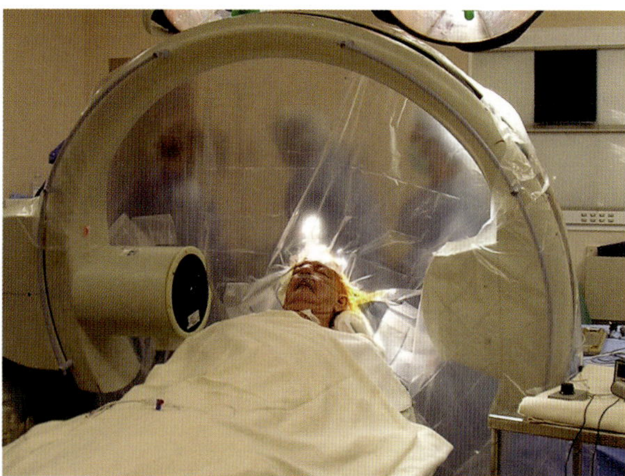

Color Plate 10.7 The C-arm fluoroscope can assist in evaluating lead placement and serves as a fixture for draping. (See **Fig. 10.7**, page 144.)

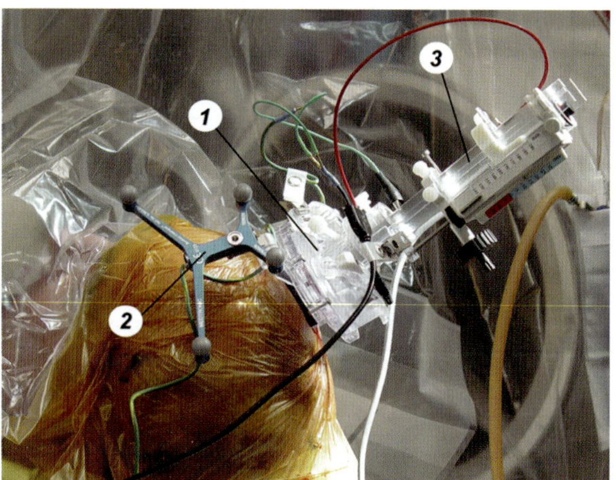

Color Plate 10.9B The Nexframe in clinical use. 1, trajectory guide platform; 2, neuronavigator reference arc; 3, microdrive. (See **Fig. 10.9B**, page 144.)

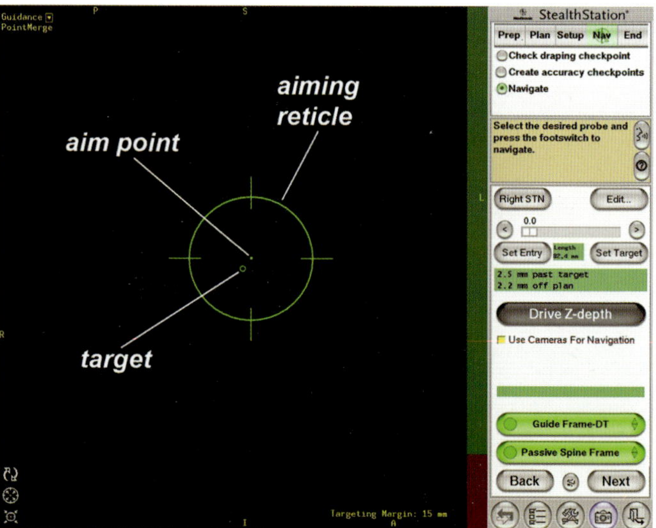

Color Plate 10.10 The StealthStation (Medtronic Navigation, Louisville, CO) display, showing the guidance view that is used to align the aim point with the target. The aiming reticle moves with the aim point, assisting the surgeon in determining the proper sweep and rotation settings. (See **Fig. 10.10**, page 145.)

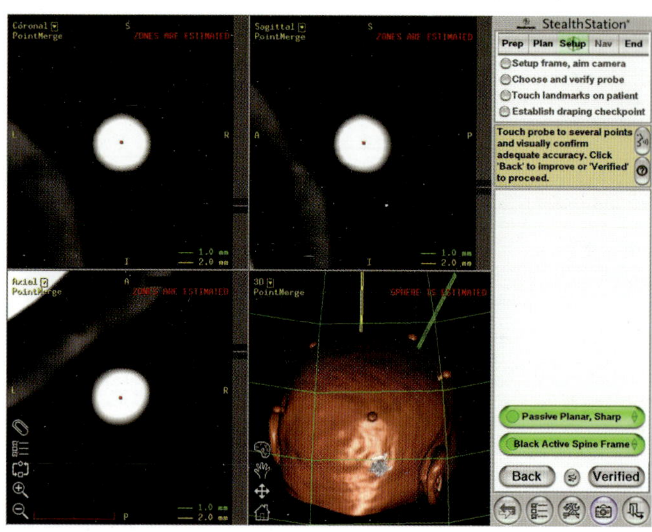

Color Plate 10.8 Relocalization of each fiducial marker verifies registration. Note the green "sphere of accuracy" within which predicted localization error is less than 1 mm. The small black dot indicates the localized position relative to the fiducial marker, showing excellent agreement. (See **Fig. 10.8**, page 146.)

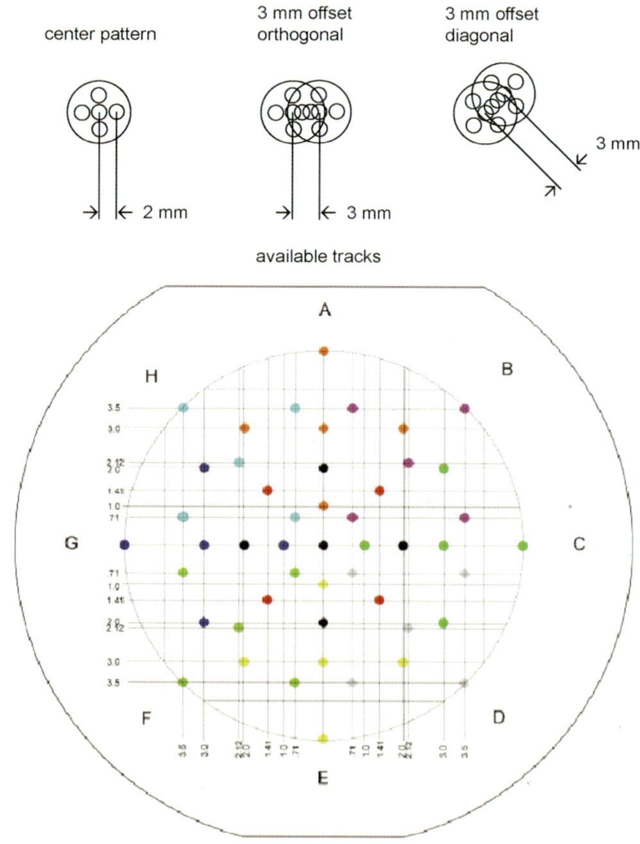

Color Plate 10.12 A diagrammatic representation of the center and 3 mm offset multilumen adapters provided with the Nexframe. By rotating the adapters to positions A through H, tracks can be made at 2 mm intervals either orthogonally or diagonally as illustrated in the lower diagram. (See **Fig. 10.12**, page 147.)

Stereotactic Surgery without Microelectrode Recording

Marwan I. Hariz and Nathalie Vayssiere

It may seem controversial to perform a functional stereotactic procedure, whether an ablation or a deep brain stimulation (DBS), without using microelectrode recording (MER). For a long time, several arguments have been presented to justify the use of MER in routine functional surgery: (1) The functional brain target could not be visualized as such on imaging studies. (2) If, however, the brain target aimed at could be visualized on magnetic resonance imaging (MRI), there was still concern about distortions in the image. (3) If brain atlas and ventricular landmarks—the anterior commissure (AC), posterior commissure (PC), and midline of the third ventricle—were used to indirectly determine the anatomical location of the brain target, there was concern about interindividual anatomical variabilities. (4) One could never be sure of the accuracy of the stereotactic frame and the probes used. (5) Functional stereotactic surgery is a physiological more than an anatomical procedure. Rather than debating these arguments,[1,2] this chapter outlines alternatives to MER for functional stereotactic procedures.

A non-MER-guided technique must obviously rely on other means than MER to achieve the success and safety of the procedure. These means may include (1) an adequate and validated preoperative stereotactic MRI method designed to visualize the individual target in the individual patient using appropriate scanning sequences to allow direct targeting without relying on brain atlas and ventricular landmarks; (2) a geometrically and mechanically accurate frame that is compatible with the imaging method used; (3) a radiofrequency (RF) machine to monitor the impedance along the track from the cortex to the target using a straight electrode with a noninsulated tip of no more than 2 mm in diameter or length; (4) a macrostimulation using standardized pulse width, frequency, and current intensity; (5) knowledge of the macroelectrophysiological response and of the functional anatomy of the target and its surrounding area so as to know where to move the electrode next in case of nonadequate response to stimulation in the awake, nonsedated patient; (6) immediate postoperative imaging performed in stereotactic conditions, with scanning sequences adapted to visualize with minimal artifacts both the target and the implanted DBS lead.

This chapter discusses these issues and their pros and cons as well as the variations in imaging, impedance, and macrostimulation parameters, according to brain target [i.e., the ventral intermediate (Vim) nucleus of the thalamus, the posteroventral pallidum (PVP), or the subthalamic nucleus (STN)].

■ Stereotactic Imaging

General Requirements

Two aspects have to be considered for MRI to be suitable as a source for direct determination of coordinates in functional neurosurgery. First, it must be able to provide good discrimination of the targeted brain structures (good structural definition); and second, the geometrical accuracy of the MRI scan has to be validated. General requirements to perform stereotactic imaging may include the following: (1) a stereotactic frame with an MRI localizer that is rigid (no possibility of deformation, or strain), and with good MRI compatibility (visibility on MRI, sensibility on image deformation, with a size as small as possible to allow for fiducials to be as close as possible to the head); (2) a suitable adapter to fix the frame in the MRI unit; (3) an adapted MRI sequence with ability to provide a good discrimination of targeted brain structures (good structure definition, see later discussion); (4) a field of view that fits the stereotactic frame; (5) a slice thickness allowing good compromise between resolution (the smallest) and signal:noise ratio (1.5 to 2.0 mm thickness is a good compromise); (6) isometric pixel size in the axial plane (x,y; square matrix, scan percentage of 100%); (7) enough slices to cover the target area with good margins, preferably without a gap between slices, and no overcontiguous slices (to avoid an interpolation of the signal between two slices); (8) a head coil to ensure maximal signal; (9) a protocol to minimize distortion through a regular check of the gradient fields (rigorous maintenance protocol); (10) control of movement during acquisition (general anesthesia if necessary); (11) weekly refills of the localizer box with new liquid ($CuSO_4$).

With few exceptions,[3,4] most functional stereotactic surgeons today do use a stereotactic MRI study to determine target coordinates. However, many workers who indeed use MRI still relate the target to its position in relation to visualized ventricular landmarks on the MRI study.[5–9] Unlike ventriculography and CT scanning, MRI is not a homogeneous imaging method. Depending on the parameters of imaging, an MRI study can visualize differently and unequally well various structures in the brain.

Ventral Intermediate Nucleus of the Thalamus

The ventral intermediate nucleus (Vim) of the thalamus is the only brain target in movement disorder surgery that still cannot be visualized as such on stereotactic thin slice MRI. Nonetheless, MRI, especially a T2-weighted MRI sequence with thicker slices, does indeed visualize the thalamocapsular border, making it easier to determine at least the laterality of the Vim target. Currently, the Vim target is used for essential tremor. The other commonly used targets in surgery for Parkinson disease and dystonia are the posteroventral pallidum and the STN. These structures can be exquisitely visualized on MRI, provided proper scanning sequences are used.

Posteroventral Pallidum

The subdivisions of the globus pallidus [globus pallidus pars interna (GPi), laminae medullaris interna and externa, globus pallidus pars externus (GPe)] and their surrounding structures (putamen, internal capsule, optic tract) can be visualized stereotactically on thin-slice axial and coronal MRI using various sequences. One such sequence[10] is a non-volumetric proton density sequence (repetition time (TR)/time to echo (TE) 4000/15, echo-train 7, field of view 250 mm, slice thickness 2 mm, gap 0, matrix 210 ◊ 256, excitations 3, imaging time 6 min, 5 sec) that depicts exquisitely the details of the pallidal target area (**Fig. 8.1**). Another sequence that has been validated by VayssiËre uses volumetric T1 sequences.[11,12] Other MRI scanning methods, based on inversion recovery sequences, have been described by Starr et al.[13] In all these cases, because the target itself is readily visualized, there is no need to refer to the landmarks of the third ventricle and to an atlas to obtain the location of the target in the individual patient, especially since it has

been shown that the individual target location may vary substantially between patients, and also between the two hemispheres in the same patient.[10,13]

Subthalamic Nucleus

In surgery on the STN, most workers who rely on MRI for targeting this structure determine its position on T1-weighted images in relation to third ventricle landmarks and brain atlases. The few publications reporting on the use of stereotactic MRI for direct visualization and targeting of the STN describe volumetric T2-weighted sequences with a rather long acquisition time,[14–18] sometimes requiring reformatting of images or additional T1-weighted sequences that are used for targeting, and often necessitating general anesthesia during imaging. These sequences do allow exquisite visualization of the STN. The present author, together with others,[19] has implemented a nonvolumetric T2-weighted MRI sequence (TR 3000–4000, TE 80–100) allowing individual visualization of the STN with fast acquisition sequences (between 3 min 5 sec and 7 min 48 sec, depending on the MRI machine) (**Fig. 8.2**). Here also, direct visualization made it possible to target the center of the visualized STN at surgery, avoiding an indirect localization based on the atlas and the AC–PC landmarks.

In all these imaging procedures, the authors have used either or both the Laitinen stereotactic apparatus[19–21] and the Leksell Stereotactic System (Elekta AB, Stockholm, Sweden),[11,12,22] together with MRI machines of various makes (Siemens, Philips, General Electric), that have undergone regular inspections for field inhomogeneity and other sources of distortions.

■ Electrophysiological Testing and Intraoperative Target Adjustment

Three methods can be used for physiological corroboration of the anatomical target in nonmicroelectrode-guided

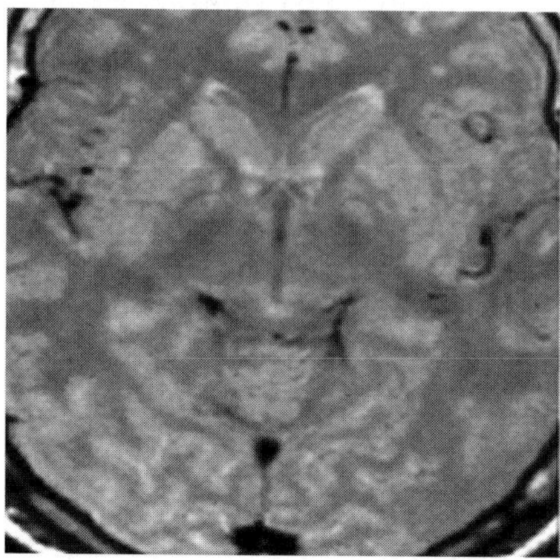
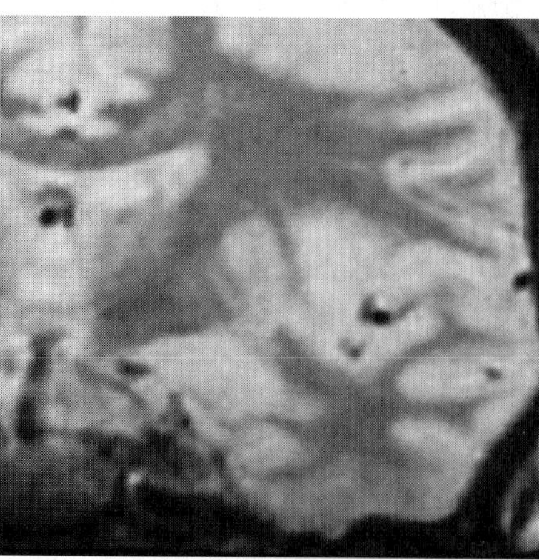

Fig. 8.1 Axial and coronal stereotactic magnetic resonance imaging showing the details of the posteroventral pallidum and its surrounding structures.

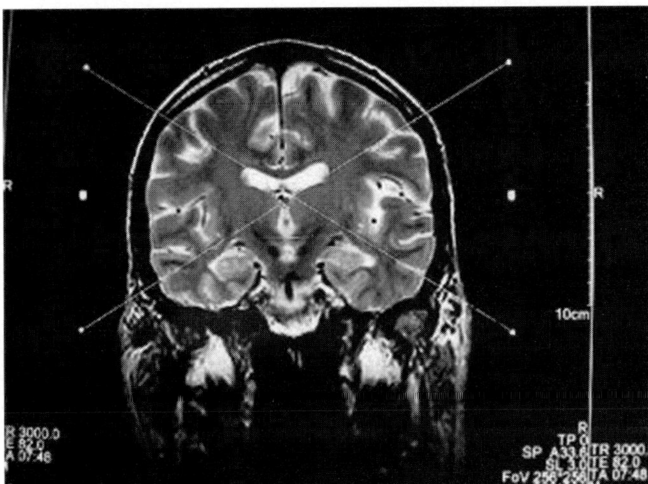

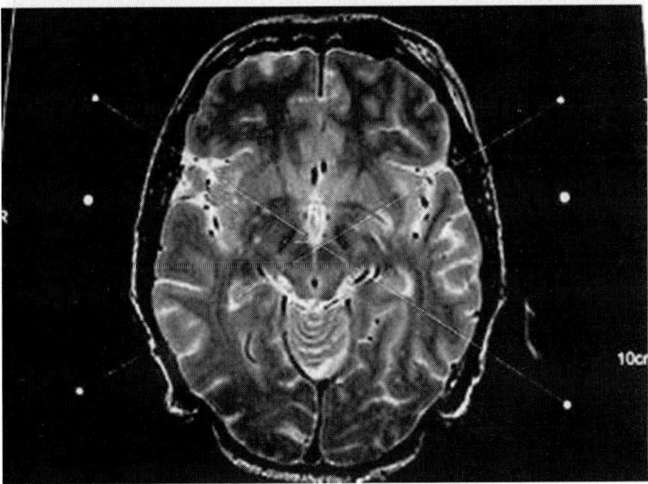

Fig. 8.2 Axial and coronal stereotactic magnetic resonance imaging showing the subthalamic nucleus. (See **Color Plate 8.2**.)

surgery: impedance recording, mechanical stunning effect when the probe reaches the target, and macrostimulation.

Impedance Recording

For impedance recording a radiofrequency (RF) electrode and RF generator are needed. Measurement of brain tissue impedance (resistance) to electrical current between a small probe tip and a large indifferent electrode is an old and excellent method to locate different structures inside the brain.[23] If the tip of the measuring probe is very small in surface area in relation to a large indifferent electrode, the impedance refers to the immediate vicinity of the probe tip. When the stereotactic probe is introduced toward the target area, the impedance is followed on a panel meter and by audio monitoring. Just by listening to the impedance pitch, the surgeon can detect the probe's location within a given structure. The Wheatstone bridge used for the impedance measurement gives the most accurate

results in the brain, when the oscillator frequency is 1 to 10 kHz. Then the impedance of the white matter is ~25% higher than that of the gray matter. The smaller the uninsulated probe tip, the more local-specific is the impedance recording. Therefore, uninsulated tips of the order of 1 to 2 mm in length and diameter are recommended. When the probe comes from the white matter perpendicularly into the gray matter of the putamen and pallidum, as for instance during pallidal procedures, the impedance fall is clearly noticed within 1 mm between white matter tracts and the anterodorsal putamen or anterodorsal pallidum, depending on angulation of the electrode trajectory. Typically, a white matter impedance of 600 to 800 ohm (depending on thickness of electrode) falls to 400 to 500 ohm into the gray matter. As the probe then approaches the base of the pallidum and the cistern between the pallidum and the temporal lobe, the impedance rapidly falls to 150 to 250 ohms. If the trajectory is such that the electrode exits the medial edge of the pallidum into the internal capsule, the impedance becomes suddenly higher again. In cases where an electrode tip of 1.0 to 1.5 mm is used, one can sometimes notice, just by listening to the impedance, when the electrode coming from the GPe toward the base of the globus pallidus internus (GPi), traverses the white matter of the internal medullary laminae.

During thalamic procedures, with a frontal approach, the probe penetrates the caudate nucleus with a low, gray matter impedance. In the white matter of the internal capsule the impedance rises again then falls again slowly toward the thalamus. As the probe comes to the vicinity of the subthalamic white matter the impedance starts rising again. The less sharp profile of impedance during ventrolateral thalamic surgery (compared with that during pallidal surgery) is due to the fact that the probe advances rather parallel to the thalamocapsular border.

When the probe is targeting the STN, one can notice, depending on angulation and trajectory of electrode toward the STN, first a rise of impedance at the immediate subthalamic area, then a decrease of impedance upon entering the STN; the impedance values here are, however, less distinctive due to the fact that the zona incerta contains small areas of mixed white matter and gray matter.

If on any trajectory the probe traverses the ventricle or any cistern or cystic cavity, there is a sharp decrease of impedance. **Fig. 8.3B** shows the impedance values in a case of pallidal surgery where the electrode (2 mm thick) ended up in capsular white matter. It was subsequently repositioned to end up in pallidal gray matter (**Fig. 8.3A**). Intraoperative stimulation at both locations confirmed in this patient the location of the electrode (see the macrostimulation section). **Fig. 8.3C** shows a cerebrospinal fluid (CSF) impedance value in a case where the electrode traverses a ventricular space. Hence, the impedance measurement, which does not require any extra time, provides an excellent method with which to check whether the probe is in gray matter, white matter, or CSF space.

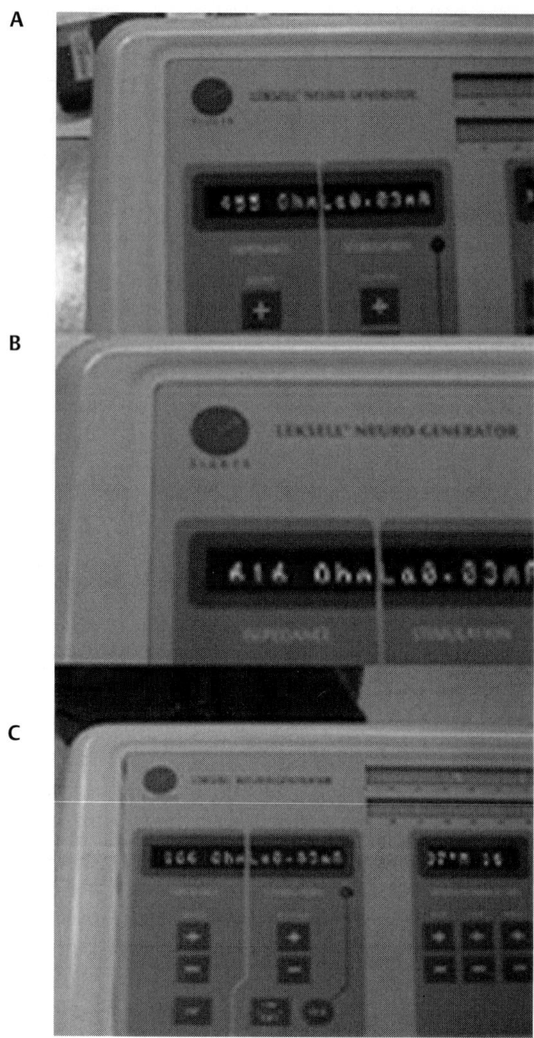

Fig. 8.3 Impedance values in **(A)** gray matter, **(B)** white matter, and **(C)** cerebrospinal fluid measured with a 2 mm thick radiofrequency electrode. (See **Color Plate 8.3**.)

Mechanical Introduction Effect

It is clinically important to observe carefully what may happen when the stereotactic probe comes to the vicinity of the surgical target. In surgery on the Vim thalamus and the STN, this mechanical effect may be very evident: In Vim surgery, tremor can sometimes be abolished just by a stunning effect when the electrode reaches the target. This stunning effect may last from a few seconds to several days. In surgery on the STN, sometimes the mere introduction of the DBS electrode provokes a sudden decrease in rigidity (assessed at the level of the wrist) and appearance of dyskinesias. The mechanical effect, also called microlesion (microthalamotomy or microsubthalamotomy) is a very good sign during surgery, suggesting accuracy in reaching the target. It may, however, not always be predictive of good and sustained long-term effect. Contrary to what some believe, this microlesioning effect does not preclude

conducting a macrostimulation of the target because, even if there are no more symptoms to stimulate (i.e., tremor or rigidity), stimulation can still be used to evaluate side-effects (see later discussion). In the pallidum, rarely do symptoms decrease by the mere introduction of the electrode to the target.

Macrostimulation

As for impedance recording, it is also important for stimulation that the probe tip is small. This guarantees that the stimulation effects are local-specific. If the uninsulated tip of the electrode is longer, for instance 4 or 5 mm, one cannot know which part of the tip generates the stimulation response. When stimulation is conducted using an RF electrode, most stereotactic surgeons use rectangular, biphasic waves, 0.2 to 1.0 millisecondsec in length. Even though some RF generators are still based on constant voltage, it is preferable to use constant current stimulators, where the current intensity is independent of tissue impedance change. In case the surgery is a DBS and not a lesional procedure, it is preferable to use the DBS lead itself for intraoperative stimulation because this is the lead that will subsequently be used for chronic stimulation; besides, one has ready access to four different contacts allowing a mapping of the stimulation response in the target area along the track of the DBS lead within the target.

Stimulation can be performed in a monopolar or bipolar fashion or both. In general, bipolar stimulation is more local-specific than monopolar but may require higher intensities and a larger pulse width. Typically, a 60 or 90 µsec pulse width is used, with a frequency of 130 Hz or more. The current intensity used varies from tissue to tissue. Depending on the nature of the brain target, intensities of 0.5 V up to 5 V can be used (see later discussion). Electrical stimulation together with observation of the mechanical introduction effect and impedance recording makes the stereotactic surgery relatively safe. If needed, the probe can be repositioned. Then the stimulation procedure is repeated. It must be stressed, however, that at the repositioning of the probe, the mechanical introduction characteristics as well as the impedance values and stimulation responses may have been modified by the first insertion of the probe. This is a drawback of macrostimulation-guided surgery.

During each intraoperative stimulation (and RF coagulation) it is important to check the patient with respect to the following: alertness, orientation, memory, speech articulation and voice strength, facial expression, limb strength, limb movements, limb dexterity, limb coordination, sensations (at fingertips, cheek, tongue and lips—paresthesias), vision and eye movements, eventual autonomic responses (sweating, heart rate, etc.), and of course eventual effect of stimulation on tremor, rigidity, akinesia, dyskinesias, and so forth. One should also maintain a conversation with the patient and ask the patient to report feeling anything special. Asking the patient to count backward or list weekdays or months backward will generate a small amount of stress, which will elicit or enhance symptoms and allow better assessment of the effect of stimulation on these symptoms. A record should be kept of the stimulation parameters and the patient's reactions during surgery.

Macrostimulation in Vim

Too low a stimulation threshold before effect or side effect (< 0.5 V, 130 Hz, 1 millisecondec) may indicate the position in the internal capsule or sensory thalamus. Even if tremor is decreased or arrested, a capsular location of the electrode may at lower voltages provoke cramps and increased difficulties in opening or closing the hand. Also, dysarthria or even speech arrest may be induced (especially during left-sided stimulation). At higher voltages, a tetanic cramp of the hand or lips may be elicited, as well as nausea. In the sensory thalamus, paresthesias at the fingertips or lips may be elicited. These features may urge repositioning of the probe in the medial or anterior direction, respectively. A too high stimulation threshold before obtaining a tremor-decreasing effect (> 3 V, 130 Hz) indicates the probe's position is too anterior, too medial, or too dorsal.

If thalamic high-frequency stimulation yields electrical feeling in the depth of the fingers, hand, or arm, and tremor arrest, with concomitant precise, fluid, and strong movements, good coordination, and good speech, then the probe must be in a good position. One can stress the patient by asking the patient to count backward to see if the tremor recurs. The same testing protocol can be applied to stimulation through the other DBS contacts to verify how many contacts would be effective for the symptoms and at what intensities, and with what side-effect profile. Intraoperative stimulation should always be conducted with rather large suprathreshold values to verify the safety window between stimulation values effective for tremor and values yielding side effects. As discussed earlier, if the mere introduction of the electrode stops the tremor, stimulation should indeed be done to detect side effects prior to permanent implantation.

If stimulation responses are not adequate, the position of the electrode has to be changed: After appropriately changing the coordinates on the frame, the electrode should be reintroduced toward the new target through a new cortical entry point within the context of the 14 mm burr hole, and the whole stimulation procedure should be repeated. In the authors' opinion, this may be done up to three times maximally, after which, if the response to stimulation is still poor, the surgery should be aborted.

Macrostimulation in the Posteroventral Pallidum

The stimulation thresholds in PVP are higher than those in the thalamus. Furthermore, the main aim of intraoperative stimulation here is not primarily to provoke an arrest of the symptoms (like tremor arrest during thalamic stimulation) but to avoid the internal capsule and optic tract. The effects of acute pallidal stimulation on the parkinsonian symptoms per se are not consistent unless one applies the stimulation for a long time (several minutes), which may not be practical during surgery. In routine intraoperative pallidal stimulation, however, sometimes nothing happens, sometimes stimulation increases the speed of movement of the leg or hand, and sometimes, more rarely, dyskinesias are elicited. This paucity of reaction in the pallidum is, however, not the case when a lesion is being performed, because, during the staged lesioning, there is almost invariably a release of rigidity and a striking amelioration of finger, hand, and leg dexterity.

To maximize the symptoms for the time of surgery, all parkinsonian medications should be stopped at least 6 hours before the operation. The burr hole should be 2.0 to 2.5 cm from the midline at the level of or slightly anterior to the coronal suture. Electrical stimulation, using a rigid RF electrode, is carried on with 5 to 6 Hz up to 8 to 10 mA and 130 Hz up to 4 to 5 mA, respectively. If, at these current intensities, stimulation does not give rise to any undesirable reactions (capsular or optic), then a coagulation is safe (if one is doing a lesional surgery) or the permanent DBS electrode can be implanted at this site, and stimulation is conducted in the same way as for thalamic surgery as far as observing the patient's reactions is concerned, but with higher thresholds to detect side effects.

It must be stressed that, at least in Europe, pallidal DBS is used much more for dystonia surgery than for PD surgery. Dystonia patients are most often operated on under general anesthesia,[24] which may preclude the use of stimulation as a means of localizing the position of the electrode. Here it is mandatory to perform an immediate postoperative stereotactic MRI to verify the exact location of the leads (see later discussion).

Macrostimulation in the Subthalamic Nucleus

At a fixed frequency of 130 Hz and pulse width of 60 μsec, the following can be obtained with monopolar stimulation of the STN through a DBS lead contact: a sudden decrease of rigidity assessed at the wrist (signe de Pollak-Limousin), a decrease or arrest of tremor, a gradual improvement of hand opening and finger dexterity, and sometimes the appearance of dyskinesias, starting typically on the contralateral foot. These responses may be obtained at amplitudes of 0.5 to 3.0 V. If none of these responses is obtained at these voltages, the probe is probably not in the STN. By increasing the voltage, one can obtain side effects that can be used to guide movement of the probe. If increased stimulation results in cramping in the hand or face together with dysarthria, the probe is probably in capsular peduncular white matter and should be moved medially and/or anteriorly or posteriorly. If paresthesias are elicited, the probe is too posterior or too medial or both. If there is a convergent eye deviation or pupil dilatation, the probe is too medial, affecting the oculomotor fibers. If there is an increase in tremor and rigidity, the probe is too close to or into the red nucleus. If there is increased rigidity associated with mood changes, the probe is probably too deep, affecting the substantia nigra.

In the STN and pallidum, it is advantageous to perform macrostimulation using the permanent DBS lead because this lead has four contacts that can be stimulated monopolarly one by one, allowing macromapping of the area along the track of the electrode. Another advantage is that the parameters of stimulation are close to those that will be ultimately used in chronic stimulation. Finally, by using the DBS lead for intraoperative macrostimulation, there is no need for replacing it once one is happy with the stimulation response: it just has to be secured to the burr hole at the level at which maximum benefit and lowest side effects are obtained.

◼ Advantages and Disadvantages of Surgery without Microelectrode Recording

In 1982, Tasker, Organ, and Hawrylyshyn published a book about the use of macro-stimulation in mapping the thalamus and midbrain in humans. In this 500-page book, entitled *The Thalamus and Midbrain of Man: A Physiological Atlas Using Electrical Stimulation,*[58] the authors provided a detailed atlas about the gross somatotopy of the subdivisions of the thalamus and midbrain, based solely on intraoperative macrostimulation. Furthermore, in a chapter published in *Neurosurgery Clinics of North America* in 1990 (pp. 846–847),[31] Tasker, who is a scientist and neurosurgeon with broad experience in both macroelectrode and MER, compared both techniques and stated the following:

> Macrostimulation is easy, requires minimal instrumentation, is quick, identifies a wide range of brain structures, even at variable distances from probe.... Microelectrode techniques are more difficult, time consuming, require more sophisticated equipment .... Microelectrode can identify only a limited repertoire of structures. The tip must be very close to a structure before it can be recognized at all.... The more limited current spread means that unless an excitable structure is very close, it will be missed; the surgeon may gain no clue from a "negative" trajectory where to seek next.

Thus macrostimulation is indeed a physiological method, simple to use, and readily available. The drawback of this technique is that sometimes it may be difficult to interpret the findings and to know in which direction one has to relocate the probe in case of unsatisfactory stimulation response, and in case no readily understandable structure, such as the sensory thalamus, the internal capsule, or the optic tract, is encountered upon macrostimulation. In surgery on the Vim during which the probe misses the Vim, unless the electrode is laterally or posteriorly misplaced,

stimulation may not give a clue as to which direction the probe should be moved. Is the probe too medial or too anterior? The same applies if, in pallidal surgery, the probe is too lateral or too anterior. The most difficult to interpret are the stimulation results in the area of the STN if the STN proper is missed upon the first introduction of the electrode. Furthermore, repeat introductions of macroelectrodes in view of finding the target may alter the physiology and anatomy of the target area, and one is lost as to what is being stimulated and how to interpret the response. In such cases, and after two to three introductions of the probe without stimulation benefit, either the surgery has to be interrupted or an intraoperative stereotactic MRI has to be performed before carrying on additional multiple penetrations to evaluate the location of the probe. This is especially the case if the STN has been missed at the first or second introduction. Hence the importance of postoperative stereotactic imaging in non-MER-guided surgery. In patients who receive DBS in general anesthesia such as patients with generalized dystonia, postoperative stereotactic MRI is simply mandatory. In these cases, no macrostimulation is possible, and even if these patients are operated on in local anesthesia, intraoperative stimulation may show nothing in terms of relief of symptoms. Therefore, one may argue that in dystonia patients MER is mandatory. However, some of the best reported results have been published by the team of Philippe AndrÈ Coubes in Montpellier, who performs pallidal DBS in general anesthesia for pediatric and adult dystonia, with neither recording nor stimulation, but using only a rigorous stereotactic imaging technique, both pre- and postoperatively.[24,59]

◼ Postoperative Stereotactic Magnetic Resonance Imaging

Stereotactic postoperative MRI is important in that it will show nonequivocally the exact location of the stereotactic lesion or the DBS electrode. This imaging should be done with the same parameters as the preoperative imaging. In cases of ablative surgery, however, it is an advantage that postoperative imaging be done several weeks after surgery to allow for postoperative edema to resolve. Unless a noninvasive frame such as the Laitinen frame has been used during surgery and repositioned on the head for the postoperative imaging,[60] the scanning can still be done with thin (2 mm thick) axial slices parallel to the AC–PC line, and thin coronal slices perpendicular to the AC–PC line. T1 or proton density sequences may be used, sometimes even T2 or inversion recovery, allowing visualization of the lesion, the target, and its boundaries (**Fig. 8.4**). In patients with DBS, postoperative imaging should be performed immediately after surgery while the frame is still on the head. If the neuropacemaker has already been implanted, MRI can still be done provided the voltage of the pacemaker is

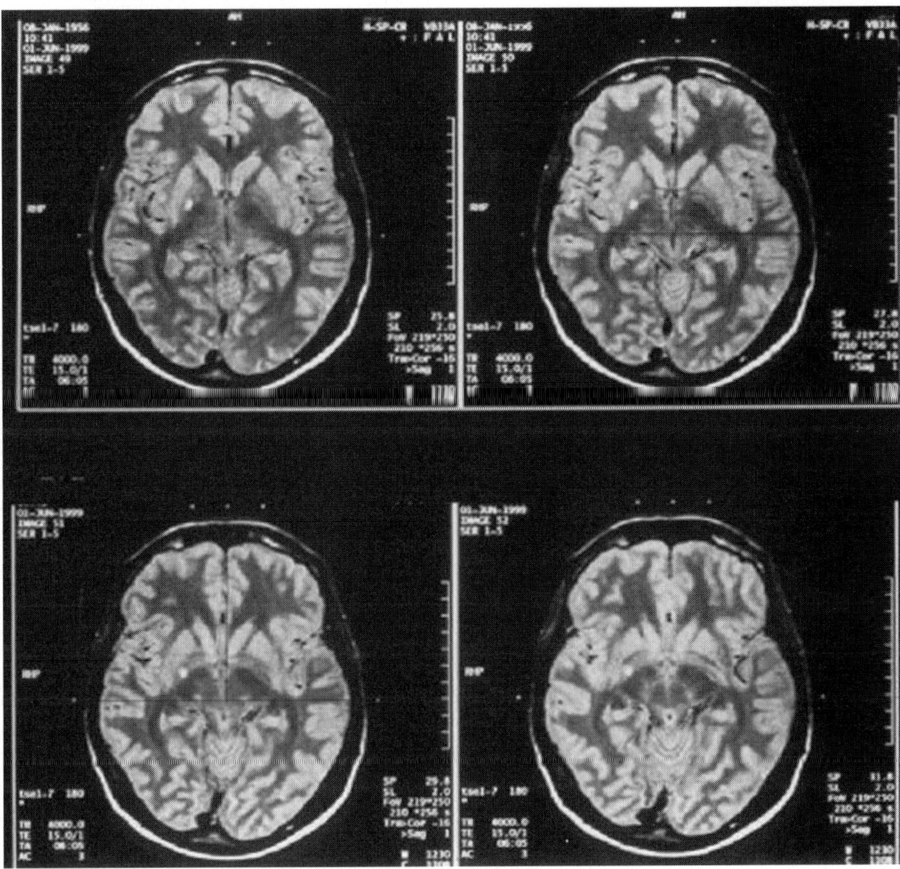

Fig. 8.4 Four contiguous axial stereotactic magnetic resonance imaging scans showing a 1-year-old, posteroventral pallidal radiofrequency lesion.

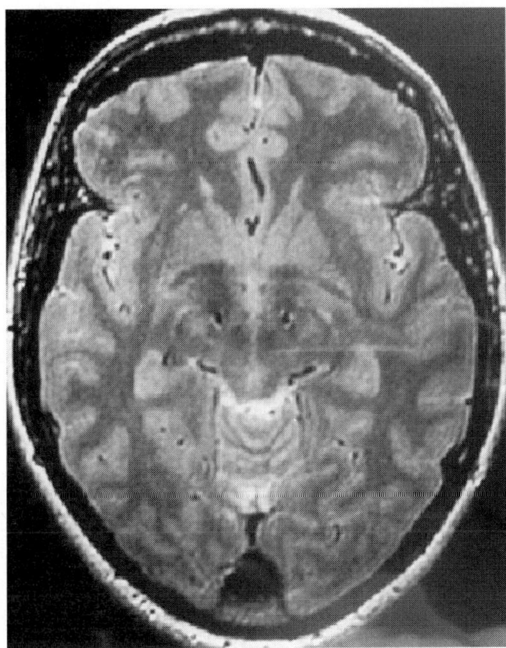

Fig. 8.5 Stereotactic thin-slice magnetic resonance imaging showing deep brain stimulation leads in the subthalamic nucleus bilaterally. (See **Color Plate 8.5**.)

set to zero and the output is off before the patient enters the MRI room. Here also, one should be able to assess the location of the lead within the visible target (**Fig. 8.5**), and if necessary, return the patient to the operating room to relocate the lead should it become misplaced.

■ Conclusion

Assuming experienced knowledge of the functional macroanatomy of the basal ganglia, a dedicated and validated stereotactic MRI method and an accurate MRI-compatible stereotactic frame are the most fundamental tools for performing a safe and precise functional procedure without MER. The precision of the technique can be enhanced if a thin, nonbent electrode is used for impedance monitoring and if the DBS lead itself is used for macrostimulation and mapping of the target area. The advantages are the safety and speed of the procedure. The disadvantages include the need for patient cooperation and the occasional difficulty to know for certain in which direction the electrode should be relocated in case of unsatisfactory stimulation response. Postoperative stereotactic imaging is mandatory to ascertain a good location of the DBS lead, especially in patients operated on under general anesthesia.

Editor's Comments

The optimal choice of adjuvant localization for stereotactic surgery for movement disorders remains controversial. It is uncommon to rely on anatomical techniques alone[17,24] except in radiosurgery (see Chapter 16). Patel and colleagues have developed a specialized technique using intraoperative cannula placement and repeat MRI to confirm targeting.[17] They report good results but do not have a recognized movement disorder neurologist to evaluate the patients with standardized instruments. Intraoperative MRI could be a wave of the future if the expense can be lowered and image quality markedly improved. Coubes and colleagues implantations are into the GPi, which is a large target for dystonia.[24] They report very good results with DYT-1 patients but so does everyone else (see Chapter 12). Patients in the same institute improve in motor scores significantly greater when under local and able to be electrophysiologically monitored than when under general anesthetic.[61] And finally there are brain shifts that are probably gravity-dependent but also may be lateral.[62,63] Because of the need for precise localization of functional targets, the vast majority of neurosurgeons are strong proponents of electrophysiological confirmation of the target and are aware of the disasters that can result when these techniques are not used.[25,26]

In attempting to compensate for the lack of direct anatomical visualization of the brain, the stereotactic and functional neurosurgeon is faced with problems of considerable magnitude: (1) errors introduced in localization of the target necessitated by the use of radiological methods, (2) errors in identifying appropriate landmarks, (3) the variability of individual anatomy, (4) lack of an appropriate stereotactic anatomical atlas, and (5) the role of human and mechanical imprecision.[27-29]

All of these factors introduce sources of error, which can be additive and can affect optimal target localization. As long as these errors exist, electrophysiological confirmation can serve as a quality assurance procedure. The question is what degree of electrophysiology localization is needed to optimize results.

Recording electrical impedance is an old method of helping define stereotactic targets for functional and biopsy cases. Macro-, semimicro-, and microelectrodes can measure impedance. The impedance measurements are highly variable depending on frequency and surface characteristics of the probe tip. Latinen et al[23] recorded the impedance and phase angle of brain tissue of 65 patients undergoing stereotactic surgery but this technique is currently rarely used. Impedance provides additional intraoperative anatomical information that is most useful in confirming the depth of a target but does not allow three-dimensional mapping, cannot differentiate among thalamic nuclei [Vim vs ventralis caudalis (Vc)], can be poor at differentiating between close nuclei (GPe vs GPi), and cannot always precisely determine the boundaries. Although it takes very little time, we stopped using it long ago.

In contrast, almost everyone uses macrostimulation. This chapter outlines the effects of macrostimulation on the standard targets. A North American survey of 36 centers that performed more than 25 procedures reported that all centers used MER, and all but two centers confirmed targets by macrostimulation.[30] Thus, for experts like Tasker[31] the choice was not MER or macrostimulation; rather, the choice was to refine the target with MER and confirm final placement with macrostimulation. The debate as to whether MER is necessary for optimal results is still actively debated between groups involved in the surgical treatment of movement disorders. Some teams consider anatomical localization by radiographic imaging with some type of adjuvant as discussed in this chapter to be sufficient, whereas most centers in the world use MER as an additional electrophysiological localization in an attempt to yield the best possible results. A few centers use semimicroelectrodes (~100 kOhm rather than 0.3 to 1.0 MOhm for MER), which record "group" activity or can record evoked movement active or tremor activity. To answer this debate it is necessary to know how accurate anatomical targeting is, how much added risk the use of MER introduces, and whether there is additional risk that is worth taking to optimize outcome.

Discrepancies between the anatomical or theoretical target and the actual physiological target when defined with MERs are of great concern and argue in favor of MER. MER allows for identification of the structural borders, localization within eloquent structures of the sensorimotor territory and somatotopic arrangement, and delineates the three-dimensional shape of the targeted nuclei that can determine spatial accuracy at each step. Multiple studies examining the impact of MER on final target selection have been performed in lesioning as well as stimulation procedures.

In a study of 160 pallidotomies, Vitek et al[9] found that the center of the lesion was located an average of 2.2 mm from the radiographically determined target. The physiological target deviated more than 4 mm in ~15% of the cases, demonstrating the need for electrophysiological correction of anatomical targeting. A learning curve was also demonstrated with direct correlation to decreasing the mean number of tracts from six to three. Azizi and Moreledge[32] compared the accuracy of anatomical targets defined by MER, and in 25% of the cases the theoretical coordinates were > 5 mm away from the lesion site. In a study by Hiner and Neal,[33] the results of MER led to a change in final pallidal lesion placement in 70% of patients. In a Toronto series, in only four of 26 pallidotomies was there a need for revision of the radiographically targeted coordinates, but 84% of the final lesions tended to be in a location more anterior and dorsal to the recommended target.[34] A study of 50 pallidotomy patients found that 55% of the lesions were placed posterior and lateral to the theoretically chosen MRI targets.[6] This suggests that individual centers may have a different targeting bias. Carlson and Iacono[35] compared standard MRI targeting, image fusion with computed tomography (CT) and MRI, and the microelectrode-refined target. Interestingly, there were no significant differences between standard MRI targeting and image fusion techniques. However, up to 80% of the pallidal lesions required physiological targeting. An even higher percentage is reported by Starr et al.[13] Nearly 90% of patients had discrepancies between the stereotactic and physiological determinants of 2 mm in 46 of 51 pallidotomies. Individual variations in the lateral coordinates correlated with third ventricular width. Alterman et al[5] performed a retrospective case study of 132 pallidotomies comparing the initial MRI-derived coordinates of the target to the final microelectrode-refined lesion coordinates, which led to targeting changes in 98% of cases. In 12% of patients, the physiologically defined target was more than 4 mm from the MRI target. One of the few studies on thalamotomy reported 75% of cases in which the theoretical target did not coincide with the final target using electrophysiological monitoring.[36]

Although anatomical localization is improving with modern technique, CT and MRI fusion was used to compare 62 patients with 28 DBS implants in multiple targets, including 51 thalamic, 10 globus pallidus, and one subthalamic nucleus. The physiological information modified the surgery in 67% of the cases.[37] Duffner and colleagues[38] documented an image fusion error (1.3 mm), which is approximately the same as that generally attributed to MRI alone (1.5 to 2.0 mm). It should also be noted that current technology is "best match" and not true three-dimensional morphing. In a study of 12 patients, Rodriguez et al[39] performed 22 subthalamic DBS implants with MER. Sixty-four percent of the time the first track was within the limits of the nucleus, but only 47% coincided with the sensorimotor region of the subthalamic nucleus. Therefore, 53% of the cases needed neurophysiological refinement. Bilateral subthalamic DBS using five parallel microelectrode tracts was studied in 12 patients for 24 subthalamic DBS implants, and intraoperative high-frequency stimulation coupled with MER corrected five of 24 implanted electrodes (21%).[14] In studies of 70 STN DBS leads implanted in 40 patients[40] and 54 leads in 27 patients,[41] MER modified the location of the final target in 58% and 90% of cases, respectively. Zonenshayn et al[42] compared direct visualization with MRI, Schaltenbrand and Wahren digitized atlases, standard midcommissural points, and a composite of all of these for targeting 30 subthalamic DBS implants. All anatomical methods yielded a statistically significant difference from the final physiological target in 2.6 mm, 1.7 mm, 1.5 mm, and 1.3 mm, respectively. Despite excellent direct MRI targeting, it still lags behind indirect targeting.[42-44] The problem may relate to brain shift that occurs as soon as the arachnoid or ventrical is violated.[45,46,62,63] In the supine position the shift will be posterior but in the semiseated position the shift will be posterior and ventral. These shifts may be as great as 4 mm.[63] The initial side may have a literal shift.[62] Finally, the type of MRI equipment used will affect precision[47] as well as the scan sequence, slice thickness, interslice spacing, slice orientation, and even the target size and location.[48]

Thus, despite excellent MRI studies, MER led to targeting changes in anywhere from 15 to 98% of the cases. Combine this with the growing evidence that even a few millimeters error may result in imperfect outcomes, incomplete improvement, or recurrence of symptoms[5,49,50] and clearly there is a need to correct anatomical targeting. Although definitive proof is lacking, it is hard not to admit that results should be improved by electrophysiological information that could correct those errors. The ability to correct errors again favors refining the target with MER and final confirmation with DBS macrostimulation. Macroelectrode probe diameters are measured in mm (1 to 2 usually), which, when introduced, frequently result in a microlesion effect that may preclude an evaluation of clinical benefits. MER tips are measured in μm, and the shaft that penetrates the target is one tenth the diameter of the macroelectrode/DBS; even with multiple tracts there may not be a significant microlesion effect. More important is that the initial placement of the probe is the best opportunity to get it right. Trying to make 1 to 2 mm adjustments with a 1 to 2 mm diameter probe is extremely difficult, and there is a strong tendency to fall back into the same hole. This assumes that after macroelectrode stimulation the direction and distance to move are known. This area of difficulty is not discussed in the macrostimulation literature.

Conversely, the additional penetrations of the brain should result in slightly more symptomatic intracranial hemorrhages. Prior to the reintroduction of pallidotomy the risk was very small (< 1%) in the hands of experts. It is the pallidotomy literature that has been used to suggest the risk is large (10 to 25%). However, this is the result of improper analysis.[51] Every report is added up; thus experts and beginners are lumped together as are those who study their patients meticulously and those who are cavalier. Looking only at series over 50 cases the difference is not significant.[52] Not included in this analysis is a report of 1116 patients that underwent a pallidotomy with only a 1.5% symptomatic hemorrhage rate.[53] Meta-analysis is of little use because the poor quality of the literature cannot support any reasonable analysis. Inexperience, poor quality, faulty equipment, and lesion effect were probably more to blame for the differences. Lesioning has a much bigger effect on the potential for hemorrhages than MER.[54] Another group found no difference between hemorrhage rates in patients who underwent MER compared with those who did not in 248 procedures.[55] Symptomatic hemorrhages in DBS series are again rare. Binder et al[56] had a 0.6% incidence of symptomatic hemorrhages following DBS using MER in 481 leads and found that patients who developed hematomas had a slightly greater number of MER tracks than those who did not; however, this difference did not reach statistical significance. They did note that there was a significantly increased incidence of hemorrhage in hypertensive patients undergoing MER versus nonhypertensive patients undergoing MER. In a study of 567 electrodes with a Charlson comorbidity scoring, hypertension and older age but not MER were correlated with increased hemorrhage.[65] In fact, there is no scientifically established evidence that the risk of hemorrhage is higher with microelectrodes or that the risk of hemorrhage increases with the number of tracts. Both are possibly true but to prove the increased risk of 1% would take over a thousand randomized patients.

If the risk is very low, there is still the question of whether MER is worth it in terms of time, expense, and outcome. Theoretically, if in fact the microelectrode is useful to localize the lesion or DBS placement more precisely, this should result in improved long-term (especially > 1 year) outcomes, fewer reoperations, and potentially fewer complications from collateral damage. Most of the outcome data in this debate over the utility of MER result from pallidotomy studies that are for the most part of very poor quality. At best, what can be said is that there are a lot of class III data suggesting that pallidotomy can be performed safely and efficaciously. This is supported by three reports with class I or II data also suggesting that this is the case. From an evidence-based perspective, the data are simply of poor quality, and no reasonable conclusions can be made. The strength of the DBS studies is from the STN data. Most investigators are microelectrode proponents. Only five of 28 centers use only macroelectrode stimulation, but, unfortunately, morbidity, complications, reoperations, and number of macroelectrode passes were not well documented; therefore, there is very little to compare and contrast. A truism is that experts can get decent results no matter what technique is used. Furthermore, not all MER techniques are the same. The single-tract technique looks for confirmation only in general terms and a second tract only if criteria are not met. This can ensure the target is reached but may result in highly variable locations within the nucleus and variable results.[7] The most common mapping approach uses multiple tracts to ensure optimal targeting.[9] And finally, there are the multiple simultaneous tracts that map a volume and pick the optimal tract for placement of the lead.[4] Benabid and colleagues use this latter technique and have the best long-term results.[57] These excellent results relate to far more than just the MER technique (Chapter 9). The problem of comparisons among centers is huge.

In a rigorous review of the literature only class IV data was found, and no conclusion could be reached as to the optimal technique.[66] The scientific answer to this debate would require conducting a randomized prospective study of the clinical outcome following surgery with or without MER by experts in both techniques. Such a study would have to be performed within the same institution, using movement disorder specialists and a large number of patients to be able to draw statistically significant conclusions. The magnitude of the difficulty can be best evaluated by calculating the number

of patients needed for a randomized study; 543 patients would be needed to show a 20% treatment difference (power 95%, λ = .05, p = .25) between patients studied with MER and those without.[52] The difference is probably smaller (in the 10–15% range), and even larger numbers would be needed. Until this type of study is done, no matter how you try to interpret bad data, no scientifically based conclusions can be reached about the role of MER in functional neurosurgery other than the clear utility in investigating the underlying pathology and effects of surgery. This aspect of the technique has contributed to the dramatic improvements that many patients have experienced as the result of improvements in a wide array of stereotactic procedures. We believe MER can be used safely and effectively in expert hands to maximize outcome, but there is no scientific proof that is essential.

References

1. Palur RS, Berk C, Schulzer M, Honey CR. A meta-analysis comparing the results of pallidotomy performed using microelectrode recording or macroelectrode stimulation. J Neurosurg 2002;96:1058–1062

2. Hariz MI, Fodstad H. Do microelectrode techniques increase accuracy or decrease risks in pallidotomy and deep brain stimulation? A critical review of the literature. Stereotact Funct Neurosurg 1999;72:157–169

3. Merello M, Cammarota A, Cerquetti D, Leiguarda RC. Mismatch between electrophysiologically defined and ventriculography based theoretical targets for posteroventral pallidotomy in Parkinson's disease. J Neurol Neurosurg Psychiatry 2000;69:787–791

4. Benabid A-L, Pollak P, Hoffmann D, et al. Chronic stimulation for Parkinson's disease and other movement disorders. In: Gildenberg PL, Tasker RR, eds. Textbook of Stereotactic and Functional Neurosurgery. New York: McGraw Hill; 1997:1199–1212

5. Alterman RL, Sterio D, Beric A, Kelly PJ. Microelectrode recording during posteroventral pallidotomy: impact on target selection and complications. Neurosurgery 1999;44:315–323

6. Guridi J, Gorospe A, Ramos E, Linazasoro G, Rodriguez MC, Obeso JA. Stereotactic targeting of the globus pallidus internus in Parkinson's disease: imaging versus electrophysiological mapping. Neurosurgery 1999;45:278–289

7. Gross RE, Lombardi WJ, Lang AE, et al. Relationship of lesion location to clinical outcome following microelectrode-guided pallidotomy for Parkinson's disease. Brain 1999;122:405–416

8. Tsao K, Wilkinson S, Overman J, Koller WC, Batnitzky S, Gordon MA. Pallidotomy lesion locations: significance of microelectrode refinement. Neurosurgery 1998;43:506–513

9. Vitek JL, Bakay RA, Hashimoto T, et al. Microelectrode-guided pallidotomy: technical approach and its application in medically intractable Parkinson's disease. J Neurosurg 1998;88:1027–1043

10. Hirabayashi H, Tengvar M, Hariz MI. Stereotactic imaging of the pallidal target. Mov Disord 2002;17(Suppl 3):S130–S134

11. Vayssiere N, Hemm S, Zanca M, et al. Magnetic resonance imaging stereotactic target localization for deep brain stimulation in dystonic children. J Neurosurg 2000;93:784–790

12. Vayssiëre N, Hemm S, Cif L, et al. Comparison of atlas- and magnetic resonance imaging–based stereotactic targeting of the globus pallidus internus in the performance of deep brain stimulation for treatment of dystonia. J Neurosurg 2002;96:673–679

13. Starr PA, Vitek JL, DeLong M, Bakay RAE. Magnetic resonance imaging-based stereotactic localization of the globus pallidus and subthalamic nucleus. Neurosurgery 1999;44:303–314

14. Bejjani BP, Dormont D, Pidoux B, et al. Bilateral subthalamic stimulation for Parkinson's disease by using three-dimensional stereotactic magnetic resonance imaging and electrophysiological guidance. J Neurosurg 2000;92:615–625

15. Zhu XL, Hamel W, Schrader B, et al. Magnetic resonance imaging–based morphometry and landmark correlation of basal ganglia nuclei. Acta Neurochir (Wien) 2002;144:959–969

16. Schrader B, Hamel W, Weinert D, Mehdorn HM. Documentation of electrode localization. Mov Disord 2002;17(Suppl 3):S167–S174

17. Patel NK, Heywood P, O'Sullivan K, Love S, Gill SS. MRI-directed subthalamic nucleus surgery for Parkinson's disease. Stereotact Funct Neurosurg 2002;78:132–145

18. Starr PA, Christine CW, Theodosopoulos PV, et al. Implantation of deep brain stimulators into the subthalamic nucleus: technical approach and magnetic resonance imaging–verified lead locations. J Neurosurg 2002;97:370–387

19. Hariz MI, Krack P, Melvill R, et al. A quick, and universal method for stereotactic visualization of the subthalamic nucleus before and after implantation of deep brain stimulation electrodes. Stereotact Funct Neurosurg 2003;80:96–101

20. Hariz MI, Laitinen LV. The Laitinen apparatus. In: Gildenberg PL, Tasker RR, eds. Textbook of Stereotactic and Functional Neurosurgery. New York: McGraw-Hill; 1997:87–94

21. Hirabayashi H, Hariz MI, Fagerlund M. Comparison between stereotactic CT and MRI coordinates of pallidal and thalamic targets using the Laitinen non-invasive stereoadapter. Stereotact Funct Neurosurg 1998;71:117–130

22. Lunsford LD, Kondziolka D, Leksell D. The Leksell Stereotactic System. In: Gildenberg PL, Tasker RR, eds. Textbook of Stereotactic and Functional Neurosurgery. New York: McGraw-Hill; 1997:51–63

23. Laitinen L, Johansson GG, Sipponen P. Impedance and phase angle as a locating method in human stereotaxic surgery. J Neurosurg 1966;25:628–633

24. Coubes P, Vayssiere N, El Fertit H, et al. Deep brain stimulation for dystonia: surgical technique. Stereotact Funct Neurosurg 2002;78:183–191

25. Okun MS, Stover NP, Subramanian T, et al. Complications of gamma knife surgery for Parkinson disease. Arch Neurol 2001;58:1995–2002

26. Jankovic J. Surgery for Parkinson disease and other movement disorders: benefits and limitations of ablation, stimulation, restoration, and radiation. Arch Neurol 2001;58:1970–1972

27. Van Buren JM, Maccubbin DA. An outline atlas of the human basal ganglia with estimation of anatomical variants. J Neurosurg 1962;19:811–839

28. Yeung D, Palta J, Fontanesi J, Kun L. Systematic analysis of errors in target localization and treatment delivery in stereotactic radiosurgery (SRS). Int J Radiat Oncol Biol Phys 1994;28:493–498

29. Maciunas RJ, Galloway RL Jr, Latimer JW. The application accuracy of stereotactic frames. Neurosurgery 1994;35:682–695

30. Ondo WG, Bronte-Stewart H. The North American survey of placement and adjustment strategies for deep brain stimulation. Stereotact Funct Neurosurg 2005;83:142–147

31. Tasker RR. Thalamotomy. Neurosurg Clin N Am 1990;1:841–864

32. Azizi A, Moreledge D. Posteroventral pallidotomy: comparison of the accuracy of anatomical targets defined by microelectrode recording. Neurology 1999;45(2):278

33. Hiner B, Madden K, Neal J. Effect of microelectrode recording on final lesion placement in pallidotomy. Neurology 1992;42:A251 A252

34. Lozano A, Hutchison W, Kiss Z, Tasker R, Davis K, Dostrovsky J. Methods for microelectrode-guided posteroventral pallidotomy. J Neurosurg 1996;84:194–202

35. Carlson JD, Iacono RP. Electrophysiological versus image based targeting in the posteroventral pallidotomy. Comput Aided Surg 1999;4:93–100

36. Kelly PJ, Derome P, Guiot G. Thalamic spatial variability and the surgical results of lesions placed with neurophysiologic control. Surg Neurol 1978;9:307–315

37. Forster A, Eljamel MS, Marma TR, Tulley M, Latimer M. Audit of neurophysiological recording during movement disorder surgery. Stereotact Funct Neurosurg 1999;72:154–156

38. Duffner F, Schiffbauer H, Breit S, Friese S, Freudenstein D. Relevance of image fusion for target point determination in functional neurosurgery. Acta Neurochir (Wien) 2002;144:445–451

39. Rodriguez MC, Guridi OJ, Alvarez L, et al. The subthalamic nucleus and tremor in Parkinson's disease. Mov Disord 1998;13(suppl 3):111–118

40. Amirnovin R, Williams ZM, Cosgrove GR, Eskandar EN. Experience with microelectrode guided subthalamic nucleus deep brain stimulation. Neurosurgery 2006; 58(1, Suppl)ONS96–ONS102

41. Hamid NA, Mitchell RD, Mocroft P, Westby GW, Milner J, Pall H. Targeting the subthalamic nucleus for deep brain stimulation: technical approach and fusion of pre and postoperative MR images to define accuracy of lead placement. J Neurol Neurosurg Psychiatry 2005;76:409–414

42. Zonenshayn M, Rezai AR, Mogilner AY, Beric A, Sterio D, Kelly PJ. Comparison of anatomic and neurophysiological methods for subthalamic nucleus targeting. Neurosurgery 2000;47:282–292

43. Breit S, LeBas J-F, Koudsie A, et al. Pretargeting for the implantation of stimulation electrodes into the subthalamic nucleus: a comparative study of magnetic resonance imaging and ventriculography. Neurosurgery 2006;58(Suppl 1):83–95

44. Cuny E, Guehl D, Burbaud P, Gross C, Dousset V, Rougier A. Lack of agreement between direct magnetic resonance imaging and statistical determination of a subthalamic target: the role of electrophysiological guidance. J Neurosurg 2002;97:591–597

45. Wester K, Krakenes J. Vertical displacement of the brain and target area during open stereotactic neurosurgery. Acta Neurochir (Wien) 2001;143:603–606

46. Winkler D, Tittgemeyer M, Schwartz J, Preul C, Stecker K, Meixensberger J. The first evaluation of brain shift during functional neurosurgery by deformation field analysis. J Neurol Neurosurg Psychiatry 2005;76:1161–1163

47. Novotny J Jr, Vymazal J, Novotny J, et al. Does new magnetic resonance imaging technology provide better geometrical accuracy during stereotactic imaging? J Neurosurg 2005;102(Suppl):8–13

48. Bucholz RD, Ho HW, Rubin JP. Variables affecting the accuracy of stereotactic localization using computerized tomography. J Neurosurg 1993;79:667–673

49. Alterman RL, Shils JL, Gudesblatt M, Tagliati M. Immediate and sustained relief of levo-dopa dyskinesias after dorsal relocation of a deep brain stimulation lead. Neurosurg Focus 2004;17:E6

50. Papavassiliou E, Rau G, Heath S, et al. Thalamic deep brain stimulation for essential tremor: relation of lead location to outcome. Neurosurgery 2004;54:1120–1129

51. Bakay RAE. Meta-analysis, pallidotomy, and microelectrodes. J Neurosurg 2002;97:1253–1256

52. Sterio DK, Bakay RAE, Israel Z, et al. Is MER necessary in movement disorder surgery: the case in favor. In: Israel Z and Burchiel KW (eds) Microelectrode Recording in Movement Disorder Surgery. New York: Thieme; 2004:189–196

53. Hua Z, Guodong G, Qinchuan L, Yaqun Z, Qinfen W, Xuelian W. Analysis of complications of radiofrequency pallidotomy. Neurosurgery 2003;52:89–99

54. Terao T, Takahashi H, Yokochi F, Taniguchi M, Okiyama R, Hamada I. Hemorrhagic complication of stereotactic surgery in patients with movement disorders. J Neurosurg 2003;98:1241–1246

55. Gorgulho A, De Salles AA, Frighetto L, Behnke E. Incidence of hemorrhage associated with electrophysiological studies performed using microelectrodes and microelectrodes in functional neurosurgery. J Neurosurg 2005;102:888–896

56. Binder DK, Rau GM, Starr PA. Risk factors for hemorrhage during microelectrode-guided deep brain stimulator implantation for movement disorders. Neurosurgery 2005;56:722–732

57. Krack P, Batir A, Van Blercom N, et al. Five-year follow-up of bilateral stimulation of the subthalamic nucleus in advanced Parkinson's disease. N Engl J Med 2003;349:1925–1934

58. Tasker RR, Organ LW, Hawrylyshyn PA. The Thalamus and Midbrain of Man: A Physiological Atlas Using Electrical Stimulation. Springfield, IL: C Thomas; 1982

59. Cif L, El Fertit H, VayssiÈre N, et al. Treatment of dystonic syndromes by chronic electrical stimulation of the internal globus pallidus. J Neurosurg Sci 2003;47:52–55

60. Hariz MI, Hirabayashi H. Is there a relationship between size and site of the stereotactic lesion and symptomatic results of pallidotomy and thalamotomy? Stereotact Funct Neurosurg 1997;69:28–45

61. Maltíte D, Navarro S, Welter ML, Roche S, Bonnet AM, Houeto JL, et al. Subthalamic stimulation in Parkinson disease: with or without anesthesia. Arch Neurol 2004;61:390–392

62. Miyagi Y, Shima F, Sasaki T. Brain shift: an error factor during implantation of deep brain stimulation electrodes. J Neurosurg 2007;107:989–997

63. Halpern CH, Danish SF, Baltuch GH, Jaggi JL. Brain shift during deep brain stimulation surgery for Parkinson's disease. Stereotact Funct Neurosurg 2008;86:37–43

64. Khan MF, Mewes K, Gross RE, Skrinjar O. Assessment of brain shift related to deep stimulation surgery. Stereotact Funct Neurosurg 2008;86:44–53

65. Sansur CA, Frysinger RC, Pouratian N, Fu KM, Bittl M, Oskouian RJ, et al. Incidence of symptomatic hemorrhage after stereotactic electrode placement. J Neurosurg 2007;107:998–1003

66. Rezai AR, Kopell BH, Gross RE, Vitek JL, Sharan AD, Limousin P, et al. Deep brain stimulation for Parkinson's disease: surgical issues. Mov Disord 2006;21:S197–S218

Implantation of Multiple Electrodes and Robotic Techniques

Alim Louis Benabid, Bradley Wallace, Dominique Hoffmann, Stephan Chabardes, Sylvie Grand, and Jean François LeBas

Advances in stereotactic methods, which are typically variations of the same basic design, entail modifications offering improved accuracy and speed while maintaining the quality of the operation. Various prototypes of robots developed during the past 10 years have permitted the fulfilment of this goal. This chapter describes the use of the NeuroMate robotic arm (Schaerer-Mayfield, Lyon, France), which has been developed in our department over the past 15 years and is currently used for all stereotactic procedures performed at our institution. The chapter also deals with the application of this methodology to the stereotactic implantation of intracerebral electrodes, particularly stimulating electrodes to be connected to implantable generators used in the treatment of movement disorders, epilepsy, obsessive–compulsive disorders, and emerging applications such as cluster headache and obesity, as well as depth recording electrodes for electroencephalography (EEG) used in the evaluation of pharmacoresistant epilepsies before the planning of resective surgery. The chapter describes the procedures, advantages, and drawbacks of robotic surgery compared with classic, frame-based surgery.

◼ Materials

The current version of the NeuroMate robotic arm (Schaerer-Mayfield, Lyon, France), which is discussed in this chapter, is the third prototype of the system, in development since 1989[1,2] and used by other teams.[3,4] It is made up of three components (**Fig. 9.1**): the robotic arm, the computer housing the software and data files, and the stereotactic frame.

Robotic Arm

The NeuroMate robotic arm (**Fig. 9.2**) is available in two versions. The first is a mobile system that can be stored in a corner of the operating room when not in use and can be accurately repositioned into a dedicated location in the operating room using a pin and plate system mounted into the floor. Our department uses the second version that is permanently fixed to the floor at the intersection of two teleradiological X-ray tubes positioned 3.5 m from the

head of the patient to minimize the magnification coefficient. The body of the system houses most of the electronics needed to activate the robot, particularly the computer called the controller. The controller translates commands given by the neuronavigation software into the six axes of the robotic arm. The trajectory to be used is a line defined by two points in space (each defined by three Cartesian coordinates). From this body, a succession of segments is articulated together by mobile joints (**Figs. 9.1** and **9.2**). The first axis is collinear to the axis of the patient in the supine position on the operating table. The second axis is perpendicular to the first and provides an additional degree of freedom to rotate from one side of the patient to the other. The third axis provides the opportunity for angulations of the rest of the system and consists of two segments of ~50 cm in length that are analogous to an arm and forearm of the robot. At the end of the forearm, an additional perpendicular axis is designed to receive a holding plate, which can also rotate by 360 degrees. This holding plate can be fitted with a tool holder compatible with a series of specific equipment needed to perform the stereotactic procedures. These tools are mainly guide tubes through which penetration of both the skull and the underlying dura can be performed along a preplanned trajectory. Additional equipment can be mounted on this tool, for example, a microdrive to advance the microrecording electrodes into the brain toward the target.

Computer

The neurosurgeon–machine interface consists of a PC powered by a 400 MHz Pentium 4 microprocessor with 512 MB of RAM, and a 40 GB hard drive. The PC is connected to the controller of the robot on one side, and on the other receives data through a digitizing scanner, or more commonly through a local area network (LAN) connection to an Ethernet network allowing the transfer of images such as a magnetic resonance imaging (MRI) study coming from the radiology department, or any other kind of digital data. This computer houses the neuronavigation software, VoXim [Integrated Visualization Systems (IVS), Chemnitz, Germany]. VoXim version 4.01 is capable of receiving three types of digital imaging data: (1) anteroposterior (AP) and lateral skull X-ray images obtained by the biorthogonal

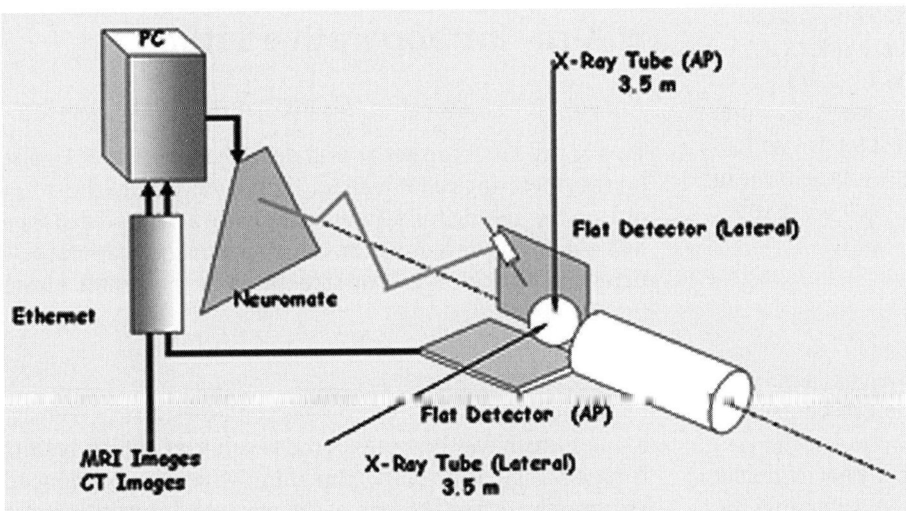

Fig. 9.1 Flow chart of the NeuroMate robotized stereotactic system. (See **Color Plate 9.1**.)

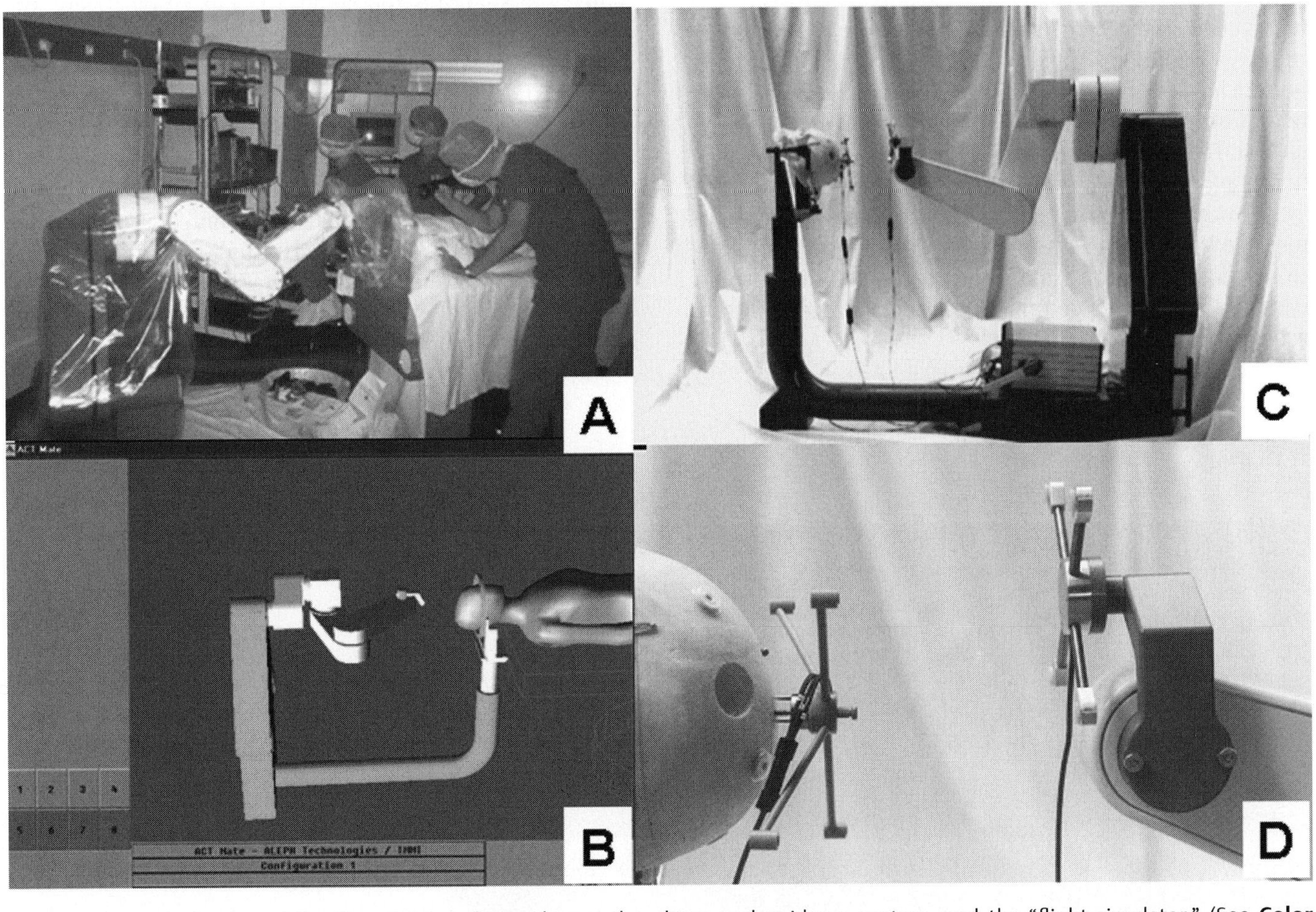

Fig. 9.2 General pictures of the NeuroMate robotized arm, the ultrasound guidance system, and the "flight simulator." (See **Color Plate 9.2**.)

teleradiological tubes. Based on ventriculographic landmarks from these images, the basal ganglia targets [ventral intermediate nucleus (Vim) of the thalamus, globus pallidus interna (GPi), or subthalamic nucleus (STN)] for functional neurosurgery of movement disorders can be defined. Avascular operative windows can be determined from angiographic images for the introduction of depth electrodes for stereoelectroencephalography (SEEG). Trajectory coordinates from these determinations provide the target points and paths for the robot motion. (2) Computed tomographic (CT) scans can also provide these data via transmission through the Ethernet image network. (3) More frequently this would be MRI studies (T1, T2, axial, sagittal, coronal) coming through the Ethernet image network. The neuronavigation tools included in this software will allow the predetermination of the best target, on the basis of statistical data banks, which could be reached by the robot when it comes into position and action.

Stereotactic Frame

The third component is the stereotactic frame (**Fig. 9.3**). Any currently available stereotactic frame can be used to rigidly fix the patient's head at the intersection of the two X-ray teleradiological beams. Frames typically have fiducial systems for use with angiography, CT, and MRI enabling the imaging data to be stereotactically registered for transfer to the robot. The frame currently used at our institution is a universal stereotactic frame derived from the Talairach frame to which an X-ray localizer, angiographic localizer, or fiducial grids (when orthogonal penetrations, frontal or lateral, are needed without the use of the robot) can be attached. This frame is mounted on a rotating circle, coaxial to the main axis of the patient allowing either partially rotated images to be obtained for stereoscopic angiograms or to place the patient in positions during ventriculography to better visualize the anterior part of the 3rd ventricle, namely the anterior commissure, which is an important stereotactic landmark.

■ X-ray Intraoperative Setup

X-ray Tubes in Teleradiological Setup

Two X-ray tubes are set at a 90 degree angle (**Fig. 9.1**), one on the operating room wall for lateral views, and the other one on the ceiling for AP views. Both are at a fixed distance of 3.5 m from the X-ray film, creating a magnification coefficient of 1.05 (i.e., 5%) for structures in the center of the brain.

Flat Digitized Detectors

X-ray films have the best spatial resolution, which results from a combination of the film grain (which can be reduced as necessary), and the size of the electron-emitting source on the X-ray tube anode, which has to be small. However, when the source is too small, the flux of electrons, and therefore of X-rays, is limited because of concern about overheating. Fortunately, the teleradiological setup decreases the apparent diameter of the source (as the reciprocal of the distance), which partially compensates for the decrease in X-ray flux (as the reciprocal of the square of the distance) resulting in increased image resolution. However, to be suitable for robotic applications and digital targeting, X-ray films must be digitized through scanning, which is time consuming and decreases quality. Digitized detectors should be much better but common light amplifiers have a strong distortion coefficient, which tends to distort the

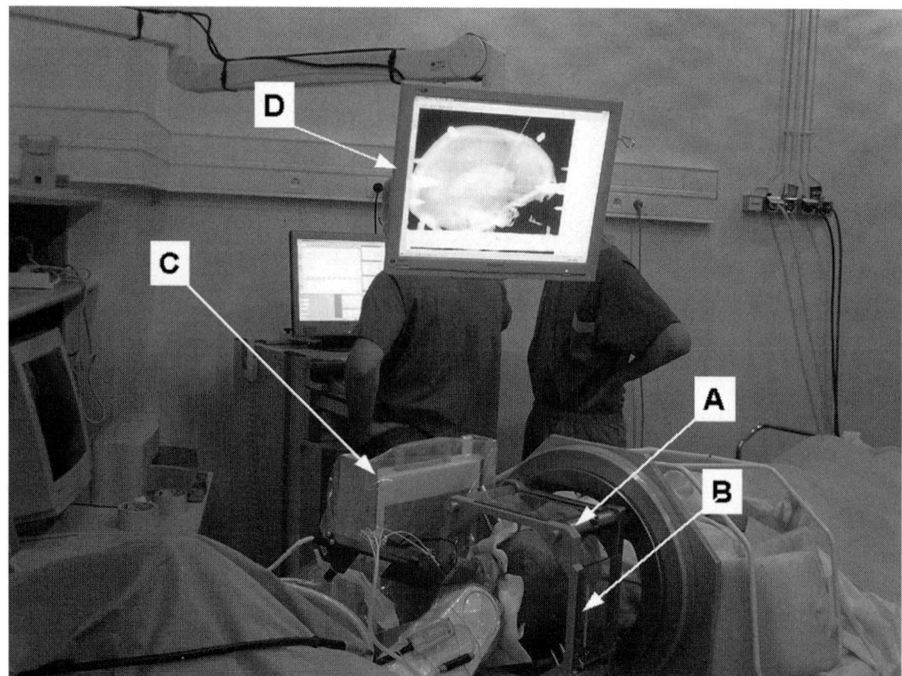

Fig. 9.3 Stereotactic frame and flat detectors. (**A**) Stereotactic frame mounted on a rotating solid-state stand. (**B**) X-ray Plexiglas localizers mounted on the stereotactic frame. (**C**) Flat angiography digitizers mounted in orthogonal setup with long-distance X-ray generators. (**D**) Display of X-ray images. (See **Color Plate 9.3**.)

image of square objects by the so-called cushion deformation, which is extremely difficult to compensate. Recent developments have made available flat digital detectors (**Fig. 9.3**) that have no planar distortion and retain an acceptable degree of spatial resolution. These flat digitized detectors (Bioscan, Geneva, Switzerland), therefore, have the major advantage of providing digitized radiographic images, which can be available online (saving significant time and expense associated with the processing of X-ray film), are able to be immediately transferred by Ethernet to the neuronavigation software, and can be subjected to image processing (filtering, subtraction, addition, measures, construction of schemes and targets).

■ Method

Acquisition of Image Data

The structure of the stereotactic setup makes it possible to perform the entire procedure in a single session, or to split it into multiple steps that can be performed at separate times, even on different days, which is typical in the current protocol at our institution.

Application of the Frame and X-ray Acquisition

Under general anesthesia, patients are secured to the stereotactic frame using four twist drill perforations of the skull. For implantation of electrodes in the basal ganglia, calvarial screws are inserted into the perforations, which allows for repositioning the frame several days late while retaining submillimetric precision over the subsequent steps (ventriculography, preimplantation MRI, electrode implantation, postimplantation MRI). For SEEG electrodes, surgery is performed relatively later (within several days to several months) requiring transparietal pins that are inserted into 2.3 mm diameter twist drill perforations with the position recorded on the frame vernier scales.

Angiography

Direct carotid puncture is performed with an 18-gauge Teflon catheter, and 6 mL of Vasobrix (Schering, Berlin) are injected using a programmable, pressure-controlled, injector. Seventy-two images are taken and stored in the digital subtraction angiography computer for further treatment, such as subtraction, and trajectory planning. Images are first obtained in orthogonal AP and lateral views (**Fig. 9.4**), in the supine position, and then again with the head tilted by 5 degrees toward the contralateral side for stereoscopic views and depth determination of the vessels.

Ventriculography

Freehand puncture of the frontal horn is performed at 9 cm from the nasion, and 2.5 cm from the midline using a

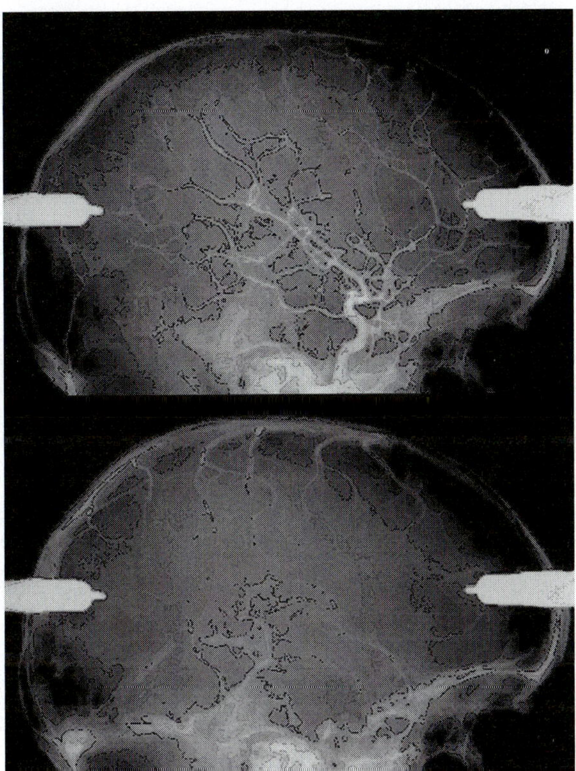

Fig. 9.4 Stereotactic angiograms: arteries and veins sampled from a continuous X-ray video sequence.

6.5 cm Cushing cannula. Air (0.5 mL) is injected to verify the location of the cannula in the frontal horn, and not in the interhemispheric fissure. Then 6.5 mL of Iopamiron (Schering) is injected over 5 to 10 seconds during which a sequence of 30 images is obtained laterally, immediately followed by AP views (**Fig. 9.5**). From the lateral sequence, a single image in which all third ventricular landmarks are visible (namely, the anterior and posterior commissures) is selected and target coordinates are calculated and superimposed.

MRI

The VoXim software of the NeuroMate allows two MRI acquisition modalities. In both cases, the T1- and T2-weighted MRI sequences are matched by the software, resulting in improved target definition. This is particularly important for implantation of the basal ganglia where the STN is visible only on T2 sequences. In the first acquisition modality (frame-based MRI), a specially designed MRI localizer (**Fig. 9.6**) is attached to the patient's head using four titanium pins inserted at the same depth as the stereotactic frame at the time of the X-ray data acquisition. The MRI data can therefore be precisely coregistered with the ventriculographic data, allowing precise targeting based on fusion of these two datasets. The second modality uses a "helicopter" frameless localizer. A base is screwed into the skull just prior to the implantation session (usually

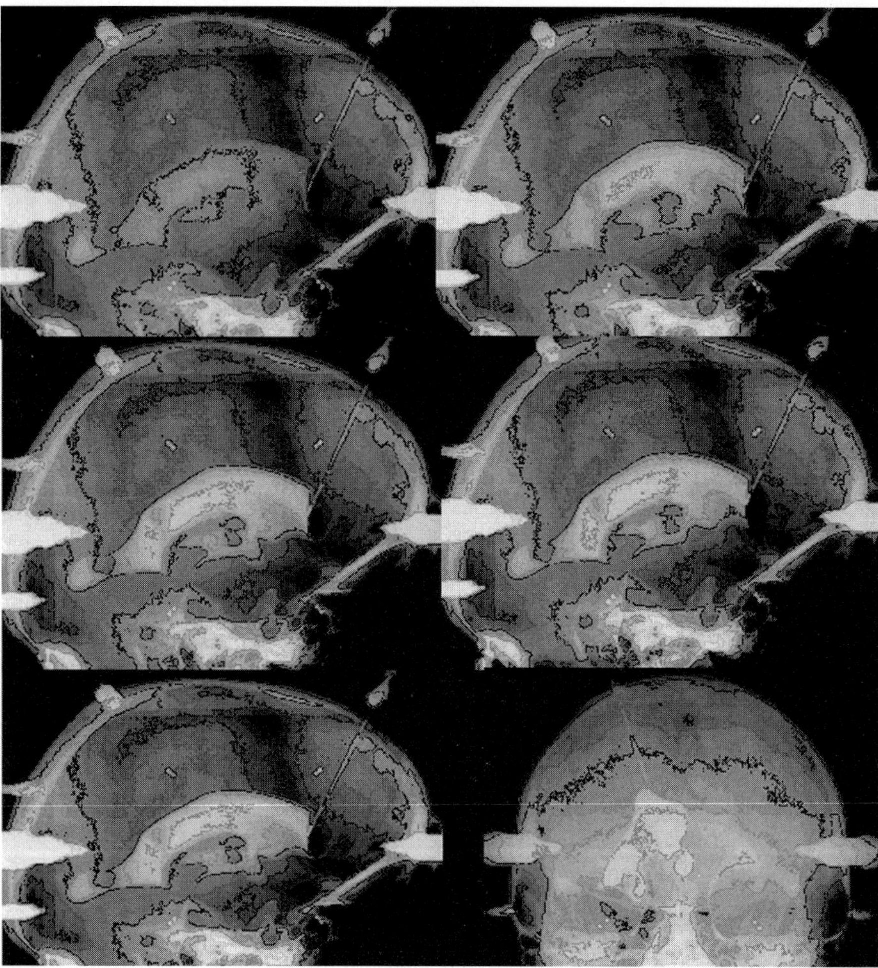

Fig. 9.5 Four frames taken from a video ventriculographic sequence (four upper images) and deep brain stimulation (DBS) target planning from the anteroposterior and lateral views of the ventriculogram, and planning of the DBS target (two lower images).

the day before surgery). On this base a four-armed localizer is mounted that bears four markers impregnated with MRI-visible gadolinium-DTPA (diethylene-triamine pentaacetate). At the time of surgery, the gadolinium localizer is replaced by a similar second localizer bearing four ultrasound emitters instead of gadolinium. The ultrasound localizer is then recognized by a set of four ultrasound detectors attached to the robotic arm. The VoXim neuronavigation software then positions the robot in front of the ultrasound emitters, allowing coregistration of the robot with the markers, and therefore to the patient's brain.

Planning of Electrode Implantation

Functional neurosurgery for movement disorders, particularly for Parkinson disease, utilizes three primary basal ganglia targets including Vim, GPi, and the most recent and most commonly used, STN. These nuclei can be targeted in different ways, including derivation of Cartesian coordinates from atlases, and validated by clinical experience. Target coordinates are based on a referential system, which is centered on an AP axis between the posterior commissure (PC) and the anterior commissure (AC), the midsagit-

tal plane bisecting the third ventricle, and laterality on an axis perpendicular to the midsagittal plane. To minimize the effect of interindividual variations, the AP coordinate is expressed as 12ths of the AC–PC distance (~27 ± 2 mm). The vertical coordinate is normalized against the height of the thalamus (~18 mm ± 2 mm) and is expressed as eighths of this value. The laterality is expressed in millimeters because there is currently no satisfactory internal standard by which it can be normalized. For the thalamic target Vim, Tasker's rule proposes using a laterality of 11 0.5 mm plus half of the width of the third ventricle.

Table 9.1 shows the numerical values of these three target coordinates, derived from our own experience. Another way to determine the position of the target is direct targeting, which involves aiming at the center of the target that is visible on the MRI (**Fig. 9.7**). Vim is not visible, but its laterality can be determined by the external limit of the thalamus abutting the internal capsule. The GPi is easily visualized on axial images, particularly on inversion recovery spin echo–weighted MRI sequences. The best GPi target point is situated at the most posterior part of the internal pallidum, medial to the external pallidum, and at the bottom of the GPi. The STN is usually well visualized on T2-weighted coronal images, which allow it to be differen-

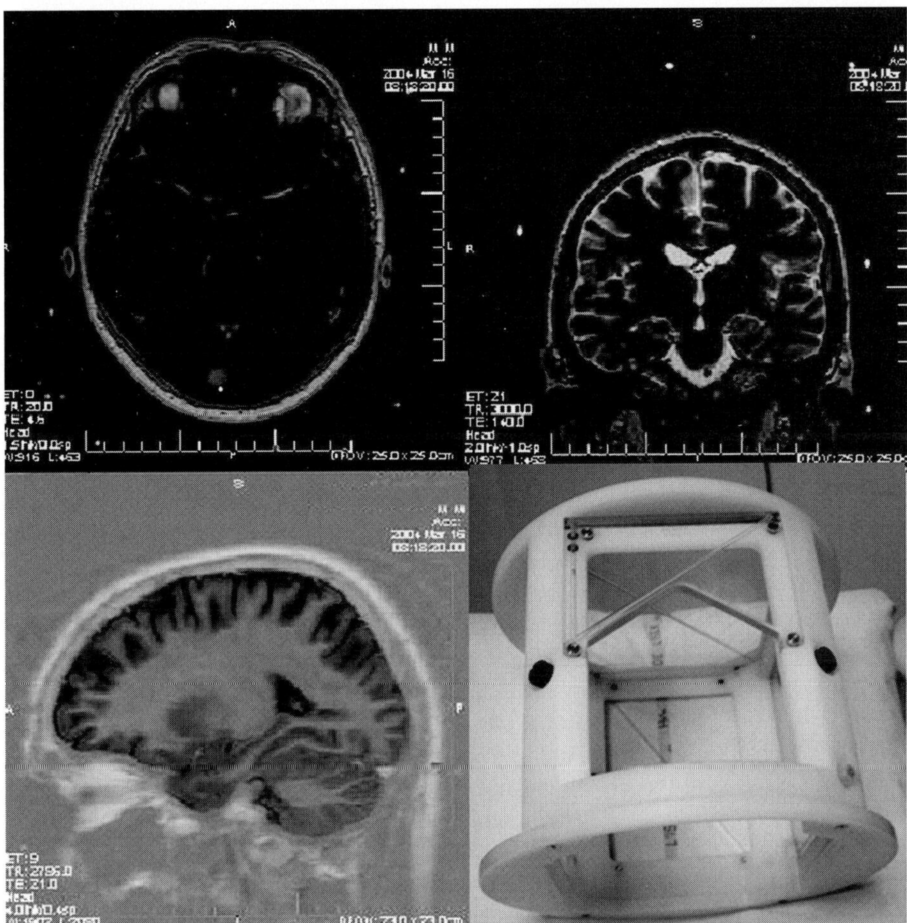

Fig. 9.6 Stereotactic magnetic resonance imaging (MRI) and MRI localizer head set. (See **Color Plate 9.6**.)

tiated from the underlying substantia nigra pars reticulata (SNr). The respective values of these various methods remain debatable. Controversy is based mainly on the distortion present in MRI that cannot be easily controlled.

Once the target has been determined, the path for implantation requires the determination of the entry point. The general direction of the track is provided by the scheme of the theoretical targets, based on Guiot's diagram (**Fig. 9.5**). The theoretical entry point is projected to the vicinity of the coronal suture, ~15 to 35 mm from the midline. The trajectory can be intraoperatively verified from the entry point to the target. The software provides a simulation of the probe, depending on the system used. At our institution, five parallel guide tubes are introduced, separated by 2 mm from center to center, creating a global diameter of 6 mms. The entry point can be modified as needed to allow a safe penetration of the guide tubes and avoid the arteries and veins on the surface of the cortex or penetrating the F1–F2

Table 9.1 Coordinates of Stereotactic Targets

	Anteroposterior	Vertical	Lateral
	1/12° AC–PC	1/8° HT	mm
Thalamic Vim	3.53 ± 1;78	1.15 ± 0.67	15.36 ± 2.7
Pallidal GPi	8.16 ± 0.71	− 0.77 ± 0.58	19.91 ± 1.73
STN	5.19 ± 0.70	− 1.25 ± 0.70	12.14 ± 1.85

Note: The coordinates used to program the NeuroMate robot for deep brain stimulation surgery are given for Vim, GPi, and STN.
Anteroposterior (AP) distance ahead of the posterior commissure (PC) is expressed in 1/12 degree of the AC–PC distance.
The vertical coordinate is expressed in 1/8 degree of the height of the thalamus (measured at the level of the floor of the lateral ventricle).
The laterality is not normalized and is expressed in millimeters as the distance from the midplane of the third ventricle.
Abbreviations; AC, anterior commissure; GPi, globus pallidus internus; PC, posterior commissure; STN, subthalamic nucleus; Vim, ventrointermedius nucleus of the thalamus.

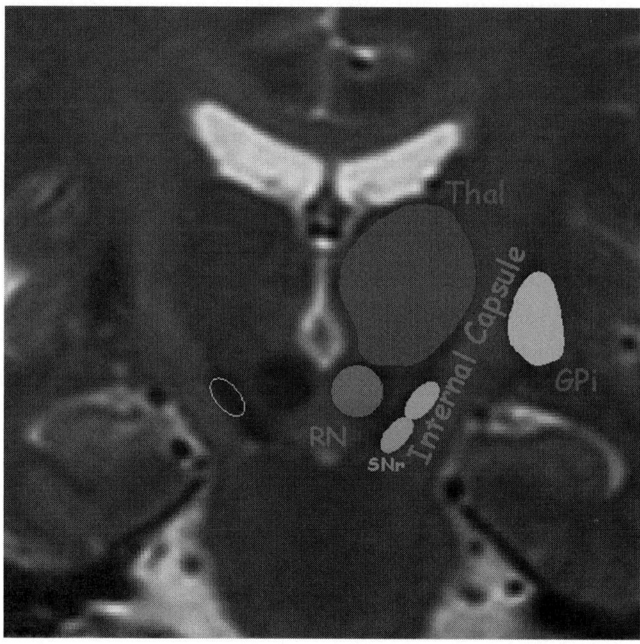

Fig. 9.7 Magnetic resonance imaging visualization of the movement disorder targets: subthalamic nucleus (SNr), thalamus (Thal), and pallidum as well as the red nucleus (RN) and the internal capsule. GPi, globus pallidus internus. (See **Color Plate 9.7**.)

sulcus. At greater depths, care should be taken to avoid the caudate nucleus because bilateral lesions may be responsible for postoperative confusion. The ventricle should also be avoided, when possible, because its penetration might result in bleeding from subependymal veins and possible deviation of the electrode during final implantation.

Electrode Implantation

Bilateral electrode implantation is usually performed in movement disorder patients, particularly those suffering from advanced stage Parkinson disease, where symptoms are usually bilateral, and often symmetrical. At our institution, bilateral implantations are performed during a single session. Although this is long and difficult for the patient, as well as for the surgical team, the overall experience is shorter, the localization is better, and common steps (installation, calibration of the robot, etc.) are performed only one time. Implantation is performed first in the hemisphere contralateral to the patient's worst symptoms. The patient is refixated to the stereotactic frame where the fixation pins are repositioned to the values recorded at the time of ventriculography. X-rays are taken to verify perfect superimposition with ventriculograms. Due to the rigidity of the system, we are normally able to superimpose X-rays corresponding to different sessions at different times without any discernible differences in alignment. If the MRI was acquired using the frameless system (the helicopter), the ultrasound version is attached to the mounting ring that remains fixed to the head of the patient.

The skin incision is performed under local anesthesia in the area of the coronal suture, with its concavity directed posterior and medially, to avoid crossing the electrodes with the skin incision at the end of the session. The skin flap is retracted after release of the periosteum from the outer table of the skull. At this time, a pouch is then prepared between the periosteum and the bone to store the external part of the electrode and the connector to protect it.

The robot is activated and comes into position. The tool holder is attached and a drill guide is inserted. A series of three progressive drill bits are used. The first one is equipped with a 1.5 mm diameter tip allowing penetration into the outer table of the skull for fixing the trajectory. AP and lateral X-rays are digitized using the Bioscan digitized angiographic system display. Graphic tools included in the Bioscan software allow for prolongation of the image of the drill and simulate the track to be performed. Manually superimposing printed X-rays, or more logically electronically superimposing digitized images, allows confirmation that the planned trajectory is correct. If corrections need to be made, the VoXim software includes a microadjustment window, which usually does not need to be performed more than once. Any adjustments in the trajectory are confirmed using AP and lateral X-rays. The first drill marks the correct position within the external table of the skull. The second drill, which also has a thin tip (to follow the trajectory of the first drill) that expands into a larger diameter, is then used to begin perforation of the final burr hole. The third drill, which has an outer diameter of 6 mm, fits into the conic precentering hole created by the second drill. Progressive and careful drilling is made by subsequent small advances of the drill bit using a motorized perforator (ELAN-E, Aesculap Inc., Center Valley, PA), until the dura is reached. Any residual bone at the inner table must be carefully removed because it may centrally deviate the subsequently placed guide tubes. Prior to insertion of the rest of the Ben-Gun system (Schaerer-Mayfield, Lyon, France), an oblique hole is drilled in the rim of the burr hole for fixation of the definitive electrode using a nylon ligature.

Electrophysiology: Microrecording and Stimulation

When the burr hole is completed, the Ben-Gun system is installed. The first component is a 6 mm diameter stainless steel cylinder containing five parallel channels of 1.3 mm internal diameter. The central channel is equidistant (center to center) by 2 mm from the four surrounding channels. The Ben-gun is inserted through the holding tool of the robot, replacing the drill guide, and is then placed into the burr hole, almost to the dura. Five guide tubes are inserted into the five channels without prior opening of the dura. Each guide tube is advanced to the dura, where a thin, sharp stylet is introduced into the guide tube and used to puncture the dura. This thin stylet can also be used to carefully puncture the arachnoid. It is replaced by

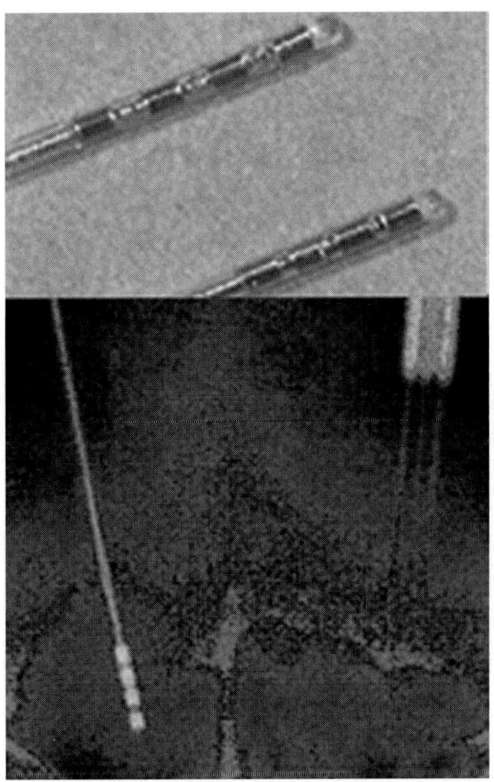

Fig. 9.8 Chronic deep brain stimulation tetrapolar electrodes and acute recording microelectrodes in a five-electrode setting. (See **Color Plate 9.8.**)

a blunt stylet that remains in the guide tube during its descent to 15 mm above the plane at which microrecording will begin. The microrecording electrode (FHC, Bowdoin, ME) is then introduced. It protrudes from the guide tube by 15 mm, and its correct alignment and positioning are confirmed by AP and lateral X-rays (**Fig. 9.8**). The remaining four guide tubes are then introduced and loaded with the microelectrodes. The Alpha Omega microdrive of

the Neurotrek system (Alpha Omega, Tel Aviv, Israel) is mounted and the bipolar microelectrodes are secured to the descending portion of the microdrive used to advance the electrodes in a precise, controlled fashion during electrophysiological explorations. Each microelectrode is connected to the preamplifier of the Alpha Omega microguide. The concentric macrocontact of each bipolar electrode, used for macrostimulation, is connected to the ground of the frame, which is itself connected to the ground of the robot and to the electrical installation of the operating room.

The Alpha Omega microguide software is turned on and, after elimination of electrical artifacts (due to surrounding electrical devices and turning machines, despite full shielding of the operating room by a Faraday cage (Medtronic, Minneapolis, MN) made of a thin layer of copper entirely surrounding all six surfaces of the stereotactic operating room), the microrecording session can start. Microrecording is performed using all five electrodes simultaneously, which are descended as a single unit (**Fig. 9.9**). Radiographic visualization of the five microelectrodes is possible (**Fig. 9.10**), and commutation permits precise investigation of each of the five tracks to measure the impedance of the electrode, the frequency of the discharge, recording of the pattern of discharge, and particularly the evoked responses to passive movements of the various joints of the patient. When the final depths of the trajectories are reached, control AP and lateral X-rays are repeated to verify that the readings on the microdrive scale correspond to the true, radiographic position of the microelectrode tips.

At this point stimulation trials are started using the parameters of stimulation, which would be used in the chronic situation (frequency: 130 Hz, pulse width: 60 μs, stimulation period duration: 10 to 30 s). During stimulation trials, the neurology team assesses for changes in the rigidity of the joints, primarily the wrist, contralateral to the side of exploration. The examining neurologist semi-

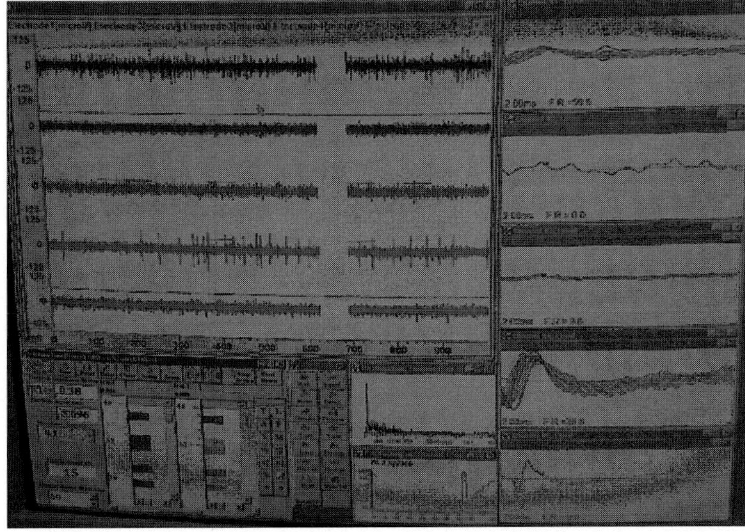

Fig. 9.9 Five microelectrode simultaneous recording traces. (See **Color Plate 9.9.**)

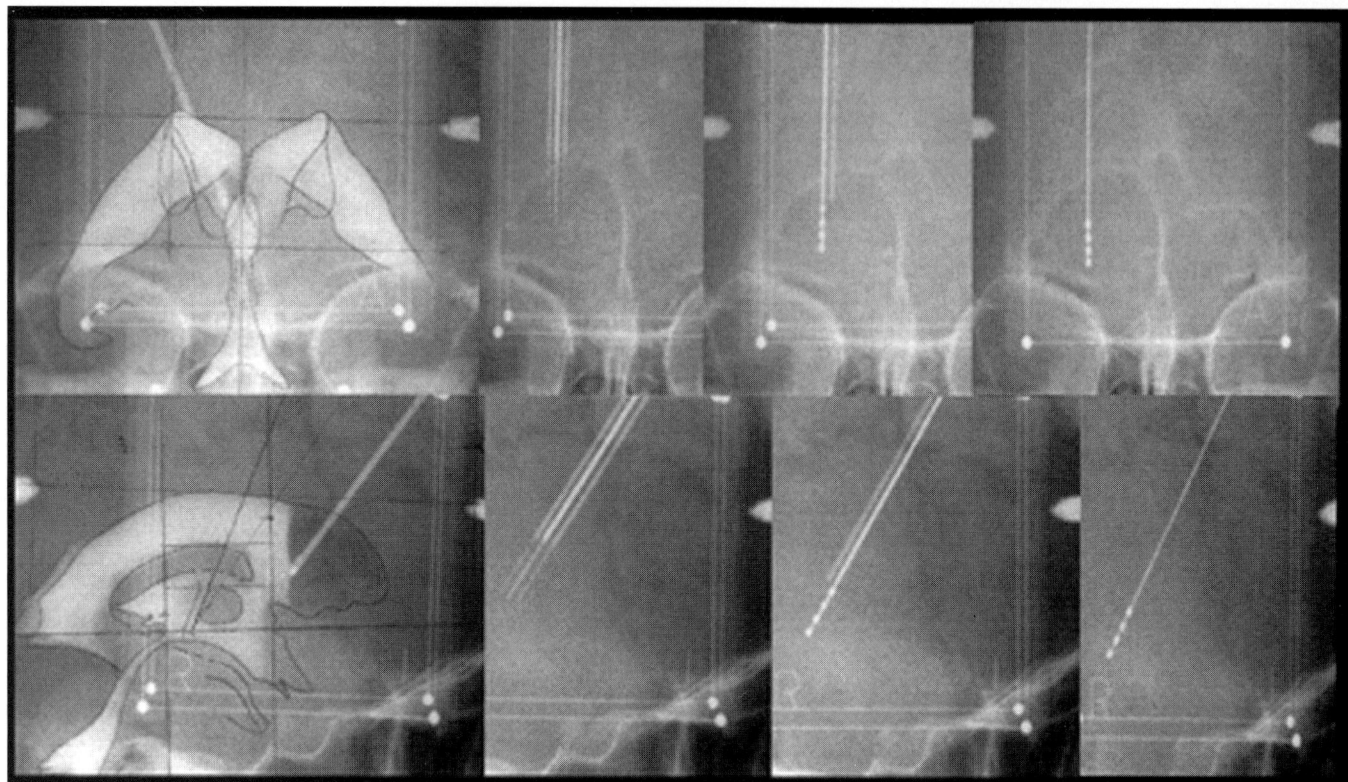

Fig. 9.10 Intraoperative X-ray control of microelectrode insertion using the five-channel Ben–Gun system (Schaerer-Mayfield, Lyon, France).

quantitatively evaluates changes in the rigidity of the wrist, and data are recorded for each individual electrode at each level. The improvement of rigidity is noted versus the intensity of stimulation, which usually varies between 1 to 3 milliamps to provide a significant improvement, which may vary from 50 to 100% of the baseline state. At high intensities, side effects may be observed that are also extremely helpful in localizing the position of the electrodes into the brain. Muscular contractions that correspond to the internal capsule are most often observed from the lateral or anterior electrodes. Stimulation-induced sensations, such as paresthesias or tingling, are generally due to the involvement of the lemniscus medialis by the posterior electrodes. Medial electrodes may induce, at deeper levels, monocular deviation of the ipsilateral eye (adduction) due to the involvement of the fibers of the oculomotor nerve. When conjugate eye movements are observed, it typically indicates the involvement of the corticopontine fibers projecting onto the nucleus para-abducens of the sixth cranial nerve. Side effects such as uncomfortable feelings, heat, fear, and sweating may be observed in multiple locations, most often in deeper and more medial areas during the exploration for STN implantation. Finally, mydriasis can be observed when exploration is close to the third nerve.

When exploring the GPi, muscular contractions are observed, mainly from the more medial electrodes, because the target is lateral to the internal capsule. Visual flashes can be induced by stimulation when the electrode reaches the bottom of the pallidum, close to the optic tract, which is one of the main anatomical surroundings of this target.

In the Vim, side effects are primarily muscular contractions from the more lateral electrodes, close to the internal capsule. Sensory paresthesias and tingling may be observed from the posterior electrodes, which are close to the ventroposterolateral (VPL) somatosensory nucleus of the thalamus.

All data concerning both the positive effects of stimulation (e.g., improvement in contralateral symptoms), and the negative effects (e.g., contractions, paresthesias, or third nerve involvement), are charted according to electrode, depth, and stimulation parameters to be analyzed during a brainstorming session whose goal is to determine which of the five trajectories is most appropriate for implantation of the chronic Medtronic tetrapolar electrode 3389 lead, known as the Reduced Space Electrode (Minneapolis, MN) (each contact is 1.5 mm long and 1.27 mm in diameter, with an intercontact distance of 0.5 mm).

The insertion of the chronic stimulating electrode is performed under digitized fluoroscopy. The depth is adjusted according to the brainstorming-based decision. The other microelectrodes as well as their guide tubes, which have prevented any deviation of the chronic electrode during insertion, are removed, and the chronic lead is secured to the bone by a nylon ligature anchored to the oblique hole drilled in the wall of the burr hole. The bottom of the burr hole is partially packed with hemostatic mesh (Sur-

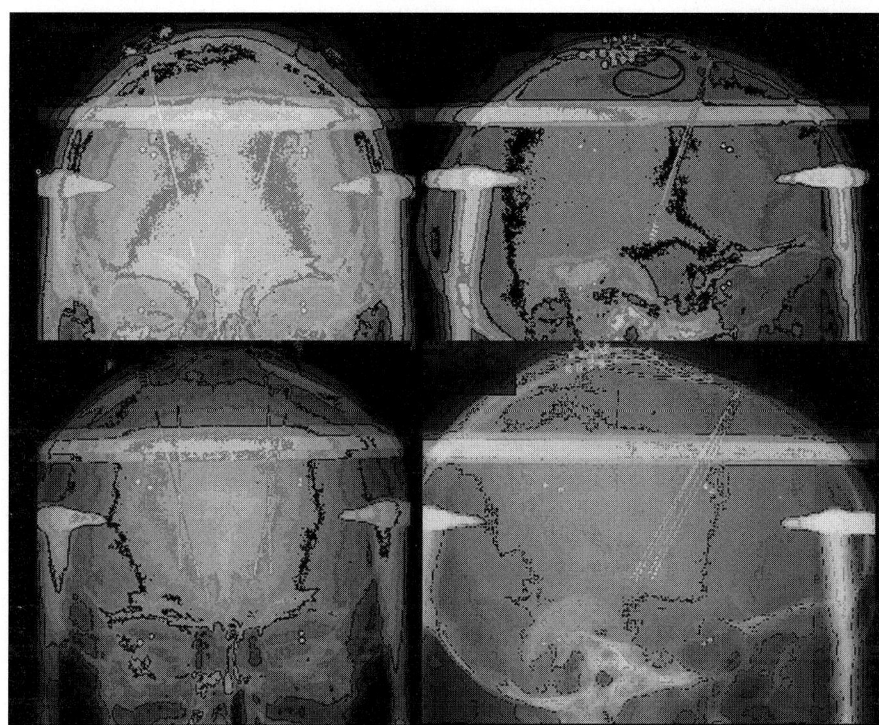

Fig. 9.11 X-ray control of deep brain stimulation electrode positioning at the end of the surgical session.

gicel, Ethicon, Inc., Somerville, NJ), and the skull opening is filled with semiliquid dental cement (CMW2, DePuy International Ltd, England), embedding the holes, the ligature, and the leads. The scalp is closed over the wires. The connection to an implantable pulse generator (IPG), either the Medtronic Kinetra 7428 or the Soletra 7426 (Medtronic, Inc., Minneapolis, MN), via extension leads is usually performed several days later.

The tool holder is dismantled from the robot arm. Final X-rays allow a check of the correct positioning of the chronic electrodes (**Fig. 9.11**). The tool holder is moved and reassembled when the robot is reactivated to execute the contralateral positioning, which is programmed prior to the beginning of the second implantation session. This change from the first to the second side is achieved in a matter of a few minutes, and the procedure is replicated similarly to that on the first side.

■ Results

Number of Cases

Since 1989, we have performed 425 deep brain stimulation (DBS) cases, 336 were implanted bilaterally, yielding a total of 761 electrodes. In the same period, 93 SEEG cases were implanted with 873 deep EEG recording electrodes (**Fig. 9.12**). Tumor biopsy has been the most frequently used application of this tool, but electrode implantation is the procedure most demonstrative of the system's full potential.

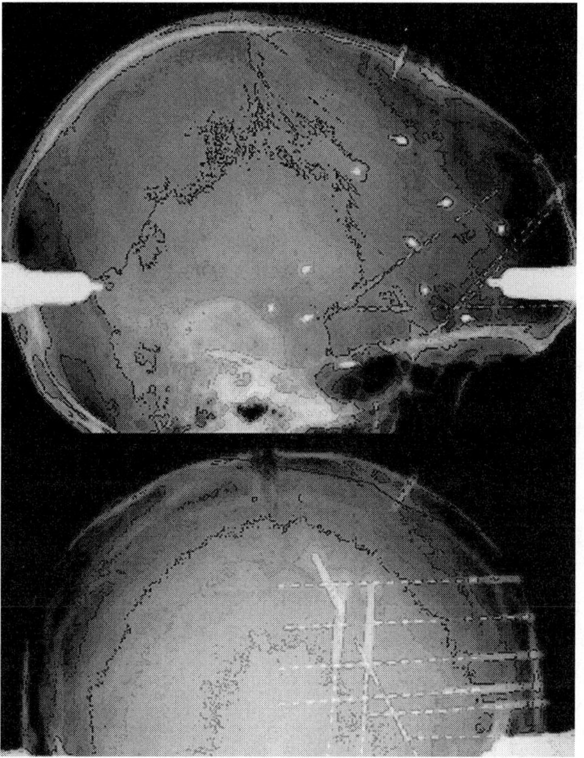

Fig. 9.12 X-ray control of the stereo-electroencephalography electrode positioning at the end of the surgical session.

Complications and Drawbacks

The major drawback of robotic procedures is that they require a robot. The cost of these systems is close to that of a complete traditional modern stereotactic system, if the frame, the goniometer and accessories, and the neuronavigation software are included. The other significant drawback is the increased time of the procedure, which, after resolution of any technical issues by dedicated teams, decreases significantly. Complications were rare, with an overall rate of 1%, none of which was attributable to the robotic aspect of the procedure. All complications were related to the nature of stereotactic surgery, including implantation of depth electrodes into the basal ganglia, or cortical areas in the case of epileptic procedures. In theory, the increased precision of robot-assisted surgery and its ability to avoid parallax errors should result in fewer complications. We cannot demonstrate this because we have not performed a controlled, prospective, randomized study. What has been done during the past 15 years is a proof of principle, a nonprospective feasibility study, which can be viewed as a research and development approach or a step along the road of robotization of neurosurgery.

Advantages

Advantages include significantly increased freedom, eliminating nearly all of the limitations of classic frames using goniometers, and facilitated execution of operative planning, particularly with multiple targets and electrodes. Double obliquity implantation is simplified by only having to determine the entry point and the target point. Planning the contralateral trajectory is rapidly achieved, eliminating the need to repeat the steps of defining a completely new trajectory.

Implantation of electrodes using orthogonal grids raises the problem of the conicity of the X-ray resulting in parallax errors. This can be particularly problematic in defining the avascular window through which the electrodes could be implanted. However, electrodes implanted through the grids are perpendicular to both the grids and the X-ray plates but are not necessarily aligned to the X-ray beams. Notably, parallax increases as the distance from the X-ray tube to the film decreases.

■ Discussion

During the past 15 years, robotic applications in surgery, in particular neurosurgery, have been increasingly performed and reported.[5–9] The predominant neurosurgical application of robotic assistance parallels the suitability of the brain for stereotactic approaches. Namely, the rigidity of the cranial vault, which provides support for immobilization of the organ; the high degree of topological organization of the brain itself, which is strongly correlated to functional diversification; and the somatotopical organization within a given function. Although the various functions controlled by the brain are also topologically organized, it is now known that the segregation between functions is apparent only in the first order, and that extremely intense cross-linking and cross-correlations are present at the anatomical, architectonic, and functional levels. The increasingly large amount of information available from the central nervous system and the necessity to display the data provided by multiple techniques to either investigate brain function or establish a diagnosis calls for methods to accurately and efficiently merge all these data. Rapid integration is imperative because such data may change over time due to their temporal nature. This is particularly true for functional investigations, such as EEG, or the increasingly frequent use of functional imaging [e.g., magnetoencephalography, positron emission tomography (PET) scan, and functional MRI]. The explosion of digital brain imaging, the increasing performance of computer techniques, and the possibility to create links between the teams or data banks of distant institutions, provide a richness that, particularly in the field of medical sciences, can no longer be ignored. Similarly, increasingly stringent standards regulating medical and surgical practices make it mandatory to employ all available technical methods in an attempt to improve medicine and particularly surgical procedures for the benefit of the patient. Improving patient care includes improved diagnostic skills and an extensive knowledge of state of the art basic science as well as reduced invasiveness, increased precision, and decreased duration of the procedures. Improvements in anatomical and functional digital imaging initiated this trend. Neuronavigation was the logical next step, integrating anatomy in its three-dimensional (3D) digitized form with different imaging modalities such as MRI, CT, and functional imaging.[10,11] Combining the use of graphic tools to define the contours of structures with the digital nature of information allowing the acquisition of 3D coordinates for points in anatomical space has provided the possibility to design targets, entry points, and therefore trajectories. The communication between neuronavigation software and various surgical tools, such as mechanical arms (beginning with the magic wand of Watanabe[12,13]), microscopes (beginning with the integrated stereomicroscopic methods of Patrick Kelly[14,15]), and finally robotized arms, represent the logical evolution toward robotization. It became evident these methods were not meant to replace surgical skills, but on the contrary, to merely provide assistance by increasing precision and speed. These benefits are particularly applicable to repetitive procedures such as multiple electrode insertion. Since 1989, this philosophy has been the foundation of our surgical methodology. Our efforts have been oriented toward the creation of a robotic arm, with skills sufficiently broad, to be adaptable to help the neurosurgeon in all stereotactic circumstances, as opposed to being dedicated to a unique single procedure.

Is this approach really useful or is it simply a poorly justified endeavor created by scientists interested in technological developments, and surgeons attracted to exotic video games? Since the completion of our first prototype in 1989, all stereotactic procedures have been systematically performed using successive versions of the NeuroMate. Progressive adaptations of tools to broaden the scope of applications of this robotic arm are continually in development. For example, spherical motion is being developed using a joystick to move the axis of the trajectory around a fixed point, which would be determined by planning, at the level of the skull, at the target point, or in between. One of the most important opportunities arising from the use of robots is that for a given technical tool available at the moment, almost limitless modifications in software can be made, and introduction of new data banks, such as digitized atlases, can be created. Any number of subroutines can be included in the software. For example, the coordinates of the basal ganglia targets for movement disorders can be preprogrammed as fixed numerical values, or formulas based on data specific to each patient, such as the spatial position of the posterior commissure, the anterior commissure, the midline, and the maximum height of the thalamus. The trajectories can be calculated based on each patient's specific anatomy. Providing the software with the position of these anatomical landmarks involves simply identifying key structures using a mouse, which are then used to automatically calculate a trajectory for the selected target. The trajectory can be edited by the surgeon, particularly when the entry point is over a critical structure.[16]

The construction of statistical atlases, such as the probabilistic functional atlas that we recently developed,[17] may be fused with other imaging modalities, such as MRI, to help determine which point has the highest probability of corresponding with the best functional target. This type of utilization of the properties of computation is only one example of how statistical data obtained by the team or coming from literature and available on Web sites might be easily integrated to the software driving robots. It might be possible to associate a given point in space with data obtained from the literature, particularly from the basic sciences, pertaining to various aspects related to this point (such as anatomy, histology, neuromediators, beneficial effects of stimulation at various frequencies, side effects, which can be expected from local lesioning or stimulation). The reverse can be done as well, such as importing into the software, at the address of this point, determined by its 3D coordinates, various features and observations gathered during the surgery and pertaining to, for instance, the pathology of the patient.[18]

Repetitive procedures such as multiple electrode insertion for deep EEG recording, bilateral insertion in one of several targets for movement disorders, or other functional indications (such as epilepsy, obsessive-compulsive disorders, cluster headache, and future indications) are particularly suited to these types of methods. Deep EEG recordings allow not only the cortical surface of the convexity, in particular, the cortex of the midline, and the deep sulci, as well as structures difficult to reach and explore, such as the orbitofrontal gyri and the insula cortex. To achieve this purpose, double oblique trajectories are determined by two points situated in the target structure. These points are chosen on the MRI (**Fig. 9.13**). Current neuronavigation software is designed to create trajectories easily from imaging modalities along multiple paths, which would be difficult to calculate and perform using the conventional goniometers of stereotactic frames. This is particularly true when boring,

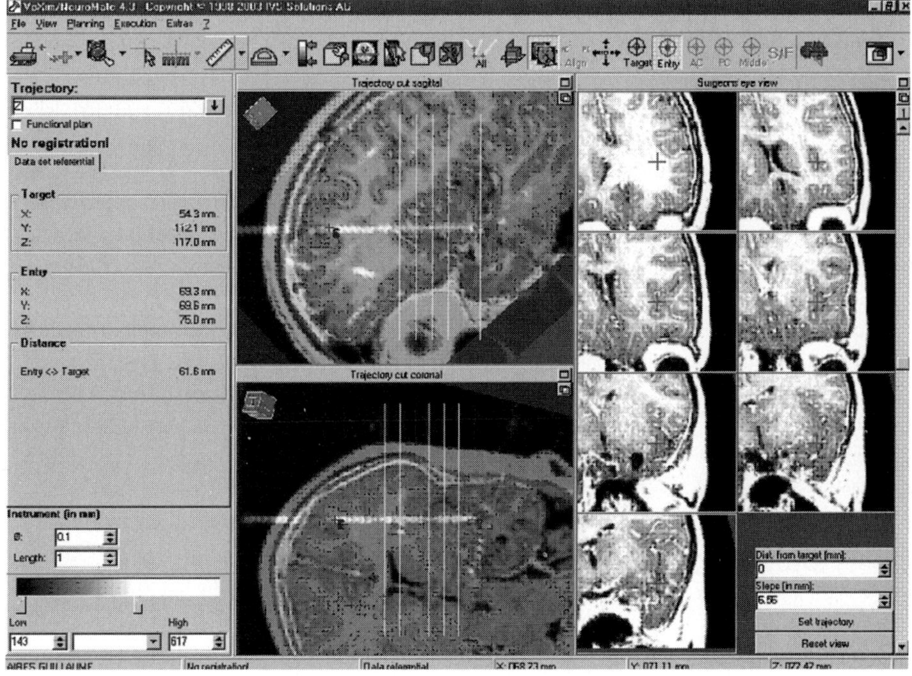

Fig. 9.13 Deep brain stimulation planning of stereoelectroencephalography electrodes on the VoXim neuronavigation software (Integrated Visualization Systems, Chemnitz, Germany). (See **Color Plate 9.13**.)

time-consuming, precision-requiring steps and manipulations might be undertaken more rapidly, efficiently, and precisely by computer-driven robotic assistance than when performed manually. Furthermore, there is the human tendency to skip steps when they become too numerous. In addition, the various trajectories can be preplanned and stored in the computer's hard drive, significantly reducing the time to change from one trajectory to the next during the surgery. This feature benefits the patient, the surgeons, and the operating room attendants because the planning is often rather time intensive.

Interestingly, the literature provides increasing examples of surgical teams devoting time and effort to developing such tools, and medical device companies including these tools in their catalogs. The application of these methods has the potential to decrease cost, determine optimal strategies, and converge toward the optimal configuration of these tools. One pitfall should be carefully avoided. For strictly commercial reasons, it is often more profitable for companies to sell a large number of items. The resultant decrease in price makes such items attainable to a large number of institutions. However, this reduced price is often associated with suboptimal performances. Putting tools in the hands of expert surgeons that are suboptimal for economical reasons alone would ultimately be contrary to the goal of all this development.

Editor's Comments

Dr. Benabid and his team in Glenoble have pioneered not only deep brain stimulation (see Chapter 1) but also robotic techniques. Functional and stereotactic procedures are a natural starting point for the introduction of robotics to neurosurgery. The father of functional neurosurgery, Sir Victor Horsley, performed the first stereotactic surgery on monkeys. This stereotactic frame was a simple machine that allowed probes to reach targets and minimally invade the brain. He in collaboration with Clarke developed the breakthrough concept of putting anatomical structure into Cartesian coordinates. However, even a bold and innovative neurosurgeon such as Sir Victor Horsley did not try this in humans. The problem was the inability to accurately identify the target, and clinical application would await developments in brain imaging. "To touch in space" you have to know where the objective is in space. Imaging has always driven progress in stereotactic neurosurgery. The introduction of the computer to imaging revolutionized neurosurgery and stereotactic neurosurgery. Now even general neurosurgeons use image-based stereotactic techniques (many without realizing it).

With computerized imaging, the potential for computerized machines to perform tasks in stereotactic space has dramatically expanded. The NeuroMate represents a highly advanced example of this technology. What it does best is integrate data, calculate, and perform repetitive tasks. When training residents and fellows, senior staff realize how often data can be misinterpreted, targets can be miscalculated, frames can be misaligned, and repetitive tasks mismanaged. Nevertheless, even the NeuroMate needs the direction and surveillance of a highly trained neurosurgeon to optimize its performance. To date the role of robots in neurosurgery is very small because they are too bulky and expensive and far too limited in their capabilities. Although excellent in performing simple, programmed, repetitive tasks, it will take a huge technological jump to allow them to perform complex tasks and even more technology before they could be considered safe to perform tasks semi-independently (forget "independently" for anyone reading this book). To perform complex tasks they need to be supplied with real-time information to evaluate the work environment to prevent them from injuring the patient or others within the workspace. The workspace is dynamic, and when things move or conditions change within the workspace the robot must be able to recognize alterations in position and stop or change directions in response. The decision capabilities are just too poor to allow independent operation. Supervisory controlled robotic systems or robotic telesurgery may be part of our future if the accuracy and precision of the robot can be controlled. Robots will act based on their programming, and their safe and effective employment will require the intellect, insight, and compassion of an experienced neurosurgeon to perform their tasks. The NeuroMate is a step toward that goal.

The other unique aspect of this team is the use of multiple simultaneous microelectrode recordings and then macrostimulation through the same electrodes. The Alpha Omega microguide (www.alphaomega-eng.com) is an excellent system for this and the Frederick Haer Company (FHC, Inc. Bowdoin, ME—www.fh-co.com) electrodes are the best available. Although several groups have added the ability to do multiple recordings, this remains a rarity among centers. The advantage is the ability to simultaneously identify neurons along parallel tracts and determine the most active tracts and the most effective locations during stimulation. Increasingly, the commercially available microdrives and recording equipment are designed to help this process. The original Axon Guideline 3000 allowed one tract to be evaluated. Then with a switching device, multiple tracts could be recorded from, but only one at a time, necessitating constant switching back and forth to find neurons. The result was tedious and could easily miss activity. Now the mT Guideline 4000 (FHC) is an update that will allow up to 10 tracts to be seen simultaneously. The problem remains that only one neuron (tract) can be effectively interrogated at a time and while doing so other neurons in other tracts can be lost. A hierarchy of testing can help but not cure this problem. Microdrive movements must be very slow, and it is debatable whether it is faster than doing a few quick tracts. With the Ben-Gun only two or three of the five microelectrodes provide significant data for STN localization.[19] We and others usually use two to four rather than five microelectrodes at one time. The ability to independently control the microelectrodes is coming and could offer greater flexibility and data collection capability. The real key is the use of the combination electrodes that allow both microelectrode recordings and macrostimulation. The stimulation is performed from separate areas of the electrode away from the microelectrode tip. This has some disadvantages of requiring deeper penetration of the electrode but the higher current density allows a much better determination of the effectiveness of stimulation in that area prior to placement of the much larger DBS lead.

References

1. Benabid AL, Cinquin P, Lavalle S, Le Bas JF, Demongeot J, de Rougemont J. Computer-driven robot for stereotactic surgery connected to CT scan and magnetic resonance imaging: technological design and preliminary results. Appl Neurophysiol 1987;50:153–154

2. Benabid AL, Hoffmann D, Lavallee S, et al. Is there any future for robots in neurosurgery? Adv Tech Stand Neurosurg 1991;18:3–45

3. Li QH, Zamorano L, Pandya A, Perez R, Gong J, Diaz F. The application accuracy of the NeuroMate robot: a quantitative comparison with frameless and frame-based surgical localization systems. Comput Aided Surg 2002;7:90–98

4. Varma TR, Eldridge PR, Forster A, et al. Use of the NeuroMate stereotactic robot in a frameless mode for movement disorder surgery. Stereotact Funct Neurosurg 2003;80:132–135

5. Cleary K, Nguyen C. State of the art in surgical robotics: clinical applications and technology challenges. Comput Aided Surg 2001;6:312–328

6. Davies B. A review of robotics in surgery. Proc Inst Mech Eng [H] 2000;214:129–140

7. Glauser D, Flury P, Durr P, et al. Configuration of a robot dedicated to stereotactic surgery. Stereotact Funct Neurosurg 1990;54–55:468–470

8. Goto T, Hongo K, Kakizawa Y, et al. Clinical application of robotic telemanipulation system in neurosurgery: case report. J Neurosurg 2003;99:1082–1084

9. Young RF. Application of robotics to stereotactic neurosurgery. Neurol Res 1987;9:123–128

10. Eisner W, Burtscher J, Bale R, et al. Use of neuronavigation and electrophysiology in surgery of subcortically located lesions in the sensorimotor strip. J Neurol Neurosurg Psychiatry 2002;72:378–381

11. Heilbrun MP, McDonald JD. The future of image-guided surgery. Clin Neurosurg 2000;46:89–101

12. Kosugi Y, Watanabe E, Goto J, et al. An articulated neurosurgical navigation system using MRI and CT images. IEEE Trans Biomed Eng 1988;35:147–152

13. Watanabe E. Neuronavigator [original in Japanese]. No Shinkei Geka 1989;17:1097–1103

14. Kelly PJ. Stereotactic surgery: what is past is prologue. Neurosurgery 2000;46:16–27

15. Kelly PJ. Neurosurgical robotics. Clin Neurosurg 2002;49:136–158

16. Roberts DW, Hartov A, Kennedy FE, Miga MI, Paulsen KD. Intraoperative brain shift and deformation: a quantitative analysis of cortical displacement in 28 cases. Neurosurgery 1998;43:749–758 (discussion 758–760)

17. Nowinski WL, Belov D, Benabid AL. An algorithm for rapid calculation of a probabilistic functional atlas of subcortical structures from electrophysiological data collected during functional neurosurgery procedures. Neuroimage 2003;18:143–155

18. Lewin JS. The neurosurgical operating room of the future: has the future arrived? AJNR Am J Neuroradiol 1999;20:1576–1577

19. Benazzouz A, Breit S, Koudsie A, et al. Intraoperative microelectrode-guided deep brain stimulator implantation for movement disorders. Neurosurgery 2002;3(Suppl 17):S145–S149

10 Frameless Functional Stereotactic Approaches

Jaimie M. Henderson

The introduction of image-guided surgical systems over the past decade has had a profound impact on neurosurgical practices. Accurate localization of intracranial targets without the use of stereotactic frames has become commonplace. For procedures such as tumor resection, where real-time feedback regarding intracranial position is helpful, image-guided surgical systems have effectively replaced stereotactic frames. However, trajectory-based functional procedures such as lesioning or stimulation of the deep nuclei for Parkinson disease (PD) and tremor are still widely performed with a frame. The benefit of real-time positional feedback in these procedures is less important than the accurate delivery of a probe to a well-defined target. In addition, functional neurosurgery requires a stable platform to support microelectrode recording and stimulation over many hours and through multiple parallel trajectories. Skin fiducials, as traditionally used for frameless localization, do not provide sufficient accuracy, and instrument holders for biopsy or other applications do not provide sufficient rigidity to meet the demands of true stereotactic localization. Thus new approaches and instrumentation are needed to adapt these systems to use in functional neurosurgery.

Although stereotactic frames have proven their utility over many decades of use, there are several theoretical advantages of a fully frameless functional surgery system. Decoupling of imaging from surgery eliminates the need for planning to be done just prior to the procedure, allowing operations to begin on schedule hours or days following planning. For PD patients undergoing deep brain stimulation (DBS) or lesioning, this translates to less time off medication, with concurrent reduction of associated discomfort. Because there is no need to restrain the head, patients are able to move and adjust their position during surgery, further improving comfort and cooperation during the procedure. Sophisticated image-guided surgery systems are employed for planning, registration, and aiming, and the possibility of real-time electrode tracking and integration of multiple information sources becomes possible, improving the situational awareness of the surgeon.[1] Because of these advances, there is the potential for a high degree of accuracy.[2] Several laboratory studies of image-guided surgical systems demonstrated localization accuracies similar to those achievable with a stereotactic frame.[3–7] Preliminary studies have shown the feasibility of using a surgical navigation system in conjunction with an image-guided microdrive to perform functional neurosurgical procedures with acceptable accuracy,[8] and a multicenter trial demonstrated equivalent accuracy between a stereotactic frame system and an image-guided, skull-mounted platform.[9]

Frameless systems are increasingly being used as an alternative to frames in stereotactic neurosurgery. There are currently two systems in use for frameless functional neurosurgery. Both rely on skull-implanted fiducials for the highest possible accuracy. Each system is designed to attach rigidly to the skull and must maintain absolute rigidity during the procedure to assure that the probe or electrode does not deviate from the planned target.

■ STarFix Platform

The STarFix platform (FHC, Inc., Bowdoin, ME) is a custom-fabricated device based on rapid-prototyping technology. Following fiducial placement and imaging, custom software is used to plan the target-entry trajectory. This plan is then submitted to the company, which manufactures a high-grade plastic platform, which attaches to the implanted fiducial markers. The finished custom platform is sent by express mail within 24 to 72 hours. On the day of surgery, the platform is attached to the implanted fiducials after sterile preparation and serves as a trajectory guide. This design trades the flexibility of real-time trajectory adjustment for simplicity and absolute rigidity.

■ Nexframe

The Nexframe from Medtronic Neuromodular IGN (www.medtronic.com/physician/activa) is an adjustable platform that uses a sweep and rotate alignment mechanism. The Nexframe requires a registration and alignment procedure with an image-guided neuronavigation system (Medtronic, BrainLAB, or Stryker). This allows for changes in trajectory should the need arise during surgery. This device has been extensively tested in both the laboratory[7] and clinical[9] settings, demonstrating equivalent accuracy to a stereotactic frame.

System Verification

The first step in preparing to perform frameless functional interventions is the verification of the image-guided navigational system. Tight quality control is required to achieve optimum accuracy. Ideally, the system should be tested in the same configuration and environment in which it will be used during actual surgery. Position of the camera array and the display screen should be optimized to provide an unobstructed field of view of the surgical field. Studies should be undertaken using a plastic skull phantom equipped with a clearly visible internal target (**Fig. 10.1**). The planning software is used to choose target and entry points as well as the center of each fiducial marker. All instruments should be checked for geometry errors, with care to verify accuracy during rotation throughout their full range of visibility. Registration and alignment should be simulated with the phantom in a position that would resemble that of a patient during surgery. A rigid probe with absolutely no bend should be used to measure localization error (**Fig. 10.1A**). Average localization accuracies should be in the 1.25 mm range, with a 99.9% confidence interval of ~4 mm.[7] The surgeon must be satisfied with the accuracy of the system during bench testing before moving to clinical use.

Operative Procedure

As with all stereotactic procedures, imaging is performed prior to the operation with the fiducial system in place (Unibody, Medtronic, Inc.). We utilize a one-piece stainless steel fiducial marker (**Fig. 10.2**)that is screwed into the skull via a small stab incision (**Fig. 10.3**) after sterile prep and infiltration of local anesthetic. Fiducials are placed in the patient while in the outpatient clinic and are generally tolerated quite well by the patients, who usually equate the experience with a visit to the dentist. The number and placement of fiducials are important to encompass the entire volume of interest. Three fiducial markers are the minimum number needed to mathematically perform a paired-point registration of two coordinate systems.[10] Most image-guided surgery systems require a minimum of four points. We place five fiducials to provide redundancy and to cover as much of the cranial volume as possible, thus providing maximum accuracy while keeping patient comfort in mind. Recommended fiducial placement is illustrated in **Fig. 10.4**. A battery-powered autodriver greatly facilitates placing the self-tapping screws and prevents wobbling during insertion, which can lead to improper seating of the screws and dislodgment of the fiducials. Properly placed

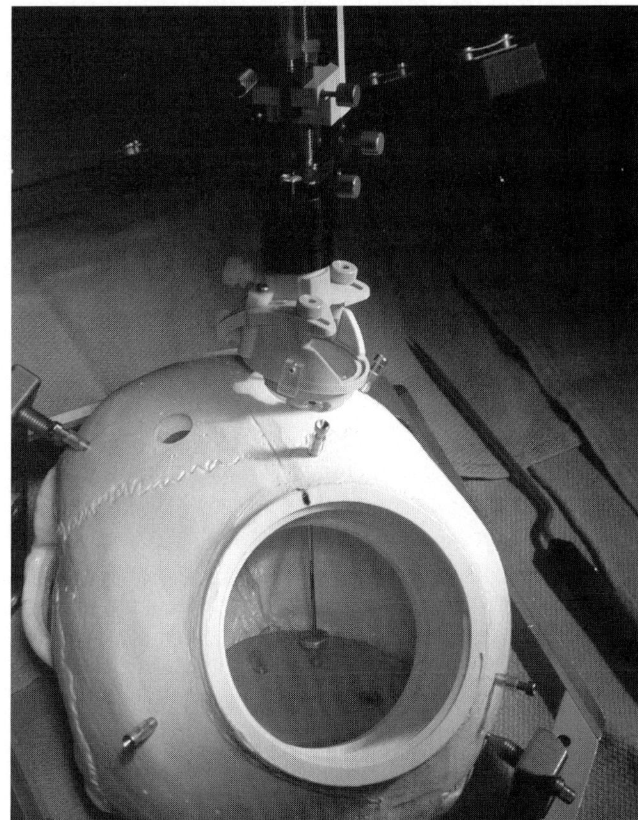

A

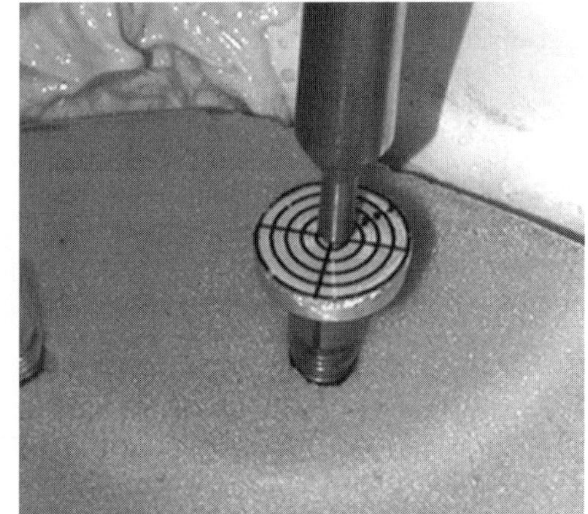

B

Fig. 10.1 **(A)** A plastic skull phantom used for verification of the image-guided navigation system. A localizing probe is being introduced to the expected target point. **(B)** A hardened steel mandrel is used to localize the target, which is marked in 1 mm increments to assess radial error in localization. (See **Color Plate 10.1A**.)

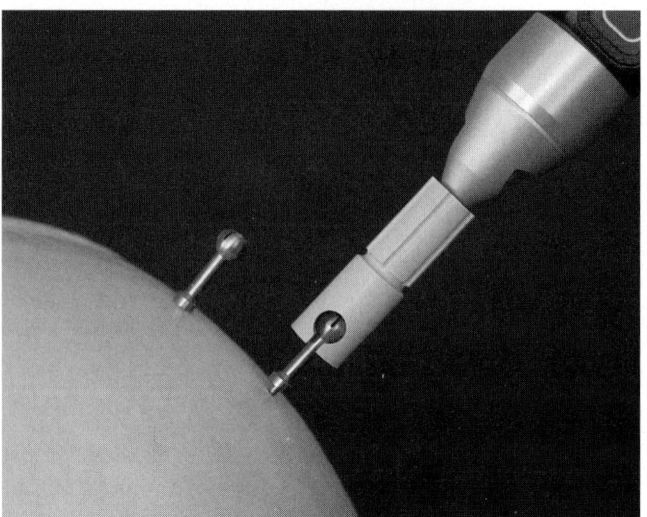

Fig. 10.2 The one-piece titanium fiducial is pictured with a battery-powered autodriver. (See **Color Plate 10.2**.)

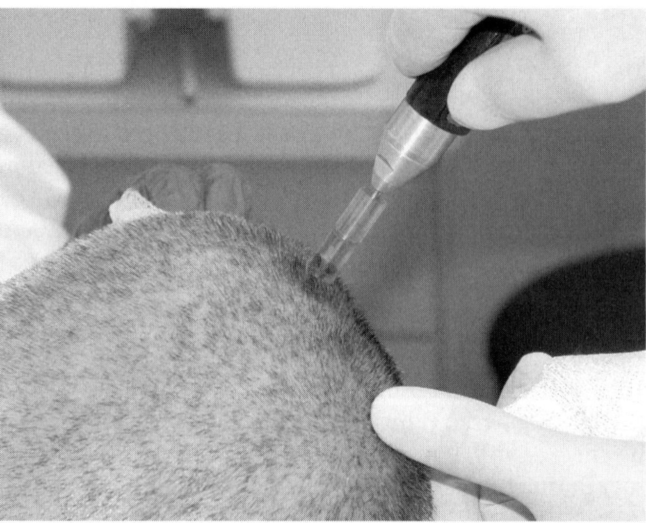

Fig. 10.3 Placement of a fiducial marker is pictured following sterile preparation, infiltration of local anesthetic, and creation of a small stab incision. (See **Color Plate 10.3**.)

fiducials do not suffer from the mechanical deformations that plague stereotactic frame systems,[11] and can provide very high levels of accuracy.[2]

Following fiducial placement, 1 mm thick computed tomographic (CT) slices are taken throughout the cranial volume. These scans are then fused with volumetric magnetic resonance (MR) scans taken several days or weeks prior to surgery (**Fig. 10.5**). Both CT and MR scanning are thus decoupled from the physical act of surgery, allowing planning to occur at any time prior to the procedure and eliminating delays on the morning of surgery related to image transfer or difficulties with frame placement. Surgical planning is performed on the image-guided workstation in a manner identical to that used with frame-based stereotaxy. Target

and entry points are selected, and the fiducials are identified. Care must be taken to locate the precise center of the fiducial marker in all three-image planes.

On the morning of surgery, the patient is brought to the operating room and placed in a lounge-chair position, which is adjusted for optimal comfort. We find that patients are better able to cooperate with the somewhat strenuous intraoperative evaluation procedure when they are comfortable and relaxed. Propofol sedation is administered. A noninvasive head holder with a cervical collar restraint (Nexframe Passive Head Rest, Medtronic, Inc.) minimizes head movement during the initial incision, burr hole placement, and initial alignment of the trajectory guide (**Fig. 10.6**). Following these steps, the collar portion is removed, allowing

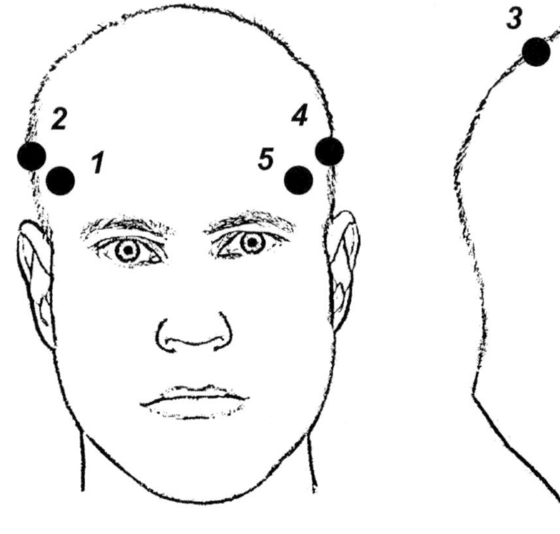

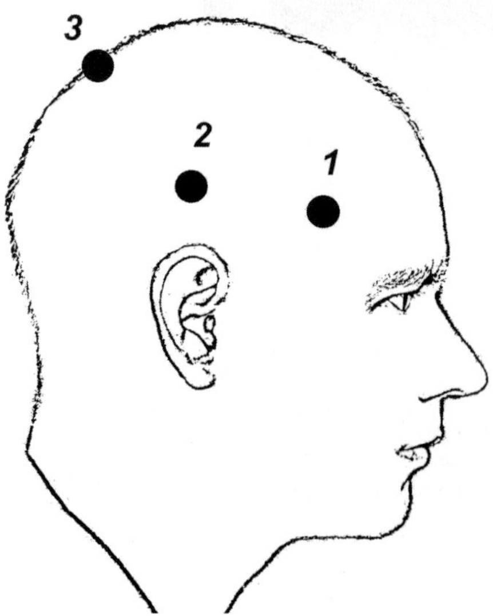

Fig. 10.4 The recommended fiducial locations for use with the Nexframe and a noninvasive head holder are illustrated.

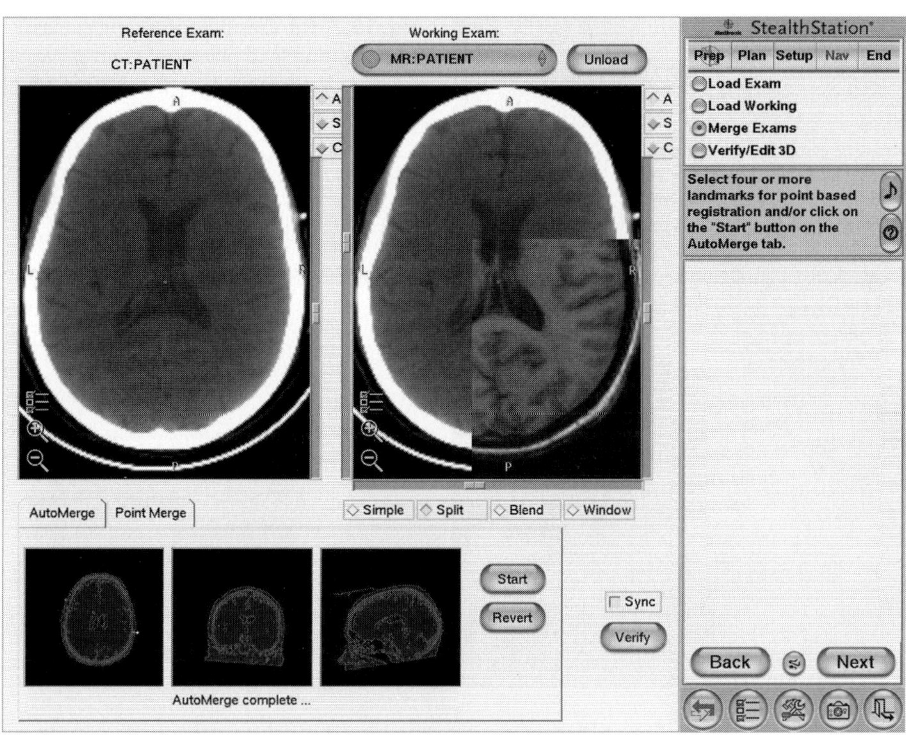

Fig. 10.5 Fusion of MR scan done 3 weeks prior to surgery with CT scan performed the day prior to surgery with fiducials in place. Note the excellent agreement of the MR and CT at the boundaries of the ventricles and in the cerebral sulci. (See **Color Plate 10.5**.)

full freedom of head movement. One unique advantage we have discovered with this method is the ability to test the cervical musculature during surgery for cervical dystonia. A C-arm fluoroscope can be used to verify electrode position and also serves as an excellent draping fixture (**Fig. 10.7**). The C-arm is brought in after patient positioning and before the initial registration phase. An initial registration is performed using a noninvasive reference frame, touching each fiducial in turn with a nonsterile probe. Pointing back to the fiducials can give the surgeon a fairly accurate estimate of the expected localization error (**Fig. 10.8**). The entry point is then localized with the image-guided surgery system and marked with a skin scratch.

The scalp is prepared using an aqueous antiseptic solution. A transparent lateral hip drape with Ioban adhesive center (3M Health Care, St. Paul, MN) is applied to the scalp, taking care to form the drape loosely around the posts of the fiducial markers. Stretching of the drape over the fiducials can inhibit accurate registration and predispose to punctures, which can lead to breaks in sterility. After draping, the planned incision is injected with a local anesthetic solution. A small stab incision is made at the marked entry

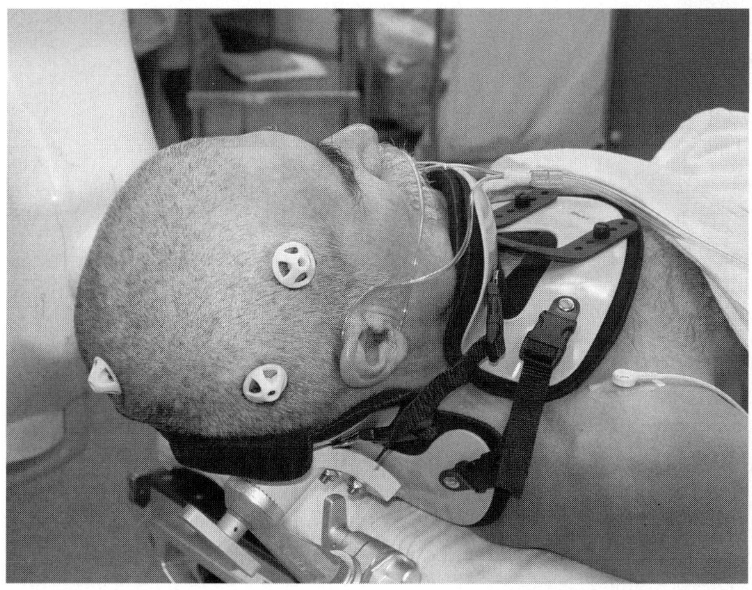

Fig. 10.6 A patient positioned for deep brain stimulator insertion. A collar attachment helps stabilize the head during the initial localization and drilling steps; this is removed once electrophysiological monitoring begins. (See **Color Plate 10.6**.)

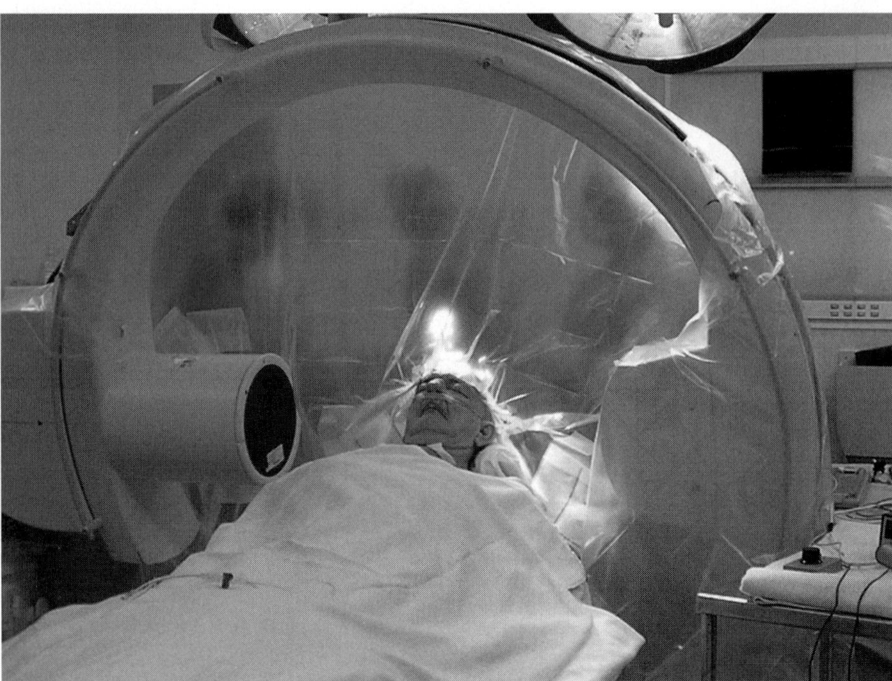

Fig. 10.7 The C-arm fluoroscope can assist in evaluating lead placement and serves as a fixture for draping. (See **Color Plate 10.7.**)

point with a no. 11 blade. A 1 mm twist drill is used to make a pilot hole in the outer table of the skull that will be used to guide accurate burr hole placement. The incision is then opened and Raney clips placed on the wound edges. A 14 mm burr hole is made using a standard automatic-releasing cranial perforator centered precisely on the pilot hole. The burr hole is initially made perpendicular to the skull, but as the diploe is reached the perforator should be angled to direct the burr hole slightly lateral. This maneuver reduces interference with the edge of the burr hole that can occur when making more medial electrode passes. We remove the small shelf of bone left by the perforator, using a Kerrison rongeur to achieve maximum working room. The bone edges are waxed, and remaining portions of the inner table are removed with a curette.

After hemostasis is achieved, a combination lead anchor/burr hole cover is placed (Stimloc, Medtronic, Minneapolis, MN). The trajectory guide platform is then attached

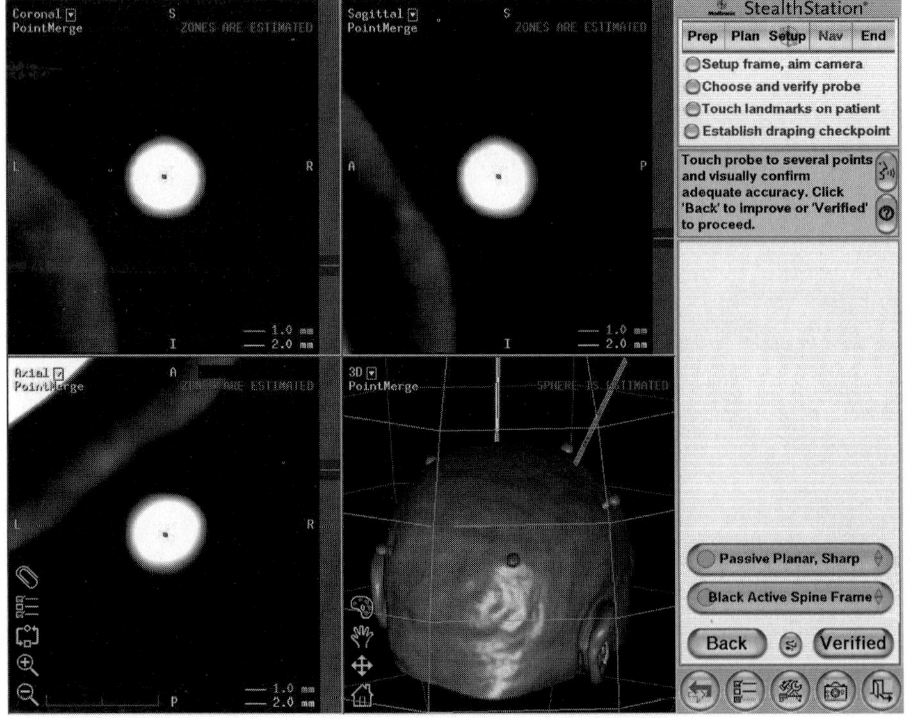

Fig. 10.8 Relocalization of each fiducial marker verifies registration. Note the green "sphere of accuracy" within which predicted localization error is less than 1 mm. The small black dot indicates the localized position relative to the fiducial marker, showing excellent agreement. (See **Color Plate 10.8.**)

to the skull using three self-drilling, self-tapping screws. It is extremely important that the coupling between the platform and the skull be completely rigid, otherwise there could be movement of the platform during surgery with displacement of the introducer cannula or electrode or both. We attempt to lift the patient's head from the table using the base of the trajectory guide, and aggressively attempt to dislodge it by rotational movements. If there is any movement of the platform whatsoever, the screws must be tightened further. Resistance to screw advancement can often be remedied by backing the screws out by a half to a whole turn to dislodge any bone chips prior to further tightening.

Once satisfied with the rigidity of the skull fixation, a reference arc is attached to the platform (**Fig. 10.9**). The fiducial markers are once again touched in sequence with the registration probe. Several subtle but important technical points can improve registration accuracy during this step. The registration probe should be aligned parallel to the long axis of the fiducial if possible to allow the tip of the probe to penetrate to the bottom of the registration "divot." The cameras of the surgical navigation system should be carefully aligned so that the probe can be "seen" throughout the localization volume. The light emitting diodes (LEDs) or reflective spheres of the probe should be squarely aligned with the camera to minimize errors, which can be introduced by viewing the instruments edge-on. Each instrument should be verified prior to use and the tip position should agree with the expected position to within less than 1 mm, and preferably within 0.5 mm or less. Pointing back to each fiducial with the registration probe once again confirms the registration. Errors greater than 1 to 2 CT voxels should prompt consideration of reregistration. Verification of system accuracy at each stage of the procedure is essential to minimize errors and achieves optimal accuracy.

The dura mater is then opened, and a cortical incision made with bipolar cautery. Gelatin sponge (Gelfoam, Pfizer,

New York, NY) and fibrin glue are placed within the burr hole to minimize loss of cerebrospinal fluid (CSF) during the alignment procedure. Careful attention should be paid to replacing the sealant promptly each time burr hole access is needed during the procedure. The greater the amount of CSF loss, the greater is the potential compromise of the recordings from brain shift or pulsatile movement of the brain.

The alignment fixture is placed on the platform and a guidance instrument is used to align the device to target. Software specifically designed for trajectory-based aiming (FrameLink (version 4.1.7 or higher) Medtronic Navigation) can aid in this task (**Fig. 10.10**). Great care should once again be exercised to assure that instrument geometry is verified and that alignment is performed precisely using the highest possible view magnification because small differences in trajectory as measured at the skull surface can translate into large errors at the target point. The trajectory guide is swept back and forth, watching the computer screen as this procedure moves the aim point along a line that will usually not intersect the target on the first attempt. The base of the guide is then rotated, repeating the sweep and observing the change in movement of the aim point across the target. Eventually, the sweep will bring the aim point through the target point, and the locking screws on the base can be tightened. This aiming procedure is graphically presented in **Fig. 10.11**. A 3 mm offset aiming fixture is provided with the Nexframe device to allow compensation for trajectories that may be affected by the burr hole edge or surface features such as cortical veins.

Once the trajectory guide has been locked into place, a distance to target measurement is made using the navigational system. Unlike frame-based stereotaxy, the configuration of each individual patient's cranial anatomy will determine the target depth, which may vary by as much as 20 mm from case to case. At this point, the multilumen adapter replaces the aiming fixture. A microdrive is mounted on the adapter and the depth to target is entered into the adjustment scale

A

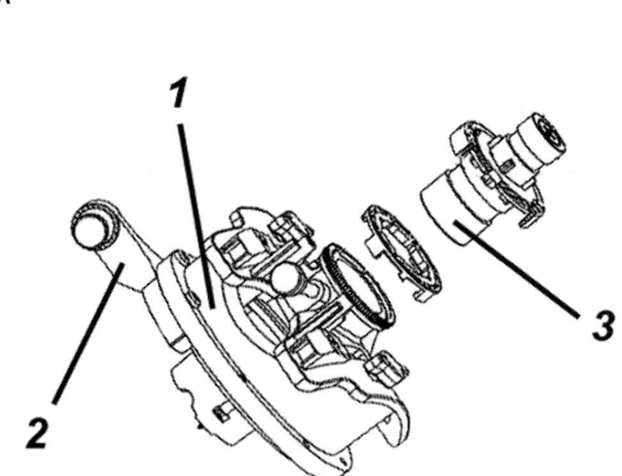

B

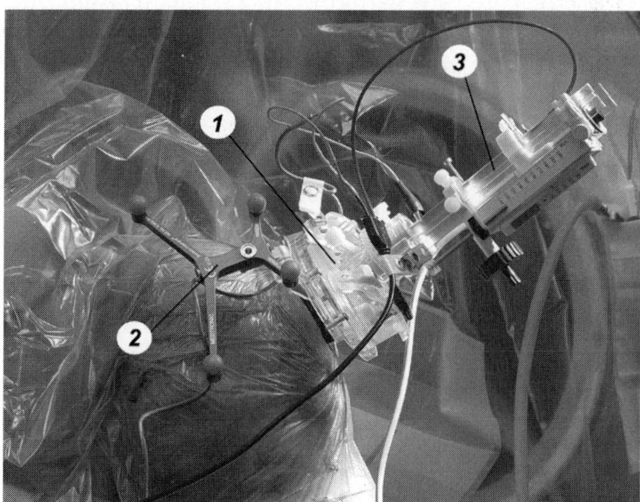

Fig. 10.9 (**A**) An exploded view of the Nexframe trajectory guide. 1, trajectory guide platform; 2, attachment point for neuronavigator reference arc; 3, multilumen adapter. (**B**) The Nexframe in clinical use. 1, trajectory guide platform; 2, neuronavigator reference arc; 3, microdrive. (See **Color Plate 10.9B**.)

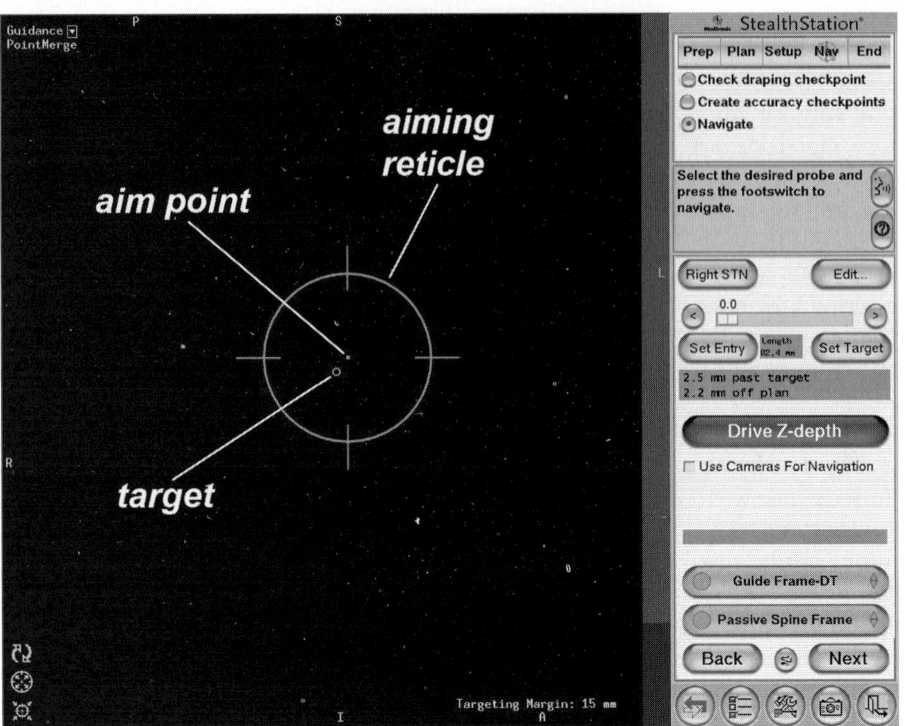

Fig. 10.10 The StealthStation (Medtronic Navigation, Louisville, CO) display, showing the guidance view that is used to align the aim point with the target. The aiming reticle moves with the aim point, assisting the surgeon in determining the proper sweep and rotation settings. (See **Color Plate 10.10.**)

(**Fig. 10.9**). The use of two individually variable depth adjustments allows a standardized microrecording paradigm without recalculation of microdrive position for each case. The fibrin glue is removed from the burr hole and the outer cannula placed into the brain. Care must be taken to avoid any deflection from bone or dural edges, and the cannula should be slowly introduced, feeling for any resistance to advancement. The gelatin sponge and fibrin glue are replaced. The stylet is then removed from the outer cannula and replaced by the reducer, through which the microelectrode is placed. The reducer is designed to allow introduction of both the microelectrode and the lesioning or stimulating electrode through the same cannula.

Microrecording is performed in a standard fashion, defining the target area electrophysiologically. Withdrawing the outer cannula and replacing it in one of the four other holes in the multilumen adapter can make parallel tracks. A 3 mm offset adapter can also be used to move the electrode up to 5 mm in any direction perpendicular to the plane of introduction. Electrode moves can be visualized using a chart of all possible positions of the center and offset adapter (**Fig. 10.12**).

Once the target has been defined physiologically, the microelectrode and inner cannula are removed. If stimulation is to be performed, the DBS electrode is measured to length using a cylindrical depth gauge, and a marker stop placed. The electrode is then placed down the outer cannula. The outer cannula is withdrawn, and the clip of the Stimloc device is placed and fastened. The cannula, electrode stylet, and Nexframe tower components are removed in a stepwise fashion, monitoring electrode position using fluoroscopy if desired. Finally, the cap is placed on the Stimloc base, firmly locking the electrode in place.

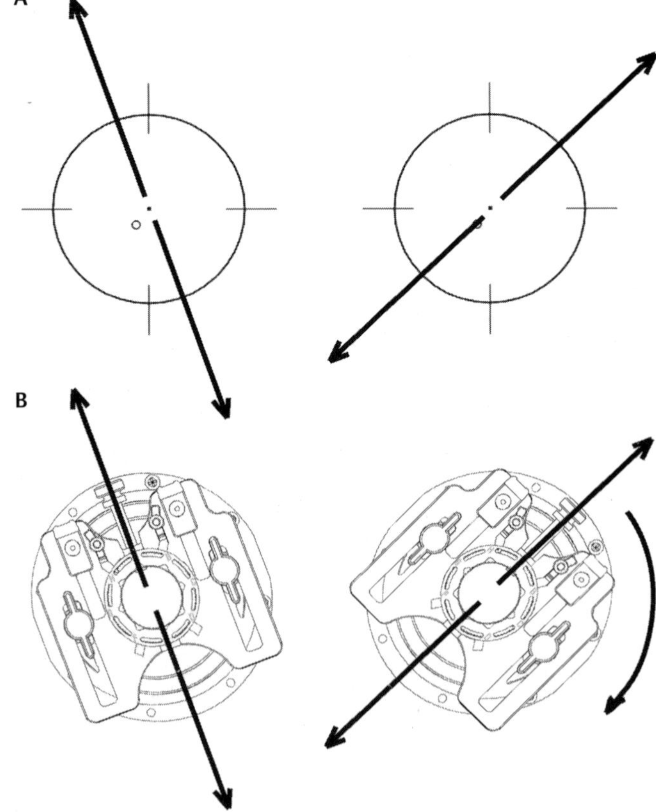

Fig. 10.11 Steps involved in aligning the trajectory guide to the target point. (**A**) The trajectory guide is swept through its full range of motion, watching the motion of the aim point and aiming reticle, which do not intersect the target. (**B**) The trajectory guide has been rotated and the aim point can now be swept through the target point. Once the aim point rests within the target circle, the thumbscrews are firmly tightened and alignment is complete.

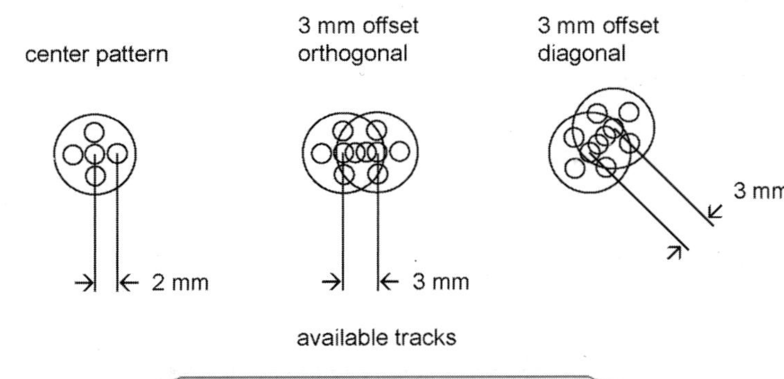

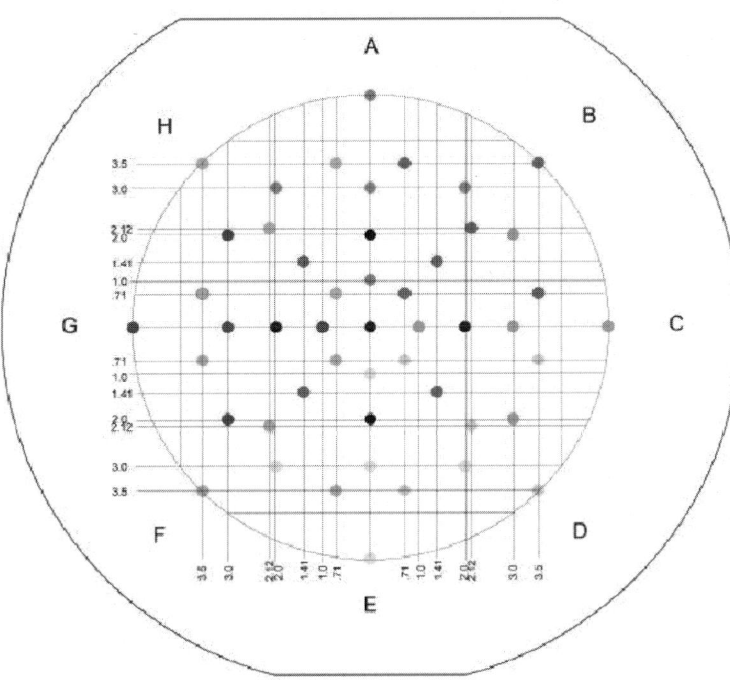

Fig. 10.12 A diagrammatic representation of the center and 3 mm offset multilumen adapters provided with the Nexframe. By rotating the adapters to positions A through H, tracks can be made at 2 mm intervals either orthogonally or diagonally as illustrated in the lower diagram. (See **Color Plate 10.12.**)

Results

In a series of 36 patients undergoing deep brain stimulation for movement disorders, the Nexframe device was used both with and without a stereotactic frame as a backup system.[9] Lead placement was evaluated with postoperative imaging and compared with the intended target. Mean localization error was 3.15 mm, which was identical to the mean localization error in a group of 76 patients implanted using a stereotactic frame.[12] The error was greatest in the z plane, 1.7 mm for the frame and 2.0 mm for the frameless system. The difference in the x and y planes was 1.4 to 1.6 mm for both techniques. There were no complications associated with the use of the device.

◼ Conclusion

Frameless techniques for functional neurosurgery confer several advantages over frame-based techniques. Foremost among these is patient comfort and cooperation. Many patients are extremely apprehensive about frame placement, and some have refused to have surgery because of this fear. In addition, rigid fixation of the patient to the operating room table can restrict mobility. The frameless approach allows the patient free movement of the head, ability to readjust position, and less claustrophobia during the procedure. The ability to apply the fiducials 1 or more days prior to surgery allows imaging and planning to be decoupled from the performance of the procedure, decreasing operating room utilization time and enhancing patient comfort due to shorter times spent off medication. As familiarity with the system has increased, actual operating time is now similar to time spent with a frame system. The net timesaving on the morning of surgery in some cases approaches 2 hours or more when compared with the use of a stereotactic frame.

Our group has found that the ability to evaluate active and passive movement of the neck is particularly valuable in cervical dystonia, where neurons responding to these movements can be directly targeted for electrode delivery. By allowing neck movement in these cases, muscular pain and fatigue can also be reduced. Finally, because the trajectory information used during the aiming procedure is stored in the image-guided system, the straightforward addition of electrode depth tracking allows for advanced software features such as direct correlation of patient anatomy with microrecording.

Along with these advantages, there are several potential pitfalls that are unique to frameless image-guided approaches. Fiducial placement must be carefully performed, with rigid fixation, non-coplanar placement, and avoidance of interference with the intraoperative headrest all taken into account. During registration, care must be taken to precisely identify the center of each fiducial marker, both on the imaging datasets and with the localizing probe. Instrument geometry and system accuracy must be meticulously verified to assure that there are no hidden sources of error. In addition, the rigid-ity of the trajectory guide should be checked at every stage to be certain that no dislodgment of the electrode occurs.

In summary, frameless approaches to functional stereotactic procedures present a viable alternative to frame-based stereotaxis. Advantages in operating room utilization and patient comfort appear to outweigh the slight inconvenience experienced by the surgeon during the learning phase. Once familiar with the procedure, operating time is equivalent, and equivalent accuracy has been demonstrated in a multicenter study. As neuronavigational technology continues to advance, frameless techniques may someday replace stereotactic frames for the delivery of therapeutic interventions to deep brain targets.

Editor's Comments

The Nexframe system has been used by several centers throughout the United States, most of which have been very pleased with its performance. One advantage of the system is the noninvasive restraint system minimally interfering with the patient. Unfortunately, it is also becoming a gimmick for marketing rather than a true tool for improved surgical outcome. Although this system has the advantage of a less claustrophobic approach, such concerns are usually grossly overstated. Most patients accept the frame quite readily, especially when that is the only alternative. Frameless surgeries can still be very long and uncomfortable. Nevertheless, the frameless approach does allow certain patients to more readily accept surgery. The lack of fixation can become a serious problem for severely tremulous or dystonic patients and for any patient where there is the potential for wild movements of the head with a probe inside the brain. The patient's mobility is improved and allows for less obstructed examination of the patient. The suggestion by some that gait can be tested is foolish and should not be attempted. It is not safe to have patients walking around with an open incision and a frame on their head.

The advantage to the surgeon is that the surgical planning can be performed at leisure. On the day of surgery, there is not the stress of a scan to be performed prior to surgery that must be of surgical quality to plan a trajectory. The efficiency of having the preoperative planning performed prior to the day of surgery speeds the operation considerably. The hospital can save money by decreased operating room time and, in addition, can obtain financial advantage by scanning long before surgery; therefore, the imaging and surgery are "unbundled." This allows the use of diagnostic codes rather than operative codes, which generate more revenue for the hospital. Although there is a claim of decreased hospital capital investment, this is only true if this is the only system available. Although purchase of a standard image-guided neuronavigation system or traditional stereotactic frame might not be needed for functional work, another system is currently required for biopsies (off-label for Nexframe) and stereotactic intracranial procedures, which this system currently cannot accommodate. Therefore, the capital gain is not really recognized in most hospital systems. The one time use then becomes a deficit because each expense limits the amount of profit the hospital can make on the procedure. The offset is that if the MRI and CT can be performed as diagnostic procedures, an overall profitability can be obtained.

The use of multiple fiducials in the Nexframe system is more robust than needed and less likely to have problems if one becomes loose. We have had an occasion that required reimaging because of multiple loose bone anchors. The suggestion of using five separate fiducials is excellent, but they need to be far away from operative sites. Although artifacts from conventional frames are removed, there are artifacts from the bone anchors. Multiple microelectrode tracks are possible. However, the displacement around the preselected trajectory is restrained as to where the microelectrode can investigate. The offset is in a circular manner, and therefore, although a microelectrode penetration 2 mm lateral to the initial trajectory is possible, a penetration 2 mm lateral and 2 mm anterior was not possible. This has been solved in the newest version. Nevertheless, the microelectrode excursion is quite adequate for mapping purposes. Another disadvantage is that it cannot be aligned strictly rectilinear to the AC–PC. Only an approximation of rectilinear registration can be obtained by aligning to the AC–PC plane but will have 2 or more degrees of error. The FHC microTargeting Drive System (FHC, Bowdoin, ME) is used and it has the advantage of being reusable and able to perform multiple simultaneous tracks while leaving the cannula in place for placement of the DBS at the optimal microelectrode-recording site. Distance to target is different with the two systems.

We like the Stimloc tabs as medial to lateral as possible so the Nexframe can be aligned as anterior to posterior as possible. Fixation of the platform to the skull is critical. If the titanium screws break by over-tightening or vigorous testing or if the bone attachment is loose, there are rescue screws of the platform that can be rotated 180 degrees and again fixated. The "A" will no longer be anterior but posterior and care must be taken not to misinterpret electrode movements. Similarly, if the offset alignment adaptor is used, the anatomy alignment feature must not be used but the 3 mm offset multilumen must match the orientation of the offset alignment adaptor to prevent trajectory errors. The lead fixation through the Stimloc anchor is not absolute. Migration can occur, especially when the lead is offset from the center. We still use an assistant with a rubber-tipped hemostat to hold the lead while the surgeon disassembles the headstage. Such migrations cannot be detected without fluoroscopy and without an accurate reticle system, the true lead deviation may be difficult to evaluate. Although there is a claim for C-arm or portable X-ray alignment, this is an attachment that is plastic and is quite flexible (**Fig. 10.13**). It is not truly rectilinear,

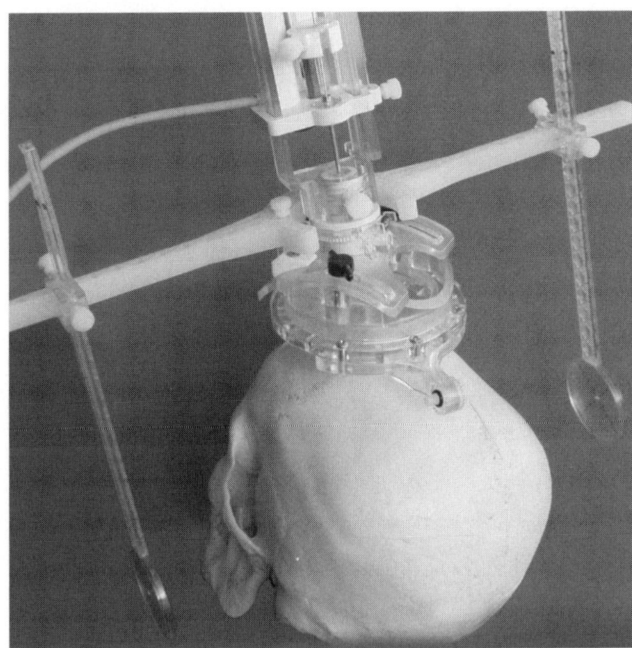

Fig. 10.13 The Nexframe reticules system is designed for intraoperative fluoroscopy to show any lead deviation and validate target depth. The cross beam attachment to the base is not rigid, and both the cross beam and the reference arms are plastic and easily deformed. The alignment marks are imprecise such that accuracy of the device is not great.

which makes verification of target depth and location unreliable. Note: the reference bracket must be attached posteriorly so the reticles can attach laterally. For bilateral procedures, the problem with the Nex-

frame system is that the entire system must be removed and reused or a second system used. Accuracy is in general very good but far too few patients have been studied to exclude a type II error. Several of us have had errors of greater than 3 mm, especially on the second side. It is recommended that the image-guided workstation be disconnected and the entire alignment procedure be repeated to prevent "software glitches." The GuideFrame DT was used early in development and has been replaced by the Nexprobe (Medtronic, Inc.) and should decrease some of these errors.

We have limited experience with the FHC microTargeting (mT) Platform (FHC, Bowdoin, ME), incorporating the STarFix guidance technology system (www.starfixtures.com). The STarFix system has very few users and is still in the process of evolution. Like the Nexframe guidance system it uses implantable fiducials and has the same financial benefits if the MR studies are performed prior to surgery. Whereas the Nexframe requires a separate registration and alignment procedure, the STarFix device is custom-manufactured to be aligned along a prechosen trajectory. We used both systems and one big advantage of the Nexframe was that the StealthStation could be employed to allow a detailed intraoperative evaluation of not only the initial trajectory but also any subsequent trajectories that might be needed to complete the mapping of the target. The STarFix software currently does not have the ability to overlay additional trajectories onto the MR images. There are plans to considerably upgrade the software (image quality and graphics are suboptimal) and become compatible with the StealthStation. Like the Nexframe system, it cannot be aligned strictly rectilinear to AC–PC. With no redundancy, it is always possible that one of the anchors will loosen and require the entire procedure to be repeated from the very beginning.

The system is based on an mT Platform that is custom made for each patient. As such, it is designed for only one side. However, a

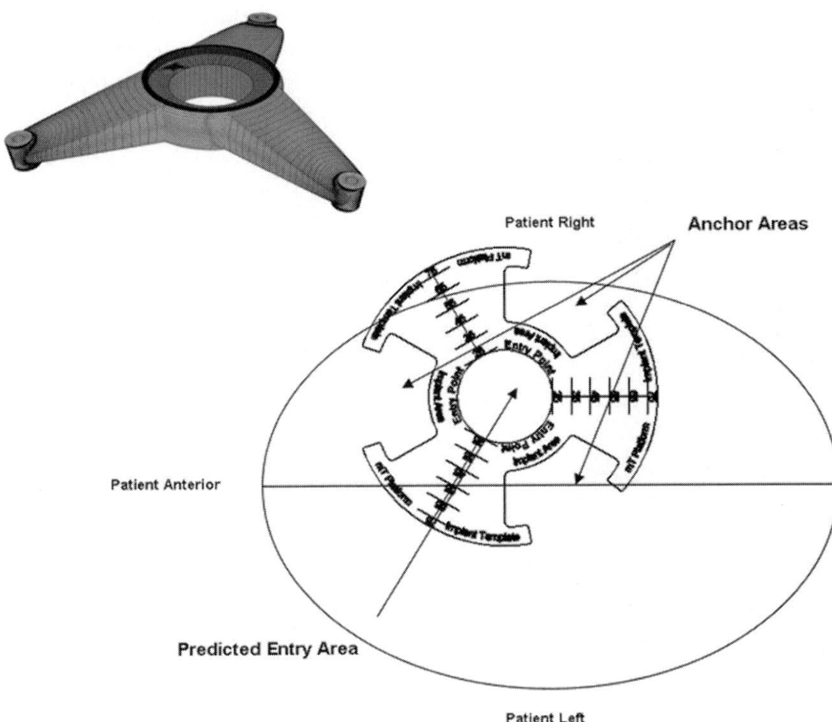

Fig. 10.14 A guide device for the STarFix (FHC, Inc., Bowdoin, ME) is used to approximate the position of the entry point and align bone anchors. One is placed in an anterior position, and two additional anchors must be set more than 120 degrees apart and in a 50 to 80 mm radius from the anticipated entry point.

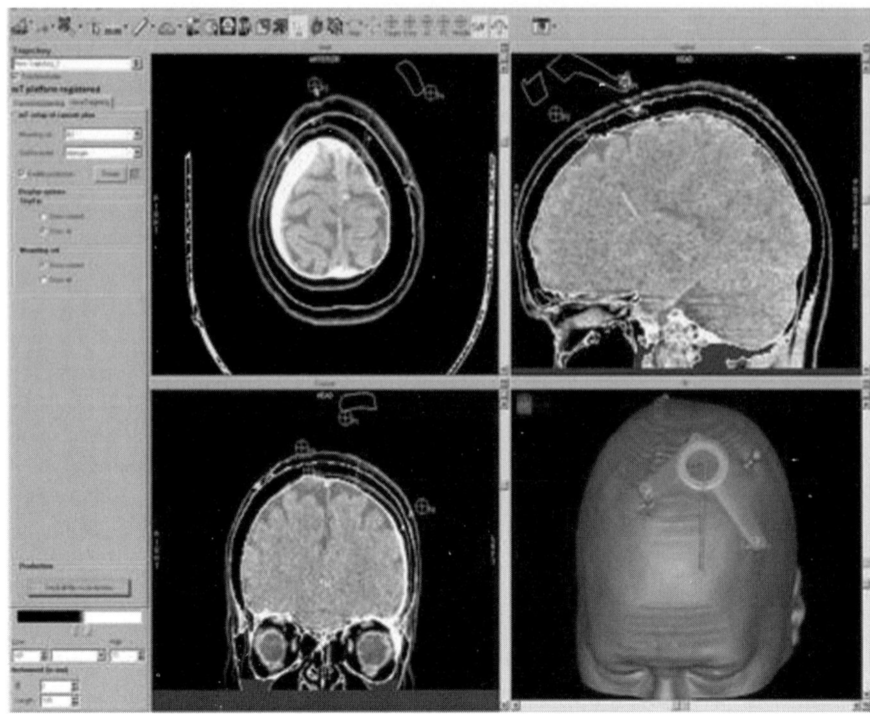

Fig. 10.15 The FHC microTargeting (mT) Drive System planning software allows selection of a target and entry point. A virtual depiction of the mT Platform and trajectory appears on the magnetic resonance and three-dimensional images. Cutaway views demonstrate the mT Platform in place.

custom made bilateral frame can be special ordered. The initial step is to approximate the position of the entry point and align bone anchors, one in an anterior position, and two additional points that must be more than 120 degrees apart and in a 50 to 80 mm radius from the anticipated entry point. An overlay model is available to help this placement (**Fig. 10.14**). At times this may require placing a fiducial marker beyond the hairline. The bone anchors (WayPoint, FHC) are stronger than those of Nexframe. The bone anchors can remain in place for 28 days if necessary. The fiducials are attached to the skull and a CT scan of the patient's entire head with 1 mm overlapping scans performed. At the conclusion of the scan, the fiducials are removed and the implanted bone anchors are covered and the skin sutured closed.

The preoperative planning is then performed on a workstation where the CT and MR are fused to obtain a functional target. The FHC computer software allows 3D rendering of the images to assist in trajectory planning after selection of target and entry points (**Fig. 10.15**). The images are then exported to FHC's fabrication facility by direct Internet connection. An mT Platform is sent by an expedited carrier within 24 to 72 hours. The mT Platform and the microdrive are sterilized along with other components of the mT system prior to surgery (www.starfixtures.com).

The patient is positioned with noninvasive restraints and the head prepped and draped in the routine manner. The assembly of the wing and center positioner of the mT Platform is then temporarily made to

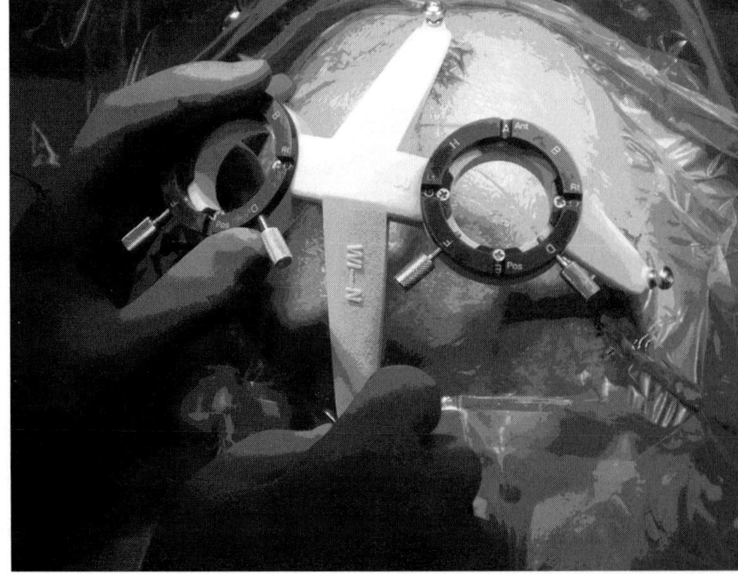

Fig. 10.16 The patient has been shaved, prepped, and draped. Bilateral STarFix (FHC, Inc., Bowdoin, ME) platform anchor sites are located and the anchors exposed with small incisions. Anchor plugs, used to protect the inner thread of the anchor head during the preimplant period are removed. The FHC microTargeting (mT) Drive System platform(s) are temporarily attached to mark entry sites on the scalp. Bilateral independent STarFix platform can now be used.

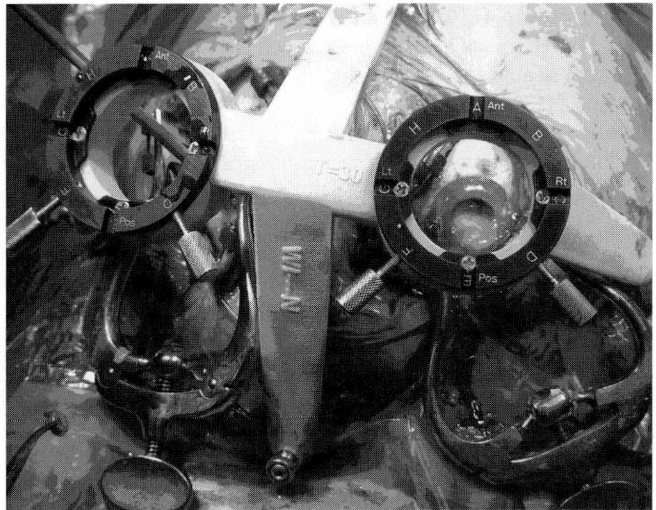

Fig. 10.17 The burr hole–marking tool is used through the platform's hub to mark the entry point. The skull is exposed. The FHC microTargeting (mT) Drive System Platform is reattached to the mount set, and the entry point is marked again, this time on the skull. The entry-marking tool scores the skull, aiding the drilling process. The burr hole may be drilled through the hub opening of the platform. The second side burr hole is drilled. Application of the Stimloc base (Medtronic, Minneapolis, MN) is performed beneath the platform before recording equipment is attached.

use the pointer to determine the entry point and center for the burr hole (**Fig. 10.16**). The mT Platform is then removed and the burr hole made and the Stimloc attached (**Fig. 10.17**). The Platform is then reattached and the microTargeting drive mounted and microelectrode recordings performed, as deemed necessary (**Fig. 10.18**). The hardware gives the surgeon the option of displacing the entry point by 3 mm in 90-degree increments, if necessary. In addition to the 10 mm diameter of the investigational area, by creating an angular offset, there are 3 mm at the entry and 6 mm at the target that can be investigated. Again, these are

limited and not truly rectilinear. When the target is confirmed, the mT Platform then allows positioning of the DBS or lesioning electrode without removal of the drive. This is a considerable advantage and one of the best aspects of both frameless systems is in that the trajectory is now fixed with the cannula. Therefore, the exact same tract that was determined to be optimal on the microelectrode can be implanted with the DBS lead without concern about loss of registration. The DBS lead is then secured with the Stimloc and disassembly of the headstage performed.

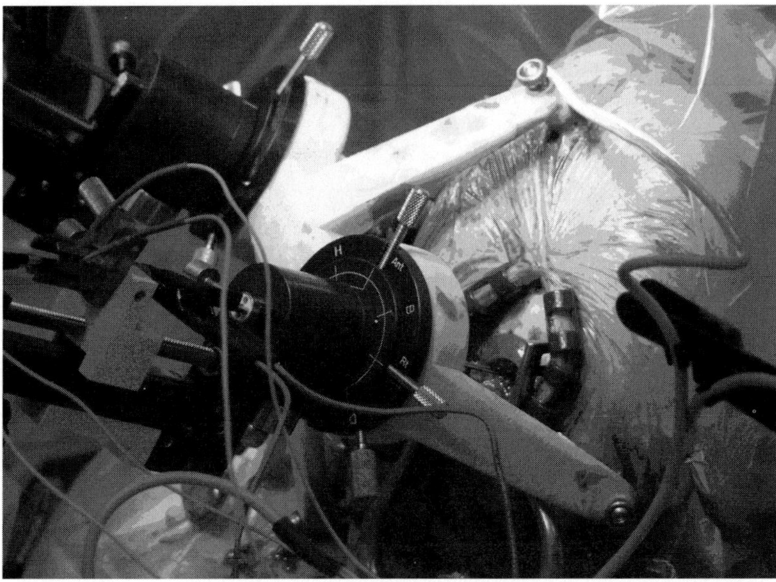

Fig. 10.18 The four-legged bilateral STarFix platform (FHC, Inc., Bowdoin, ME) can hold two drives for simultaneous recording.

References

1. Henderson JM. The role of computer-assisted image-guided techniques. Semin Neurosurg 2001;12:175–181.
2. Maciunas RJ, Fitzpatrick JM, Galloway RL, Allen GS. Beyond stereotaxy: extreme levels of application accuracy are provided by implantable fiducial markers for interactive image guided neurosurgery. In: Maciunas RJ, ed. Interactive Image Guided Neurosurgery. Park Ridge, IL: AANS Publications; 1993:259–270.
3. Helm PA, Eckel TS. Accuracy of registration methods in frameless stereotaxis. Comput Aided Surg 1998;3:51–56, 9784952.

4. Dorward NL, Alberti O, Palmer JD, Kitchen ND, Thomas DGT. Accuracy of true frameless stereotaxy: in vivo measurement and laboratory phantom studies. J Neurosurg 1999;90:160–168, 10413173.

5. Benardete EA, Leonard MA, Weiner HL. Comparison of frameless stereotactic systems: accuracy, precision, and applications. Neurosurgery 2001;49:1409–1416.

6. Steinmeier R, Rachinger J, Kaus M, Gansalndt O, Huk W, Fahlbusch R. Factors influencing the application accuracy of neuronavigation systems. Stereotact Funct Neurosurg 2000;75:188–202.

7. Henderson JM, Holloway KL, Gaede SE, Rosenow JM. The application accuracy of a skull mounted trajectory guide for image-guided functional neurosurgery. Comput Aided Surg 2004;9:155–160, 16192055.

8. Henderson JM. Frameless localization for functional neurosurgical procedures: a preliminary accuracy study. Stereotact Funct Neurosurg 2004;82:135–141, 15467380.

9. Holloway KL, Gaede SE, Starr PA, Rosenow JM, Ramakrishnan V, Henderson JM. Frameless stereotaxy using bone fiducials for deep brain stimulation. J Neurosurg 2005;103:404–413, 16235670.

10. Roberts DW. The mathematics of Cartesian coordinates. In: Tasker RR, ed. Textbook of Stereotactic and Functional Neurosurgery. New York: McGraw Hill; 1998:21–27.

11. Rohlfing T, Maurer CR, Dean D, Maciunas RJ. Effect of changing patient position from supine to prone on the accuracy of a Brown-Roberts-Wells stereotactic head frame system. Neurosurgery 2003; 52:610–618, 12590686.

12. Starr PA, Christine CW, Theodosopoulos PV, et al. Implantation of deep brain stimulators into the subthalamic nucleus: technical approach and magnetic resonance imaging-verified lead locations. J Neurosurg 2002;97:370–387, 12186466.

11 Deep Brain Stimulation for Tremor

Jorge L. Eller and Kim J. Burchiel

Tremor is the most prevalent of the movement disorders and is defined as an involuntary, rhythmic, oscillatory contraction of agonist and antagonist muscles that exhibits a regular frequency. Tremor is further categorized as rest or action (postural, kinetic tremor, task-specific, etc.), depending on when it occurs.[1] Resting tremor is defined as tremor occurring in an extremity fully supported against gravity. Postural tremor is defined as tremor occurring when the extremity is maintaining position against gravity. Kinetic (the preferred term over intentional) tremor is defined as tremor occurring with voluntary movement from one point in space to another. Task-specific tremor describes tremor that increases in amplitude during movement directed at a particular goal (e.g., writing tremor). Moreover, tremor can be further characterized objectively with electromyography, accelerometry, and Fourier analysis.[2,3] The differential diagnosis of tremor divides it into specific clinical entities, the most common being essential tremor (ET), parkinsonian tremor, cerebellar outflow tremor, Holmes tremor (also called rubral tremor), and dystonic tremor (**Table 11.1**). These can be differentiated based upon features in the history and physical exam as well as electrophysiological characteristics.[4]

Epidemiological studies of ET confirm that it is the most common movement disorder. A 45-year retrospective analysis of medical records from Rochester, Minnesota, revealed the incidence and prevalence of ET were 23.7 and 305.6 per 100,000 cases, respectively. Mean age of diagnosis was 58 years, with men and women being equally affected. The investigators noted that age-specific incidence increased after 49 years of age and peaked in the 80s.[5-7] Although a gene variant (HS1-BP3) on chromosome 2 is associated with familiar ET, the pathophysiology of ET remains unknown. No obvious histopathologic abnormalities are associated with ET; therefore, no animal models are available that conclusively replicate human ET.

An aberrant central oscillator in the inferior olive is hypothesized as one possible cause of ET. The rationale is that the olivocerebellar oscillations are transmitted via the cerebellothalamocortical pathway, thus encompassing the cerebellum, thalamus, and brainstem areas that are known to be involved in ET.[8,9]

The early days of functional neurosurgery involved destruction of parts of the motor system.[10-12] Surgery to treat movement disorders became popular following Spiegel and Wycis's 1947 development of the first stereotactic apparatus that enabled minimally invasive surgery on deep nuclei in the human brain.[12] Further refinement eventually led to the determination that Hassler's ventrointermedius (Vim) nucleus of the thalamus is the optimal surgical target (**Fig. 11.1**). Regardless of tremor etiology, Vim is the preferred target of surgery to treat tremor except dystonic tremor (see Chapter 12) and of course psychogenic tremor. The Vim is the major termination of cerebellar efferents of the cerebellothalamocortical pathway (**Fig. 11.2**) and projects to the motor cortex.[14] This area contains the greatest concentration of tremor cells or neurons that fire in bursts synchronous with the patient's tremor (**Fig. 11.3**). In addition to the anatomical connection revealed in primate tracing studies, positron emission tomography (PET) has demonstrated an increase in blood flow to the ipsilateral motor cortex with stimulation of the thalamic Vim, suggesting a functional connection between these structures.[15] The surgical repertoire available to treat tremor includes either ablation of the contralateral thalamic Vim by means of radiofrequency lesion (thalamotomy) or placement of a deep brain stimulation (DBS) electrode in the contralateral thalamic Vim.

In 1991, Benabid et al published an article that described tremor suppression with chronic high-frequency stimulation of the thalamic Vim nucleus.[16] Although it had been known since the 1950s that high-frequency stimulation of the Vim nucleus could arrest tremor acutely, this

Table 11.1 Differential Diagnosis of Tremor

Postural tremor	8–12 Hz	Limb supported against gravity	Essential tremor may have some kinetic elements but not rest elements; usually upper extremities and bilateral
Kinetic tremor	< 5 Hz	Finger to nose movement	Cerebellar (intention) tremor that may have some postural elements but not rest; multiple sclerosis is a frequent etiology
	2–4 Hz	Finger to nose movement	Holmes tremor (rubral or midbrain) has elements of rest tremor; stroke is a frequent etiology
Dystonic tremor	Variable; mostly 4–7 Hz	Frequently "trick maneuvers" are able to reduce tremor	Tremulous torticollis in dystonic patient; combined postural and kinetic elements; usually focal

introduced the first practical technique for chronic brain stimulation as an alternative to lesioning (thalamotomy) in the treatment of tremor. Indications for both procedures are similar. Basically, patients must have tremor that is refractory to medical therapy and represents the predominant manifestation of the disorder. The ideal candidates

for thalamic surgery are patients with ET and those with tremor-predominant Parkinson disease (PD), although surgery may also be considered for tremor secondary to multiple sclerosis, stroke, or trauma. The remainder of this chapter describes our surgical technique and experience with placement of DBS electrodes to treat tremor.

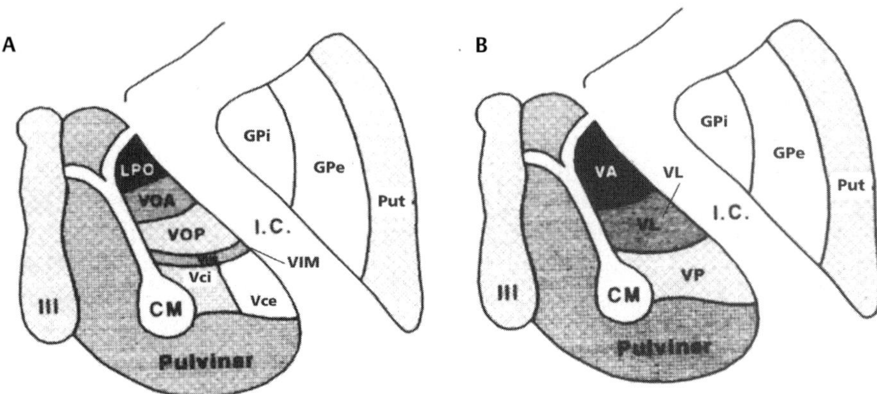

Fig. 11.1 Terminology of the thalamic nuclei. **(A)** Hassler classification system. **(B)** Anglo-American classification system. LPO, lateral polaris; VOA, ventral oral anterior; VOP, ventral oral posterior; VIM, ventral intermediate; Vci, ventral caudal internal; Vce, ventral caudal external; CM, centrum medianum; VA, ventral anterior; VL, ventral lateral; VP, ventral posterior; GPi, internal segment of the globus pallidus; GPe, external segment of the globus pallidus; put, putamen; I.C., intercommissural region; III, third ventricle. (From Burchiel KJ. Thalamotomy for movement disorders. Neurosurg Clin N Am 1995;6:55–71.)

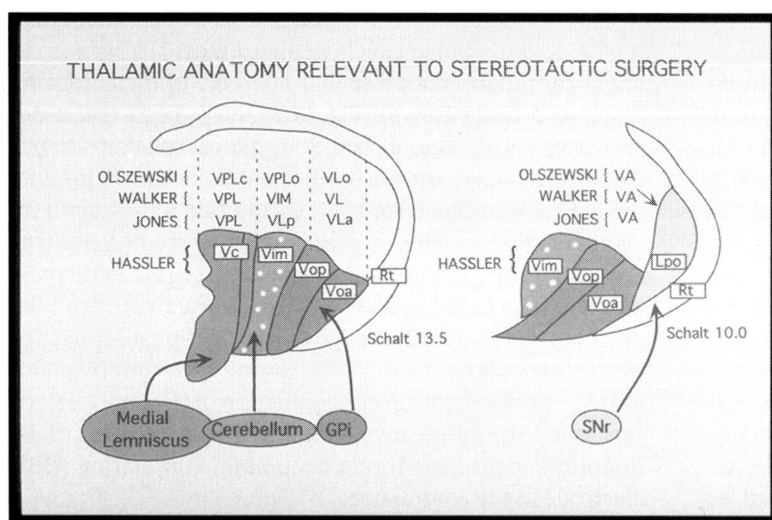

Fig. 11.2 Thalamic neuroanatomy relevant to neurosurgery. The major inputs to the sensory and motor thalamus are illustrated using Hassler's nomenclature and alternative nomenclature. The ventral lateral (VL) nucleus is roughly the equivalent of Hassler's nucleus ventralis oralis anterior (Voa), nucleus ventrali oralis posterior (Vop), and ventral intermediate (Vim). Vim receives both vestibulothalamic and cerebellothalamic afferents. Vop may also receive cerebellothalamic afferents. Both Vop and Voa receive pallidothalamic fibers from the medial globus pallidus interna (Gpi).

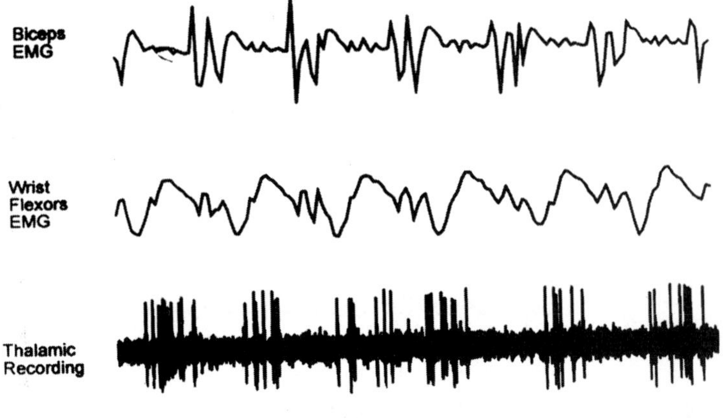

Fig. 11.3 Tremor cells recorded from the VIM (bottom). Note the correlation between the neuronal discharges from the tremor cells and the electromyogram. These discharges stop when the tremor ceases. (Modified from Bakay RAE, Vitek JL, Delong MR. Thalamotomy for tremor. In: Rengechary SS, Wilkins RR, eds. Neurosurgical Operative Atlas. Vol 2. Park Ridge, IL: American Association of Neurological Surgeons; 1992:299–312.)

Editor's Comments

The Walker nomenclature of the ventral lateral (VL) thalamus is less precise than the Hassler terminology (**Table 11.2**). The VL nucleus is roughly the equivalent of Hassler's nucleus ventralis oralis anterior (Voa), nucleus ventralis oralis posterior (Vop), and Vim. Vim receives both vestibulo-thalamic and cerebellothalamic afferents and projects to the primary motor cortex (area 4) but not to area 3a of the sensorimotor cortex as suggested by Hassler. Vop may also receive cerebellothalamic afferents. Both Vop and Voa receive pallidothalamic fibers from the medial globus pallidus (GPi), and project to the precentral motor cortex and the supplementary motor cortex. Empirically, lesioning of the Voa/Vop is considered a target for control of rigidity and dyskinesia, whereas Vim is the best target for control of tremor. Despite multiple attempts to modify Hassler's nomenclature to a more contemporary and accurate reflection of the neuroanatomy, functional neurosurgeons have kept it because the sensory and motor subdivisions matched what has been observed anatomically, electrophysiologically, and physiologically.[17]

These subnuclei are differentiated electrophysiologically (**Fig. 11.4**). Although most neurons in Vop and Vim fire in the 10 to 20 Hz range, there are tremor-synchronous neurons with rhythmic 5 to 7 Hz bursts. These tremor cells are recorded primarily in Vim, and to a limited extent in Vop. In PD, these tremor cells occur approximately four times as often as in ET and five times more often than in Holmes or cerebellar tremors.[18] The highest percentage of non-tremor bursting neurons occurs in Vop, but also occurs frequently in Voa. Neurons that alter their firing rate with joint movement or deep muscle pressure are called kinesthetic cells. These are very common in Vim (44%), but uncommon in Vop (16%),[19] whereas neurons that change their firing rate with active movements are called voluntary cells and are common in Vop (70%) and less so in Vim (49%), but are rare in Voa. When transitioning into the thalamic sensory ventralis caudalis nucleus (Vc), there is a "shell" of deep sensory (proprioceptive) neurons (Vcae) that respond to deep pressure (66%) prior to the cutaneous responsive neurons (Vcpe).[20] Identifying these subdivisions then facilitates lead placement (**Fig. 11.5**).

There are multiple potential targets for DBS to affect tremor, including the pallidothalamic cells in the GPi,[21,22] the point where the pallidal and cerebellar fibers cross the subthalamic area around the zona incerta, the fields of Forel (subthalamic lesion or campotomy),[23–25] at their termination in Vim,[26–42] or downstream projections to the GPi from the subthalamic nucleus (STN).[21,22,43,44] Vim DBS is currently believed to be the best procedure for treating all forms of tremor and is the focus of this chapter. There have been several optimal thalamic locations for tremor suppression described in the past: anterior to where evoked potentials can be recorded in response to cutaneous stimulation of the thumb,[45] where there are hand kinesthetic cells and where electrical stimulation produces effects on tremor,[46] where electrical stimulation effects tremor and anterior to where electrical stimulation evokes sensations,[47] or where there is tremor cell activity.[48] These all appear to describe the same site. However, the optimal thalamic DBS site may be more anterior and dorsal[49] and is probably more medial[50] (i.e., the Vim/Vop boarder). DBS stimulation, unlike lesioning, alters the characteristics of the tremor.[51–53] PET consistently demonstrates Vim DBS tremor suppression is associated with decreased regional blood flow in multiple ipsilateral motor-related cortical and cerebellar areas suggesting modulation of the cerebellothalamocortical pathways.[11,54] Where the tremor (pathological or physiological) originates is unknown.

The focus of stereotactic surgeons in the past was primarily on tremor, especially parkinsonian tremor. Tremor, however, is usually not the most disabling symptom of PD. Akinesia is the most disabling feature of the disease and is not ameliorated by Vim DBS. The combination of both resting and intention tremors is not uncommon in severely affected PD patients and is likely to be disabling. However, at this point in the disease process, the other symptoms of PD often require treatment and would likely be better treated with stimulation of the STN or GPi. Re-evaluation of appropriate targets has led to targeting of the STN or GPi more commonly to treat parkinsonian akinesia, rigidity, and gait disturbance of PD in addition to the tremor. Thalamotomy remains an option in the treatment of tremor for well-informed patients who decide against stimulation, in cases where DBS fails, where the cost is prohibitive, or in remote areas where mandatory follow-up for adjustments of pulse generators is not possible.[55]

Table 11.2 Nomenclature Related to Electrophysiological and Stimulation Properties of Thalamic Targets

	Pallidal Territory	Cerebellar Territory	Sensory Territory
Hassler	Voa, Vop	Vim	Vc
Walker	VL	VL	VPL
Jones	VLa	VLp	VPL
Electrophysiology	Highest number of cells	Highest number of cells	Highest number of cells
	responding to active movement (voluntary cells)	responding to passive joint movement (kinesthetic cells)	responding to focal cutaneous stimuli
	Higher number of nontremor bursting cells	Highest number of tremor cells	
Stimulation	May have an effect on rigidity and/or tremor	Low frequency increases tremor High frequency arrests tremor	Paresthesias in same focal cutaneous area
DBS target	Used for rigidity	Used for tremor	Used for pain

Abbreviations: DBS, deep brain stimulation; Vc, ventralis caudalis; Vim, ventrointermedius; VL, ventral lateral; VLa, ventral lateral anterior; VLp, ventral lateral posterior; Voa, ventralis oralis anterior; Vop, ventralis oralis posterior; VPL, ventral posterior laterial.

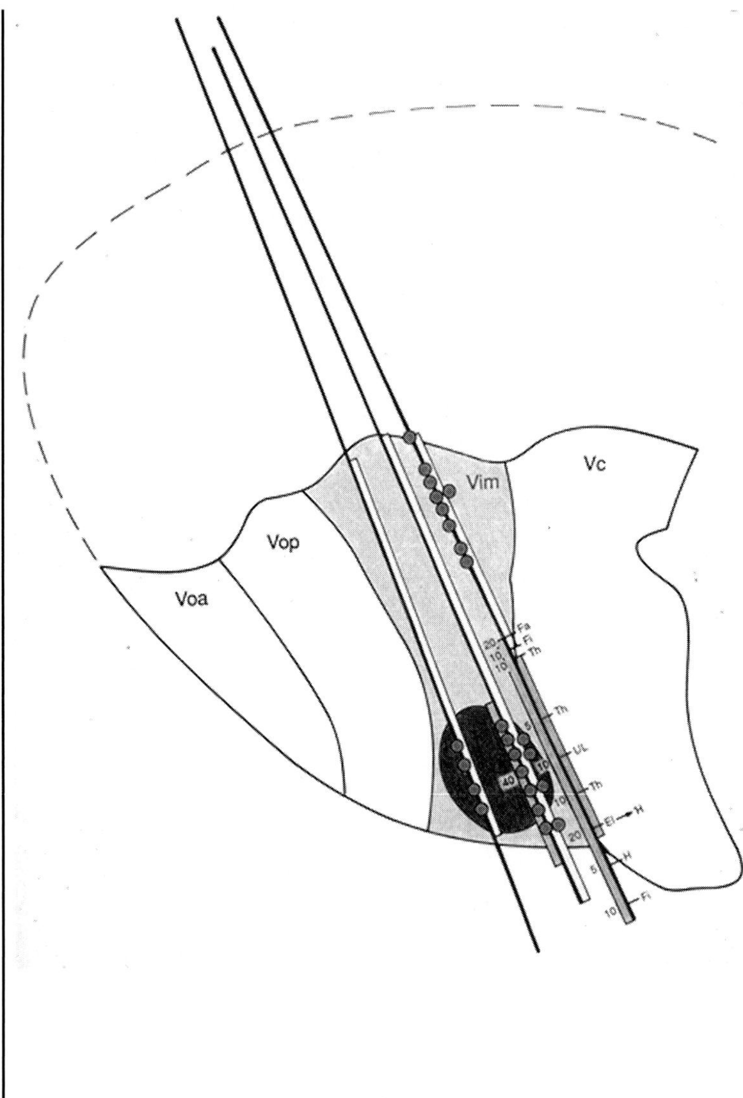

Fig. 11.4 Three representative microelectrode tracts through the ventrolateral thalamus. The labeled nuclei are ventralis oralis anterior (Voa), ventralis oralis posterior (Vop), ventrointermedius (Vim), and ventralis caudalis (Vc). The electrode tracts are depicted by the three straight lines entering the thalamus from the anterodorsal border and proceeding in a caudoventral direction. Neurons were isolated using standard electrophysiological techniques, and the sensory modality and somatotopic specificity were assessed for each neuron. Neuronal responses to somatosensory examination are coded by letters depicting the body part and the color of the bar along the right side to the electrode tract, which depicts the sensory modality. Portions of the tract in which tactile responses were found are in green; those with deep proprioceptive responses are colored yellow. Body regions are depicted by the letter along the right side of the tract: El, elbow; Fa, face; Fi, finger; H, hand; L, leg; M, mouth; S, shoulder; Th, thumb; UL, upper lip; W, wrist. Along the left side of the tract, the purple bar depicts the response to microstimulation; the numbers are the thresholds in microamps required to elicit a sensory response. The solid red circles denote cells with a tremor-related firing pattern. The shaded region encompasses the greatest concentration of tremor-related cells found in the ventral portion of the Vim. The penetrations through the thalamus in this orientation in the parasagittal plane generally proceed through the leg area into the arm area. Proximal limb regions are encountered before distal limb regions (e.g., shoulder regions are encountered first, followed by progressively more distal arm regions). The relatively greater number of neuronal responses related to the arm and face area reflect the somatotopic organization (homunculus) in the Vim with face, arm, and leg areas oriented in a medial-to-lateral direction. Deep pressure responses are found through the Vim, giving way to tactile responses as one proceeds into the Vc. Responses to microstimulation are generally similar to those found on somatosensory examination; the thresholds decrease as one moves closer toward the Vc.

However, there are very few comparative studies and little randomized data upon which to scientifically base clinical practice.[29,33,38]

For patients with other types of disabling tremor, thalamic stimulation remains a viable option. Approximately a third of ET patients will be refractory to medical therapy and are potential candidates for thalamic stimulation. There is no effective medication for cerebellar or Holmes tremors. These result from several etiologies, including multiple sclerosis, stroke, or head injury. Nevertheless, all of these pathological tremors may respond to some degree to thalamic stimulation. These patients must be evaluated very carefully because damage to the brain may result in a less predictable surgical result. Surgical success is diminished and the risk of complications increased in the presence of severe generalized brain atrophy, ataxia, and significant memory or speech abnormalities.

If the tremor is unilateral or dramatically asymmetrical, the surgical recommendation is straightforward. If the tremor is bilateral but asymmetrical, there is more uncertainty as to the most effective method of treatment. Some stereotactic neurosurgeons would prefer treating the more severely affected side and hope postoperatively that medications will optimize the effectiveness. Others would concentrate on the dominant side to allow maximum rehabilitation from a unilateral procedure. In our opinion, the best choice depends on the degree of asymmetry. Patients with dramatic differences in side-to-side tremor should be operated on the more severely affected side. In those where asymmetry is less marked, we prefer operating on the dominant hemisphere to restore function to the dominant side. If the patient has symmetrical bilateral tremor, there is again less controversy, with the dominant side being operated on first to provide a unilateral procedure, which would be functionally beneficial. If at all possible, a second procedure should be avoided because the risk of complications increases, even with DBS. When a second-side procedure is unavoidable due to the severity of the symptoms, then we prefer to wait 3 to 6 months before the second side is operated upon. This will ensure that the second operation is necessary and allows one to better assess the potential for complications.

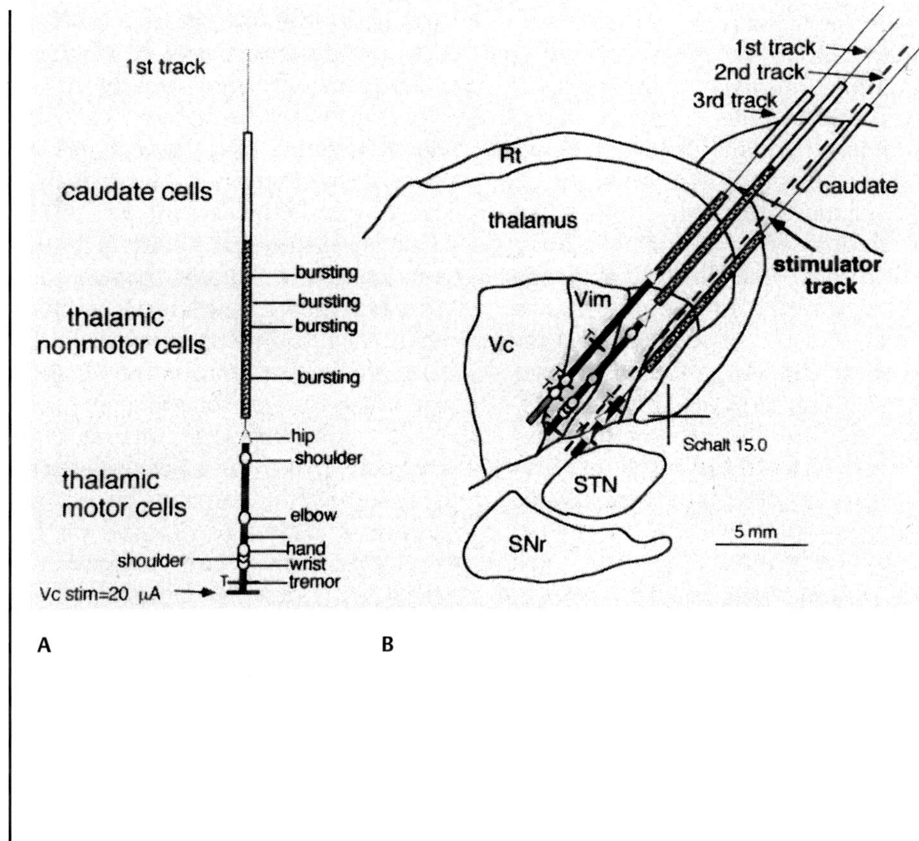

Fig. 11.5 Method of microelectrode mapping of the motor and sensory thalamus before placement of a stimulator for essential tremor. Segments of the track reconstructions are shaded to indicate caudate cells (*open segment*), nonmotor thalamus (*stippled segment*), motor thalamus (*black segment*), or sensory thalamus (*gray segment*). Locations of movement-related cells are indicated by triangles (leg), or circles (arm). (**A**) Detail of the first microelectrode track. The microstimulation threshold for sensory activation, marked "Vc stim," was measured at the bottom of this track (frequency = 300 Hz, pulse width = 200 µs). (**B**) Three microelectrode tracks are superimposed on a scaled map of the thalamus and basal ganglia in a parasagittal plane (*Schaltenbrand and Bailey Atlas* parasagittal 15 plane) according to the surgical team's judgment of the best fit of the tracks to the atlas. As illustrated here, the fit of actual microelectrode tracks to a standard atlas map is frequently not perfect. The eventual location of the stimulator is shown as a dotted line. (Starr PA, Vitek JL, Bakay RAE. Deep brain stimulation for movement disorders. Neurosurg Clin N Am 1998;9:381–402.)

■ Stereotactic Frame Placement

The surgical implantation of DBS electrodes involves sequential steps, and optimal results require careful performance. Placement of a stereotactic frame is the first step and sets the stage for magnetic resonance imaging (MRI)-guided stereotactic localization. At our institution, we use the Leksell Stereotactic System (Elekta Inc., Norcross, GA, www. elekta.com/healthcareus.nsf). To obtain images that easily correlate with standard brain neuroanatomical atlases, this frame requires placement orthogonal to the anatomical planes of the brain. The frame has ear bars to prevent lateral tilt or rotation. The anteroposterior axis of the frame should be placed parallel to a line connecting the glabela to the inion, which places the frame parallel to the anterior commissure–posterior commissure (AC–PC) line.[56]

■ Anatomical Targeting

Anatomical targeting of the Vim is the next step and employs a combination of indirect and direct targeting. Indirect targeting is based upon fixed distances from the midpoint of a line connecting the AC to the PC to the Vim nucleus. The locations of the AC and PC can be determined by MRI, CT, or ventriculography. MRI is slightly less accurate than CT, with average errors of ~2 mm due to artifacts related to inhomogeneities in the magnetic field. In an attempt to decrease such errors, imaging fusion, or overlapping of CT and MRI data, is often used.[57–59] Targeting of the Vim nucleus is then accomplished with the use of computer programs such as the FrameLink Stereotactic Linking System software (Medtronic Neuro Navigation, Louisville, CO, www.MedtronicNavigation.com) that relate a standard atlas[10] to the patient's radiological anatomy, as measured by CT or MRI.[60] In this manner the radiological location of the Vim nucleus is converted to Cartesian coordinates on the Leksell frame. In an attempt to compensate for individual variations in nuclear location, direct targeting is based upon direct visualization of nuclear boundaries in an MRI T2 fast spin echo (FSE) sequence. Unfortunately, it is not always possible to clearly visualize target borders in MRI sequences.

■ Surgical Exposure and Trajectory

The patient is brought to the operating room and positioned supine, with the head slightly elevated. The Leksell frame is fixated to the Mayfield headholder with an adapter. Standard prepping and draping are performed and local anesthetic injected. A single bifrontal semicurve C-shaped incision is performed, anterior to the coronal suture. Burr holes are placed anterior to the coronal suture and 2.5 cm from the midline on either side. Dura and pia are coagulated and opened sharply. The Leksell arc is positioned for a standard trajectory of 60 degrees from the AC–PC line.

■ Physiological Targeting

Due to limitations inherent to mechanical properties of the stereotactic frame and the imaging technique employed, anatomical targeting alone is insufficient for optimal electrode placement. Standard stereotactic frame system precision has been measured to be approximately within 1.5 mm (95% confidence interval).[61] Furthermore, MRI distortion effects, imperfect visualization of the anatomical target, potential brain shift, and variability of physiological function within any specific anatomical target further decrease the accuracy of anatomical targeting.[62] Therefore, physiological methods for localization are important to confirm and if necessary adjust the final placement of the DBS lead.

Two physiological methods to refine anatomical targeting are microelectrode recording (MER) and macrostimulation. MER isolates single neuronal action potentials using platinum-iridium or tungsten microelectrodes with an impedance greater than 500 KΩ.[63,64] The microelectrode is attached to a microdrive and mounted on the stereotactic frame. The microelectrode tip is retracted into a protective cylindrical sheath and inserted to a standard depth, from which the microdrive is used to drive the microelectrode toward the target,[65] and the signal from the microelectrode is amplified and filtered. Neuronal discharges are viewed on an oscilloscope and sound is heard through an audio monitor. Distinguishing characteristic patterns of spontaneous discharge within the nuclei of the basal ganglia are then used for localization. Macrostimulation is employed to identify the target area in the Vim nucleus by a high-frequency stimulation-evoked decrease in tremor. Similarly macrostimulation can be used to identify the internal capsule (by stimulation-evoked contractions of skeletal muscle), and the thalamic sensory ventralis caudalis (Vc) nucleus (by stimulation-evoked paresthesias).

■ Deep Brain Stimulation Lead Placement and Anchoring

At our institution, once the target is defined bilaterally using anatomical and physiological techniques, we proceed to implant the DBS leads. There are two US Food and Drug Administration (FDA)-approved lead models (Medtronic Minneapolis, MN, www.medtronic.com/physician/activa/

techmanuals.html). Both are quadripolar with four platinum-iridium contacts at the distal end. Each contact is 1.5 mm in length and separated by wide (1.5 mm) spacing (model #3387) or narrow (0.5 mm) spacing (model #3389). The lead is implanted along the desired MER trajectory with the second contact from the tip (#1 contact) positioned at the target. The lead is then secured in place using the Stimloc ring and cap lead anchor system (Medtronic, Inc., Minneapolis, MN). Intraoperative lateral fluoroscopy is used to confirm that the DBS lead remains in position after being detached from the stereotactic frame and secured in the Stimloc device. The procedure is repeated for the DBS lead on the other side. The DBS leads are then tunneled under the subgaleal tissue, and the surgical wound is closed with special care to avoid damaging the leads. The stereotactic Leksell frame is then removed.

■ Internal Pulse Generator Placement

To finalize the procedure the patient is placed under general anesthesia, positioned supine with the head turned away from the side of the implant. An internal pulse generator (IPG) is usually placed in a subcutaneous pocket below the clavicle. Therefore, the bifrontal incision, as well as the ipsilateral retroauricular, cervical, and subclavicular areas, are prepped and draped in sterile fashion. To accommodate the IPG an incision is performed 2.5 cm below the clavicle, and a subcutaneous pocket is created over the pectoralis fascia. A second incision is created 2.5 cm posterior to the ipsilateral ear for placement of the connectors between the distal ends of the DBS leads and the extension cables that will connect the DBS leads to the IPG. Care is taken to assure that these connectors will sit over the periosteum, in a subgaleal pocket created to accommodate them, and not in the neck, where excessive movement may cause lead fracture. The extension cables are tunneled from the subclavicular pocket to the retroauricular incision. In a similar fashion, the distal ends of the DBS leads are retrieved and tunneled from the bifrontal incision (which is reopened carefully so as not to damage the leads) to the retroauricular incision. The DBS leads are connected to the extension cables using a standard four-screw connector, which is protected by a Silastic (Dow Corning, Midland, MI) sheath and placed in the subgaleal pocket mentioned earlier. The distal ends of the extension cables are then connected to the IPG. All wounds are irrigated with antibiotic irrigation and closed in layers.

■ Deep Brain Stimulation Programming

The DBS IPG is programmed using an external programming device. Adjustable stimulation variables include amplitude, frequency, pulse width, and choice of active contacts (see Chapter 13).

Editor's Comments

For initial target coordinates for stereotactic procedures, we use serial 1.5 mm contiguous, nonoverlapping, contrast-enhanced three-dimensional (3D) volumetric 1.5T MRI studies,[66] which are performed through the entire brain (for our technique see Chapter 7). Direct identification of the Vim target remains very difficult but possible on occasion (**Fig. 11.6**). Use of planning stations allows calculation not only of the target but also of the entry point and trajectory to the target. Contrast allows cortical veins to be easily visualized, and trajectories can be customized for each patient to avoid deep blood vessels in the ventricle en route to the desired target. Many times, the ventricular system may be avoided as well by choosing a more lateral entry point. Proponents of this technique argue that penetration of the ventricular system causes increased brain shift due to excess cerebrospinal fluid (CSF) loss, potential damage to blood vessels, and alteration of microelectrode trajectory by passing through matter of variable densities. Opponents make the points that stereotactic atlases have been based upon rectilinear approaches to the deep brain targets, placing the guide tube through the ventricle avoids deflection, and blood vessels can be avoided. We prefer minimal angulations (1 to 8 degrees) to allow the most rectilinear approach possible (offset error of 1 mm through Vim) while avoiding the lateral ventricle most of the time. The entry point generally correlates to a ring angle of 60 to 70 degrees relative to the AC–PC line if the approach is applied in a rectilinear fashion to parallel the borders of the Vim.[67] An overlay of a Guiot derivation of the thalamic subnuclei location based on the AC–PC line and the height of the thalamus on MRI of a DBS lead illustrates this point (**Fig. 11.7**).

The target coordinates should be considered as only the initial starting point; physiological confirmation is required. Because the initial target point for many surgeons will vary from Vop to Vim, recommended target coordinates may vary from 1 to 7 mm posterior to the midpoint of the AC–PC line. Similarly, the lateral coordinates from the midline vary from 12 to 15 mm and the vertical coordinates vary from 0 to 3 mm above the AC–PC line. We measure 4 mm anterior to the PC along the intercommissural line to identify the border of the Vc. We prefer to use MER and neurological examination intraoperatively to identify the Vc nucleus first, and then move anteriorly to the

appropriate position in the Vim (**Fig. 11.8**). The DBS lead needs to be placed 3 to 4 mm anterior to the Vc hand area. For direct targeting, the lateral distance depends on the observed location of the internal capsule on MRI, which is more accurate than ventriculography.[68] The lateral coordinate is selected as 3 mm from the edge of the internal capsule. For indirect targeting, the thalamotomy target is 14 to 16 mm lateral to the midline or 11.5 mm plus half the width of the third ventricle from midline and depth is at the level of the AC-PC plane. For DBS, the target (Vim/Vop border) is 11 to 14 mm or 10 mm plus half the width of the third ventricle from midline because the thalamic-capsular border moves medially. For predominantly head and neck tremor a more medial approach is used.

Because of the inherent variability in biological systems, radiographic determination of the target may be inaccurate, varying as much as several millimeters from physiologically determined sites. By combining MER and macroelectrode stimulation techniques with conventional radiographic methods, we believe accurate localization of the optimal target site can be greatly improved. Precise localization allows restriction of the size of the electrical field (lower voltage and longer battery life) while maintaining its effectiveness and minimizing potential complications. If electrophysiological recordings are initiated greater than 30 mm above target, identification of the caudate nucleus may be useful in plotting the tract on an atlas. Passage through the caudate nucleus will yield insertional activity (action potentials stimulated by MER movement that rapidly abates at rest) that would not be identified if the tract were too posterior or very lateral or if the nucleus were markedly atrophic.

The dorsal thalamus is then encountered 15 to 20 mm above target and is characterized by occasional low amplitude neuronal firing, often in a 4 Hz bursting pattern. Lateral and ventral boundaries of the Vim and the anterior border of the Vc are determined based on microstimulation effects and neuronal response properties. Because of the lateral convexity of the thalamus, penetrations through its more lateral border are characterized by neuronal responses that occur at deeper locations and over shorter distances. There is a gradation of cell responses to sensorimotor examination as one moves posterior from the Voa and Vop to the Vim; cells in the Vop tend to respond

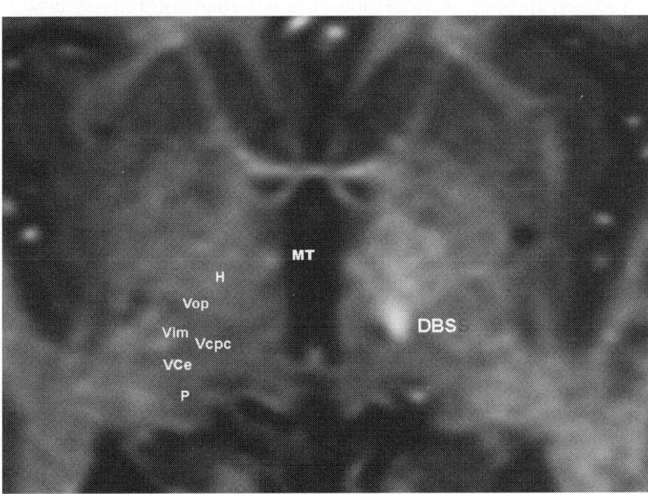

Fig. 11.6 An axial inversion recovery IR magnetic resonance imaging scan at the level of the anterior and posterior commissures showing the localization of the ventralis caudalis (Vc) at the level of the posterior commissure. The Vce extends out like a finger (dark) separated from the pulvinar (P) by the fibers of the thalamic peduncle (white) and the fiber-rich ventral Vim. Note the relationship of the internal capsule lateral to the Vim appears indistinct. The Vc extends as a dark band medially toward the ventricle (Vcpc). Vop appears like a finger (dark) between the Vim and Forel fields (H). The exact position of the DBS lead is impossible to determine due to the artifacts. Excellent tremor relief was produced at 1.5 V and no side effects were observed until 3 V (speech) and no paresthesias until greater than 3.5 V. VOP, ventralis oralis posterior; Vim, ventralis intermedius; Vce, ventralis caudalis externus; Vcpc, ventralis caudalis parvocellularis; MT, mammillothalamic tract.

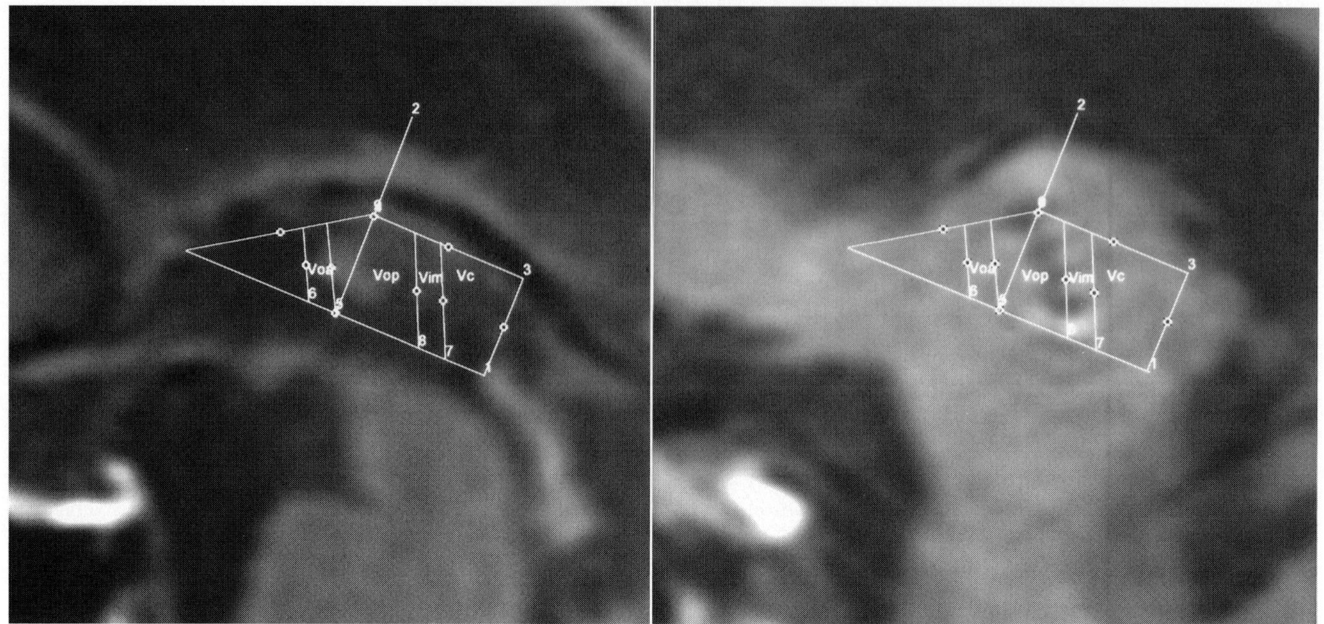

Fig. 11.7 The relative location of a ventralis intermedius (Vim) lead is shown in the midsagittal plane. The Guiot geometric construct is made at the midsagittal plane (left) and then carried to the parasagittal plan of the DBS lead (right). The construct divides the anterior–posterior commissural (AC–PC) line into 12th and construction of a perpendicular at the midpoint to the height of the thalamus (2). A rectangle is formed with half the thalamic height. The bottom of the Vim is 3/12 to 2/12th AC–PC line from PC and the top is 1/12 to 2/12th from half the thalamic height construct. The lead straddles the Vop and Vim.

more selectively to voluntary movement and less to passive kinesthetic manipulation, whereas cells in Vim respond readily to passive kinesthetic manipulation (**Fig. 11.4**). It is also in this location where rhythmic grouped discharges time locked to the tremor frequency of the contralateral limbs may be identified. Voa cell firing does not correlate to limb movement. Because of the somatotopic arrangement of the Vim and Vc, penetrations made too medial or lateral are characterized by the microstimulation-induced paresthesias or somatosensory responses predominantly restricted to the face or leg, respectively. Furthermore, the lateral border of the thalamus is adjacent to the internal capsule where microstimulation results in intense short-latency muscle contractions that generally involve a small area of the contralateral body. The anterior border of the Vc is characterized by low-threshold (2 to 10 µA), microstimulation-induced paresthesias, and the presence of neurons with small, well-defined receptive fields to tactile sensation in a body area in which the stimulation-induced paresthesias occurred.

Posterior and inferior to the thalamus, the fibers of the medial lemniscus are ascending and entering the thalamus. Stimulation of these fibers will produce paresthesias as well but frequently widespread, including the hemibody. This is a useful finding for orientation if the Vc has not been identified. The ideal location for the DBS lead is at the Vim/Vop boarder anterior to where induced somatosensory responses from movement of the contralateral thumb and by a lack of microstimulation-induced paresthesias, even at current intensities of 100 µA. It is important to explore below the target with microelectrode recording to ensure placement of the lead at the ventral boundary of the nucleus. Below the target is the zona incerta, a nucleus that is surrounded and penetrated by fiber tracts. Here isolated neurons may be encountered within a generally quiet background and should not be confused with the high background and high amplitude activity in either the thalamus above or the subthalamic nucleus below.

Careful monitoring and continuous evaluation of speech, strength, and tremor need to be performed throughout the entire procedure. Once the electrode is believed to be in the proper position, tremor frequently resolves following placement of the DBS probe. This is a very good sign, but failure to diminish the tremor with lead placement does not mean that chronic stimulation will not succeed. Histology studies show little tissue damage from either MER or the lead, and long-term improvements are attributable to stimulation.[69,70] Nevertheless, the minilesion or microthalamotomy effect is real and can temporarily or permanently alter tremor. Having the patient count backward or recite the months of the year backward still may exacerbate resting tremor. Having the ET patient draw spirals can monitor the effect on their tremor. Low-voltage stimulation (1 to 3 V, 140 Hz, and 100 µs) should eliminate any residual tremor. If the voltage required to achieve control is greater than 5 V, the placement may be too anterior. Any suggestion of persistent dysarthria, muscle contractions, or paresthesias at less than 3 V is a strong indication to move the lead.

Separating sensory and motor effects can be very difficult in some patients, and the Medtronic test stimulator 3625 (www.medtronic.com/physician/activa/techmanuals.html) is very limited in its abilities

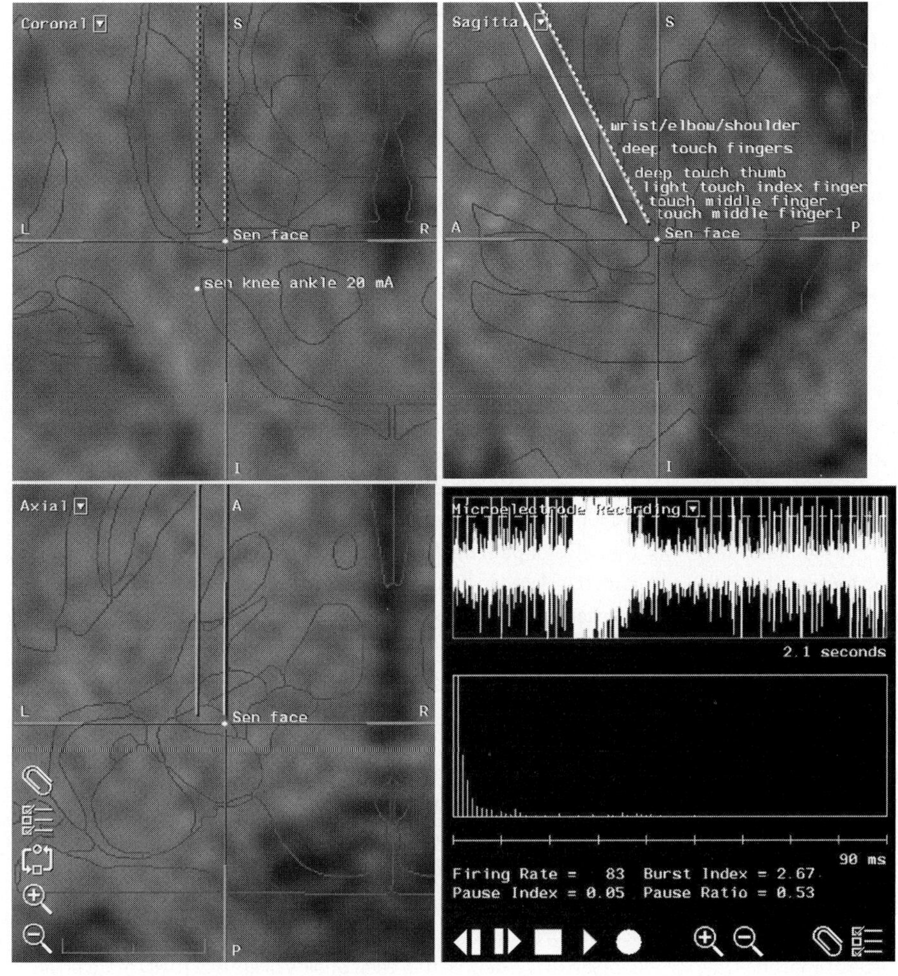

Fig. 11.8 Sagittal, coronal, and axial views as well as microelectrode electrophysiology are demonstrated on the StealthStation (Medtronic Navigation, Louisville, CO) using FrameLink 4.0 software. The *Schaltenbrand and Bailey Atlas* overlay is shown in three planes. The analysis of the firing pattern is shown in the lower right-hand corner. There is a progression through the Vim from kinesthetic cells of the upper extremity to deep touch (shell) in the fingers and thumb to light touch in the fingers and then face ventralis caudalis (Vc). Note the marked increase in firing with light touch to the face (center of the microelectrode recording).

to test at low frequencies to help differentiate the response. If stimulation could be made at 2 Hz, clear separation would be possible. Instead we evaluate at threshold and superthreshold voltages. At threshold, a patient might confuse motor stimulation for paresthesia, but with a slight increase in voltage, contractions should be present. Be sure to warn the patient! Repeat with both slow and rapid increases until you are convinced. Also, test the higher leads because too deep a placement can create confusion (stimulation of sensory fibers or mesencephalon: fear, dizziness, or oculomotor activity). Remember when moving in the medial direction the Vc border moves anterior and when moving in the anterior direction the capsule moves medially. Here prior MER mapping is extremely valuable in determining the best move. As a general rule, if too lateral, move medially 2 mm and possibly anteriorly 1 to 2 mm; if too posterior, move anteriorly 2 to 3 mm if near sensory hand, but anterior 2 to 3 mm and laterally 0 to 1 mm if near sensory face. It is impossible to move the lead 1 mm and may be difficult to move 2 mm without "falling" into the prior tract. Use X-ray to confirm the move because stimulation after a move is far less reliable. Multiple moves of the DBS lead are to be avoided. If the move is confirmed and electrophysiological confirmation is not possible, it is probably best to leave the lead in place and work hard on programming it postoperatively. Following completion of the pro-

cedure, we like to continue tight blood pressure control and intensive care monitoring until follow-up MRI the next day to confirm DBS location and to evaluate the accuracy of targeting (see Chapter 7).

For treatment of parkinsonian tremor, benefits appear to remain stable over time, although the disease process will continue to progress, and symptoms not improved by DBS will worsen.[16,27–39] Complete arrest or major tremor improvement in the first year is in the 70 to 90% range. Continued benefit is reported for up to 8 years but with a decrease in percentage of significantly improved patients with time. Tremor relief is similar to thalamotomy but only DBS is associated with functional status improvement.[29] Although writing and other functions may improve, there is no improvement in activities of daily living.[27] Some investigators report minor improvements in rigidity or lowering of dopaminergic medications, but most do not observe benefit to anything but tremor. If the lead is anterior in Voa/Vop or medial in the centromedial/parafascicular complex,[32] additional benefit may be observed. Women and men do equally well but women present far less often for surgery.[71] Vim DBS should not be performed with the primary anticipation of improving speech, gait, or vegetative or emotional function. Tolerance has not been reported in most series but can occur.[72] Distal hand areas are well defined and respond best to stimulation. Proximal areas are more diffuse with shoulder and elbow extending over considerable distance anteroposterior (AP) and medial–lateral so that correspondingly proximal tremors are harder to control. Axial and trunkal tremors are difficult to locate and least likely to respond.

Vim DBS is also very effective for ET.[16,27–30,33,39] Complete arrest or major tremor improvement in the first year is in the 70 to 90% range but is often reported less than that for PD. Unlike PD, there is significant improvement in activities of daily living.[27,73,74] Head, orofacial, and vocal areas are very medial and can be improved, but side effects from midline nuclei, including dysphonia, may limit effectiveness.[39,40,75] Tolerance is a much bigger problem in ET, with recurrences in the 20% range.[26,30,36,41,42] Late ET failures with Vim DBS may relate to volume effect. Failed thalamotomies for ET were common (~10 to 20%) and frequently needed reoperation to expand a thalamotomy. When increasing stimulation voltage fails to control the tremor (mean of 25% in 12 months),[30] a second lead[76] or a lesion[77,78] or another target[43] has been successful in some cases. Ipsilateral tremor is occasionally but not reliably improved and may worsen with stimulation.[36]

Cerebellar tremors from multiple sclerosis[25,79–82] or Holmes tremors from posttraumatic injury or stroke[83–88] can be improved significantly and initially respond well to Vim DBS. Ataxia, however, does not respond to DBS and may limit success. Long-term results are much less consistent than those in PD and not cost-effective.[89] Historically, cases of PD required a small lesion (30 to 60 mm³) for successful treatment, whereas secondary tremor due to infarct or trauma often required large lesions (100 to 200 mm³) that included the Voa, Vop, and Vim.[90] DBS stimulation probably also requires widespread current to be effective in these cases.[91] But the addition of a second lead may not always help.[92] There is also the suggestion that STN DBS may be as effective or more effective in ET and multiple sclerosis.[93]

The complication rate is very difficult to determine because the literature is limited to small case studies and inconsistent reporting. The complication profile is the same as for thalamotomy but less frequent and many times is reversible.[29,94] Only one operative death from DBS placement has been reported, but there have been late postoperative deaths due to pulmonary embolism, myocardial infarction, and

so forth that have not been reported. The general consensus is that mortality should be less than 0.5%. The most common source of mortality and severe morbidity is hemorrhage, which is an unavoidable complication from stereotactic surgery.[29,95] With current techniques, an incorrectly placed lead should be a rare source for complications, but collateral damage from incorrectly placed leads is possible. Major complications (2 to 3%) that result from hemorrhage or misplaced leads include cognitive disturbances, paralysis, dysarthria, dystonia, balance disturbance, dysphagia, paresthesias, and ataxia. It is very common for stimulation to induce these same side effects, but they are potentially reversible and by adjustments are usually well tolerated by patients.[36] Some cognitive problems relate to stimulation and can be improved by programming.[96,97] The combined complication rate would be anticipated to be 15 to 20%, with permanent disability at ~5%. Hardware-related complications include erosions, infections, lead migrations, wire fractures, or malfunctions, which are long-term sources of complications. The Toronto group reported that 25% of patients followed for at least a year had complications directly related to hardware.[98] Bilateral thalamotomy is no longer recommended given the higher risk of morbidity, but bilateral DBS can be performed effectively and with only modest increases in complications.[36–39] There is a significant risk of stimulation-induced dysarthria especially if is a contralateral thalamotomy.[36,37,99,100] Left Vim DBS may decrease verbal performance. These rates can quadruple when high-risk patients are included. The infection rate is less than 5% and seizures occur in the 1% range. Hemiballism is rarely seen with DBS, and certainly would be anticipated at less than a 0.1% rate. Additionally, kinetic tremors may have unique complications. Although these tremors are often improved, the other symptoms may prevent significant improvement in function, and the overall clinical condition may worsen to the degree that their quality of life is actually reduced after the procedure. Multiple sclerosis patients who undergo surgery may have an increased risk of acute exacerbation of their disease shortly after surgery. Careful patient selection is critical in these subsets of patients to achieve satisfactory outcomes.

■ Efficacy of Deep Brain Stimulation in the Treatment of Tremor

Many studies have demonstrated the efficacy of DBS stimulation in the treatment of tremor, for both PD and ET patients. In Benabid's report with 13 ET patients who underwent DBS placement, a major benefit in 68% of the patients was recorded.[26] Ondo et al reported on 14 ET patients who underwent unilateral thalamic DBS and demonstrated an 83% reduction in contralateral arm tremor.[27] Koller et al published results of a multicenter study of unilateral thalamic stimulation in 53 patients with both PD and ET. At 3-month follow-up, 23 of 29 ET patients reported marked improvement, three patients reported moderate improvement, one reported mild improvement, and two patients were unchanged.[28]

■ Complications Associated with Deep Brain Stimulator Placement

Complications associated with thalamic stimulation can be divided into those that are common to any stereotactic procedure and those that are specific to implanted hardware. The first category includes complications primarily from intracranial hemorrhages, speech or cognitive dysfunction, or superficial wound infections. The risk of intracranial hemorrhage for thalamic stimulation is similar to that for thalamotomy and varies from 2 to 5%.[29] Infection of pin sites and meningitis have been reported in ~1% of all stereotactic surgeries.[101] Specific risks associated with implanted hardware include hardware malfunctions, migrations, erosions, or hardware infections. In the study by Koller et al,[28] complications included two perioperative hemorrhages, one perioperative seizure, two wound infections, and one instance of hardware erosion. In another multicenter trial, 111 patients were treated with thalamic stimulation. The complications related to the surgery in these patients included three subdural hematomas, one thalamic hematoma, two infections, and one patient with transient cognitive deficits.[30]

■ Conclusion

The decision to perform thalamotomy or place DBS electrodes for treatment of tremor is not clear-cut. The advantages of DBS over thalamotomy include reversibility, adaptability (change in stimulus variables to increase efficacy or reduce side effects), and the ability to place bilateral DBS electrodes. Due to the high risks of hypophonia, dysarthria, and cognitive deficits,[99,100] bilateral thalamotomies are rarely performed. Disadvantages of stimulation include the increased expense, the need to implant a foreign body (with the concomitant higher risk of infections), and the need for future operations to replace the IPG and other hardware due to malfunction or fracture. Moreover, there is more effort and cost involved in continuous adjustment of the stimulation variables.

In a retrospective comparison of 19 thalamic stimulator implants and 26 thalamotomies (for both ET and PD), Tasker reported similar results regarding tremor control but a higher incidence of side effects in the thalamotomy group.[94] Tremor was "completely abolished" (42%) in both groups and "almost abolished" in 79% the thalamic stimulation and 69% in the thalamotomy group. Complications such as ataxia and dysarthria were more common in the thalamotomy group (42%) than in the thalamic stimulation group (26%). There were some limitations to this study, such as retrospective analysis, lack of randomization, and mixed diagnosis groups.

Further prospective, randomized studies are required to assess which procedure may prove most beneficial in treating tremor of specific patient populations.

References

1. Findley LJ. Classification of tremors. J Clin Neurophysiol 1996;13: 122–132
2. Deuschl G, Bain P, Brin M. Consensus statement of the movement disorder society on tremor: ad hoc Scientific Committee. Mov Disord 1998;13:2–23
3. Schwalb JM, Lozano AM. Surgical management of tremor. Neurosurg Q 2004;14:60–68
4. Elble RJ. Diagnostic criteria for essential tremor and differential diagnosis. Neurology 2000;54:S2–S6
5. Rajput AH, Offord KP, Beard CM, Kurland LT. Essential tremor in Rochester, Minnesota: a 45-year study. J Neurol Neurosurg Psychiatry 1984;47:466–470
6. Haerer AF, Anderson DW, Schoenberg BS. Prevalence of essential tremor: results from the Copiah County study. Arch Neurol 1982;39:750–751
7. Louis ED, Ottman R. How familial is familial tremor? The genetic epidemiology of essential tremor. Neurology 1996;46:1200–1205
8. Deuschl G, Elble RJ. The pathophysiology of essential tremor. Neurology 2000;54:S14–S20
9. Hallett M. Overview of human tremor physiology. Mov Disord 1998;13:43–48
10. Hassler R. Anatomy of the thalamus. In: Bailey P, ed. Introduction to Stereotaxis with an Atlas of the Human Brain. Stuttgart: Thieme; 1959:230–290
11. Ceballos-Baumann AO, Boecker H, Fogel W, et al. Thalamic stimulation for essential tremor activates motor and deactivates vestibular cortex. Neurology 2001;56:1347–1354
12. Gildenberg PL. The history of surgery for movement disorders. Neurosurg Clin N Am 1998;9:283–294
13. Cooper IS. Ligation of the anterior choroidal artery for involuntary movements; parkinsonism. Psychiatr Q 1953;27:317–319
14. Cooper IS, Bravo GJ, Riklan M, Davidson NW, Gorek EA. Chemopallidectomy and chemothalamectomy for parkinsonism. Geriatrics 1958;13:127–147
15. Spiegel EA, Wycis HT, Marks M, Lee AJ. Stereotaxic apparatus for operations on the human brain. Science 1947;106:349–350
16. Benabid AL, Pollak P, Gervason C, et al. Long-term suppression of tremor by chronic stimulation of the ventral intermediate thalamic nucleus. Lancet 1991;337:403–406
17. Krack P, Dostrovsky J, Ilinsky I, et al. Surgery of the motor thalamus: problems with the present nomenclatures. Mov Disord 2002;17 (Suppl 3):S2–S8
18. Brodkey JA, Tasker RR, Hamani C, McAndrews MP, Dostrovsky JO, Lozano AM. Tremor cells in the human thalamus: differences among neurological disorders. J Neurosurg 2004;101:43–47
19. Lenz FA, Kwan HC, Dostrovsky JO, Tasker RR, Murphy JT, Lenz YE. Single-unit analysis of human ventral thalamic nuclear group: activity correlated with movement. Brain 1990;113:1795–1821
20. Lenz FA, Dostrovsky JO, Tasker RR, Yamashiro K, Kwan HC, Murphy JT. Single-unit analysis of human ventral thalamic nuclear group: somatosensory responses. J Neurophysiol 1988;59:299–316
21. Volkmann J, Allert N, Voges J, et al. Safety and efficacy of pallidal or subthalamic nucleus stimulation in advanced PD. Neurology 2001;56:548–551
22. DBS Study Group. Deep-brain stimulation of the subthalamic nucleus or the pars interna of the globus pallidus in Parkinson's disease. N Engl J Med 2001;345:956–963
23. Murata J, Kitagawa M, Uesugi H, et al. Electrical stimulation of the posterior subthalamic area for the treatment of intractable proximal tremor. J Neurosurg 2003;99:708–715
24. Plaha P, Patel NK, Gill SS. Stimulation of the subthalamic region for essential tremor. J Neurosurg 2004;101:48–54
25. Nandi D, Chir M, Liu X, et al. Electrophysiological confirmation of the zona incerta as a target for surgical treatment of disabling involuntary arm movements in multiple sclerosis: use of local field potentials. J Clin Neurosci 2002;9:64–68
26. Benabid AL, Pollak P, Seigneuret E, et al. Chronic VIM thalamic stimulation in Parkinson's disease, essential tremor and extra-pyramidal dyskinesias. Acta Neurochir Suppl (Wien) 1993;58:39–44

27. Ondo W, Jankovic J, Schwartz K, Almaguer M, Simpson RK. Unilateral thalamic deep brain stimulation for refractory essential tremor and Parkinson's disease tremor. Neurology 1998;51:1063–1069

28. Koller W, Pahwa R, Busenbark K, et al. High-frequency unilateral thalamic stimulation in the treatment of essential and parkinsonian tremor. Ann Neurol 1997;42:292–299

29. Schuurman PR, Bosch DA, Bossuyt PM, et al. A comparison of continuous thalamic stimulation and thalamotomy for suppression of severe tremor. ([see comment]) N Engl J Med 2000;342:461–468

30. Limousin P, Speelman JD, Gielen F, Janssens M, and study collaborators. Multicentre European study of thalamic stimulation in parkinsonian and essential tremor. J Neurol Neurosurg Psychiatry 1999;66:289–296

31. Putzke JD, Wharen RE, Wszolek ZK, Turk MF, Strongosky AJ, Uitti RJ. Thalamic deep brain stimulation for tremor-predominant Parkinson's disease. Parkinsonism Relat Disord 2003;10:81–88

32. Caparros-Lefebvre D, Blond S, Feltin MP, Pollak P, Benabid AL. Improvement of levodopa induced dyskinesias by thalamic deep brain stimulation is related to slight variations in electrode placement: possible involvement of the centre median and parafascicularis complex. J Neurol Neurosurg Psychiatry 1999;67:308–314

33. Rehncrona S, Johnels B, Widner H, et al. Long term efficacy of thalamic deep brain stimulation for tremor: double-blind assessments. Mov Disord 2003;18:163–170

34. Kumar R, Lozano AM, Sime E, Lang AE. Long-term follow up of thalamic deep brain stimulation for essential and parkinsonian tremor. Neurology 2003;61:1601–1604

35. Yamamoto T, Katayama Y, Kano T, Kobayashi K, Oshima H, Fukaya C. Deep brain stimulation for the treatment of parkinsonian, essential and post stroke tremor: a suitable stimulation method and changes in effective stimulation intensity. J Neurosurg 2004;101:201–209

36. Benabid AL, Pollak P, Gao D, et al. Chronic electrical stimulation of the ventralis intermedius nucleus of the thalamus as a treatment of movement disorders. J Neurosurg 1996;84:203–214

37. Siegfried J, Lippitz B. Chronic electrical stimulation of the VL–VPL complex and of the pallidum in the treatment of movement disorders: personal experience since 1982. Stereotact Funct Neurosurg 1994;62:71–75

38. Ondo W, Almagaur M, Jankovic J, et al. Thalamic deep brain stimulation: comparison between unilateral and bilateral placement. Arch Neurol 2001;58:218–222

39. Taha JM, Jenszen MA, Favre J. Thalamic deep brain stimulation for the treatment of head, voice, and bilateral limb tremor. J Neurosurg 1999;91:68–72

40. Koller WC, Lyons KE, Wilkinson SB, Pahwa R. Efficacy of unilateral deep brain stimulation of the Vim nucleus of the thalamus for essential head tremor. Mov Disord 1999;14:847–850

41. Koller WC, Lyons KE, Wilkinson SB, Troster AL, Pahwa R. Long-term safety and efficacy of unilateral deep brain stimulation of the thalamus in essential tremor. Mov Disord 2001;16:464–468

42. Sydow O, Thobois S, Alesch F, Speelman JD. Multicentre European study of thalamic stimulation in essential tremor: a six year follow-up. J Neurol Neurosurg Psychiatry 2003;74:1387–1391

43. Stover NP, Okun MS, Evatt ML, Raju DV, Bakay RA, Vitek JL. Stimulation of the subthalamic nucleus in a patient with Parkinson disease and essential tremor. Arch Neurol 2005;62:141–143

44. Diamond A, Shahed J, Jankovic J. The effects of subthalamic nucleus deep brain stimulation on parkinsonian tremor. J Neurol Sci 2007;260:199–203

45. Kelly PJ, Derome P, Guiot G. Thalamic spatial variability and the surgical results of lesions placed with neurophysiologic control. Surg Neurol 1978;9:307–315

46. Tasker RR, Organ LW, Hawrylyshyn P. The Thalamus and Midbrain in Man: A Physiologic Atlas Using Electrical Stimulation. Springfield, IL: Charles C Thomas; 1982

47. Ohye C, Fukamachi A, Miryazaki M, et al. Physiologically controlled selective thalamotomy for the treatment of abnormal movement. Acta Neurochir (Wien) 1977;37:93–104

48. Lenz FA, Normand SL, Kwan HC, et al. Statistical prediction of the optimal lesion site for thalamotomy in parkinsonian tremor. Mov Disord 1995;10:318–328

49. Kiss ZH, Wilkinson M, Krcek J, et al. Is the target for thalamic deep brain stimulation the same as for thalamotomy? Mov Disord 2003;18:1169–1175

50. Papavassiliou E, Rau G, Heath S, et al. Thalamic deep brain stimulation for essential tremor: relation of lead location to outcome. Neurosurgery 2004;54:1120–1129

51. Vaillancourt DE, Sturman MM, Verhagen Metman L, Bakay RA, Corcos DM. Deep brain stimulation of the VIM thalamic nucleus modifies several feature of essential tremor. Neurology 2003;61:919–925

52. Sturman MM, Vaillancourt DE, Metman LV, Bakay RA, Corcos DM. Effects of subthalamic nucleus stimulation and medication on resting and postural tremor in Parkinson's disease. Brain 2004;127:2131–2143

53. Rubin JE, Terman D. High frequency stimulation of the subthalamic nucleus eliminates pathological thalamic rhythmicity in a computational model. J Comput Neurosci 2004;16:211–235

54. Fukuda M, Barnes A, Simon ES, et al. Thalamic stimulation for parkinsonian tremor: correlation between regional cerebral blood flow and physiological tremor characteristics. Neuroimage 2004;21:608–615

55. Okun MS, Vitek JL. Lesion therapy for Parkinson's disease and other movement disorders: update and controversies. Mov Disord 2004;19:375–389

56. Tamas LB, Tcheng TK. Selective thalamotomy for tremor: a new look at an old procedure. Tech Neurosurg 1999;5:65–72

57. Hardy PA, Barnet GH. Spatial distortion in magnetic resonance imaging: impact on stereotactic localization. In: Gildenberg PL, Tasker RR, eds. Textbook of Stereotactic and Functional Neurosurgery. New York: McGraw-Hill; 1998:271–280

58. Holtzheimer PE III, Roberts DW, Darcey TM. Magnetic resonance imaging versus computed tomography for target localization in functional stereotactic neurosurgery. Neurosurgery 1999;45:290–297

59. Alexander E III, Kooy HM, van Herk M, et al. Magnetic resonance image–directed stereotactic neurosurgery: use of image fusion with computerized tomography to enhance spatial accuracy. ([see comment]) J Neurosurg 1995;83:271–276

60. Hawrylyshyn P, Rowe IH, Tasker RR, Organ LW. A computer system for stereotaxic neurosurgery. Comput Biol Med 1976;6:87–97

61. Maciunas RJ, Galloway RL Jr, Latimer JW. The application accuracy of stereotactic frames. Neurosurgery 1994;35:682–694

62. Starr PA. Placement of deep brain stimulators into the subthalamic nucleus or globus pallidus internus: technical approach. Stereotact Funct Neurosurg 2002;79:118–145

63. Lenz FA, Dostrovsky JO, Kwan HC, et al. Methods for microstimulation and recording of single neurons and evoked potentials in the human central nervous system. J Neurosurg 1988;68:630–634

64. Hubel DH. Tungsten microelectrode for recording from single units. Science 1957;125:549–550

65. Vitek JL, Bakay RA, Hashimoto T, et al. Microelectrode-guided pallidotomy: technical approach and its application in medically intrac-

table Parkinson's disease. ([see comment]) J Neurosurg 1998;88:1027–1043

66. Starr PA, Vitek JL, Bakay RAE. Deep brain stimulation for movement disorders. Neurosurg Clin N Am 1998;9:381–402

67. Taira T, Speelman JD, Bosch DA. Trajectory angle in stereotactic thalamotomy. Stereotact Funct Neurosurg 1993;61:24–31

68. Kawashima Y, Chen HJ, Takahashi A, Hirato M, Ohye C. Application of magnetic resonance imaging in functional stereotactic thalamotomy for the evaluation of individual variations of the thalamus. Stereotact Funct Neurosurg 1992;58:33–38

69. Gross RE, Jones EG, Dostrovsky JO, Bergeron C, Lang AE, Lozano AM. Histological analysis of the location of effective thalamic stimulation for tremor: case report. J Neurosurg 2004;100:547–552

70. Henderson J, Rodriguez M, O'Sullivan D, et al. Partial lesion of thalamic ventral intermediate nucleus after chronic high-frequency stimulation. Mov Disord 2004;19:709–711

71. Hariz GM, Lindberg M, Hariz MI, Bergenheim AT. Gender differences in disability and health related quality of life in patients with Parkinson's disease treated with stereotactic surgery. Acta Neurol Scand 2003;108:28–37

72. Hariz MI, Shamsgovara P, Johansson P, et al. Tolerance and tremor rebound following long-term chronic thalamic stimulation for Parkinsonian and essential tremor. Stereotact Funct Neurosurg 1999;72:208–218

73. Fields JA, Troster AI, Woods SP, et al. Neuropsychological and quality of life outcomes 12 months after unilateral thalamic stimulation for essential tremor. J Neurol Neurosurg Psychiatry 2003;74:305–311

74. Bryant JA, DeSalles A, Cabatan C, Frysinger R, Behnke E, Bronstein R. The impact of thalamic stimulation on activities of daily living for essential tremor. Surg Neurol 2003;59:479–484(discussion 484–485), 12826348.

75. Putzke JD, Uitti RJ, Obwegeser AA, Wszolek ZK, Wharen RE. Bilateral thalamic deep brain stimulation: midline tremor control. J Neurol Neurosurg Psychiatry 2005;76:684–690

76. Yamamoto T, Katayama Y, Fukaya C, Oshima H, Kasai M, Kobayashi K. New method of deep brain stimulation therapy with two electrodes implanted in parallel and side by side. J Neurosurg 2001;95:1075–1078

77. Raoul S, Faighel M, Rivier I, Verin M, Lajat Y, Damier P. Staged lesions through implanted deep brain stimulating electrodes: a new surgical procedure for treating tremor or dyskinesias. Mov Disord 2003;18:933–938

78. Giller CA, Dewey RB. Ventralis intermedius thalamotomy can succeed when ventralis intermedius thalamic stimulation fails: report of 2 cases for tremor. Stereotact Funct Neurosurg 2002;79:51–56

79. Schulder M, Sernas TJ, Karimi R. Thalamic stimulation in patients with multiple sclerosis: long-term follow up. Stereotact Funct Neurosurg 2003;80:48–55

80. Hooper J, Taylor R, Pentland B, Whittle IR. A prospective study of thalamic deep brain stimulation for the treatment of movement disorders in multiple sclerosis. Br J Neurosurg 2002;16:102–109

81. Minneboo A, Barkhof F, Polman CH, Uitdehaag BM, Knol DL, Castelijns JA. Infra-tentorial lesions predict long term disability in patients with initial findings suggestive of multiple sclerosis. Arch Neurol 2004;61:217–221

82. Berk C, Carr J, Sinden M, Martzke J, Honey CR. Thalamic deep brain stimulation for the treatment of tremor due to multiple sclerosis: a prospective study of tremor and quality of life. J Neurosurg 2002;97:815–820

83. Foote KD, Okun MS. Ventralis intermedius plus ventralis oralis anterior and posterior deep brain stimulation for posttraumatic Holmes tremor: two leads may be better than one: technical note. Neurosurgery 2005;56:E445

84. Deuschl G, Bain P. Deep brain stimulation for tremor [correction of trauma]: patient selection and evaluation. Mov Disord 2002;17(Suppl 3):S102–S111

85. Goto S, Yamada K. Combination of thalamic Vim stimulation and GPi pallidotomy synergistically abolishes Holmes tremor. J Neurol Neurosurg Psychiatry 2004;75:1203–1204

86. Nikkhah G, Prokop T, Hellwig B, Lucking CH, Ostertag CB. Deep brain stimulation of the nucleus ventralis intermedius for Holmes (rubral) tremor and associated dystonia caused by upper brain stem lesions: report of two cases. J Neurosurg 2004;100:1079–1083, 15200125.

87. Romanelli P, Bronte-Stewart H, Courtney T, Heit G. Possible necessity for deep brain stimulation of both the ventralis intermedius and subthalamic nuclei to resolve Holmes tremor: case report. J Neurosurg 2003;99:566–571

88. Umemura A, Samadani U, Jaggi JL, Hurtig HI, Baltuch GH. Thalamic deep brain stimulation for posttraumatic action tremor. Clin Neurol Neurosurg 2004;106:280–283

89. Hooper J, Whittle IR. Costs of thalamic deep brain stimulation for movement disorders in patients with multiple sclerosis. Br J Neurosurg 2003;17:40–45

90. Hirai T, Miyazaki M, Nakajima H, et al. The correlation between tremor characteristics and predicted volume of effective lesions in stereotaxic Vim-thalamotomy. Brain 1983;106:1001–1018

91. Foote KD, Seignourel P, Fernandez HH, Romrell J, Whidden E, Jacobson C, et al. Dual electrode thalamic deep brain stimulation for the treatment of posttraumatic and multiple sclerosis tremor. Neurosurgery 2006;58:280–285

92. Lim DA, Khandhar SM, Heath S, Ostrem JL, Ringel N, Starr P. Multiple target deep brain stimulation for multiple sclerosis related and poststroke Holmes' tremor. Stereotact Funct Neurosurg 2007;85:144–149

93. Hamel W, Herzog J, Kopper F, Pinsker M, Weinert D, Muller D, et al. Deep brain stimulation in the subthalamic area is more effective than nucleus ventralis intermedius stimulation for bilateral intention tremor. Acta Neurochir (Wien) 2007;149:749–758

94. Tasker RR. Deep brain stimulation is preferable to thalamotomy for tremor suppression. Surg Neurol 1998;49:145–153

95. Binder DK, Rau GM, Starr PA. Risk factors for hemorrhage during microelectrode-guided deep brain stimulator implantation for movement disorders. Neurosurgery 2005;56:722–732 (discussion 722–732)

96. Woods SP, Fields JA, Lyons KE, Pahwa R, Troster AI. Pulse width is associated with cognitive decline after thalamic stimulation for essential tremor. Parkinsonism Relat Disord 2003;9:295–300

97. Loher TJ, Gutbrod K, Fravi NL, Pohle T, Burgunder JM, Krauss JK. Thalamic stimulation for tremor: subtle changes in episodic memory are related to stimulation per se and not to a microthalamotomy effect. J Neurol 2003;250:707–713

98. Oh MY, Abosch A, Kim SH, et al. Long-term hardware-related complications of deep brain stimulation. Neurosurgery 2002;50:1268–1274

99. Hood TW, Yap JC. A survey of infections in stereotactic surgery. Appl Neurophysiol 1981;44:314–319

100. Burchiel KJ. Thalamotomy for movement disorders. Neurosurg Clin N Am 1995;6:55–71

101. Bakay RAE, Vitek JL, Delong MR. Thalamotomy for tremor. In: Rengechary SS, Wilkins RR, eds. Neurosurgical Operative Atlas. Vol 2. Park Ridge, IL: American Association of Neurological Surgeons; 1992:299–312.

Deep Brain Stimulation for Dystonia

Brian Harris Kopell, Craig I. Horenstein, and Ali R. Rezai

What is the basic feature of the disease I have detailed? We find no indication of paralysis and the patient can move about freely. However, there is a certain clumsiness, especially of the upper extremities, and the movements are neither graceful nor elastic but rather stiff and disjointed . . . there is no athetosis . . . if the patient is fully at rest, the extremities are also quiet. . . . If involuntary movements are present, they show rhythmic, clonic features. . . . Upon detailed inspection, it becomes obvious that isolated muscles have a tendency to a moderate tonic tension . . . we are surprised to encounter rather a hypotonia upon passive movement of the lower extremities. . . . The salient feature of this disease is an alteration of muscle tone.[1]

In 1911, Hermann Oppenheim, a German neurologist, introduced the term *dystonia* to designate the coexistence of muscular hypotonia and hypertonia.[1] Dystonia is a heterogeneous group of disorders that encompasses a wide range of manifestations and etiologies. The hallmark of dystonia is involuntary twisting movements and postures, which may be exacerbated by voluntary movements. Most dystonias are treatable with medication and botulinum toxin. However, refractory dystonia may also cause severe functional handicap, debilitating pain, and progress to life-threatening stages. It is for these cases of intractable dystonia that deep brain stimulation (DBS) should be considered.

■ Classification of Dystonia

Traditionally, dystonia was classified according to the distribution of symptoms, etiology, and age of onset. In *focal* dystonia a single body region is affected, which includes writer's cramp (arm), blepharospasm (eyes), cervical dystonia/torticollis (neck), and spasmodic dysphonia or laryngeal dystonia (larynx). In *segmental* dystonia, two or more adjacent areas are affected. Examples include cranial–cervical dystonia, crural dystonia (one leg plus trunk or both legs), and brachial dystonia (one arm with trunk or both arms). *Multifocal* dystonia refers to cases where two or more noncontiguous body regions are affected. *Generalized* dystonia refers to crural dystonia with at least one other body part involved. When dystonia is confined to one side of the body, it is termed *hemidystonia*.

Historically, age of onset was perhaps the most important classification feature because it was the most significant prognostic indicator of whether focal symptoms would spread to other body parts. Early-onset dystonias typically present around age 9. They begin focally, usually in an arm or leg, and often spread to the trunk, resulting in a generalized dystonia producing severe disability. Adult-onset dystonia commonly presents in the fourth and fifth decades and manifests with focal symptoms of the cranial or cervical areas.[2] Symptoms usually remain localized though they can still cause significant disability. Generalization nevertheless does occur in 15 to 30% of patients with adult-onset primary facial, cervical, or upper extremity dystonia.[3] Dystonic tremor is sometimes difficult to distinguish from other forms of tremor, especially essential tremor (ET). It is characterized as irregular and slow (4 to 7 Hz) tremorlike movements that are frequently associated with focal dystonia such as torticollis or writer's cramp.

As our understanding of the molecular genetics and pathophysiology of dystonia has increased, more clinically useful classification schemes have been developed. Fahn et al[4] proposed classifying dystonias into one of four categories: primary dystonias, dystonia-plus syndromes, heredodegenerative dystonias, and secondary dystonias.

Primary dystonia refers to syndromes where there is no history of a brain injury (e.g., trauma or anoxia), brain imaging and laboratory studies do not suggest an etiology, and the symptoms are unresponsive to low dose L-dopa. The most common form of inherited primary generalized dystonia is DYT-1 dystonia. *Dystonia musculorum deformans* (Oppenheim's dystonia) was the original name of what is now known as DYT-1 dystonia. With an autosomal dominant inheritance pattern and variable penetrance, it accounts for 90% and 60% of early-onset primary dystonia in Jewish and non-Jewish children, respectively. The gene in question encodes the protein *torsion A* and has been mapped to a GAG deletion on chromosome 9q34.1.

Dystonia-plus category encompasses dystonic syndromes associated with clinical and laboratory findings suggestive of a neurochemical disorder without evidence of neurodegeneration, such as the L-dopa responsive dystonias.

Heredodegenerative dystonias include neurodegenerative disorders that often produce dystonia as a prominent clinical feature, but other neurological features are usually present. The class of heredodegenerative dystonias includes Parkinson disease (PD), Wilson disease, Huntington disease, and GM1 and GM2 gangliosidosis.

The fourth category, *secondary* dystonia, refers to syndromes where dystonia occurs as a result of an environmental insult to the brain. Focal dystonia can occur after direct injury to an extremity and is not unique to brain insult. Common causes include perinatal cerebral injury/anoxia, encephalitis, trauma, hypoxia, and L-dopa–induced dystonia.

■ History of Treatment for Dystonia

Pallidotomy and Thalamotomy

In the 1930s, Russell Meyers first performed selective basal ganglia lesions via craniotomy for the treatment of extrapyramidal movement disorders, including dystonia. Although he found that pallidal lesions abolished abnormal movements without causing weakness, his high rate of side effects resulted in pallidal targets being abandoned by the surgical community.[5,6]

In the 1950s, surgeons began revisiting Meyers's pallidotomy using stereotactic techniques.[7–10] Early stereotactic pallidotomies targeted the anterodorsal portion of the globus pallidus, and though the surgeries could be performed with less morbidity and mortality, the clinical outcomes were poor.[11] For the next several decades, thalamic targets, including the ventral lateral thalamus [ventral intermediate (Vim), ventro-oralis anterior (Voa), ventro-oralis posterior (Vop), ventral caudal (Vc)], centromedian nucleus (CM), pulvinar, and subthalamic region were the preferred sites for surgical intervention in dystonia.[12–15]

Cooper performed thalamotomies on 226 patients with primary or secondary generalized dystonia between 1953 and 1976.[12] He initially targeted the ventral lateral thalamus (Voa/Vop) and CM, but he refrained from simultaneous bilateral interventions due to the high risk of speech disturbances. If a further operation was required, Cooper lesioned the pallidal and cerebellar efferent fibers to the thalamus. If a patient was still disabled following this surgery, he performed a pulvinotomy. Cooper reports that improvement of dystonia was progressive and occurred up to 6 months postoperatively. Furthermore, a larger lesion was needed to treat dystonia than was necessary to suppress parkinsonian tremor. After an average follow-up of 8 years, 25% of Cooper's patients had "good" and 45% had "moderate" improvement. There was no change in 18% of patients, and symptoms worsened in 12%. Cooper's best results were in Jewish patients with early-onset hereditary dystonia.

In 1952, Leksell noticed improved outcomes following pallidotomy for movement disorders when he modified the anterodorsal pallidotomy to a more posteroventral target, where the ansa lenticularis emerges.[16] This work was largely overlooked until Laitinen's efforts in the late 1980s.[11] Leksell's posteroventral pallidotomy (PVP) was particularly successful in treating tremor, rigidity, and bradykinesia, as well as on-period dyskinesias and off-period dystonias. The beneficial effects on dystonic symptoms in PD encouraged neurosurgeons to attempt the PVP for the treatment of dystonia, and in recent years, the PVP has been performed for the treatment of dystonia with good results.[17,18,19,20,21] Although still controversial, *bilateral* PVP has been associated with increased risks of dysphagia, speech difficulty, and cognitive disturbance compared with unilateral interventions.[22] This increased risk makes DBS for dystonia more attractive than PVP due to the often needed bilateral aspect of intervention.

Peripheral Denervation Procedures

Peripheral denervation procedures for focal cervical dystonia have been largely replaced by botulinum toxin injections but may still be considered in medically refractory patients. Various selective peripheral denervation procedures have been used for treating cervical dystonia, including rhizotomy with intradural sectioning of anterior cervical roots C1–C3, posterior ramisectomy with extradural sectioning of the dorsal rami, microvascular decompression of the spinal accessory nerve, and myotomy. Krauss et al[23] used a combination of denervation procedures tailored to each patient's specific symptoms and reported mild to excellent improvement in 41 of 46 patients.

Electrostimulation

In 1960, Hassler et al[24] reported that low-frequency (4 to 8 Hz) stimulation of the pallidum in a patient with primary cervical dystonia and athetosis elicited abnormal movements, whereas higher-frequency stimulation eventually suppressed them. However, no other reports of electrical stimulation for the treatment of dystonia appear in the literature until 1977, when Mundinger[25] reported encouraging short-term results for seven patients with cervical dystonia who underwent unilateral, low-frequency (2 to 12 Hz), intermittent (30-minute, several times per day) electrical stimulation of the thalamus (Voa, Voi, and subthalamic areas). However, no long-term results were ever published, and the technique was abandoned due to difficulty with the hardware.

In the 1980s, several groups reexamined thalamic stimulation for dystonia. Andy, stimulating in the motor thalamus, demonstrated that intermittent 50 Hz thalamic stimulation improved symptoms in two patients with cervical dystonia.[26] Targeting the sensory (Vc) thalamus, Siegfried[27] reported a reduction of dystonic symptoms in four patients treated with 33 Hz stimulation, and Sellal et al[28] showed a dramatic improvement in a patient with secondary hemidystonia with intermittent 60 Hz stimulation.

The modern era of continuous high-frequency deep brain stimulation (DBS) began when Benabid et al[29] stimulated ventral Vim in PD or ET patients. The procedure was later performed in the globus pallidus internus (GPi) and in the subthalamic nucleus (STN).[30,31] The ensuing success of high-frequency DBS in treating ET, PD, and related L-dopa–induced on-dyskinesias and off-dystonias encouraged surgeons to expand the indications for DBS. Pollak et al[32] first applied high-frequency DBS for generalized dystonia when they stimulated Vim in 12 patients with generalized dystonia. The following year, three groups reported short-term results of pallidal DBS in the treatment of dystonia.[33–35] The positive outcomes encouraged other groups to attempt DBS in dystonic patients of varying etiologies, and GPi soon became the preferred target for DBS for dystonia.

■ Deep Brain Stimulation for Dystonia

Indications and Patient Selection

The indications for DBS for the treatment of dystonia are starting to emerge, though large, prospective, randomized trials are lacking.[36,37] Patients who are considered for surgery must have severe motor symptoms and/or pain refractory to medical therapy and resulting in significant functional disability. A variety of medications are utilized before a patient is considered refractory. Patients with primary dystonia initially undergo a therapeutic trial with L-dopa. If this is unsuccessful, anticholinergic therapy with trihexyphenidyl is instituted, and benefit is typically seen in 40 to 50% of patients.[38–40] Baclofen and benzodiazepines are generally considered useful as adjunctive therapies. Baclofen has been reported to be more effective in children and adolescents, and intrathecal baclofen is used in patients with dystonia associated with spasticity and pain.[41,42] Clozapine, an atypical neuroleptic that primarily blocks D4 receptors, has shown a 30% improvement in subjective ratings and dystonia scales.[43] Other commonly used medications for treating dystonia include mexiletine (an antiarrhythmic related to lidocaine), anticonvulsants, muscle relaxants, and riluzole (a glutamine antagonist).[41]

Botulinum toxin injections have become one of the main medical therapies, with response rates of 70 to 100%, depending on the type of dystonia.[44] Single injections range from $100 for focal dystonia to $2500 for generalized dystonia.[45] There are many different subtypes of botulinum toxins, but only type A (BOTOX, Allergan, Inc., Irvine, CA) and type B (Myobloc/Neurobloc, Solstice Neurosciences, Inc., South San Francisco, CA) have been approved by the U.S. Food and Drug Administration (FDA) for use in dystonia.[41] Approximately 4 to 10% of patients, however, do not respond to botulinum toxin injection, either primarily or secondarily, due to development of neutralizing antibodies.[46]

Clinical evaluation of dystonia is essential for patient selection prior to surgery and for documenting outcomes postoperatively. Currently accepted rating scales include the Global Dystonia Rating Scale (GDRS), the Burke-Fahn-Marsden (BFMDRS), and the United Dystonia Rating Scale (UDRS) for generalized dystonia, and the Toronto Western Spasmodic Torticollis Rating Scale (TWSTRS) for cervical dystonia.[37,47,48] A large, multicenter study conducted by the Dystonia Study Group critically assessed the BFMDRS, GDRS, and UDRS, confirming their internal consistency, validity, interrater reliability, and ease of use, concluding that the BFMDRS and GDRS were appropriate for use in clinical trials and the UDRS was appropriate for use in an office setting.[47]

Traditionally, only patients with generalized, segmental, or hemidystonia were considered for stereotactic neurosurgical procedures. Focal dystonia usually responds to botulinum toxin injections and, in most cases, does not produce significant enough disability to warrant the risks of surgery. Furthermore, published outcomes have shown that patients with primary generalized dystonia have the best surgical outcomes, and patients with appendicular symptoms are believed to respond better than patients with axial disease. The literature also suggests that the subset of patients with DYT-1 dystonia has the best results following stereotactic lesioning or DBS.[49–51] However, the reported safety of bilateral GPi stimulation has encouraged various groups to attempt to expand the indications for DBS in dystonia. The results from the literature suggest that many patients with severe focal dystonia and secondary dystonia may also benefit from chronic DBS therapy.

Targets

Stereotactic neurosurgery has traditionally been considered the last option in treating severe dystonia. However, recent reviews have shown bilateral DBS to be safe and highly effective in treating adults and children with various types of dystonia and PD. Because of its safety and reversibility, DBS is replacing brain lesioning as the preferred stereotactic procedure.[52,53] Currently, thalamic and pallidal targets have been the focus for DBS intervention for dystonia, with pallidal stimulation dominating the investigative literature both by frequency performed and by efficacy.

The pallidal target is the sensorimotor portion of the GPi as initially described by Leksell and popularized by Laitinen.[11,16] Though the exact lead placement varies from institution to institution, it is generally agreed to be 18 to 21 mm lateral to midline, 2 to 3 mm anterior to the midcommissural point (MCP) and 3 to 6 mm ventral to the intercommissural plane. The DBS tip is ideally 4 to 5 mm anterior to the internal capsule border and 2 mm dorsal to the optic tract. Many authors favor placing the leads laterally within this territory to avoid complications secondary to DBS effects on the internal capsule. An additional variable has been the higher voltages used to achieve therapeutic benefits. This has necessitated a more anterior placement of the DBS lead to reduce the current spread to the internal capsule.

Thalamic interventions have been mainly described in the Voa/Vop and Vim thalamus. Such coordinates have been as follows: Voa—2 mm anterior to the MCP, 10 mm lateral to the MCP, and 5 mm dorsal to the intercommissural plane[54]; Vim—6.0 to 6.5 mm anterior to the posterior commissure, 13.8 to 14.0 mm lateral to the MCP, and 1 mm dorsal to the intercommissural plane.[55]

Because most published reports for DBS for dystonia have focused on the internal pallidum, the following sections discuss physiology and localization methods from the perspective of the pallidal target. Key aspects of thalamic intervention are also given.

Target Acquisition, Headframe Placement, and Anesthesia Management

Although DBS for dystonia shares many common features with DBS for other movement disorders, there are several unique considerations. The first issue concerns target acquisition. Preoperative target localization is performed utilizing magnetic resonance imaging (MRI). MRI sequences such as inversion recovery can directly visualize the borders of the GPi and allow modification of the initial target based on the anatomical variations of individual patients.[56] These images are often merged with a concurrent computed tomographic (CT) scan because CT presently produces less spatial distortion of localizing fiducials than does MRI.

Vayssiere et al[57] reported that accurate DBS lead placement with good clinical outcome can be achieved based solely on MRI localization. Postoperative MRIs, obtained immediately after surgery with the patient still under general anesthesia, should confirm precise lead placement. The actual lead placement was not statistically (mean 2 to 3 mm) different from the theoretical target chosen preoperatively. These authors also report a mean improvement of 83.8% in the BMFDRS score at a mean follow-up of 1 year. Another method utilizes "semimicroelectrode" guidance and tissue impedance monitoring to guide final targeting of the DBS electrode.[58]

Most institutions, however, utilize intraoperative microelectrode recording (MER) to confirm accurate lead placement. MER is still highly recommended for several reasons.[56] First, the borders of target nuclei are not always perfectly visualized on MRI. Despite the use of CT fusion, there may still be image distortion effects, and shifting of brain tissue may occur intraoperatively due to cerebrospinal fluid (CSF) leakage and air entering the cranial cavity. Second, there is not always a perfect correlation between structure and function, especially in patients with pathophysiologi-

cal changes.[56,59] Reports of DBS placement have shown that the first trajectory chosen does not usually result in optimal lead placement, and that based on the results of MERs, the optimal lead placement varies by 1.27 mm or greater from the initial target in 25% of cases.[60] Finally, microstimulation enables the surgeon to confirm that the lead placement will allow stimulator settings to be increased to higher voltages without causing pyramidal side effects via activation of fibers in the internal capsule, intolerable paresthesias via activation of the Vc nucleus/medial lemniscus, or visual scotomas from optic tract activation.

Anesthesia management is particularly important during DBS interventions for dystonia. Often patients with dystonia, especially severe generalized and cervical dystonias and the pediatric population, will present with challenges regarding airway management, headframe placement, and comfort during the procedure itself. Unlike PD patients, who in their off state are often rigid and immobile, the dystonic patient can have violent, uncontrolled movements. Initially this can make accurate headframe placement extremely difficult. In these patients, careful coordination with anesthesia colleagues to obtain propofol intravenous (IV) sedation or light general anesthesia with laryngeal mask airway (LMA) can be helpful during this phase.

During the surgical implantation of DBS electrodes, IV sedation, especially propofol, can confound MER data by lowering the firing rate of the globus pallidus externus and internus (GPe, GPi).[61] Although many adults can tolerate awake-surgery in this state, the pediatric population may not. Starr et al[62] reported the use of ketamine and opiate sedation in pediatric dystonia patients that seemed to interfere least with MER data. Such combinations and others such as the 2 agonist, dexmedetomidine may prove useful in providing sedation and pain control for dystonia patients while allowing electrophysiological mapping to occur.

Some of these challenges may be overcome with the use of frameless stereotactic equipment. A frameless stereotactic system may potentially obviate the need for the dystonia patients, with their attendant abnormal and sometimes violent movements, to be constrained by a headframe. This freedom of movement would necessarily afford the patient greater comfort and the anesthesiology personnel a greater degree of control over airway function. The issue of accuracy of these systems compared with the standard frame-based placement is still being evaluated by several centers.

Editor's Comments

Several drugs are used to treat dystonia. Unfortunately, they are often ineffective and can cause serious side effects, including confusion, memory and attention disorders, blurred vision, constipation, and urinary retention. In an open-label trial, it was reported that only 38% of adults and 50% of children gain moderate to marked benefit from medical therapy.[39] In a double-blind crossover study of 31 patients with generalized dystonia, only 42% obtained good benefit, and many patients were unable to continue therapy due to side effects

from the medication.[38] As a result, considerable effort has been spent to develop alternative treatment strategies. Historically, a variety of surgical approaches have been tried for the treatment of dystonia. The results were highly variable and associated with a very high rate of complications. These have included surgical approaches such as peripheral surgical denervation, electrical dorsal column stimulation, pallidotomy, and thalamotomy. Cervical rhizotomy has played a small role in the treatment of dystonia. It is not useful for hemi- or generalized dystonia due to the multiple muscle groups involved in these dystonias; therefore, it has been used predominantly for focal or segmental dystonia, in particular for spasmodic torticollis. Although effective in some cases, results are unpredictable and may often be associated with severe weakness, dysphagia, and sensory disorders. Ablation of various portions of the cerebellum has met with mixed success and is not currently used to treat dystonia.

Thalamotomy has been the most widely used procedure for the treatment of dystonia. There are four major studies of thalamotomy for dystonia (see references 12, 15, 50, 63). All reported that thalamotomy was effective in alleviating both primary and secondary dystonia; however, the benefits to individual patients varied from none to marked, with approximately one third showing marked benefit, one third mild to moderate, and one third no or little benefit.[50] No one could replicate Cooper's results. This could be related to the high number of genetic dystonia patients (possibly DYT-1) or overly enthusiastic evaluations. Many patients who initially experienced improvement in symptoms following surgery gradually lost benefit over the ensuing months. These patients were often reoperated and the lesion was gradually expanded with the hope of regaining lost benefit. An average of two surgeries per patient was reported by Cooper in his seminal work of surgery for dystonia published in 1976, with some patients undergoing as many as seven operations.[12] The lack of a common target and the selection of patients with different pathophysiological mechanisms for their dystonia may account for some of the variability in outcomes reported across studies. There was no consensus as to the thalamic target, and surgeons often targeted various combinations of thalamic subnuclei, including the Vim, Vop, Voa, CM, Vc, or pulvinar. The variable outcome, gradual loss of benefit in some patients, and high incidence of side effects associated with bilateral thalamotomy gradually blunted the enthusiasm for this approach to the treatment of dystonia.

Historically the pallidum was also targeted for the treatment of dystonia. Compared with thalamotomy, however, pallidotomy for dystonia was performed infrequently due to the inconsistent benefits associated with this procedure. Although the signs of dystonia frequently responded acutely to surgery, similar to that reported following thalamotomy, many patients suffered a regression or worsening of signs over the ensuing weeks to months. The underlying basis for these variable results remains speculative because there is little histological or radiographic evidence as to the lesion site, nor were there rigorous and comprehensive pre- and postoperative evaluations of motor, cognitive, and emotional changes. It is highly likely that the reasons for this variability relate to patient selection, problems with target localization, and lesioning techniques. With the more recent reintroduction of pallidotomy for PD it has become apparent that the outcome depends on the site of the lesion.[64–67] In our experience, lesions involving the caudal portions of the GPi are more effective in alleviating parkinsonian motor signs than more rostrally placed lesions, and lesions only a few millimeters apart may have vastly different long-term results. Recent observations of marked improvement in patients with primary dystonia with lesions in the posterolateral "sensorimotor" portion of the GPi, confirmed using high-resolution MRI, would suggest that lesions in this region of the pallidum can be highly effective in the alleviation of dystonia and that the inconsistency of earlier studies of pallidotomy for dystonia may have been

due, at least in part, to differences in lesion location.[68] In addition to lesion location, other factors such as lesion size, disease progression and/or plasticity of neuronal pathways mediating the development of dystonia could also play a role in the return of dystonic symptoms over time.

The concerns over the development of permanent side effects related to surgical lesioning have led many to consider DBS as the preferred surgical option, over ablative procedures for the treatment of primary generalized dystonia. Earlier ablative studies often required reoperation to expand the lesion, whereas with DBS adjustment of stimulation parameters may allow one to accomplish the same goal without reoperation. Chronic DBS in the GPi has emerged as the surgical therapy of choice due to the encouraging results of initial studies, reversibility of side effects, and ability to perform bilateral procedures without the associated high incidence of side effects associated with bilateral ablative procedures. As of April 15, 2003, the Medtronic Activa (Medtronic, Inc., Minneapolis, MN) was approved for humanitarian device exception (http://www.fda.gov/cdrh/ode/hdeinfo.html) for uni- or bilateral GPi or STN DBS placement for chronic, intractable primary dystonia, including generalized or segmental dystonia for patients 7 years or older. It requires an institutional review board (IRB)-approved protocol.

Rush Inclusion Criteria

1. Clinical diagnosis of primary dystonia from a movement disorder specialist.
2. Age range up to 70 years, but more important is the physiological condition of the patient to undergo surgery.
3. Unsatisfactory clinical response to maximal medical management, including high-dose anticholinergics, baclofen, benzodiazepines, and where appropriate, botulinum toxin. All individuals with dystonia will have undergone a trial of L-dopa to a total dose of 600 mg per day to exclude patients with dopa-responsive dystonia.
4. The presence of dystonia for greater than 36 months.
5. No other neurological deficit to suggest other diseases (see below) and no fixed contractures.
6. Normal perinatal and developmental history.
7. Clinical diagnosis of secondary acquired dystonias (e.g., perinatal brain injury, stroke, drug-induced or focal cerebral pathology) is evaluated on an individual basis.
8. Clinical diagnosis of dystonia-plus syndromes (e.g., dopa-responsive dystonia, myoclonus dystonia, rapid-onset dystonia-parkinsonism), inherited degenerative disorders [e.g., Wilson disease, Parkin-associated parkinsonism, spinocerebellar ataxias, gangliosidoses, glutaric aciduria, neurodegeneration with brain iron accumulation/pantothenate-kinase-associated neurodegeneration (PKAN), amino and organic acidurias] or with degenerative disorders of unclear etiology (PD, progressive supranuclear palsy, corticobasalganglionic degeneration, etc.) as a cause of dystonia unless part of a study should be avoided.

Rush Exclusion Criteria

1. Abnormal MRI based on evidence of intracranial pathology, including extensive white matter changes, cortical atrophy, evidence of large lacunes, or lesions in the basal ganglia.

2. Ongoing botulinum toxin therapy or a botulinum toxin injection within 3 months of study entry. This interval was chosen to allow sufficient time to recover from botulinum toxin treatment to allow adequate examination and evaluation.
3. Psychogenic dystonia.
4. Clinically significant medical disease that would increase the risk of developing pre- or postoperative complications (e.g., unstable cardiac or pulmonary disease, uncontrolled hypertension).
5. Dementia (based on DSM-IV criteria) or severe cognitive impairment (e.g., IQ < 70) that in a neuropsychologist's clinical judgment would preclude the patient's ability to comply with the demands of surgery or would adversely affect the reliability of subsequent follow-up evaluations.
6. Patients with clinically significant depression or anxiety that causes or contributes to increasing symptoms of dystonia are not to be included unless the psychiatric condition is assessed, treated, and deemed stable by a psychiatrist prior to study entry. These patients would include those diagnosed with generalized anxiety disorder, social phobia, minor depression, and dysthymia.

Most patients with generalized dystonia will undergo bilateral simultaneous implantation in the internal segment of the GPi. If for technical reasons bilateral implantation cannot be performed or at the time of operation it is decided by the surgeon or patient not to proceed with the second side, a second surgery can be planned within 3 to 6 months from the first procedure. The preferred anesthetic protocol for focal dystonic or mildly symptomatic general dystonic patients is to have patients awake (local anesthesia with intermittent IV sedation) for the part of the procedure involving physiological mapping. Most patients under 14 years of age will not tolerate awake surgery; therefore, patients under 14 are offered a general anesthetic for the entire procedure. Nevertheless, we have done patients as young as 9 under local and have had to do some adults under general. Preoperative evaluation is critical. How well patients can tolerate a diagnostic MRI is a clue to whether general anesthesia, IV sedation, or awake surgery should be planned. Following placement of a stereotactic headframe, an MRI scan is obtained to define both the target and the trajectory through the brain. The anterior commissural–posterior commissural (AC–PC) line is defined. Using the AC–PC line for reference, our initial target for the pallidum is the posterior region of the GPi at 21.5 mm lateral to the midline, 3 mm anterior, and 5 mm below the MCP, per the Schaltenbrand and Bailey Human Brain Atlas. We will adjust these coordinates to account for individual anatomical variations evident on direct targeting from the MRI using StealthStation (Medtronic Navigation, Louisville, CO) image guidance.

Once the stereotactic frame is placed and the initial target is identified by MRI, MER is used to map the pallidal region.[69] A motorized microdrive is used to advance the microelectrode. MER is performed in the parasagittal plane; the angle of entry may vary slightly from parasagittal based on preoperative planning and the need to vary the angle of entry to avoid blood vessels along the trajectory. The microelectrode is advanced in the anterodorsal to posteroventral direction at an angle of ~30 degrees from vertical. The microelectrode is lowered within a protective guide tube. As the microelectrode is advanced, patterns of neural activity are noted throughout the track, and the depths from the starting position are recorded. The major structures that are identified using this plane of approach are the white matter, striatum (caudate and putamen), GPe and GPi, internal and external medullary laminae, optic tract, and internal capsule as has been discussed in Chapter 7. The nucleus basalis may be encountered with anteriorly placed penetrations. In PD patients, each cellular region has a characteristic pattern of neural activity.[64] In patients with dystonia, neural activity in the GPi is typified by grouped irregular discharges of varying frequency and may sound similar to that in GPe. Although it is argued that the use of anesthetic agents may have lowered these rates in humans undergoing stereotactic surgery,[61] our data in patients with and without propofol and studies in multiple other centers in patients without the use of anesthetic agents[21,65,70–72] all support the original hypothesis that rates are lower in patients with dystonia. Because in dystonia the rates and patterns are very similar, differentiating GPe and GPi under general anesthesia is difficult. Therefore, special attention to the location of laminae (quiet regions) is particularly important for these patients and provides a landmark for identification of the border between nuclei. Within the laminae of the pallidum (i.e., between the GPe and GPi and within the GPi), neurons with slower rates of tonic neural activity ("border" cells) may be encountered. Their pattern of spontaneous activity is distinct and helpful in identifying the laminae and borders of the pallidal segments. The pattern of discharge of those neurons is the same as those found in the nucleus basalis (these are probably the same neuronal types). The lack of cellular activity and the frequent presence of "border" cells can identify the lamina between the GPe and GPi and the accessory lamina within the GPi. To determine the location of the sensorimotor territory of the GPi, neurons are examined in awake patients for their response to passive manipulations and active movement of the extremities and orofacial structures. The posterior portion of the GPi (sensorimotor) contains neurons whose discharge is related to passive or active movement of either or both the limbs and the orofacial structures. The responses of neurons to passive and active manipulations in dystonia are robust and help to locate the sensorimotor portion of the GPi. There is a general somatotopic organization within the GPi, with the preponderance of cells representing the leg found medial and dorsal to those representing the arm and face, which are predominantly ventral and lateral.[64] The jaw representation is found more ventral. Sensorimotor responses are found predominantly in the posterolateral portions of the GPi. Neurons in regions more anterior and medial do not generally respond to active or passive manipulations. These anteromedial regions are likely related to nonmotor "associative" functions and should be avoided.[68] General anesthesia will also render these discharge pattern determinations impossible. This may necessitate more microelectrode tracts and greater dependency on finding the optic tract and corticospinal tract.

After passing through the pallidum, the electrode may enter either the optic tract or the internal capsule. The optic tract can be identified in the vast majority of patients by flashing a strobe light in the patient's eyes and listening for high-frequency modulation of the background audio signal coincident with the light stimulus. In awake patients, the optic tract can also be identified in most cases by microstimulation. For microstimulation we use balanced biphasic pulses at 300 Hz of 0.2 msec duration with currents from 5 to 40 µA. Patients typically report seeing brief speckles or flashes of light of various colors in the contralateral visual field in a localized region, which is most often lateral to or near the midline. The internal capsule can be identified by observing stimulation-induced (60 to 90 µA, 300 Hz) movement of the limbs or orofacial structures. The relative proximity of these structures (i.e., optic tract and internal capsule) can be ascertained by the stimulation threshold at which muscle contraction occurs or the patient reports seeing speckles or flashes of light.

Once the sensorimotor portion of the GPi and its borders are defined, the site for lead implantation is selected based on the physiological map. The DBS lead (Medtronic DBS 3387, Medtronic, Inc., Minneapolis, MN) is placed in the sensorimotor pallidum, at approximately lateral 21.5 mm, 4 mm anterior to the posterior border with the bottom contact placed at the ventral border of the GPi. The DBS 3387 lead has four metal contacts, each 1.5 mm in diameter, separated from each other by 1.5 mm. The total distance from the top of the first contact to the bottom of the last is 10.5 mm. Macrostimulation with the DBS lead is used to further confirm the distance of the lead from the optic and corticospinal tracts to insure activation thresholds for these structures are significantly higher than those generally required for improvement in dystonia. Intraoperatively, there is often little or no improvement (decrease tone) in motor function observable in dystonia patients at the time of stimulation. Improvement in dystonic symptoms is often gradual occurring over days to weeks and months following the onset of stimulation and adjustment of stimulation parameters. Thus the decision to move the lead will be based primarily on the ability to stimulate at parameters necessary to obtain relief from dystonic symptoms without inducing side effects. Dystonia patients require wider pulse widths (> 210 µs) and higher voltages (> 3.0 V) than patients with PD. Therefore, macrostimulation with the DBS lead should be free of side effects at 8 V for standard 90 Ms or at 5 V with pulse widths 210 µs and a frequency of up to 250 Hz.

Following implantation and screening macrostimulation with the DBS lead, prior to removing the equipment holding the lead in place, a fluoroscopic image is taken and stored to monitor the anteroposterior and dorsoventral location of the lead. The protective guide tube and anchoring equipment are removed, leaving the lead in place. Fluoroscopy will again be used to confirm that the lead has not moved, and screening thresholds will be reconfirmed. Following satisfactory test stimulation, the guide tubes holding the lead are removed, and the lead is anchored to the skull with a lead-anchoring device (Stimloc, Medtronic, Inc., Minneapolis, MN). The excess lead is coiled below the galea and the wound closed. Placement of the extension head and implantable pulse generator (IPG) are performed within 2 weeks following lead placement, under general anesthesia as described in Chapter 7. Due to the potential of a transient lesion effect following placement of the DBS lead as well as the presence of edema in the region, initial programming occurs 2 to 4 weeks following lead implantation. A pulse width of 210 µs is one used most commonly by centers currently performing DBS for dystonia. Each lead contact will be tested using monopolar stimulation, with the contact as the cathode and the case (IPG) as the anode. For each contact the voltage will be increased in intervals while assessing the patient for beneficial effects and for side effects indicating spread to the optic tract or internal capsule. The effect of stimulation on speech is also assessed. The deepest contact in the GPi that permits a voltage of at least 3.0 V and pulse width of 210 µs without associated side effects is used for stimulation. Depending on the degree of benefit derived from stimulation using this contact, other contacts are explored for effectiveness, and the most effective contact or combination of contacts is used. Various lead combinations (bipolar stimulation, use of two contacts as cathodal), voltage and pulse durations can be used to maximize the clinical benefit while minimizing any potential side effects. Due to the delay in benefit often reported with stimulation, programming dystonic patients will require careful and thorough evaluations over multiple visits. Once benefit is achieved, however, it has been our experience that stimulation parameters remain stable, and little change is required other than small increases in voltage.

Frameless systems are a less encumbering method of performing stereotactic surgery.[73] It is a misnomer in that the frame is attached around the entry point rather than by four-point fixation around the entire calverium. There are unique limitations of the frameless system in targeting the GPi nuclei. Because the Nexframe (Medtronic, Inc., Minneapolis, MN) base sits on the skull, the convexity of the calverium makes alignment difficult for lateral targets. The approach to target must be within a 12-degree angle, or an offset must be used. In these cases, we have had to either drill a second burr hole or use the restricted trajectories available to map the target. In addition, the head is steadied by a restraining device, most commonly a cervical collar attached to the operating table. It offers no help for a patient with significant movement of the neck. Patients will rub themselves raw against the restraints, compromise their airway, and render the recordings worthless. In these cases, we prefer a frame and heavy sedation or general anesthesia. We are still struggling to define the role of frameless stereotactic surgery for dystonia.

Microelectrode Recording

Typical structures encountered along a recording tract during the implantation of GPi electrodes include the corona radiata, striatum (caudate/putamen), external pallidal lamina, GPe, medial pallidal lamina, GPi, internal pallidal lamina, GPi, ansa lenticularis, and optic tract, which is located ~2 mm ventral to the border of the GPi. The technique of MERs and the basic electrophysiological findings have been published in detail.[56,69] However, there are several important physiological findings in the basal ganglia and the thalamus that distinguish dystonia from other clinical syndromes and from normal nonhuman primates.

Microelectrode Recordings in the Basal Ganglia

In dystonia, most groups have found that GPe neurons have a mean firing rate of 30 to 60 Hz, which is similar to the rates in PD.[56,74] However, a large number of investigators report a decrease in mean firing rate of GPi neurons in dystonia compared with PD (**Fig. 12.1**). Lenz et al[74] report a mean firing rate of 40.8 Hz (range 20 to 53 Hz), whereas Vitek et al[75] reported a rate of 50 ± 20.5 Hz in dystonia patients without tremor and a rate of 63.8 ± 21 Hz in dystonia patients with tremor. This is significantly lower than the mean firing rate of GPi neurons in patients with PD (60 to 100 Hz) and in normal nonhuman primates (average 63 Hz).[56,74,76] Border cell activity, which appears regular and tonic, remains unchanged in dystonia, ranging from 20 to 40 Hz.[56] In dystonia, there may be such an overall similarity in the tonic activity rates from GPe and GPi that border cells become a critical landmark for navigation.

Another commonly reported finding is that a greater than normal percentage of GPi neurons respond to somatosensory input. Lenz et al[74] report that 53% of GPi neurons had somatosensory responses (SSRs) compared with 34% in PD. Similarly, Vitek et al[75] report that 43% of GPi neurons had SSRs, and of these neurons, 68% showed widened receptive fields including abnormal ipsilateral responses. Finally, the same groups reporting rate modulation have documented an altered pattern of GPi neural activity in dystonia. Consistent with Lenz et al,[74] findings that low-frequency modulation and pauses in the spike train are more pronounced in GPi of dystonia compared with PD, Vitek et al[75] report increased bursting index in dystonia as-sociated with tremor, and increased dispersion (irregularity) in dystonia without tremor.

A publication by Hutchison et al[61] refutes the notion that the GPi in dystonia has a decreased rate of firing and widened receptive fields compared with that in PD (**Fig. 12.2**). They report that in three dystonia patients who received propofol anesthesia, the firing rate of the GPi, 31 Hz, was indeed reduced. However, in seven dystonia patients who underwent surgery with local anesthesia only, and no propofol sedation, the mean firing rate of the GPi was 77 Hz. This rate was not statistically different than the rate of 74 Hz the authors observed in PD patients. They also report that the slower firing rates under propofol anesthesia were associated with long pauses and increased bursting. Propofol anesthesia also decreased the mean firing rate of neurons in the GPe, but not border cells. Contrary to other published findings, the authors report that in this study, GPi neurons responded mainly to passive movements of single joints, and there was no evidence of widened receptive fields.

Hutchison et al[61] propose that decreased pallidal firing rates are not the sine qua non of dystonia, but rather a consequence of propofol anesthesia. In support of this theory the authors report that one patient who had low-dose propofol had a mean GPi firing rate that was intermediate between the two groups. They also report two siblings with DYT-1 dystonia. One sibling received propofol and had a mean firing rate of 27 ± 15 Hz. The other did not receive propofol and had a mean firing rate of 70 ± 21 Hz. Furthermore, the first sibling who had low firing rates on propofol was reoperated on 2 years later without propofol anesthesia, and the mean firing rate of the GPi was 62 ± 14 Hz.

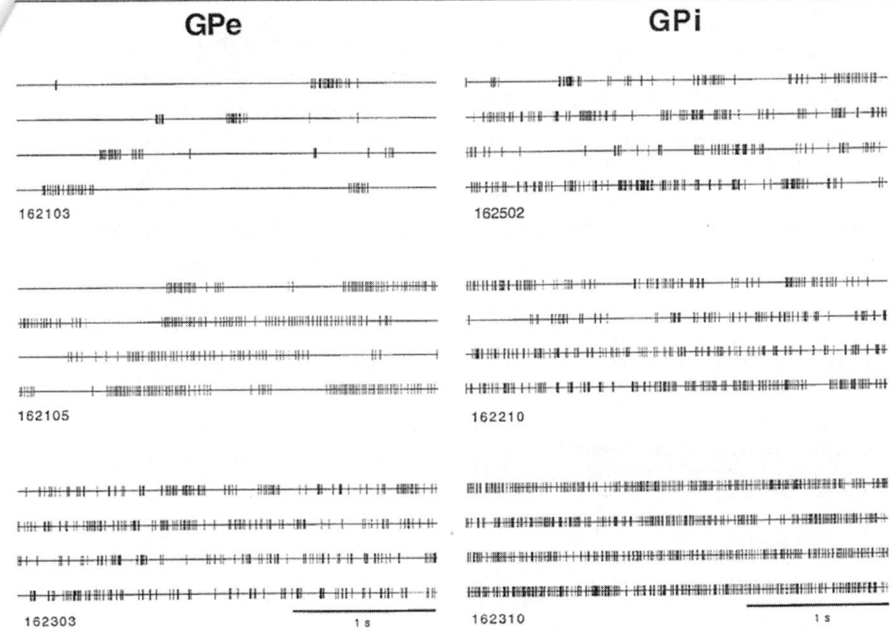

Fig. 12.1 Typical microelectrode recording data gathered from neurons from the external and internal segments of the globus pallidus (GPe and GPi, respectively) in patients with dystonia.

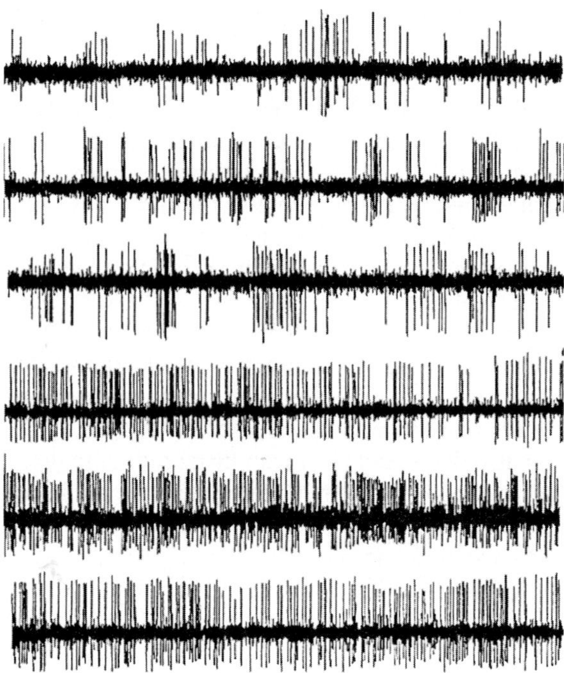

Fig. 12.2 Microelectrode recording data gathered from neurons from the internal globus pallidus (GPi) in a patient with dystonia. The set of data above was gathered while the patient was under propofol anesthesia. The lower set of data was from the same patient once the anesthesia was withdrawn. Such data may refute the notion that there exists a strict frequency difference between the firing rates of GPi neurons in Parkinson disease and dystonia. (From Hutchison WD, Lang AE, Dostrovsky JO, et al. Pallidal neuronal activity: implications for models of dystonia. Ann Neurol 2003;53:480–488. Reprinted by permission.)

Microelectrode Recordings in the Thalamus

MER data from the thalamus of dystonia patients also show alterations in neuronal activity. Lenz and Byl[77] demonstrated significant somatotopic reorganization in the thalamic sensory nucleus Vc, including widened receptive and widened projection fields. In dystonia, 29% of Vc neurons responded to multiple body parts compared with 11% in control patients with ET, and widened projection fields were found in 71% of neurons in dystonia compared with 41% in ET. There was also significantly increased mismatch of receptive and projection fields in dystonia.

Lenz and colleagues[78] also recorded thalamic neuronal signals from the Vim and Vop during thalamotomy and compared dystonia patients with control patients without motor abnormality who were undergoing thalamic surgery for treatment of chronic pain. The results showed that neurons in the Vop had increased power at the dystonia frequency as measured on electromyography (EMG). The activity of these Vop neurons was correlated with and phase-advanced to EMG activity during dystonia, suggesting that this neuronal activity was causally related to dys-

tonic movements. This same group also elicited dystonic muscular activity with microstimulation within the boundaries of the Vim that did not occur in surrounding areas.

■ Models of Pathophysiology of Dystonia

Models of pathophysiology underlying the development of dystonia are not as well elucidated as the ones for PD. Much of this is due to the somewhat ill-defined etiology and widespread phenotypic manifestations of the disease. Nevertheless, some common elements have emerged. Dystonia appears to be mediated by striatopallidal dysfunction that is reflected by abnormal activity in the thalamus and sensorimotor cortex. Several pathological features are evident at each anatomical level.

Pathologic Features of the Basal Ganglia and Thalamus

Striatal, pallidal, and thalamic abnormalities have been implicated in the expression of dystonia. MER data from the GPi and thalamus in dystonia, as discussed earlier, have demonstrated altered patterns of neuronal activity. Evidence of basal ganglia and thalamic dysfunction has also been seen on positron emission tomography (PET). Early PET studies showed hypermetabolism in the lentiform nucleus that was dissociated from thalamic activity.[79] PET studies of [^{18}F]-spiperone binding, a dopamine agonist, has shown decreased binding of dopamine to the D2 receptor within the striatum.[80]

Pathologic Features of the Cortex

Abnormalities in the motor and sensory systems at the cortical level have been demonstrated in dystonia. Cortical electroencephalographic (EEG) studies have also demonstrated abnormalities in movement-related cortical potentials (MRCPs)[81,82] that are consistent with the notion of abnormal inhibition at the cortical level.[83,84] Investigations using transcranial magnetic stimulation (TMS) have demonstrated increased motor cortex excitability that is due to deficits in intracortical inhibitory interneurons.[85–87]

The literature suggests that increased cortical excitability in dystonia results from a defect in cortical inhibition that is associated with altered gamma-aminobutyric acid (GABA)ergic activity in cortical interneurons. Direct evidence from magnetic resonance (MR) spectroscopy showed that GABA expression is diminished in the motor cortex region in patients with hand dystonia.[88] It is plausible that genetically defined changes in GABA expression may be important in determining the phenotypic expression of dystonia, as well as the variable penetrance of disease.

Functional imaging studies utilizing PET have revealed a wide range of metabolic abnormalities in cortical areas. The most consistent findings are increased activation in premotor cortex (PMC) and rostral supplementary motor areas (rSMAs) associated with joystick movements.[89,90] Hypometabolism in caudal SMAs and the primary sensorimotor cortex has also been consistently reported.[89,91] However, PET studies in patients with acquired hemidystonia showed hypermetabolism of the primary motor cortex suggesting there may be a different pathophysiological mechanism in secondary dystonia.[89] Interestingly, DYT-1 carriers, who do not frankly exhibit the phenotypical symptoms of dystonia, have hypermetabolism in the PMC and rostral SMA, but do not show the corresponding decreased metabolism of the primary sensorimotor cortex.[92]

Dystonia is also associated with changes in the sensory-related cortex. This is consistent with MER data showing abnormal SSRs and widened receptive fields in pallidal and thalamic neurons. Magnetoencephalography (MEG) and functional MRI (fMRI) investigations have demonstrated blurring of the individual digit representations in the hand area of the primary somatosensory cortex in dystonic patients.[93–95] PET studies have also showed decreased metabolism of the primary sensorimotor cortex during vibrotactile stimulation.[96]

These abnormalities can be fit together in a framework to understand the pathophysiology of dystonia. Original pathophysiological models of dystonia focused on the "rate hypothesis" that decreased pallidal output results in overactivity of thalamic motor nuclei and an increase in cortical motor activity. This theory was supported by MER data showing a decreased mean firing rate of GPi neurons and early PET studies that revealed hypermetabolism of the lentiform nucleus that was dissociated from metabolic activity of the thalamus and associated with overactivity in the SMA and primary motor cortex.

Several recent literature reviews have criticized the rate hypothesis as a pathophysiological model for dystonia.[61,68,82] A major flaw in rate hypothesis is its inability to explain how pallidotomy and pallidal stimulation, both of which inhibit pallidal output, can improve dystonia. Furthermore, the results of Hutchinson et al[61] suggest that decreased GPi firing rates may not even be a consistent feature of dystonia.

It is becoming more apparent that changes in the pattern, degree of synchronicity, and somatosensory responsiveness of sensorimotor network neurons must be incorporated into models of this disease. In his model for dystonia, Vitek[68] suggests that dysfunction in the thalamus, cortex, brainstem, and spinal cord occurs secondarily to changes in the globus pallidus. Vitek argues that the increased synchronization and the noncontinuous bursting pattern of pallidal neurons could alter the afferent signals sent to the cortex, contributing to defects in sensorimotor integration and the generation of pathological motor signals. Hutchinson et al state that proprioceptive information is underrepresented in the pallidum of dystonia patients and suggest that dystonia may primarily be a sensory disorder at the level of the basal ganglia.

Future research needs to investigate how specific changes in the globus pallidus and thalamus relate to cortical dysfunction, and it is not yet clear how changes in cortical excitability are related to abnormal movements of dystonia. Proper brain function requires a balance between cortical inhibition and excitation. Ridding et al[97] proposed that cortical inhibition helps focus motor commands so that, during any movement, individual muscles contract with the proper amount of force. Hallet[84] states that the brain activates a specific movement and simultaneously suppresses other possible movements. Deficits in intracortical inhibition could result in pathological overflow activity, causing unwanted muscle contractions in dystonia.

The corticostriatopallidothalamocortical networks that control motor function receive convergent and divergent input from the entire neural axis. Changes in excitation or inhibition to a certain population of neurons are likely to have more subtle effects then simply increasing or decreasing the firing rate of those neurons. Clinical pathology such as unwanted movements and perceptual deficits seen in dystonia may likely be due to subtle changes in temporal coding that affects neuronal responsiveness to specific inputs, and affects the neuron's ability to synchronize with or desynchronize from specific populations of neurons. It has been hypothesized that pathological changes in neural activity resulting in changes in bursting activity and synchronization of thalamic neurons represent a common pathophysiological mechanism in a diverse set of neurological disorders, including movement disorders, psychiatric illnesses, tinnitus, epilepsy, and central pain syndromes.[99,99] The ability of pallidal or thalamic DBS to improve the cardinal symptoms of dystonia, as well as other movement disorders, suggests that these procedures have complex effects on neuronal excitability, synchronization, and firing patterns that modulate the activity in large-scale networks extending well beyond the basal ganglia and thalamus.

■ Results of Deep Brain Stimulation for Dystonia

Currently, the most utilized surgical target for dystonia is the GPi. Thalamic DBS has also been studied, but results have been more variable than pallidal interventions.

Focal Dystonia

There are reports in the literature (**Table 12.1**) of GPi DBS for patients with focal cervical dystonia who suffered from severe disability and pain, and nonsatisfactory response to botulinum toxin injections. Krauss et al[33] report three patients with primary cervical dystonia who underwent bilateral

Table 12.1 Results of Deep Brain Stimulation for Dystonia

Authors	Patients/Diagnosis	Target	Outcomes
Krauss et al 1999	3 patients with adult-onset complex cervical dystonia, ages 42–53	Bilateral posteroventral lateral GPi	Cervical dystonia improved gradually over 3 months with decrease in TWSTRS total severity, total pain, and total functional disability scores
Kumar et al 1999	49-year-old woman with adult-onset primary generalized dystonia and mild dystonic tremor	Bilateral posteroventral lateral GPi	67% improvement in dystonia on BMFDRS score; PET study of joystick movement showed DBS reduced the overactivity in primary motor, lateral premotor, SMA, anterior cingulate, and prefrontal motor cortex bilaterally and ipsilaterally in the lentiform nucleus.
Coubes et al 1999 (French)	8-year-old girl with DYT-1 generalized dystonia, sedated and on a ventilator	Bilateral	Patient was able to return to school and neurological examination was near normal at 30-month follow-up
Islekel et al 1999	42-year-old woman with focal cervical dystonia causing contraction of left sternocleidomastoid	Unilateral stimulation of right GPi	With stimulation, the patient's symptoms were relieved and she was able to rotate her head in all directions without limitation
Coubes et al 2000	7 patients with DYT-1-generalized dystonia (mean age 14 years, 6 months)	Bilateral, posteroventral portion of GPi	60–100% (mean 90.3%) improvement in BMFDRS score at a minimum follow-up of 1 year
Angelini et al 2000	13-year-old, cerebral palsy, secondary dystonia with life-threatening symptoms requiring intubation and sedation in an ICU	Bilateral GPi stimulation	Stimulation resulted in marked improvement of dystonia; at 7 months follow-up patient had regained ability to walk and eat independently and to speak audibly
Tronnier and Fogel 2000	1 patient (age 18, onset age 10) with DYT-1 generalized dystonia, 1 patient (age 27, onset age 8) with non-DYT-1 primary generalized dystonia,1 patient (age 28, onset age 12) with secondary dystonia after birth asphyxia	Bilateral GPi stimulation (3 mm anterior to MCP, 20 mm lateral to mid-line, 4 mm below IC line)	The 2 patients with primary dystonia had marked relief of axial and limb dystonia. DYT-1 patient walked for the first time in several years and had significant speech improvement; the patient with secondary dystonia had subjective improvement that exceeded objective change in BMFDRS score
Loher et al 2000	1 patient (age 24) with left-sided hemidystonia and tremor secondary to a closed head injury. Prior thalamotomy provided only transient amelioration of symptoms	Unilateral stimulation of right posteroventral GPi	At 4-year follow-up, patient had remarkable improvement of dystonia-associated pain, phasic dystonic movements, and dystonic posture (this was a retrospective report and authors did not use standardized rating scales)
Kulisevsky et al 2000	2 patients with primary cervical dystonia and severe pain in neck and shoulders	Bilateral, posteroventral GPi	17–24-month follow-up, minimal or no improvement in dystonia, but marked improvement in pain scores
Andaluz et al 2001	61-year-old male, 10-year history of progressive and disabling secondary cervical and truncal dystonia following trauma to head and neck	Bilateral stimulation of GPi	At 8-month follow-up, 80% subjective improvement. TWSTRS score decreased by 50% with complete resolution of dystonic neck tremor, rare occurrence of upper limb dystonia, and correction of kyphoscoliosis
Gill et al 2001	11-year-old male with cerebral palsy, secondary generalized dystonia and hyperkinetic (ballistic) movement disorder	Bilateral, posteroventral GPi	Extreme flailing movements were abolished; he could initiate movements more easily, but found it more difficult to stop a movement or hold a position; there was overall improvement in quality of life

Table 12.1 (*continued*)

Authors	Patients/Diagnosis	Target	Outcomes
Parkin et al 2001	3 patients with secondary (posttraumatic) focal cervical dystonia (ages 23, 36, 67)	Bilateral, posteroventral GPi	Authors report progressive improvement in pain, voluntary head movement and posture over several months, but residual cervical dystonia and tremor remained
Trottenberg et al (2001a)	70-year-old woman with tardive dystonia (orrobuccolingual dyskinesia, blepharospasm, painful opisthotonic posturing of neck, retropulsive twisting movements of both arms) secondary to neuroleptic medications	Simultaneous implantation of bilateral posteroventrolateral GPi and bilateral Vim stimulators	At 6-month follow-up, the patient showed an improvement in her BMFDRS (73%) and AIMS (54%) scores with bilateral GPi stimulation. Bilateral Vim stimulation alone or simultaneously with pallidal stimulation did not provide any benefit to the patient
Trottenberg et al (2001b)	60-year-old man with inherited myoclonus dystonia syndrome	Bilateral Vim stimulation	Patient myoclonus improved by 80% but there was no significant change in his dystonic symptoms
Muta et al 2001	61-year-old woman, Meige syndrome (blepharospasm and oromandibular dystonia beginning at age 43), s/p bilateral thalamotomy (Voa + Vop) with no improvement	Bilateral GPi stimulation	Stimulation produced 80% improvement on BFMDRS with complete resolution blepharospasm and oromandibular symptoms
Vercueil et al 2001	19 consecutive patients (mean age 24.8); first 12 (4 primary, 8 secondary dystonia) treated with VLp DBS; 3 of these patients had subsequent pallidal DBS after first procedure failed; last 7 patients (5 primary, 2 secondary) underwent pallidal DBS	Bilateral or unilateral stimulation of VLp or GPi	In VLp patients, long-term results were satisfactory for 6/12 patients (especially those with tremor); in GPi patients, long-term results were satisfactory for 7/10 patients (2 patients with GPi electrodes implanted did not have stimulators internalized for chronic stimulation, one b/c of extracranial infection, the other b/c of no response during external test stimulation)
Loher et al 2001	37-year-old with dystonic paroxysmal nonkinesigenic dyskinesia following, pharyngitis and high fever	Unilateral Vim stimulation	At 4-year follow-up, there was significant reduction in the frequency and duration of attacks and the intensity of pain was reduced
Bereznai et al 2002	1 patient with DYT-1 generalized dystonia and 5 patients with primary (adult-onset) cervical (2 patients) or segmental (3 patients) dystonia	Bilateral GPi stimulation (3 mm anterior to MCP, 18–22 mm lateral to midline, 3–6 mm below IC line)	5 patients showed progressive improvement within 7 days; one patient (cervical dystonia and Meige syndrome) showed no improvement at 3 months but beneficial effects were observed at 1 year; overall, BFMDRS scores improved by 72.5% and Tsui scale scores improved by 63%
Krauss et al 2002	5 patients with primary cervical dystonia (ages 28–53)	Bilateral, posteroventral GPi (2–3 mm anterior to MCP, 20–22 mm lateral to midline, 4 mm below IC line)	At 20 months, modified TWSTRS improved by 63% in total severity scores, 50% in total pain scores, and 69% in total functional disability scores
Liu et al 2002	1 patient with familial myoclonic dystonia and primarily cervical symptoms	Bilateral DBS of medial pallidum	At 20-month follow-up, the patient's persistent lateral/horizontal tilt of the neck was abolished; the spontaneous jerking movements and movement-induced myoclonus were also reduced
Ghika et al 2002	Secondary (hypoxic coma following drug overdose) generalized dystonia with necrosis of the globus pallidum bilaterally	Bilateral Voa stimulation after bilateral GPi DBS had failed	After 4–5 months, the patient, who had been wheelchair bound, had decreased dystonic movements, developed independent gait and complete; patient committed suicide soon after

(*continued*)

Table 12.1 (*continued*)

Authors	Patients/Diagnosis	Target	Outcomes
Coubes et al 2002	32 patients all with primary generalized dystonia	Bilateral posteroventrobasal GPi	BMFDRS scores improved 65% at 3 months, 71% at 1 year, and 93% at 2 years in DYT-1+ patients; BMFDS scores improved 65% at 3 months, 74% at 1 year, and 84% at 3 years in non-DYT-1 patients
Goto et al 2002	3 patients with cervical dystonia	Bilateral posteroventral GPi stimulation	Low-frequency stimulation (50–60 Hz) with wide pulse width (500 µs) and high amplitude (4.5–8 V) produced immediate improvement of dystonia and pain that was still present at 1-year follow-up in all 3 patients; stimulation of anterodorsal portion or dorsal border of GPi resulted in significant worsening of symptoms
Vesper et al 2002 (German)	26-year-old with primary generalized dystonia	Bilateral GPi	> 90% improvement on BFMDRS scores at 2 years; patient continued intrathecal baclofen at reduced rate
Krauss et al 2003	2 patients with non-DYT-1 primary generalized dystonia and 4 patients with choreoathetosis secondary to infantile cerebral palsy	Bilateral, posteroventral lateral GPi	In 2 patients with generalized dystonia, BMFDRS improved by 78 and 70% at 2 years; in choreoathetosis, mean improvement was 23% at 2 years which was not significant; 2 patients had subjective improvement that exceeded clinical measures; all patients had improved pain
Yianni et al 2003	14 patients with generalized dystonia and 6 patients with focal cervical dystonia	Bilateral GPi stimulation	In generalized dystonia group (mean follow-up 8.6 months) BMFDRS scores improved 45.8% and in the cervical dystonia group (mean follow-up 19 months), TWSTRS scores improved by 59.5%; analysis of time course of improvement predicts maximum improvement at 1 year for generalized dystonia patients and 2 years for cervical dystonia patients
Cif L et al 2003	Group 1 (15 patients with DYT-1 dystonia); Group 2 (17 patients with non-DYT-1 primary generalized dystonia); Group 3 (21 patients with secondary dystonia)	Bilateral stimulation of posteroventral portion of GPi	Follow-up 1 year: BFMDRS clinical score improved by 71% in DYT-1, 74% in non-DYT-1 primary and 31% in secondary dystonia; the BFMDRS functional score improved by 63% in DYT-1, 49% in non-DYT-1 primary and 7% in secondary dystonia; there was no difference between adults and children

Abbreviations: AIMS, Assessment Instrument for Mental Health Systems; BFMDRS, Burke-Fahn-Marsden Dystonia Rating Scale; DBS, deep brain stimulation; GPi, globus pallidus internus; IC, intracommissural line; ICU, intensive care unit; MCP, midcommissural point; PET, positron emission tomography; SMA, secondary motor area; TWSTRS, Toronto Western Spasmodic Torticollis Rating Scale; Vim, ventral intermediate nucleus; VLp, ventral lateral posterior; Voa, ventro-oralis anterior.

GPi DBS with improvement in TWSTRS scores over 3 months. Islekel et al[100] report that unilateral GPi DBS in a woman with cervical dystonia relieved the patient's symptoms, allowing her to rotate her head in all directions without limitation. However, the outcome was not presented in terms of standardized rating scales. Kulisevsky et al[101] report that bilateral GPi DBS in two patients with primary cervical dystonia and severe pain in the neck and shoulders produced no improvement in dystonia, but a marked decrease in pain scores improved the patients' quality of life. Parkin et al[58] report on three patients with secondary cervical dystonia following traumatic head injuries. Bilateral GPi stimulation resulted in mixed results with improvement in pain, pos-

ture, and voluntary head movement, but residual cervical dystonia and tremor remained. Bereznai et al[102] report two patients with primary cervical dystonia who underwent DBS. One patient initially had complete resolution of symptoms, but they recurred at 3 months in a less severe form. This patient was also able to decrease his daily dose of lorazepam. The other patient had severe retrocollis, which disappeared completely after surgery; however, a clinically insignificant head tremor remained. This patient's pain was also markedly reduced, but analgesic use continued because of dependency issues, and his postoperative course was complicated with a depressive episode. Krauss et al[103] report on five patients with idiopathic focal dystonia who underwent bilateral GPi stimulation. All three patients had a progressive improvement in all categories of the TWSTRS over the course of 1 year, and at a mean follow-up of 20 months, the authors report overall improvements of 63% in the severity score, 69% in the disability score, and 50% in the pain score. Goto et al[104] report immediate improvement of dystonia and pain in three patients with primary cervical dystonia who underwent bilateral GPi stimulation with a low stimulation frequency (50 to 60 Hz), a wide pulse width (500 µs), and a high amplitude (4.5 to 8 V). Yianni et al[105] reported six patients with cervical dystonia who underwent bilateral GPi DBS. These authors report that TWSTRS scores improved by 59.5% at a mean follow-up of 19 months. The authors also studied the time course of improvement and predict that maximal benefit in patients with focal cervical dystonia will not occur for 2 years. Eltahawy et al[113] reported four patients with primary cervical dystonia and mean follow-up period of 15 months with 73% mean reduction in TWSTRS scores. Finally, Bittar et al[106] report 59% improvement in TWSTRS scores of six patients with spasmodic torticollis followed for 2 years after GPi DBS.

There have also been case reports of bilateral GPi DBS for patients with Meige syndrome, a focal dystonia consisting of involuntary chin thrusting, grimacing, and forceful blinking that is also know as hemifacial spasm.[107] Muta et al[108] report on a 61-year-old patient with an 18-year history of Meige syndrome with prior ineffective bilateral thalamotomy (Voa and Vop). She demonstrated an 80% improvement in the BFMDRS with complete resolution of blepharospasm and oromandibular symptoms following bilateral GPi stimulation. Bereznai et al[102] report a 78-year-old woman with segmental dystonia (cervical dystonia and Meige syndrome). This patient had no initial improvement during the first 6 months of bilateral GPi DBS, but a clear decrease in the patient's symptoms was seen at 1 year, after her stimulation parameters were increased. Houser and Waltz[109] reported 75% and 85% improvement in BFMDRS and UDRS scores, respectively, following bilateral DBS of GPi in a 44-year-old female with Meige syndrome.

The foregoing results suggest that there is a role for bilateral GPi stimulation in the treatment of medically refractory focal dystonia that causes severe disability and pain. The wide range of improvement is probably a result of differences in symptoms and etiology of disease, variations in the exact target location within the GPi, and the lack of standardized stimulation parameters for DBS therapy. Prospective trials are needed to develop clear indications, selection criteria, and stimulation parameters for focal dystonia.

Secondary Dystonia

For secondary dystonia, the reported results of DBS therapy have been mixed, reflecting the heterogeneity of the patient population. Some patients demonstrate significant improvement, whereas others have no benefit at all. It has been speculated that the pathophysiology is different in secondary dystonia than in primary dystonia, which could explain the variability of outcomes that have been reported. Angelini et al[110] report on a 13-year-old boy with cerebral palsy, severe dysarthria, and mild cognitive impairment. At the age of 5, the child achieved an autonomous gait. He was stable for many years, but at age 12 he developed severe dystonic spasms associated with ballismus. He lost the ability to walk and his speech worsened. The child eventually developed respiratory failure secondary to dystonic spasms and required artificial respiration and continuous propofol sedation in an intensive care unit setting. The patient underwent bilateral GPi stimulation and by 4 months he had regained autonomous gait and audible speech and was off all medications. Tronnier and Fogel[111] report one patient with secondary generalized dystonia caused by birth asphyxia. At 6 months follow-up, the patient had subjective improvement that exceeded the objective change in his BFMDRS (70 preop and 60 postop). Loher et al[112] report a patient with secondary hemidystonia and a low-frequency tremor of the left arm following a closed head injury suffered during a motor vehicle accident. The patient had no structural lesion on CT or MRI. Three years postinjury, the patient had a thalamotomy, which improved his tremor but not his dystonia. Six years postthalamotomy, the patient underwent unilateral, right GPi stimulation and had "remarkable improvement of dystonia-associated pain, phasic dystonic movements, and dystonic posture, which was accompanied by function gain." These improvements persisted after 4 years of follow-up. Andaluz et al[113] report a case of a 62-year-old male with secondary cervical and trunk dystonia following trauma to the head and neck. Bilateral GPi stimulation of this patient resulted in an 80% subjective improvement and a 50% decrease in TWSTRS scores at 8 months. The patient had complete resolution of dystonic neck tremor and only rare occurrence of upper limb dystonia. The patient had marked kyphoscoliosis preoperatively, which improved with DBS therapy. Trottenberg et al[55] describe a woman with segmental dystonia secondary to neuroleptic medications. At 6 months follow-up, the patient had 73% improvement in her BFMDRS with bilateral GPi stimulation. Gill et al[114] report mixed results in an 11-year-old boy with cerebral palsy and secondary generalized dystonia associated with ballismus. With pallidal stimulation, the boy's flailing arm movements were abolished. He could initiate movements more easily but found it more difficult to stop a movement or hold a fixed position. His overall quality of life was reported to improve. Parkin et al[58] also report mixed results with bilateral GPi stimulation in three patients with secondary (traumatic) cervical dystonia. The patients showed progressive improvement in pain, voluntary head movement, and posture, but residual dystonia and tremor remained. Vercueil et al[115] report mixed results in four patients with secondary dystonia. One patient with postanoxic multifocal dystonia and myoclonus affecting both upper extremities had no improvement following thalamic Vim stimulation, and minimal improvement following bilateral GPi stimulation. A patient with generalized dystonia and bilateral striatal necrosis, with severe and painful rigidity, also had no improvement following thalamic Vim stimulation but had improvements in the BFMDRS of 28% on the movement scale and 41% on the disability scale at 18 months following bilateral GPi stimulation. The third patient, with postanoxic generalized dystonia, had test stimulation but permanent leads were never implanted because there was no initial response. The authors concluded on hindsight that this was a mistake because of reports that maximal improvement with bilateral pallidal stimulation may take 3 months or longer in patients with dystonia. The final patient in this report had posttraumatic hemidystonia. He demonstrated improvements in the BFMDRS of 72% on movement scale and 60% on the disability scale at 1 year following unilateral GPi stimulation. Interestingly, simultaneous GPi and Vim stimulation in this patient did not produce any added benefit. More recently, Cif et al[51] reported on their experience with DBS for dystonia. Their results show that patients with secondary dystonia received the least benefit as a group; however, some individual patients did show significant improvement. The authors also note that pain associated with spasms is significantly decreased, and they conclude that because of pain control plus partial symptomatic improvement, DBS is recommended in select patients with secondary dystonia.

It is difficult to make recommendations based on the few case reports of pallidal stimulation for treatment of secondary dystonia; however, patients without any structural lesions seem to have better outcomes. In addition, those with tardive dystonia seem to have a better outcome. A case report by Ghika et al[54] indicated that bilateral thalamic Voa DBS was effective in alleviating symptoms in a patient with postanoxic generalized dystonia and necrosis of the pallidum, who had failed prior attempts at bilateral pallidal (GPi) DBS. However, there are no other reports of DBS stimulation of this target. Based on the literature, some patients with secondary dystonia do have marked improvement following DBS therapy. However, patients must be selected with care because results are highly variable, and patients with secondary dystonia are more likely to receive no improvement in their functional status following GPi stimulation.

Primary Generalized Dystonia

The literature shows that pallidal DBS on patients with primary generalized dystonia, especially DYT-1 subtypes, yields the best results. Kumar et al[34] first reported a 67% improvement on the BFM scores following bilateral posteroventral lateral GPi stimulation. PET studies in this patient showed that, during joystick movements, DBS therapy reduced the overactivity in cortical motor

areas bilaterally and the lentiform nucleus ipsilaterally. Coubes et al[35] reported an excellent outcome in a patient with DYT-1 dystonia. In 2000, they reported seven patients with DYT-1 dystonia and a 90.3% improvement at 1 year.[116] They also published a retrospective review of 32 patients with primary generalized dystonia. At a mean of 2 years, BFM scores had improved by 93% for DYT-1 and 84% for non-DYT-1 primary generalized dystonia patients. Furthermore, there was no significant difference in outcomes between adults and children.[51,1217] In a case series by Tronnier and Fogel[111] one patient with non-DYT-1 primary generalized dystonia had marked relief of axial and limb symptoms, but his laryngeal dystonia remained. His functional status improved enough that he could learn to drive. A second patient with DYT-1 dystonia was able to walk for the first time in several years, and his speech improved. Vercueil et al[115] reported a 49-year-old woman with primary generalized dystonia who had primarily dystonic tremor of the right upper limb successfully treated with unilateral Vim stimulation. Three years following her first procedure she had generalization of her dystonia with torsion movements involving limbs and trunk. She showed improvements in the BFMDRS of 67%/81% at 1 year. Two other patients, one with DYT-1 dystonia and one with non-DYT-1 primary generalized dystonia, received an 86% and 41% improvement in the BFM movement scores, respectively. Bereznai et al[102] report that one patient with DYT-1 dystonia involving mainly the legs experienced a significant reduction in lower-extremity spasticity, was able to walk without the aid of a cane, and could run for longer distances. Krauss et al[118] report two patients with non-DYT-1 dystonia, who at 2 years follow-up had improvements on BFM scores of 78% and 70% and improvements on the UDRS of 70% and 65%, respectively. Finally, Yianni et al[107] report that 14 patients with primary generalized dystonia received an improvement of 46% on BFM scores on a mean follow-up of 8.6 months. However, the authors comment that, based on the time course of improvement, patients with generalized dystonia would not reach maximal benefit until 1 year.

Thalamic Dystonia

Reports of Vim stimulation for treatment of dystonia have not demonstrated good clinical outcomes. Pollak et al[32] reported the results of 12 patients undergoing Vim DBS for treatment of dystonia. Five patients experienced mild to moderate improvement of limb dystonia, whereas axial symptoms were not improved. Seven patients had no benefit. Trottenberg et al[119] report that Vim stimulation in a patient with inherited myoclonus dystonia improved the patient's myoclonus without any change in dystonic symptoms. A retrospective study by Vercueil et al[115] also demonstrates that the Vim is an inferior target to the GPi.

Editor's Comments

Observations of significant amelioration of dystonic symptoms in patients with primary dystonia undergoing DBS in GPi strongly suggest that this procedure may offer an effective and reliable treatment for patients with dystonia. However, there is only one randomized, blinded stimulation study comparing surgery to medical therapy, and there are only two open-label studies that have reported the effect of bilateral GPi DBS in a reasonably large series of patients using standardized rating scales. Vidailhet et al[120] performed a prospective, controlled, multicenter study assessing the efficacy and safety of bilateral pallidal stimulation in 22 patients with primary generalized dystonia. The dystonia movement score improved from a mean ($\pm$ SD) of 46.3 $\pm$ 21.3 before surgery to 21.0 $\pm$ 14.1 at 12 months ($p <$ .001). The disability score improved from 11.6 $\pm$ 5.5 before surgery to 6.5 $\pm$ 4.9 at 12 months ($p <$ .001). General health and physical functioning were significantly improved at 12 months without significant changes in measures of mood and cognition. During the 3-month randomization, dystonia movement scores were significantly better with neural stimulation than without neural stimulation (24.6 $\pm$ 17.7 vs 34.6 $\pm$ 12.3, $p <$ .001). There is also an ongoing Canadian multicenter trial of pallidal DBS for cervical dystonia.[121]

Of all the remaining studies documenting the benefit of GPi DBS for dystonia, most included only a few patients, many included patients with both primary and secondary dystonia, most provided little long-term follow-up, and many did not use standardized rating scales (**Table 12.1**). Very little data have been provided regarding lead location or optimal stimulation parameters, and little attention has been paid to the role of these variables in predicting clinical outcome. The number of patients is not large enough to allow for the assessment of the role of different clinical variables such as age, genetic status, and lead location and stimulation parameters in determining clinical outcome. It is likely that long-term outcome will be difficult to assess due to loss of patients to follow-up from an already small sample size. Even if such follow-up is obtained, the small sample size precludes determination of clinical variables in predicting long-term outcome. There are few studies assessing the relationship between etiology and inheritance patterns with outcome. Nevertheless, the literature shows that pallidal DBS is very effective for patients with primary generalized dystonia, especially DYT-1 subtypes. Coubes et al[117] reported excellent long-term outcomes in patients with DYT-1 dystonia. Zorzi et al[122] reported the results of bilateral GPi DBS in 12 patients with childhood-onset generalized dystonia refractory to medication, including three patients with status dystonicus. Dystonic postures and movements of the axis and limbs responded to DBS to a greater extent than oromandibular dystonia and fixed dystonic postures. These findings give strong open-label evidence that pallidal stimulation is an effective treatment for intractable childhood-onset dystonia, including status dystonicus, and suggest that GPi DBS should be considered the treatment of choice for these conditions. Although there is general agreement that secondary dystonia is not as responsive as primary,[123] dramatic success has been reported with dystonia-plus syndrome,[72,124] dystonia associated with inherited disorders,[125,126] and drug-induced dystonia.[127,128] There is only one published study addressing the psychiatric and neuropsychological variables associated with GPi DBS in dystonia. Halbig et al[129] reviewed 15 patients treated with bilateral GPi DBS for primary dystonia and at 3 months to 1 year found no deterioration in cognitive scores and neuropsychiatric measures.

The Kinetra (Medtronic, Inc., Minneapolis, MN) provides the best IPG for dystonia because of its expanded parameters and extended battery life (see Chapter 13). However, most neurosurgeons in the United States place the Soletra (Medtronic, Inc., Minneapolis MN) because the Kinetra is not FDA approved for dystonia. Generally stimulation frequencies > 130 Hz and pulse widths > 210 μs have been reported as the most beneficial for patients with dystonia; however, parameters can be modified to obtain the desired benefit, and in many cases larger pulse widths, greater voltages, and the use of two contacts may be necessary.[32,34,39,65,105,130] A study reported a progressive benefit of stimulation at frequencies greater than 130 Hz up to 250 Hz, with a loss of benefit at frequencies of 50 Hz or less.[131] This is in contrast to recent observations[130] and personal observations (Alterman, Vitek, Bakay) of marked improvement in dystonic symptoms with 60 Hz stimulation, comparable with that reported at frequencies $\geq$ 130 Hz; age and duration of symptoms may be critical factors. The ideal stimulation parameters for dystonia remain unclear. In general a trial-and-error approach has been used when programming patients to obtain optimal benefit from the surgical therapy while minimizing side effects. There have been no studies of DBS for dystonia that have evaluated the effect of changing stimulation parameters on clinical outcome. The choice of stimulation frequency has historically been based on previously published reports that stimulation frequencies below 100 Hz were not effective for the treatment of tremor. In Parkinson's disease STN DBS was most effective when frequencies of greater than 130 Hz were used, and a worsening of clinical effect can be seen at a frequency of 5 Hz.[132] The authors concluded that frequency itself is at the origin of the mechanism by which stimulation can mimic ablation. They hypothesized that low-frequency stimulation synchronously activates a large population of STN neurons, whereas higher frequencies lead to either a neuronal blockage or a hypersynchronized activation patterned activity that disrupts the neuronal message. Thus stimulation frequencies > 100 Hz, generally in the range of 130 Hz or higher, have been typically used for the treatment of tremor and PD.

As a result of these observations, most physicians working with DBS have focused on maximizing clinical benefit from adjustments in voltage and pulse width stimulation settings. In most cases of GPi DBS programming in dystonia, a higher pulse width and voltage are needed compared with STN stimulation in PD, perhaps due to stimulating a relatively larger structure. This leads to earlier battery replacements in these patient compared with patients implanted for PD and ET. The effects of various frequencies of stimulation have been studied very little, and most published series have used high-frequency settings (> 150 Hz). Although the use of anesthetic agents may lower GPi firing rates in some cases, there is very strong support for the original observation that rates are lower in patients with dystonia. However, although altered mean discharge *rates* are likely to contribute to the pathogenesis of dystonia and PD, more importance has been given to the role of altered discharge *patterns* and the development of oscillatory synchronization of pallidal neurons in the development of dystonia and PD. Transmission of altered patterns of neuronal activity through the basal ganglia thalamocortical network is disrupted by subthalamic or pallidal stimulation.[133] The observation that stimulation frequencies must be > 100 Hz to be effective for PD may be accounted for by the fact that pallidal neurons in PD are discharging at a mean of 80 to 90 Hz. Effective stimulation frequencies would have to be greater than this to effect a change in the pattern of neuronal activity throughout the network. Similarly, we have observed in dystonia mean discharge rates of 56 ± 20 Hz. Thus we would hypothesize that stimulation frequencies ≥ 60 Hz would be effective in regulating activity in the pallidothalamocortical circuit and would result in an improvement in dystonic symptoms. If 60–90 Hz stimulation is effective for the treatment of dystonia, it will significantly increase the battery life, doubling and even tripling it compared with 130 or 180 Hz stimulation, and will in turn improve the quality of life and reduce the cost for patients undergoing DBS for the treatment of dysto-

nia by reducing the number of battery replacements required over their lifetime. Clearly more research is needed to optimize the IPG settings.

Because most dystonic patients are young, the pallidotomy versus pallidal stimulation arises. Despite the belief that there is a much lower complication rate with DBS, there has been no comparison study with or without randomization. Some have argued that the lifetime of maintenance of bilateral DBS with frequent fractures, almost yearly IPG replacements, and the potential at any time for infection could shift the risk:benefit ratio in favor of pallidotomy.[134] Without data against long-term DBS use, we would definitely continue with DBS because the empirical evidence suggests that the complications are much fewer and less severe. The primary problem with pallidotomy is the lesion-induced (thermal) hemorrhages that are a major source of morbidity that we just have not seen with pallidal DBS. And while there has been a question of loss of efficiency with pallidotomy, long-term (3-year) follow-up with pallidal DBS has shown sustained benefit.[135]

■ Complications

DBS for movement disorders often requires multiple programming sessions to yield the most optimal outcome. In general, the complication rate of DBS therapy for dystonia is believed to be similar to the complication rate of DBS therapy for other indications. A review of the literature demonstrates that DBS therapy can be performed safely in the vast majority of dystonia patients. However, complications of therapy do occur. There have been no reports of perioperative mortality; however, surgical complications included two patients with transient hemiparesis caused by edema of the internal capsule, and a subdural hematoma following headframe placement that did not result in any neurological deficits.[103,115] Reported hardware complications include lead migration, electrode fracture, skin erosions, and infection.[104,107,115–117] The most common complication in DBS for dystonia reported is accidental deactivation of the IPG with immediate return to baseline dystonic symptoms.[103,104,107,116] In all cases, the symptoms resolved within a few hours of stimulation being resumed. Also, side effects of GPi stimulation, including dysarthria, hypophonia, cough, paresthesias, and shuffling gait, have been reported.[55,100,103,118] Two reports of suicide after DBS placement in the GPi have been reported.[136,137] With regard to stimulation side effects, a particular case must be considered separately. In 2003, Pralong et al[136] reported a patient who committed suicide after placement of bilateral GPi and Voa DBS electrode for secondary postanoxic dystonia. Although this patient did have a significant premorbid psychiatric history, it must be considered that stimulation itself may have contributed to this outcome. The motor, limbic, dorsolateral prefrontal, and orbitofrontal loops all pass through the GPi.[138] It is possible that the stimulation needed to affect dystonia symptoms could also have modulated these other loops, resulting in exacerbation in a patient with a predisposition for depression. Therefore, particular weight must be given to the presence of a significant psychiatric history in the perioperative evaluation of dystonia patients for DBS.

A recent article by Umemura et al reviewed the complications of DBS therapy for movement disorders.[139] At the University of Pennsylvania, 109 consecutive patients were implanted with 179 electrodes for various movement disorders. The mortality rate was 1.8%, and the permanent morbidity rate was 4.6%. The overall complication rates were similar to previous reports. At other institutions, mortality ranged from 0 to 2.9%. Reported causes of perioperative death include pulmonary embolism, intracranial hemorrhage, and aspiration pneumonia. Other surgical complications included intracranial hemorrhage (0 to 5%), cerebral contusion (0 to 3%), venous infarction (0 to 0.9%), seizures (0 to 4.5%), pulmonary embolism (0 to 1.8%), and CSF fluid leak (0 to 0.9%). Hardware complication rates at the University of Pennsylvania also compared favorably with those reported at other institutions, including lead migration (0 to 5.1%), electrode fracture (0 to 2.3%), and skin erosion/infection (0 to 15.2%). Stimulation-induced side effects are common, but actual rates have not been reported. For pallidal DBS, stimulation-induced side effects include confusion, depression, increased akinesia, and induction of speech and gait disturbances. These effects are usually mild and are reversible with proper adjustment of the stimulation parameters. There have been multiple reports of patients with borderline cognitive status preoperatively who experienced irreversible dementia following bilateral STN stimulation for PD. However, no cases of DBS-induced dementia have been reported in dystonia.

■ Intermittent Pulse Generator Programming Considerations

DBS for movement disorders often requires multiple programming sessions to yield the best results. This is even more pronounced in DBS for dystonia where benefits may take months or years to manifest. A careful review of the literature suggests a variable pattern of benefit onset from a few hours to several months. Maximal benefit may not be seen for 1 to 2 years.[97] There is a suggestion that the abnormal phasic movements of dystonia may resolve more quickly than the other symptoms such as abnormal posturing and gait disorders, sometimes within minutes or hours.[106] Whether this is due to the inherent nature of DBS on dystonic networks or the result of inexperience with the necessary parameters for dystonia symptoms remains to be seen.

Because the effects of GPi DBS on dystonia may be delayed and gradual, it is generally quite useful to allow at least 24 hours of continuous stimulation on any one setting before assessing the efficacy of stimulation. Therefore, in patients who do not exhibit a relatively quick response, sessions can be relatively brief with assessment of settings put into place during the last session and instituting new settings to be assessed during the next session. Despite this heterogeneity, some useful guidelines can be proposed following many of the same principles used for PD.[111]

Generally, DBS for dystonia requires higher voltages, pulse widths, and frequencies than corresponding PD patients. Bipolar stimulation should be assessed initially, followed by unipolar stimulation if the former is suboptimal. If higher-frequency settings are ineffective, a trial of low-frequency stimulation at 50 Hz can be considered.[111] In our experience, a typical PD patient has best results with 3 to 3.5 V, 90 μs, and 100 to 130 Hz. The dystonia patients generally require 4 to 5.5 V, 210 to 240 μs, and 160 to 185 Hz.

■ Conclusion

DBS for dystonia is a promising but emerging therapy. Although the disease itself consists of a heterogeneous population, in terms of both etiology and phenotypic expression, the patients that fail conservative therapy are all severely disabled without means of relief. These patients may benefit from DBS surgery. As our understanding of the pathophysiology and the underlying neural network of dystonia improves, the optimal target for surgical intervention will emerge. This along with enhanced insights into DBS mechanisms and studies assessing benefits of DBS for specific groups of dystonias will improve the variable results seen in today's efforts.

References

1. Oppenheim H. Uber eine eigenartige Krampfkrankheit des Kindlichen Alters (Dysbasia lordotica progressive. Dystonia musculorum deformans). Neurol Centrabl 1911;30:1090–1107
2. de Carvalho Aguiar PM, Ozelius LJ. Classification and genetics of dystonia. Lancet Neurol 2002;1:316–325
3. Greene P, Kang UJ, Fahn S. Spread of symptoms in idiopathic torsion dystonia. Mov Disord 1995;10:143–152
4. Fahn S, Bressman S, Marsden CD. Classification of dystonia. Adv Neurol 1998;78:1–10
5. Meyers R. Surgical procedure for postencephalitic tremor with notes on the physiology of premotor fibers. Arch Neurol Psychiatry 1940;44:455–459
6. Meyers R. The present state of neurosurgical procedures directed against extrapyramidal disease. N Y State J Med 1942;42:317–325
7. Guiot G, Brion S. Traitement neurochirurgical des syndromes choreo-athetosique et parkinsonien. Sem Hop Paris 1952;28:2095–2099
8. Hassler R, Riechert T. Indikationen und Lokalisationmethode der gezielten Hirnoperationen. Nervenarzt 1954;25:441–447
9. Cooper IS. Dystonia musculorum deformans: natural history and neurosurgical alleviation. J Pediatr 1969;74:585–592
10. Bertrand C, Molina NP, Martinez SN. Combined stereotactic and peripheral surgical approach for spasmodic torticollis. Appl Neurophysiol 1978;41:122–133
11. Laitinen LV, Bergenheim AT, Hariz MI. Leksell's posteroventral pallidotomy in the treatment of Parkinson's disease. J Neurosurg 1992;76:53–61
12. Cooper IS. 20-year follow-up of the neurosurgical treatment of dystonia musculorum deformans. Adv Neurol 1976;14:423–452
13. Gros C, Frerebeau PH, Perez-Dominguez E, et al. Long-term results of stereotactic surgery for infantile dystonia and dyskinesia. Neurochirurgia (Stuttg) 1976;19:171–178
14. Kandel EI. Functional and Stereotactic Neurosurgery. Watts G, trans. New York: Plenum; 1989
15. Andrew J, Fowler CJ, Harrison MJD. Stereotaxic thalamotomy in 55 cases of dystonia. Brain 1983;106:981–1000
16. Svennilson E, Torvik A, Lowe R, et al. Treatment of Parkinsonism stereotactic thermolesions in the pallidal region: a clinical evaluation of 81 cases. Acta Psychiatr Scand 1960;35:358–377
17. Iacono RP, Kuniyosji SM, Lonser RR, et al. Simultaneous bilateral pallidoansotomy for idiopathic dystonia musculorum deformans. Pediatr Neurol 1996;14:145–148
18. Lozano AM, Kumar R, Gross RE, et al. Globus pallidus internus pallidotomy for generalized dystonia. Mov Disord 1997;12:865–870
19. Lin JJ, Lin GY, Shih C, et al. Benefit of bilateral pallidotomy in the treatment of generalized dystonia. J Neurosurg 1999;90:974–976
20. Ondo WG, Desaloms JM, Jankovic J, et al. Pallidotomy for generalized dystonia. Mov Disord 1998;13:693–698
21. Vitek JL, Zhang J, Evatt M, et al. GPi pallidotomy for dystonia: clinical outcome and neuronal activity. Adv Neurol 1998;78:211–219
22. Hua Z, Guodong G, Qinchuan L, et al. Analysis of complications of radiofrequency pallidotomy. Neurosurgery 2003;52:89–99 discussion 99–101

23. Krauss JK, Toups EG, Jankovic J, et al. Symptomatic and functional outcome of surgical treatment of cervical dystonia. J Neurol Neurosurg Psychiatry 1997;63:642–648

24. Hassler R, Reichert T, Mundinger F, et al. Physiologic observations in stereotaxic operations in extrapyramidal motor disturbances. Brain 1960;83:337–356

25. Mundinger F. Neue stereotaktisch-funktionelle Behandlungsmethode des torticollis spasmodicus mit Hirnstimulatoren. Med Klin 1977;72:1982–1986

26. Andy OJ. Thalamic stimulation for control of movement disorders. Appl Neurophysiol 1983;46:107–123

27. Siegfried J. Effets de la stimulation du noyau sensitive du thalamus sur les dyskinesies et la spasticite. Rev Neurol (Paris) 1986;142:380–383

28. Sellal F, Hirsh E, Barth P, et al. A case of symptomatic hemidystonia improved by ventrolateral thalamic stimulation. Mov Disord 1993;8:515–518

29. Benabid AL, Pollak P, Louveau A, et al. Combined (thalamotomy and stimulation) stereotactic surgery of the Vim thalamic nucleus for bilateral Parkinson's disease. Appl Neurophysiol 1987;50:344–346

30. Pollak P, Benabid AL, Gross C, et al. Effet de la stimulation du noyau sous-thalamique dans la maladie de Parkinson. Rev Neurol (Paris) 1993;148:175–176

31. Siegfried J, Lippitz B. Bilateral chronic electrostimulation of ventroposterolateral pallidum: a new therapeutic approach for alleviating all parkinsonian symptoms. Neurosurgery 1994;35:1126–1130

32. Pollak P, Benabid AL, Krack P, et al. Deep brain stimulation. In: Jankovic J, Tolosa E, eds. Parkinson's Disease and Movement Disorders. Baltimore: Williams and Wilkins; 1998:1085–1101

33. Krauss JK, Pohle T, Weber S, et al. Bilateral stimulation of the globus pallidus internus for treatment of cervical dystonia. Lancet 1999;354:837–838

34. Kumar R, Dagher A, Hutchinson WD, et al. Globus pallidus deep brain stimulation for generalized dystonia: clinical and PET investigation. Neurology 1999;53:871–874

35. Coubes P, Echenne B, Roubertie A, et al. Traitement de la dystonie generalisee a debut precoce par stimulation chronique bilaterale des globus pallidus internes: a propos d'un cas. Neurochirurgie 1999;45:139–144

36. Bronte-Stewart H. Surgical therapy for dystonia. Curr Neurol Neurosci Rep 2003;3:296–305

37. Volkmann J, Benecke R. Deep brain stimulation for dystonia: patient selection and evaluation. Mov Disord 2002;17(Suppl 3):S112–S115

38. Burke RE, Fahn S, Marsden CD. Torsion dystonia: a double-blind, prospective trial of high-dosage trihexyphenidyl. Neurology 1986;36:160–164

39. Greene P, Sable H, Fahn S. Analysis of open-label trials in torsion dystonia using high dosages of anticholinergics and other drugs. Mov Disord 1988;3:46–60

40. Jabbari B, Scherokman B, Gunderson CH, et al. Treatment of movement disorders with trihexyphenidyl. Mov Disord 1989;4:202–212

41. Goldman JG, Comella CL. Treatment of dystonia. Clin Neuropharmacol 2003;26:102–108

42. Albright AL, Barry MJ, Fasick P, et al. Continuous intrathecal baclofen infusion for symptomatic generalized dystonia. Neurosurgery 1996;38:934–939

43. Karp BI, Goldstein SR, Chen R, et al. An open trial of clozapine for dystonia. Mov Disord 1999;14:652–659

44. Jankovic J, Schwartz K, Donovan DT. Botulinum toxin treatment of cranial-cervical dystonia, spasmodic dysphonia, other focal dystonias, and hemifacial spasm. J Neurol Neurosurg Psychiatry 1990;53:633–639

45. Ondo WG, Desaloms M, Krauss JK, et al. Pallidotomy and thalamotomy for dystonia. In: Krauss JK, Jankovic J, Grossman RG, eds. Surgery for Parkinson's Disease and Movement Disorders. Philadelphia: Lippincott Williams & Wilkins; 2001:299–306

46. Jankovic J. Treatment of dystonia. In: Watts RL, Koller WC, eds. Movement Disorders: Neurologic Principles and Practice. New York: McGraw-Hill; 1997:443–454

47. Comella CL, Leurgans S, Wuu J, et al. Rating scales for dystonia: a multicenter assessment. Mov Disord 2003;18:303–312

48. Comella CL, Stebbins GT, Goetz CG, et al. Teaching tape for the motor section of the Toronto Western Spasmodic Torticollis Scale. Mov Disord 1997;12:570–575

49. Cooper IS. 20-year follow-up of the neurosurgical treatment of dystonia musculorum deformans. Adv Neurol 1976;14:423–452

50. Tasker RR, Doorly T, Yamashiro K. Thalamotomy in generalized dystonia. Adv Neurol 1988;50:615–633

51. Cif L, El Fertit H, Vayssiere N, et al. Treatment of dystonic syndromes by chronic electrical stimulation of the internal globus pallidus. J Neurosurg Sci 2003;47:52–55

52. Schuurman PR, Bosch DA, Bossuyt PM, et al. A comparison of continuous thalamic stimulation and thalamotomy for suppression of severe tremor. N Engl J Med 2000;342:461–468

53. Krack P, Batir A, Van Blercom N, et al. Five-year follow-up of bilateral stimulation of the subthalamic nucleus in advanced Parkinson's disease. N Engl J Med 2003;349:1925–1934

54. Ghika J, Villemure MD, Miklossy J, et al. Postanoxic generalized dystonia improved by bilateral Voa thalamic deep brain stimulation. Neurology 2002;58:311–313

55. Trottenberg T, Paul G, Meissner W, et al. Pallidal and thalamic neurostimulation in severe tardive dystonia. J Neurol Neurosurg Psychiatry 2001;70:557–559

56. Starr PA. Placement of deep brain stimulators into the subthalamic nucleus or globus pallidus internus: technical approach. Stereotact Funct Neurosurg 2002;79:118–145

57. Vayssiere N, Hemm S, Zanca M, et al. Magnetic resonance imaging stereotactic target localization for deep brain stimulation in dystonic children. J Neurosurg 2000;93:784–790

58. Parkin S, Aziz T, Gregory R, et al. Bilateral internal globus pallidus stimulation for the treatment of spasmodic torticollis. Mov Disord 2001;16:489–493

59. Lozano AM, Hutchinson WD. Microelectrode recordings in the pallidum. Mov Disord 2002;17(Suppl 3):S150–S154

60. Starr PA, Christine CW, Theodosopoulos PV, et al. Implantation of deep brain stimulators into the subthalamic nucleus: technical approach and magnetic resonance imaging verified lead locations. J Neurosurg 2002;97:370–387

61. Hutchison WD, Lang AE, Dostrovsky JO, et al. Pallidal neuronal activity: implications for models of dystonia. Ann Neurol 2003;53:480–488

62. Starr PA, Marks WJ, Lindsey N, et al. Pallidal deep brain stimulation for dystonia: technical approach and magnetic resonance imaging-verified electrode locations. Abstract presented at: Annual Meeting of the Congres of Neurological Surgeons; 2003; Denver, Colorado

63. Cardoso F, Jankovic J, Grossman RG, Hamilton WJ. Outcome after stereotactic thalamotomy for dystonia and hemiballismus. Neurosurgery 1995;36:501–508

64. Vitek JL, Bakay RA, DeLong MR. Microelectrode-guided pallidotomy for medically intractable Parkinson's disease. Adv Neurol 1997;74:183–198

65. Gross RE, Lombardi WJ, Lang AE, et al. Relationship of lesion location to clinical outcome following microelectrode-guided pallidotomy for Parkinson's disease. ([see comments]) Brain 1999;122(Pt 3): 405–416

66. Eskandar EN, Cosgrove GR, Shinobu LA, Penney JB. The importance of accurate lesion placement in posteroventral pallidotomy: report of two cases. J Neurosurg 1998;89:630–634

67. Bronte-Stewart H, Hill B, Molander M, et al. Lesion location predicts clinical outcome of pallidotomy. Mov Disord 1998;13:300

68. Vitek JL. Pathophysiology of dystonia: a neuronal model. Mov Disord 2002;17(Suppl 3):S49–S62

69. Vitek JL, Bakay RAE, Hashimoto T, et al. Microelectrode-guided pallidotomy: technical approach and application for medically intractable Parkinson's disease. J Neurosurg 1998;88:1027–1043

70. Steigerwald F, Hinz L, Pinsker MO et al. Effect of propofol on pallidal neuronal discharges in generalized dystonia. Neurosci Lett 2005;386:156–159

71. Starr PA, Rau GM, Davis V, et al. Spontaneous pallidal neuronal activity in human dystonia: comparison with Parkinson's disease and normal macaque. J Neurophysiol 2005;93:3165–3176

72. Magarinos-Ascone CM, Regidor I, Martinez-Castrillo JC, Gomez-Galan M, Figueiras-Mendez R. Pallidal stimulation relieves myoclonus-dystonia syndrome. J Neurol Neurosurg Psychiatry 2005;76:989–991

73. Holloway KL, Gaede SE, Starr PA, Rosenow JM, Ramakrishnan V, Henderson JM. Frameless stereotaxy using bone fiducial markers for deep brain stimulation. J Neurosurg 2005;103:404–413

74. Lenz FA, Suarez JI, Metman LV, et al. Pallidal activity during dystonia: somatosensory reorganization and changes with severity. J Neurol Neurosurg Psychiatry 1998;65:767–770

75. Vitek JL, Chockkan V, Zhang JY, et al. Neuronal activity in the basal ganglia in patients with generalized dystonia and hemiballismus. Ann Neurol 1999;46:22–35

76. DeLong MR. Activity of pallidal neurons during movement. J Neurophysiol 1971;34:414–427

77. Lenz FA, Byl NN. Reorganization in the cutaneous core of the human thalamic principal somatic sensory nucleus (ventral caudal) in patients with dystonia. J Neurophysiol 1999;82:3204–3212

78. Lenz FA, Jaeger CJ, Seike MS, et al. Thalamic single neuron activity in patients with dystonia: dystonia-related activity and somatic sensory reorganization. J Neurophysiol 1999;82:2372–2392

79. Eidelberg D. Abnormal brain networks in DYT1 dystonia. Adv Neurol 1998;78:127–133

80. Perlmutter JS, Stambuk MK, Markham J, et al. Decreased [18F] Spiperone binding in putamen in idiopathic focal dystonia. J Neurosci 1997;17:843–850

81. van der Kamp W, Rothwell JC, Thompson PD, et al. The movement related cortical potential is abnormal in patients with idiopathic torsion dystonia. Mov Disord 1995;10:630–633

82. Kaji R, Ikeda A, Ikeda T, et al. Physiologic study of cervical dystonia: task specific abnormality in contingent negative variation. Brain 1995;118:511–522

83. Tinazzi M, Rosso T, Fiaschi A. Role of the somatosensory system in primary dystonia. Mov Disord 2003;18:605–622

84. Hallett M. Dystonia: abnormal movements result from loss of inhibition. Adv Neurol 2004;94:1–9

85. Ikoma K, Samli A, Mercuri B, et al. Abnormal cortical motor excitability in dystonia. Neurology 1996;46:1371–1376

86. Filipovic SR, Ljubisavljevic M, Svetel M, et al. Impairment of cortical inhibition in writers cramp as revealed by changes in electromyographic silent period after transcranial magnetic stimulation. Neurosci Lett 1997;222:167–170

87. Rona S, Berardelli A, Inghilleri M, et al. Alterations of motor cortical inhibition in patients with dystonia. Mov Disord 1998;13:118–124

88. Levy LM, Hallett M. Impaired brain GABA in focal dystonia. Ann Neurol 2002;51:93–101

89. Ceballos-Baumann AO, Brooks DJ. Activation positron emission tomography scanning in dystonia. Adv Neurol 1998;78:135–152

90. Filipovic SR, Siebner HR, Rowe JB, et al. Modulation of cortical activity by repetitive transcranial magnetic stimulation (rTMS): a review of functional imaging studies and the potential use in dystonia. Adv Neurol 2004;94:45–52

91. Playford ED, Passingham RE, Marsden CD, et al. Increased activation of frontal areas during arm movement in idiopathic torsion dystonia. Mov Disord 1998;13:309–318

92. Ghilardi MF, Carbon M, Silvestri G, et al. Impaired sequence learning in carriers of the DYT1 dystonia mutation. Ann Neurol 2003;54:102–109

93. Bara-Jimenez W, Catalan MJ, Hallet M, et al. Abnormal somatosensory homunculus in dystonia of the hand. Ann Neurol 1998;44:828–831

94. Elbert T, Candia V, Atenmuller E, et al. Alteration of digital representations in somatosensory cortex in focal hand dystonia. Neuroreport 1998;9:3571–3575

95. Butterworth S, Francis S, Kelly E, McGlone F, Bowtll R, Sawle G. Abnormal cortical sensory activation in dystonia: an fMRI study. Mov Disord 2003;18:673–682

96. Tempel LW, Perlmutter JS. Abnormal vibration-induced cerebral blood flow responses in idiopathic dystonia. Brain 1990;113:691–707

97. Ridding MC, Sheean G, Rothwell JC, et al. Changes in the balance between motor cortical excitation and inhibition in focal task specific dystonia. J Neurol Neurosurg Psychiatry 1995;59: 493–498

98. Llinas R, Ribary U, Jeanmonod D, et al. Thalamocortical dysrhythmia, I: Functional and imaging aspects. Thalamus Relat Syst 2001;1: 237–244

99. Jeanmonod D, Magnin M, Morel A, et al. Thalamocortical dysrhythmia, II: Clinical and surgical aspects. Thalamus Relat Syst 2001;1:245–254

100. Islekel S, Zileli M, Zileli B. Unilateral pallidal stimulation in cervical dystonia. Stereotact Funct Neurosurg 1999;72:248–252

101. Kulisevsky J, Lleo A, Gironell A, et al. Bilateral pallidal stimulation for cervical dystonia: dissociated pain and motor improvement. Neurology 2000;55:1754–1755

102. Bereznai B, Steude U, Seelos K, et al. Chronic high-frequency globus pallidus internus stimulation in different types of dystonia: a clinical, video, and MRI report of six patients presenting with segmental, cervical, and generalized dystonia. Mov Disord 2002;17:138–144

103. Krauss JK, Loher TJ, Pohle T, et al. Pallidal deep brain stimulation in patients with cervical dystonia and severe cervical dyskinesias with cervical myelopathy. J Neurol Neurosurg Psychiatry 2002;72:249–256

104. Goto S, Mita S, Ushio Y. Bilateral pallidal stimulation for cervical dystonia. Stereotact Funct Neurosurg 2002;79:221–227

105. Yianni J, Bain PG, Gregory RP, et al. Post-operative progress of dystonia patients following globus pallidus internus deep brain stimulation. Eur J Neurol 2003;10:239–247

106. Bittar RG, Yianni J, Wang S, et al. Deep brain stimulation for generalised dystonia and spasmodic torticollis. J Clin Neurosci 2005;12: 12–16

107. Meige H. Les Convulsions de la face: une forme clinique de convulsion faciale, bilaterale et mediane. Rev Neurol 1910;10: 437–443

108. Muta D, Goto S, Nishikawa S, et al. Bilateral pallidal stimulation for idiopathic segmental axial dystonia advanced from Meige syndrome refractory to bilateral thalamotomy. Mov Disord 2001;16: 774–777

109. Houser M, Waltz T. Meige syndrome and pallidal deep brain stimulation. Mov Disord 2005;20:1203–1205

110. Angelini L, Nardocci N, Estienne M, et al. Life-threatening dystonia-dyskinesias in a child: successful treatment with bilateral pallidal stimulation. Mov Disord 2000;15:1010–1012

111. Tronnier VM, Fogel W. Pallidal stimulation for generalized dystonia. J Neurosurg 2000;92:453–456

112. Loher TJ, Hasdemir MG, Burgunder JM, et al. Long-term follow-up study of chronic globus pallidus internus stimulation for posttraumatic hemidystonia. J Neurosurg 2000;92:457–460

113. Andaluz N, Taha JM, Dalvi A. Bilateral pallidal deep brain stimulation for cervical and truncal dystonia. Neurology 2001;57:557–558

114. Gill S, Curran A, Tripp J, et al. Hyperkinetic movement disorder in an 11-year-old child treated with bilateral pallidal stimulators. Dev Med Child Neurol 2001;43:350–353

115. Vercueil L, Pollak P, Fraix V, et al. Deep brain stimulation in the treatment of severe dystonia. J Neurol 2001;248:695–700

116. Coubes P, Roubertie A, Vayssiere N, et al. Treatment of DYT1-generalized dystonia by stimulation of the internal globus pallidus. Lancet 2000;355:2220–2222

117. Coubes P, Cif L, El Fertit H, et al. Electrical stimulation of the globus pallidus internus in patients with primary generalized dystonia: long-term results. J Neurosurg 2004;101:189–194

118. Krauss JK, Loher TJ, Weigel R, et al. Chronic stimulation of the globus pallidus internus for treatment of non-DYT1 generalized dystonia and choreoathetosis: 2-year follow up. J Neurosurg 2003;98:785–792

119. Trottenberg T, Meissner W, Arnold G, et al. Neurostimulation of the ventral intermediate thalamic nucleus in inherited myoclonus-dystonia syndrome. Mov Disord 2001;16:769–771

120. Vidailhet M, Vercueil L, Houeto JL, et al. Bilateral deep-brain stimulation of the globus pallidus in primary generalized dystonia. N Engl J Med 2005;352:459–467

121. Kiss ZH, Doig K, Eliasziw M, Ranawaya R, Suchowersky O. The Canadian multicenter trial of pallidal deep brain stimulation for cervical dystonia: preliminary results in three patients. Neurosurg Focus 2004;17:E5

122. Zorzi G, Marras C, Nardocci N, et al. Stimulation of the globus pallidus internus for childhood-onset dystonia. Mov Disord 2005;20:1194–1200

123. Eltahawy HA, Saint-Cyr J, Giladi N, et al. Primary dystonia is more responsive than secondary dystonia to pallidal interventions: outcome after pallidal deep brain stimulation. Neurosurgery 2004;54:613–619

124. Cif L, Valente EM, Hemm S, et al. Deep brain stimulation in myoclonus dystonia syndrome. Mov Disord 2004;19:724–727

125. Castelnau P, Cif L, Valente EM, et al. Pallidal stimulation improves pantothenate kinase-associated neurodegeneration. Ann Neurol 2005;57:738–741

126. Umemura A, Jaggi JL, Dolinskas CA, Stern MB, Baltuch GH. Pallidal deep brain stimulation for longstanding severe generalized dystonia in Hallervorden-Spatz syndrome: case report. J Neurosurg 2004;100:706–709

127. Trottenberg T, Volkmann J, Deuschl G, et al. Treatment of severe tardive dystonia with pallidal deep brain stimulation. Neurology 2005;64:344–346

128. Franzini A, Marras C, Ferroli P, et al. Long-term high-frequency bilateral pallidal stimulation for neuroleptic-induced tardive dystonia: report of two cases. J Neurosurg 2005;102:721–725

129. Halbig TD, Gruber D, Kopp UA, Schneider GH, Trottenberg T, Kupsch A. Pallidal stimulation in dystonia: effects on cognition, mood, and quality of life. J Neurol Neurosurg Psychiatry 2005; 76:1713–1716

130. Kumar R. Methods for programming and patient management with deep brain stimulation of the globus pallidus for the treatment of advanced Parkinson's disease and dystonia. Mov Disord 2002;17(Suppl 3):S198–S207

131. Kupsch A, Klaffke S, Kuhn AA, et al. The effects of frequency in pallidal deep brain stimulation for primary dystonia. J Neurol 2003;250:1201–1205

132. Moro E, Esselink RJ, Xie J, Hommel M, Benabid AL, Pollak P. The impact on Parkinson's disease of electrical parameter settings in STN stimulation. Neurology 2002;59:706–713

133. Hashimoto T, Elder CM, Okun MS, Patrick SK, Vitek JL. Stimulation of the subthalamic nucleus changes the firing pattern of pallidal neurons. J Neurosci 2003;23:1916–1923

134. Okun MS, Vitek JL. Lesion therapy for Parkinson's disease and other movement disorders: update and controversies. Mov Disord 2004;19:375–389

135. Vidailhet M, Vercueil L, Houeto JL, Krystkowiak P, Lagrange C, Yelnik J, et al. Bilateral, pallidal, deep-brain stimulation in primary generalised dystonia: a prospective 3 year follow-up study. Lancet Neurol 2007;6:223–229

136. Pralong E, Debatisse D, Maeder M, et al. Effect of deep brain stimulation of GPI on neuronal activity of the thalamic nucleus ventralis oralis in a dystonic patient. Neurophysiol Clin 2003;33:169–173

137. Foncke EM, Schuurman PR, Speelman JD. Suicide after deep brain stimulation of the internal globus pallidus for dystonia. Neurology 2006;66:142–143

138. Alexander GE, DeLong MR, Strick PL. Parallel organization of functionally segregated circuits linking basal ganglia and cortex. Annu Rev Neurosci 1986;9:357–381

139. Umemura A, Jaggi JL, Hurtig HI, et al. Deep brain stimulation for movement disorders: morbidity and mortality in 109 patients. J Neurosurg 2003;98:779–784

13 Deep Brain Stimulation Programming

Erwin B. Montgomery Jr.

Deep brain stimulation (DBS) is already standard therapy for several chronic neurological conditions, including Parkinson disease (PD), essential tremor, cerebellar outflow tremor such as that due to multiple sclerosis, and dystonia.[1-4] Clinical trials are under way or planned for epilepsy, obsessive-compulsive disorder, depression, and minimally conscious state patients. With regard to PD, DBS has helped patients for whom the most aggressive pharmacological interventions[1] and fetal cell transplants have failed.[5] Yet, despite the remarkable efficacy, fewer than anticipated numbers of patients are being referred for DBS. There are many factors contributing to this underutilization. One of them is the perceived difficulty in managing these patients postoperatively.

The central theme of this chapter is that effective postoperative DBS adjustments are not happenstance or the result of random chance. Nor should programming be based solely on historical precedent, which risks perpetuating misconceptions. "Cookbooks" are ineffective given the variability among patients and the over 4000 possible combinations of stimulation parameters (active contacts, voltage, pulse width, and frequency). There are principles that guide DBS management. These principles are based on electrophysiological properties and the regional functional anatomy surrounding the DBS lead. DBS management is primarily science with a little art. As a science, it can be learned by a rational approach that does not depend solely on the experience of the DBS adjuster. A programmer has to decide whether to invent a sufficiently large cookbook with the potential to address the multitude of programming problems, or to invest in learning a handful of principles that can be recombined and tailored to any number of patients. Efficient strategies for DBS programming are important for cost-effective and timely care.

An important concept is that the therapeutic benefit of DBS is related to adequate activation of target structures. Factors include the volume of brain stimulated and the number of neuronal elements activated within that volume. Generally, the volume of brain activated is related to the size of the electrical field generated by DBS. The number of neuronal elements within the volume activated is related to the current density, which is the concentration of electrons (ions) within the electrical field. Thus effective activation is a complex interaction of electrical field size and strength and the unique properties of the neuronal elements affected.

DBS injects electrical charge into the brain. With metallic conductors, charge is in terms of electrons. In the brain, charge is mediated by ions. To facilitate use of the analogy of DBS to electronics, electrons and ions will be used interchangeably. We can manipulate the size of the electrical field by adjusting the voltage and the combinations of active DBS contacts. We can manipulate the current densities within the electrical field by changing the configuration of the active DBS contacts. For example, monopolar stimulation, where a single contact on the DBS lead acts as the cathode (negative contact) and the impulse generator case acts as the anode (positive contact), generates less concentrated current densities compared with bipolar where the anode and cathode are on the DBS lead.

The side effects of DBS are directly related to stimulation of unintended structures. This will depend on the unique regional anatomy of the individual patient and the orientation of that patient's DBS lead to the regional anatomy. This means that the shape, size, and strength of the electrical field will be critical. We can manipulate the shape, size, and strength of the electrical field by changing the configurations of the active contacts on the DBS lead.

◾ Basic Electrophysiology

There is clear evidence that DBS excites a variety of neuronal elements and that it does not inhibit neuronal activity, at least directly.[6,7] We use the term *neuronal elements* because we do not know which specific elements, such as axon initial segments, internodes, cell bodies, and/or dendrites, mediate the DBS effect. How are neuronal elements excited?

The Action Potential

Neuronal activation requires generation of an electrical impulse across the cell membrane that is transmitted down the axon to the next neuron.[8] Electrical impulses generated are in the form of electrically charged ions that flow across the cell membrane. For electrically charged ions to flow, there must be a force that will move the ions. This force is called the membrane voltage and is the difference between the forces on each side of the membrane. This difference in force across the membrane is generated by pumping sodium (Na^+) out of the cell and in exchange moving potassium (K^+) ions in. The resulting difference in Na^+ and K^+ (and other ions as well) creates a chemical concentration difference (gradient) that will tend to move ions, for example, Na⁺ into the cell and K⁺ out. When these ions flow across the cell membrane in sufficient quantity, there is an electrical impulse called the action potential (**Fig. 13.1**).

The cell membrane resists the flow of ions and therefore, the generation of an electrical impulse or action potential. However, channels in the cell membrane can open allowing ions to flow across the cell membrane and generate an electrical impulse. One way to open these channels is to change the voltage inside the cell relative to the voltage outside. If the inside of the cell becomes less negative (called depolarization) to a certain threshold, then the channels open and allow the flow of ions and the creation of an electrical impulse or action potential. DBS acts to depolarize the cell membrane, to open the channels and create an electrical impulse (**Fig. 13.1**).

To depolarize the neuronal cell membrane, DBS has to drive electrical current, which is the flow of electrical charges, into the neuron across the cell membrane. The voltage of the DBS pulse is what drives the current into the neuron. Thus, by controlling the voltage we can control which and how many neurons are depolarized to generate action potentials. Also, the longer the duration of the DBS pulse (pulse width) the more current will be driven into the neuron, and there will be greater depolarization and greater probability of generating an axon potential. Thus we can see that already we have two means to control the generation of action potentials, voltage and pulse width.

Voltage

The size and shape of neuronal elements can vary greatly. We can take advantage of this variability to control which neuronal elements are activated by DBS. Smaller-diameter neuronal elements such as axons are excited at lower voltages than large elements such as neuronal cell bodies. However, larger-diameter axons are excited at lower voltages than small-diameter axons. Thus, by controlling the voltage we can control which neuronal elements are activated. Also, the voltage generated in the brain tissue

decreases the further the distance from the electrode. By controlling the voltage we can control the volume of tissue that experiences sufficient voltage to generate action potentials.

Pulse Width

Controlling the pulse width also controls which neuronal elements are activated. Small elements, such as axons, can be activated by smaller pulse widths than large elements such as neuronal cell bodies (**Fig. 13.2**). One could imagine the DBS electrical stimulus driving electrons (ions) into a neuronal element. The amount of electrons (ions) will depend on how long the electrical pulse is applied (pulse width). The longer the pulse width, the more electrons (ions) are pumped into the neuronal element. However, once the electrons (ions) enter the neuronal element such as cell body compared to axon, they are diluted by the intracellular contents. The larger the neuronal element, such as cell body compared to axon, the more the intracellular contents, and the new electrons (ions) that have entered the neuronal element will be more dilute. This will result in less depolarization; therefore, this will have a lower probability of generating an electrical impulse. However, there will be less dilution of the electrons (ions) in smaller-size neuronal elements and, therefore, higher probability of generating an action potential. Note that considerable license has been taken here. The electrical charge is not actually diluted in a chemical sense, but charge is affected by the resistance of the cell membrane and intracellular contents and the capacitance of the cell membrane. All of these are affected by the neuronal elements' size and geometry.[9]

By controlling the voltage we can control the volume of tissue subjected to effective stimulation and by controlling the pulse width we can control how many and which neuronal elements within the volume of voltage will be stimulated. This difference can be exploited. For example, consider a DBS contact that is placed too close to a structure, such as the internal capsule. Stimulation produces

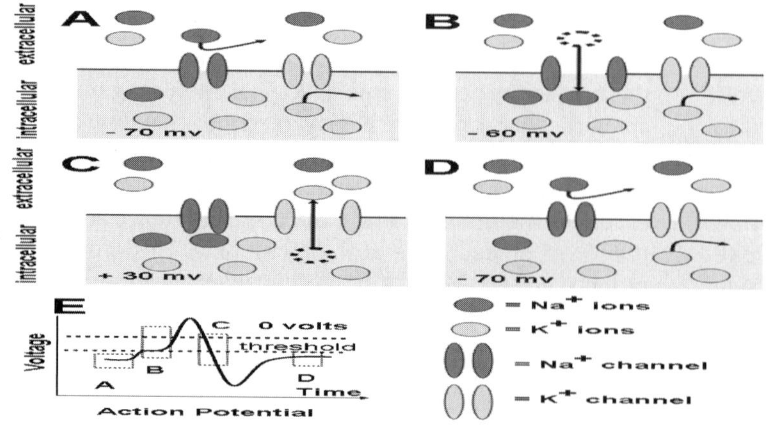

Fig. 13.1 Schematic representation of an action potential generation. **(A)** At rest, there are more Na⁺ ions outside compared with inside the cell and there are more K⁺ ions inside compared with outside. As a result, the interior of the cell is at –70 mV relative to the outside in this hypothetical example. **(B)** When the cell membrane is depolarized (becomes less negative inside the cell) to –60 mV by the DBS pulse, Na⁺ channels open up and let Na⁺ into the cell to initiate the action potential. **(C)** When the cell membrane reaches a certain voltage K⁺ channels open to allow K⁺ ions to exit the cell and reverse the action potential. **(D)** At a certain voltage both the Na⁺ and K⁺ close and the neuronal membrane returns to its resting condition. **(E)** The shape of the action potential and the time course where each event occurs.

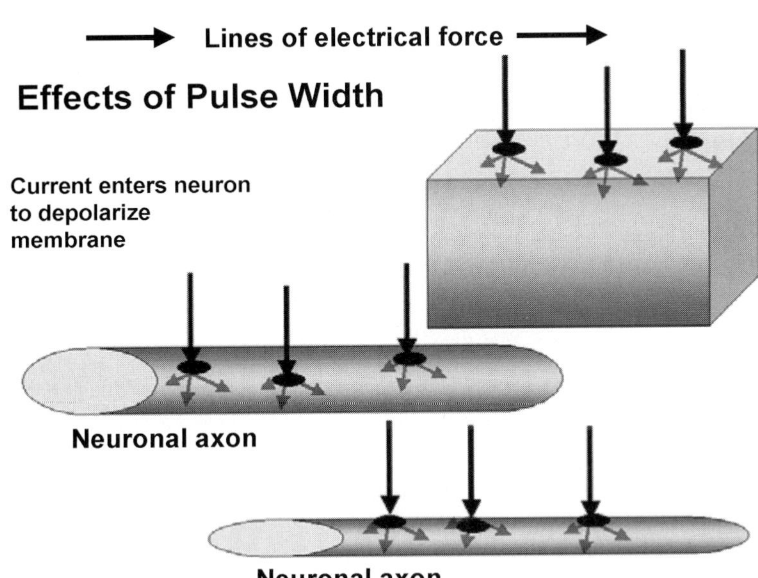

Fig. 13.2 Effects of pulse width on activation of different-sized neuronal elements. During the stimulation pulse, electrical charge is injected into the neuronal element. The wider the pulse width, the more charge that is injected. Smaller neuronal elements are activated at lower pulse widths than larger elements, such as cell bodies compared to axons; however, larger axons are activated at lower current densities than small axons.

intolerable side effects, such as tonic muscle contraction. We can lower the voltage to pull the effective electrical field away from the internal capsule but that could result in insufficient activation of the target neuronal elements. We can then increase the pulse width to excite more neuronal elements in the smaller restricted electrical field (**Fig. 13.3**).

Orientation of the Electrical Field

In order for the DBS pulse to activate the neuronal element, the pulse must drive electrons (ions) across the cell membrane. Therefore, the lines of electrical force generated by DBS must be directed into the cell membrane. The lines of electrical force run from the cathode (negative contact) to the anode (positive contact). Lines of electrical force must be perpendicular to the cell membrane (**Fig. 13.4**). If the lines of electrical force run parallel to the cell membrane, then no electrons (ions) will be driven into the neuronal element and it will not be depolarized to activation.

We can control the direction of the lines of electrical force by controlling the electrode configuration, which is how the anodes and cathodes are programmed on the DBS lead by the impulse generator. In the case of monopolar

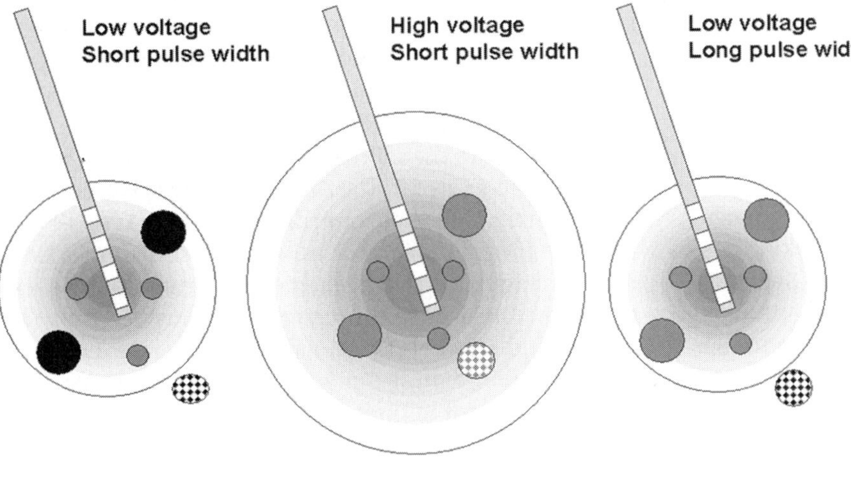

Fig. 13.3 Schematic representation of how pulse width can be used to selectively activate intended target elements when just increasing the voltage activates unintended neuronal elements. Low voltage and low pulse width does not activate all the intended neuronal elements but does not activate the unintended elements. Increasing the voltage then increases the size and strength of the electrical field, and all the intended target elements are activated. However, in this case unintended neuronal elements are also activated. Using low voltage keeps the electrical field small, but the wider pulse width activates more of the intended neuronal elements.

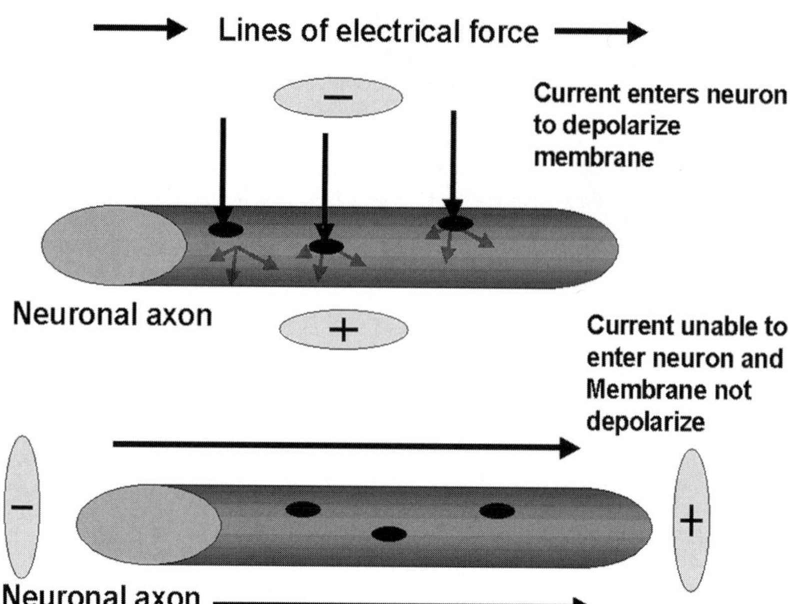

Fig. 13.4 The orientation of the cathode (negative contact) and anode (positive contact) determines the direction the lines of electrical force run. The lines of electrical force must be perpendicular to the cell membrane to drive electrons (ions) into the neuronal element to depolarize it to activation.

stimulation, the lines of electrical force radiate outward from the cathode on the DBS lead (**Fig. 13.5**). This may not be symmetrical due to inhomogeneity of the electrical conductivity of the tissue around the DBS lead. The radiation of the electrical lines of force will differ if the DBS lead is near white matter such as the internal capsule or near the cerebrospinal fluid (CSF)-filled ventricle. The directions of the electrical lines of force change dramatically in the case of bipolar stimulation (**Fig. 13.5**) and with reversing the contacts, which are anodes and cathodes.

Deep Brain Stimulation Frequency

The frequency, in pulses per second (pps) is an important factor in DBS efficacy. Typically, high-frequency stimulation (> 130 pps) is more effective, and, in fact, low-frequency stimulation can worsen symptoms. The mechanisms whereby DBS frequency improves symptoms are unknown. However, high-frequency stimulation is important in propagating stimulation effects across multiple synapses. Synaptic efficiency is very low. Only a small fraction of action potentials that arrive at the synaptic terminal result in action potentials in the postsynaptic neuron. High-frequency stimulation can increase synaptic efficiency by taking advantage of temporal summation of excitatory postsynaptic potentials (EPSPs). Thus, before the EPSP from one stimulus pulse has faded, a second EPSP occurs and is added to the remaining EPSP of the first pulse (**Fig. 13.6**). This additive effect increases the probability that the postsynaptic neuron will generate an action potential.

Another mechanism by which high-frequency DBS may be more effective relates to resonance effects. This assumes that the DBS pulse sets up a reentrant oscillation. The first pulse sets up activation that traverses the closed basal ganglia–thalamic–cortical loop to arrive back at the

site of the initial DBS activation.[10] If this occurs just as the next DBS pulse is delivered, then there will be an additive effect that will increase the probability of generating an action potential (**Fig. 13.6**).

■ Deep Brain Stimulation Electronics

Now that we have seen how electrical energy can activate neuronal elements, we need to understand how we can control that process. We need to understand how the various stimulation parameters (voltage, pulse width, frequency) and particularly electrode configuration can shape the electrical field in both size and strength.

It is probable that the therapeutic benefit may relate, at least in part, to the volume of brain tissue activated. However, the size of the electrical field that can be tolerated is related to the distance of the active DBS contacts to structures that should not be activated. For example, the medial lemniscus runs posterior to the subthalamic nucleus (STN). If the electrical field generated by the DBS is too large or too posterior, the patient may develop intolerable paresthesias to DBS that limit the programmer from using sufficient stimulation to control symptoms. Thus the regional anatomy and the relation of the DBS lead to the regional anatomy determine the efficacy and, particularly, the side effects.

At the minimum, an understanding of the regional anatomy is important in understanding the patient's response to DBS. An understanding of the regional anatomy can provide important information used to change the electrical field. For example, realizing that the internal capsule lies ventral to the ventral intermediate nucleus of the thalamus (Vim) means that if tonic contraction limits the therapeutic efficacy of Vim DBS, for example, with contact 0 the

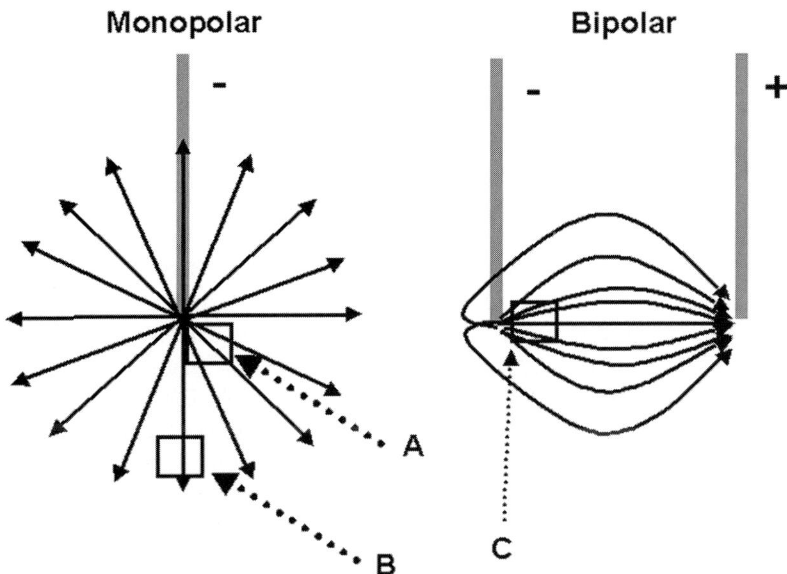

Fig. 13.5 Orientation of the lines of electrical force can be changed by changing the configuration of cathodes (negative contacts) and anodes (positive contacts). In addition, different configurations also affect the strength of the field (current densities) at different locations relative to the cathode. This can be appreciated by describing a box and counting the number of lines of electrical force that pass through the box. The number of lines of electrical force going through the box is proportional to the strength of the electrical field within the box. The number of lines of electrical force going through box A near the monopolar cathode is greater than the number passing through box B further away. Thus the current densities near the monopolar cathode are greater than those further away. However, the number of lines of electrical force going through box C in the bipolar configuration is even greater than that for the box near the monopolar cathode (box A), suggesting a stronger electrical field.

cathode and contact 3 as the anode, the electrical field can be moved dorsally by the proper selection of the more dorsal contacts, such as contact 2 being the cathode and contact 3 the anode.

Understanding the regional anatomy and the relation of the patient's DBS to the regional anatomy is key to successful DBS. The ability to shape the electrical field corresponding to the regional anatomy specific to the DBS lead location allows compensation for DBS leads not optimally placed and compensation for those patients whose regional anatomy is such that there would be significant risk of stimulation side effects with any DBS placement. As will be seen, the programmer can control to a significant degree the shape and densities of the electrical fields. However, to do so, it is important for the programmer to understand some of the basic electronics of the DBS system.

Ohm's Law

The critical factor in activation of neuronal elements is driving electrical current into the neuronal element. Cur-

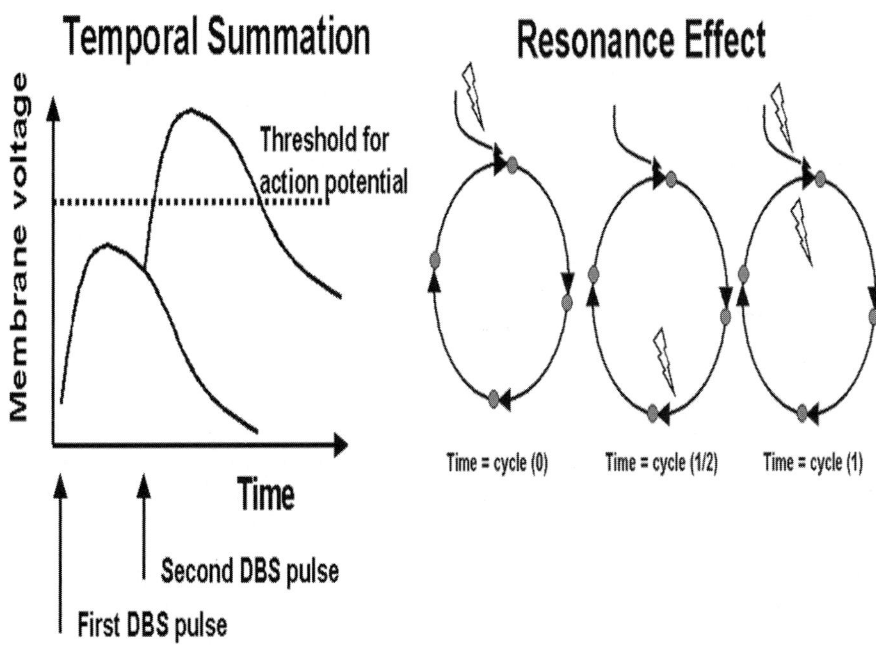

Fig. 13.6 Possible effects of high-frequency deep brain stimulation (DBS). One mechanism is temporal summation where the second excitatory postsynaptic potential (EPSP) induced by the second DBS pulse occurs before the effect of the EPSP from the first pulse has worn off; thereby, having an additive effect. DBS frequencies with interstimulus intervals (period of the DBS frequency) greater than the duration of EPSP will not have an additive effect. An alternative mechanism may be a resonance (amplifying) effect, where the effect of the first DBS pulse is propagated through a closed loop to return to the original site of activation. If the second pulse is delivered to coincide with the return pulse, there will be a synergistic or additive effect.

rent is defined as the number of electrons (or the equivalent ions) flowing per second. The force behind the flow of electrons is the voltage. However, the effects of voltage on the current depend on the resistance to the flow of electrons (ions). In the case of DBS, this resistance is called impedance. Impedance is the resistance to varying current frequencies and increases with increasing frequency of the changing current. The relationship between voltage, current, and impedance is given by Ohm's law (**Fig. 13.7**).

For those not familiar with electronics, a good analogy is given by plumbing and the flow of water. We can imagine water flowing from a reservoir through a valve into a bucket (brain) as shown in **Fig. 13.7**. The valve controls the amount of water flowing per unit time (current) by offering more or less resistance (impedance) to the flow. The amount of water flowing out the valve per second is the current, which in electrons (ions) is measured as amperes (amps). The impedance is measured in ohms. The amount of water flowing (current) is going to be determined by the impedance and the hydrostatic water pressure (voltage) based on the height of the reservoir. The higher the reservoir, the greater the force (volts or V) pushing the water (electrons) through the value (impedance) into the bucket (brain). The actual amount of water is analogous to the amount of electrons (ions) dumped into the brain and is measured in coulombs. One amp is equal to one coulomb per second.

Constant Voltage versus Constant Current Stimulators

To activate neuronal elements, we must move current in the electrons (ions) across the cell membrane to depolarize and activate the neuronal element. Thus the current generated across the cell membrane is the critical factor. As described earlier, the currently commercially available impulse generators (Soletra or Kinetra, Medtronic, Inc., Minneapolis, MN) provide only constant voltage, which is only indirectly related to the most important factor, which is current. The amount of current is determined by both the voltage and the tissue impedance (resistance). After the acute tissue changes associated with the implantation of the DBS lead have subsided, the tissue impedance generally remains constant for any constant electrode configuration. Therefore, the amount of current remains correlated directly with the stimulation voltage, assuming no changes in the electrode configuration. Consequently, we will discuss how the impulse generator controls the electrical voltage field and not the current density field; however, the distinction between voltage and current is important to keep in mind. As we shall see, changing the electrode configurations can greatly change the impedance, leading to significant changes in stimulation current for the same voltage.

Electrode Configurations and the Size and Strengths of the Electrical Fields

The usual practice is to keep the electrode configurations the same while a series of voltages, frequencies, and pulse widths are manipulated. One reason is that the configuration is often determined principally by the regional anatomy and the orientation of the DBS lead relative to the regional anatomy. We will discuss the electrical field generated by DBS in terms of the spatial distribution of the voltages. Neuronal elements further from the active DBS contact will experience a lower voltage than those elements closer to the active DBS contact. Thus we can control the spread of the

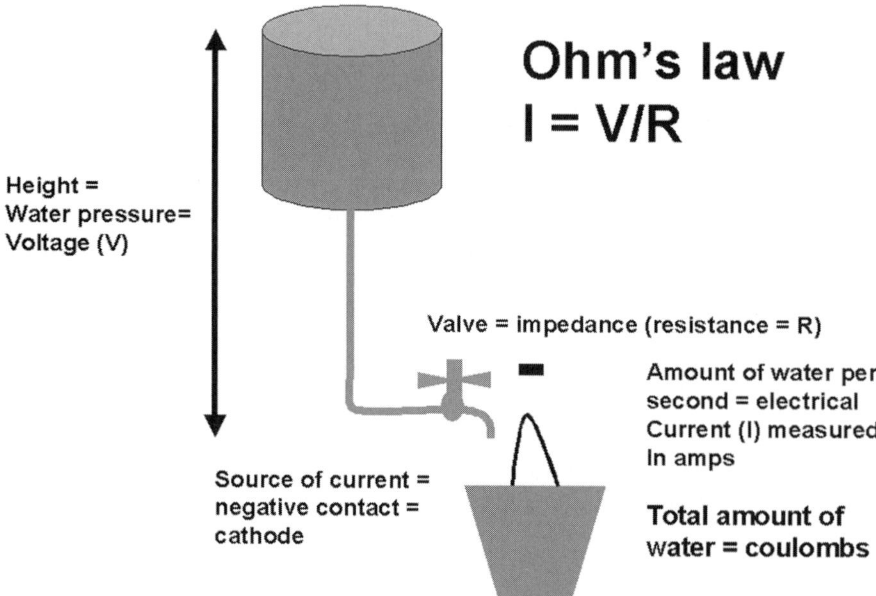

Fig. 13.7 Ohm's law, which relates voltage, current, and impedance (resistance). The relationships can be intuitively appreciated by analogy to plumbing. Voltage (and hydrostatic pressure) is the force that drives current (water flow) through the impedance (water valve) to deliver electrical charge in coulombs (amount of water).

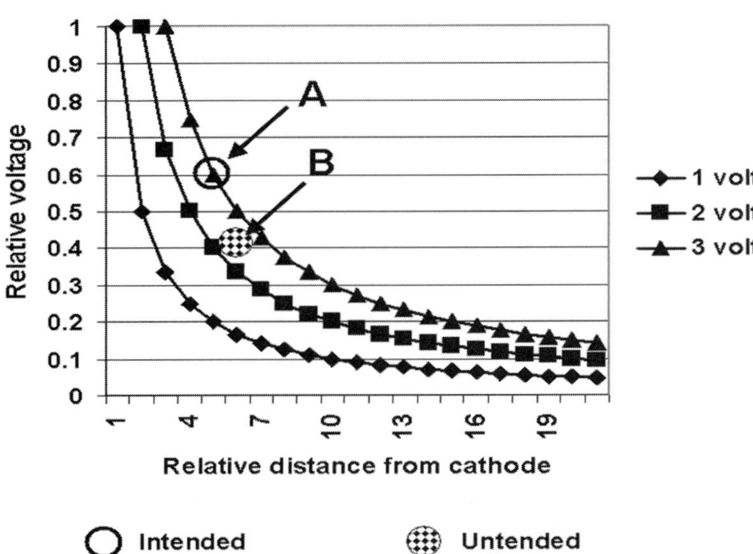

Fig. 13.8 A hypothetical schematic of the drop in voltage experienced by a neuronal element as it moves further from the cathode. This model is based on a monopolar electrode configuration. Also represented are two elements, **(A)** an intended element that when stimulated results in clinical improvement and **(B)** an unintended element that if stimulated produces limiting side effects. The height of the elements indicates the voltage necessary to excite the element, and the location on the horizontal axis represents the distance of the neuronal element from the cathode contact. Note that it takes 3 V of deep brain stimulation to produce sufficient voltage at the intended element, but this also results in excitation of the unintended element.

electrical field by controlling the voltage of the stimulation pulse. We may need to increase the spread of the electrical field to activate intended target neuronal elements but at the risk of activated unintended elements (**Fig. 13.8**). We need other ways to control the spread of the voltage.

Fortunately, there are other ways to change the shape, size, and strength of the electrical fields by changing the configuration of the active contacts. For example, a monopolar configuration has a cathode (negative contact) on the DBS lead, and the impulse generator acts as the anode (positive contact) as represented in **Fig. 13.9**. Other configurations include bipolar and tripolar (**Fig. 13.9**). The voltage in the monopolar falls off by the radius ($V \propto 1/r$ where r = distance from the cathode), in bipolar the voltage drops off by the square of the radius ($V \propto 1/r^2$), and in the tripolar configuration the voltage drops off by the cube of the radius ($V \propto 1/r^3$). These relationships are shown schematically in **Fig. 13.10**.

As can be seen in **Fig. 13.10**, monopolar stimulation produces the widest spread of the voltage, while the tripolar configuration produces the lowest spread. These different shapes of the electrical fields can be exploited as shown in **Fig. 13.10C**. In this hypothetical example, the empty circle D represents the intended target while the checkerboard filed circle E represents the unintended element. The voltages are adjusted so as to produce the threshold voltage for the intended target at D. In the monopolar configuration, the unintended element threshold will be less than the voltage produced at that site by the monopolar configuration. This would result in activation of the unintended element producing side effects. However, the voltage at the unintended site by the bipolar and tripolar configuration would be less than the threshold voltage necessary to activate the unintended element and consequently, bipolar or tripolar stimulation would not produce side effects.

For bipolar (and any multipolar) configuration, the distance between the cathode and anode also affects the size and strength of the electrical field. In this case the voltage generated increases as the distance between cathode and anode increases by the square of the distance ($V \propto d^2/r^2$, were r = distance from the cathode and d = distance between the cathode and anode). **Fig. 13.11** schematically shows how the distance between the cathode and anode for a bipolar configuration affects the falloff in voltage as the distance from the cathode increases.

By controlling the voltage and electrode configurations, an enormous number of electrical fields can be generated with different sizes and strengths. This has the advantage of allowing the DBS electrical field to be tailored to the

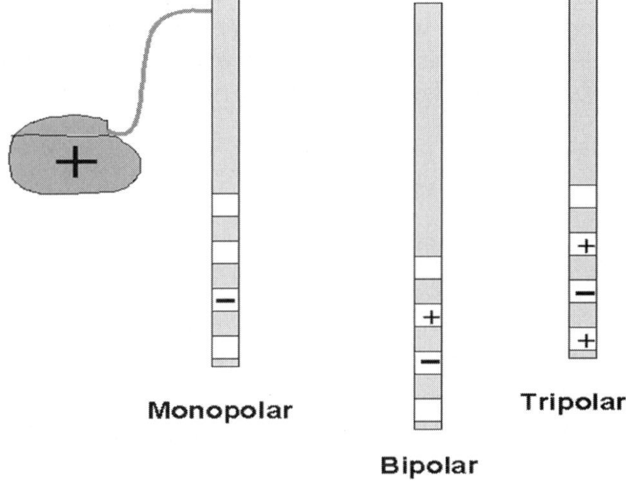

Fig. 13.9 A few of the many possible electrode configurations. Monopolar has the cathode (negative contact) on the deep brain stimulation (DBS) lead while the impulse generator acts as the anode (positive contact). In the bipolar configuration, the cathode and anode are on the same DBS lead. In the tripolar configuration, two anodes flank a single cathode.

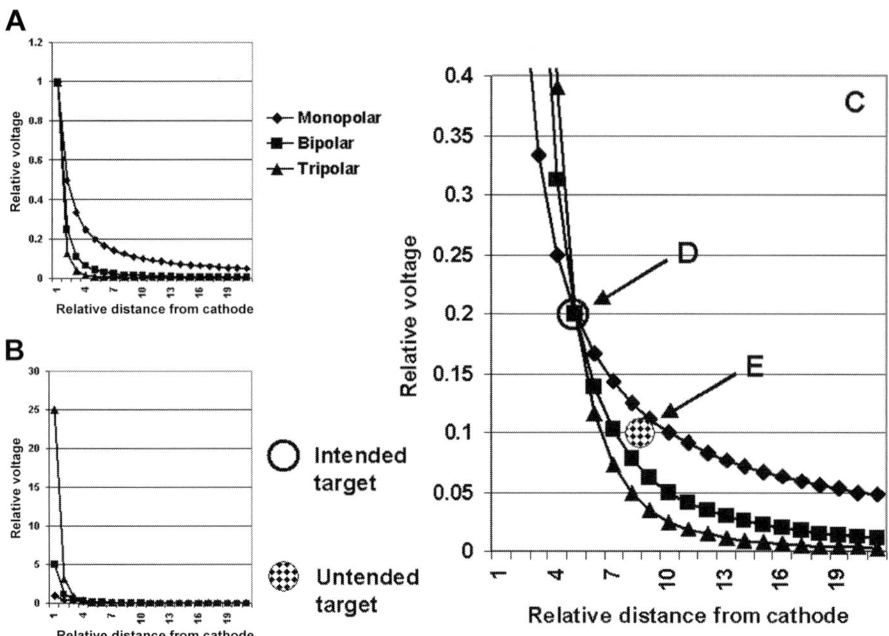

Fig. 13.10 Schematic representation of the voltage at distances from the cathode. **(A)** The different falloffs in voltage over distance for monopolar, bipolar, and tripolar configurations. **(B)** A hypothetical case where the voltages in the different configurations are adjusted to produce the same relative voltage (0.2 V) at the same distance from the cathode (5 units). As can be seen, the tripolar configuration produces the largest voltages close to the cathode, and bipolar produces larger voltage than the monopolar configuration. **(C)** However, the opposite is the case at distances greater than 5 units as shown here. The tripolar produces the least voltage at distances greater than 5 units, whereas bipolar produces less voltage compared with monopolar stimulation. These differences can be exploited. For example, raising the voltage in the monopolar configuration necessary to reach the threshold of the intended target (D) also raises the voltage experienced by the unintended neuronal element (E) above threshold, thereby producing side effects. However, with bipolar or tripolar, it is possible to have voltages at threshold for the intended target (D) but below threshold for activation of the unintended neuronal element (E).

unique regional anatomy of each patient and the unique relationship of the DBS lead to the patient's regional anatomy. This flexibility can mean the difference between DBS success and failure. The disadvantage is that there are an enormous number of different DBS settings that can and may need to be tried to help some patients. **Table 13.1** describes some of the advantages and disadvantages of the various configurations. Note that the bipolar configurations are divided into close and far bipolar. *Close bipolar* refers to when adjacent contacts are the cathodes and an-

odes, whereas *far bipolar* means that there is at least one inactive DBS contact between the cathode and anode.

The distance between the cathode and anode is a factor in deciding which DBS lead to use. There are two commercially available DBS leads. Each has contacts that are 1.27 mm in diameter and 1.5 mm in height. In one model the contacts are spaced 1.5 mm apart (Medtronic model 3387, Medtronic, Inc., Minneapolis, MN), and the other has contacts spaced 0.5 mm apart (Medtronic model 3389). As shown schematically, the wider-spaced DBS lead can produce more voltage

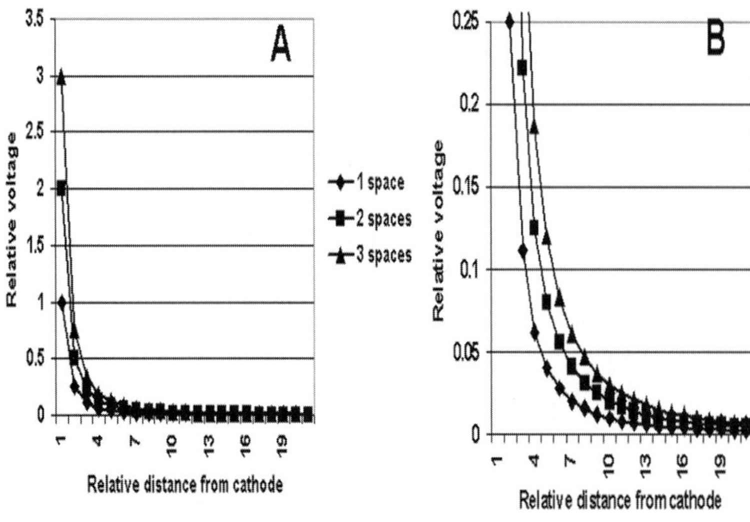

Fig. 13.11 Schematic representations of the voltages at various distances from the cathode with the deep brain stimulation (DBS) lead in bipolar configuration. There are three graphs; one for DBS leads with one, two, and three spaces between the cathode and anode. **(A)** Three spaces between the cathode and anode produces the largest voltages, whereas a single space produces the least voltage. **(B)** An expanded view of **(A)**.

Table 13.1 The Relative Advantages and Disadvantages of Various Deep Brain Stimulation Lead Active Contact Configurations

Configuration	Advantages	Disadvantages
Monopolar	1. Produces the widest spread of the electrical field at the same relative voltages 2. More effective if large volumes of brain need to be activated	1. Wider spread increases risk of activation of unintended neuronal elements 2. Tends to require higher stimulation voltages and consequently could increase the drain from the battery
Far bipolar	1. Produces a more intense electrical field for the same relative volume 2. May be an advantage if DBS lead near unintended neuronal elements	1. Produces a smaller spread of the electrical field at the same relative voltages 2. More effective if moderate volumes of brain or more neuronal elements within the target volume need to be activated
Close bipolar	1. Produces a moderately intense electrical field for the same relative volume 2. May be an advantage if DBS lead near unintended neuronal elements	1. Produces the least spread of the electrical field at the same relative voltages 2. Least effective if large volumes of brain or more neuronal elements within the target volume need to be activated

than the narrower-spaced lead, and there is less current drain from the impulse generator battery (**Fig. 13.12**). Consequently, this author recommends the use of the wider-spaced DBS lead. This is particularly true with thalamic and globus pallidus interna (GPi) DBS where therapeutic efficacy may require larger volumes of brain to be activated.

The question arises, Why would anyone want to use the narrow-spaced DBS lead? This lead is thought to better correspond to the anatomical dimensions of the STN. However, there is considerable evidence that stimulation of the STN may have little to do with the clinical efficacy[11] and that stimulation of the pallidal-fugal fibers (lenticular fasciculus and thalamic fasciculus) may be most important for efficacy.[12–14]

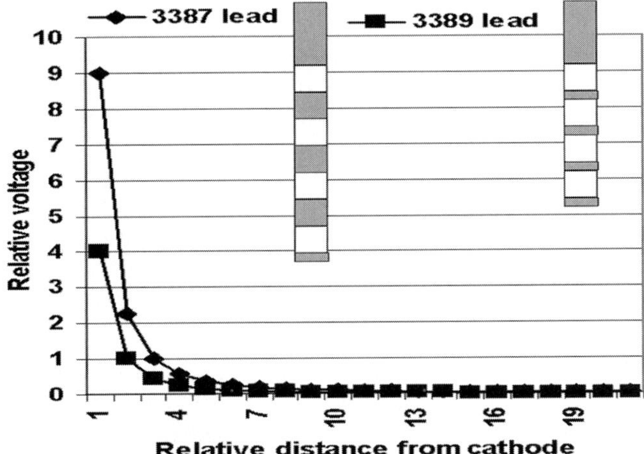

Fig. 13.12 Schematic representation of the relative voltage distributions created by the wide-spaced deep brain stimulation (DBS) lead (Medtronic model 3387, Medtronic, Inc., Minneapolis, MN) and the narrow-spaced DBS lead (Medtronic model 3389). As can be seen, the wider-spaced DBS lead can produce more intense voltage fields. Further, the wider-spaced DBS leads can produce all the same electrical field produced by the narrow-spaced DBS lead.

Deep Brain Stimulation Active Contact Configuration, Safety, and Battery Life

As described earlier, different active contact configurations can have a marked impact on the electrical voltage field. In addition, the different configurations can have a marked impact on the amount of electrical energy dumped into the brain, which has safety consequences. There is a limit to how much electrical energy can be safely given, and that is 30 μC per cm² per phase. *Thirty microcoulombs* refers to the amount of electrons (ions) passed into the brain with each stimulation pulse. *Per cm²* refers to the surface area of the active contact. *Per phase* refers to one component of the stimulation pulse (**Fig. 13.13**). Note that the description of contact being cathode (negative) or anode (positive) is a misnomer. All contacts are cathode during the first phase and then anode during the second phase or vice versa (**Fig. 13.13**). This is because the stimulation pulse is biphasic; that is, it contains two phases where the polarity (negative and positive) reverses.

Unfortunately, the operator does not directly control the amount of energy (in coulombs) injected into the brain with each stimulation pulse. Rather, the operator controls the voltage, which is indirectly related to the amount of energy injected into the brain per unit time (current measured in amps) through Ohm's law (**Fig. 13.7**). The relationship of the current to the voltage is mediated by the impedance (resistance). Thus, if the voltage is kept constant but the impedance is markedly reduced, then there will be a marked increase in the current being delivered to the brain.

Changing the DBS active contact configurations can have a marked effect on the impedances. For example, the impedance going through any single contact may be quite high, thereby limiting the amount of current for any given voltage. However, if multiple active contacts are used, such

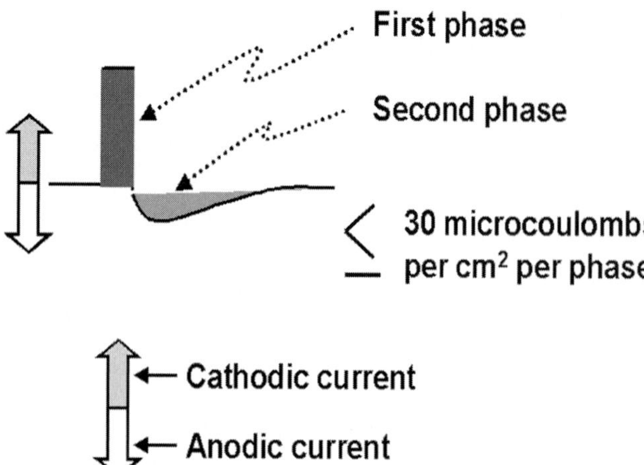

Fig. 13.13 Schematic representation of the stimulus pulse of currently commercially available impulse generators (Soletra and Kinetra, Medtronic, Inc., Minneapolis, MN). The initial phase has a high voltage (that voltage set by the programmer) of a short duration (the pulse width set by the programmer), whereas the second phase has a lower voltage and longer duration.

as multiple cathodes or multiple anodes, the overall impedance can become very low (**Fig. 13.14**). For example, using the computer simulator of the currently commercially available DBS programmer (8840 N'Vision Clinician Programmer, Medtronic, Inc., Minneapolis, MN) configured as bipolar with contact 0 the cathode and contact 3 the anode, voltage of 4, and a pulse width of 270 produces an impedance of > 2000 ohms, and DBS is within safety limits. Increasing the number of cathodes to contacts 0, 1, and 2 and keeping contact 3 as the anode results in the impedance becoming 75 ohms and the electrical charge injected into the brain exceeds the safety limit. Thus it is important to know the impedance of any configuration to assure that the amount of current being delivered to the brain is within safety limits. The manufacture of the currently commercially available devices (ww.medtronic.com) provides a nomogram that relates pulse width, voltage, and impedance to the amount of electrical energy injected into the brain with DBS and defines regions that are within the safety limits (**Fig. 13.15**).

The Model 8840 N'Vision Clinician Programmer provides a warning if the selected stimulation parameters exceed the safety limit. However, the programming device does not measure the current densities nor can it calculate them based on the voltage because the programming device does not know what the impedances are. The warnings provided by the programming device are based on the assumption that the impedance is 500 ohms. This means that if the actual impedance of the DBS configuration is 500 ohms, the warnings are accurate. However, if the impedances are significantly greater than 500 ohms, then the device will give a false-positive warning. Indeed the foregoing example where the DBS was configured as bipolar with contact 0 the cathode and contact 3 the anode, voltage of 4, and a pulse width of 270 producing an impedance of > 2000 ohms would give a safety warning although the normogram indicates being within safety limits. Although this may be the safer situation for the patient, it does risk not using higher DBS voltage and pulse widths that could be necessary to achieve symptomatic control and provide the patient with optimal benefit from DBS. Alternatively, the actual impedances may be lower than the estimate of 500 ohms, for example, where there are several active DBS contacts as already described.

The programmer can determine whether the current densities being delivered by a specific DBS configuration and parameter set are within the safety limits by consulting a nomogram (**Fig. 13.15**) that relates pulse width and voltage to the amount of current delivered at a given

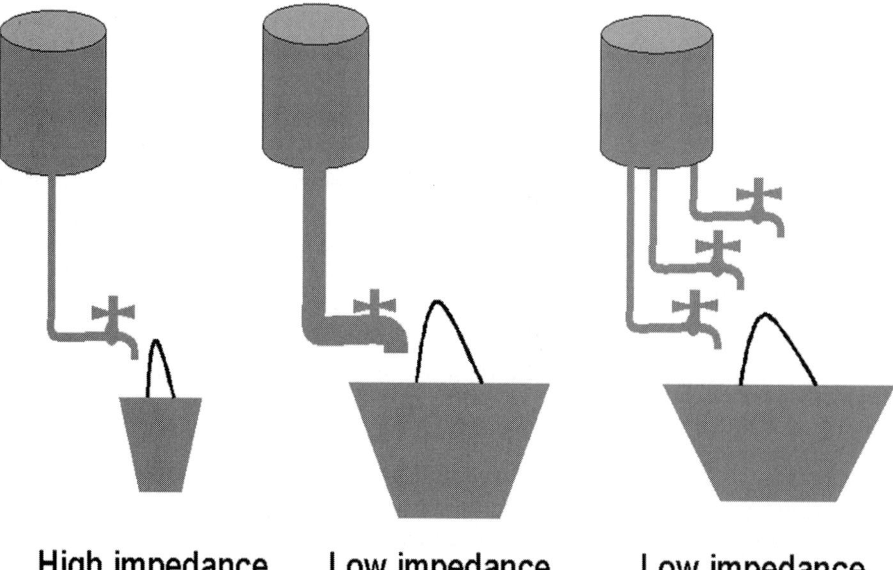

Fig. 13.14 Analogy describing how multiple active contacts can lower the impedance. The lower the impedance (or more open the water valve) the greater the amount of current delivered to the brain. However, when multiple contacts are active (multiple valves open) the overall impedance is lower even though the impedances of the individual contacts are high. This will result in significant increases in the amount of electrical charge injected into the brain.

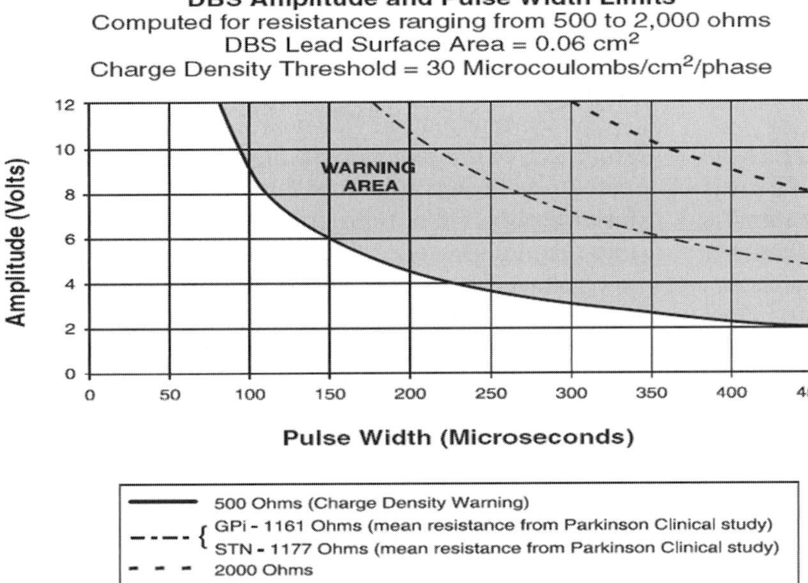

Fig. 13.15 Nomogram that relates deep brain stimulation (DBS) voltage, pulse width, and impedances to determine whether the particular DBS contact configuration and parameter set specific to the individual patient is within the safe operating range. The programmer first determines the impedances by using the therapeutic measurements function and *not* the electrode impedance function on the programming device (Model 8840 N'Vision Clinician Programmer, Medtronic, Inc., Minneapolis, MN).

impedance. The programmer must first determine the impedances of the specific therapeutic DBS configuration and stimulation parameter set unique to the patient by using the "therapeutic measurements" function and *not* the "electrode impedance" function on the Model 8840 N'Vision Clinician Programmer.

As already described, there are two methods for determining impedances of the DBS contacts for the N'Vision Clinician Programmer. The electrode impedance function tests the impedances (and current) through all possible pairwise combinations of DBS lead contacts and the impulse

generator case (**Fig. 13.16**). The particular DBS frequency, voltage, and pulse widths used to measure the impedances and current flows are based on a user-modifiable factory default set. This particular configuration and parameter set is unlikely to be relevant to the patient's configurations and stimulation parameter sets that are used therapeutically. Therefore, the impedances measured during the electrode impedance function are not relevant to the safety of the configurations and stimulation parameter sets that are needed by the patient. The impedances and current flows measured during the therapeutic measurements function

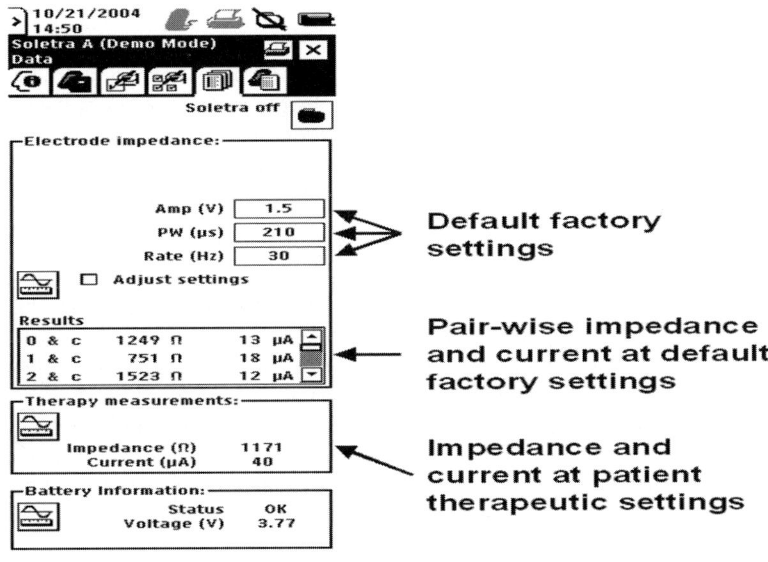

Fig. 13.16 Example of the panel for the currently commercially available deep brain stimulation (DBS) programming device showing the menu and data for the electrode impedance and the therapy measurement functions (N'Vision Clinician Programmer, Medtronic, Inc., Minneapolis, MN). As can be seen, the electrode impedance function reports the impedance and current for each possible pair of DBS contacts and the case. Note that the rate is 30 Hz, which is different from the rates typically used for therapy. Because impedance varies with the rate and the rate is different in therapy, the impedances from the electrode impedance function are not likely to be relevant to the patient during therapeutic DBS. Also, the configuration of the DBS active contacts will greatly change the impedances. The impedances measured from the therapeutic measurements function are related to the individual patient's unique therapeutic DBS active contact configuration and stimulation parameter set. (From the N'Vision Clinician Programmer simulation software, Medtronic, Inc., Minneapolis, Minnesota. Reproduced with permission).

utilize the specific DBS contact configuration and stimulation parameter sets that are programmed into the impulse generator for the patient's therapy (**Fig. 13.16**). It is this impedance that can be used with the nomogram above to assess DBS electrical safety.

The electrode impedance function is used to test the electrical integrity of the implanted DBS system. If there is a break in the electrical connection between the impulse generator and the DBS contact, the impedance will be over 2000 ohms and the current low. Occasionally, the impedance of a particular contact may be over 2000 ohms in systems that are operating properly, but the current will not be low. However, if there is a change in the impedance from a lower value, the programmer must suspect an electrical discontinuity in the system. If there is a marked reduction in the impedance or increase of current of a particular DBS contact or set of contacts, there may be a short-circuit in the DBS system. It is important to obtain baseline impedance measurements after the patient has stabilized following DBS surgery.

The electrical safety of DBS depends on the amount of current passed into the brain during any DBS stimulation pulse as described earlier. However, another aspect of DBS electrical safety has to do with charge balanced biphasic stimulation pulses (**Fig. 13.17**). If more electrical charge is passed into the brain by the cathodal (negative) current than is taken out by the anodal (positive) current, then there will be a buildup of electrical charge on the DBS contact. This residual electrical charge can cause chemical reactions at the DBS contact surface that can be dangerous to tissue. For example, a constant charge can cause water to hydrolyze to oxygen and hydrogen gas, which forms

bubbles that can tear or damage tissue or can cause other injurious chemical reactions. Therefore, the cathodic and anodic phase must deposit and remove equal amounts of electrons (ions).

The waveform of the DBS pulse in either the Soletra or Kinetra is not symmetrical. The first phase uses a high voltage (the voltage programmed into the impulse generator) for a short period of time (the pulse width programmed into the impulse generator) and the second phase uses a low voltage for a longer period of time. This has advantages and disadvantages. The disadvantage is that if the second phase is incomplete there could be a buildup of dangerous residual electrical charge on the DBS contact surface. This could happen if the DBS impulse generator is placed into cycling mode (**Fig. 13.17**). Consequently, cycling mode stimulation should not be used under usual circumstances.

The asymmetric DBS pulse has an advantage. The cathodal (negative) pulse is the current that is most effective for exciting neuronal elements. In a multipolar configuration, each active DBS contact acts as both a cathode and an anode because of the biphasic design of the DBS pulse. If the waveforms of the DBS pulse were symmetric, all the neuronal elements would be subject to a large (for example suprathreshold) cathodic phase regardless of whether it is the first or second phase. With the asymmetric pulse, it is possible that only the first phase produces a response because it is above the voltage threshold, and the second phase, being below threshold, does not produce a response. This allows specific DBS contacts to be effectively only cathodal (negative) or anodal (positive) as shown in **Fig. 13.18**.

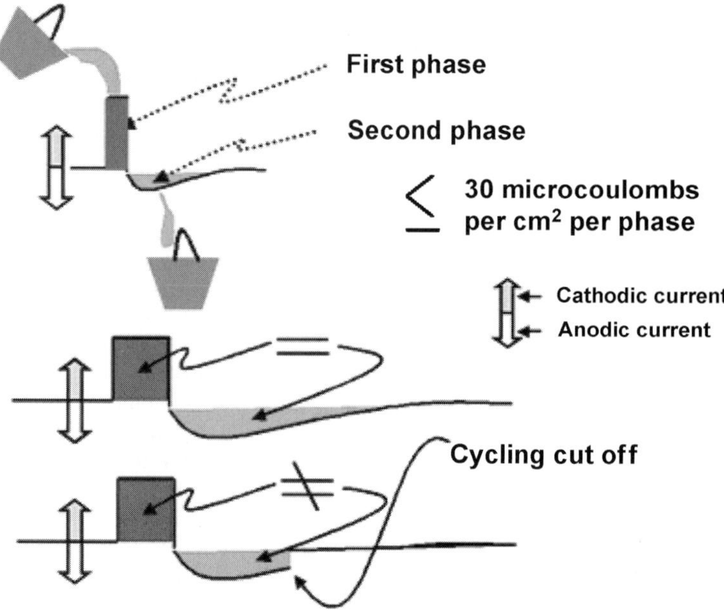

Fig. 13.17 A schematic representation of the deposition and removal of electrical charge, electrons (ions), by the first phase (cathodic) and its removal by the second phase (anodic). Note that if these are not equal, there will be a residual charge that can cause dangerous tissue chemical reactions. The current commercially available impulse generator does not deliver symmetric biphasic pulses. The first phase uses high voltage for a short period of time, whereas the second phase uses a low voltage for a longer period of time. This can be dangerous if the impulse generator is used in cycling mode where the stimulation is started and stopped at periodic intervals. If the stimulation is stopped before the second phase is completed, dangerous residual charge could build up. This is a concern because the second phase is prolonged relative to the first phase; therefore, the second phase is more likely interrupted than the first phase, increasing the risk of charge buildup.

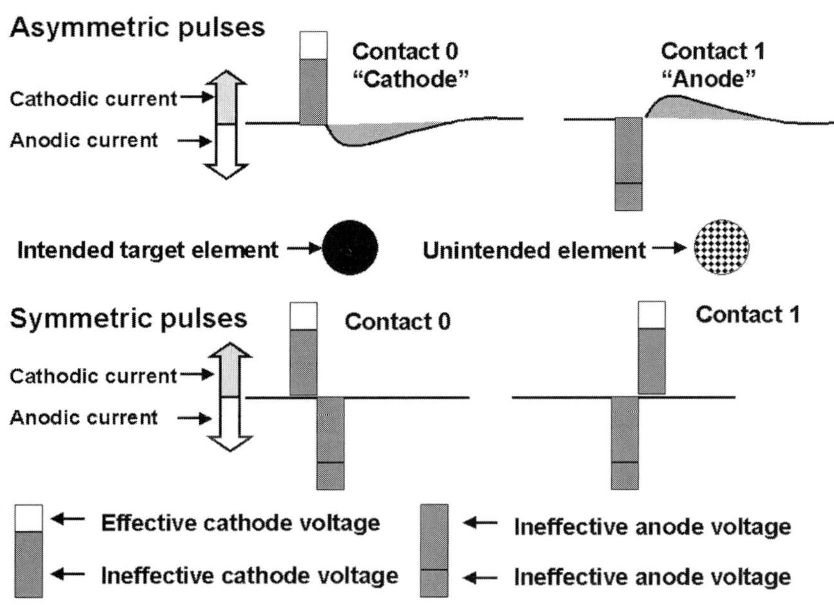

Fig. 13.18 Schematic representation of the advantage of asymmetric deep brain stimulation (DBS) pulses. This is based on the notion that cathodal (negative) DBS current is the most effective for exciting neuronal elements. The representation is that of bipolar stimulation where contact 0 is configured as the cathode (initial phase negative) and contact 1 is configured as the anode (initial phase positive). Note that all contacts have both a cathodal (negative) and an anodal (positive) phase. With the asymmetric DBS pulse only contact 0 exceeds the cathodal threshold to activate neuronal elements. The intended target element will be activated because it is sufficiently close to contact 0, whereas the unintended element will not be activated. However, with the symmetric pulses both contact 0 and contact 1 exceed threshold cathodal (negative) current, and both the intended and unintended elements will be activated. This could produce intolerable side effects that would limit therapeutic efficacy.

◼ Importance of Regional Anatomy in Deep Brain Stimulation Effects

The programmer has many tools available to control the size and strengths of the electrical fields as already described. The programmer then uses these tools to optimally excite the intended neuronal elements in the target and to avoid activation of unintended elements that are usually adjacent to the intended target. For example, for STN DBS, the programmer will want to optimally excite either the STN output axons or those axons passing to or in the vicinity of the STN. However, the programmer will not want to stimulate the medial lemniscal fibers that pass posterior to the STN, the oculomotor nerve fibers that pass medial to the STN, or the corticospinal and corticobulbar fibers that pass lateral, anterior, and inferior to

the STN. This will depend on the regional anatomy specific to the individual patient and the relation of that patient's DBS lead relative to the specific regional anatomy. Consequently, it is very important for the programmer to understand the regional anatomy and how the surgical placement trajectory affects the orientation of the DBS lead to the regional anatomy.

Subthalamic Nucleus Deep Brain Stimulation Effects

Figs. 13.19 and **13.20** show schematics of the sagittal and coronal views of the regional anatomy around the STN. In the sagittal plane, the STN is bordered by the internal capsule containing corticospinal and corticobulbar fibers anteriorly and ventrally. The ascending fibers of the medial lemniscus are posterior to the STN. In the coronal plane,

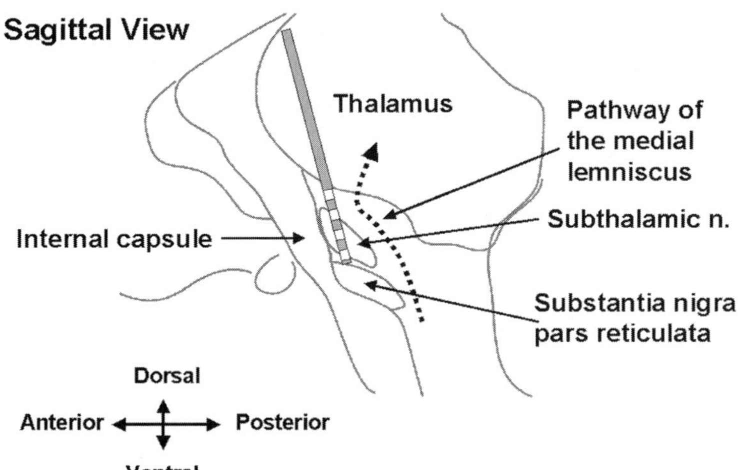

Fig. 13.19 Schematic representation of the regional anatomy about the subthalamic nucleus in the sagittal plane.

Coronal View

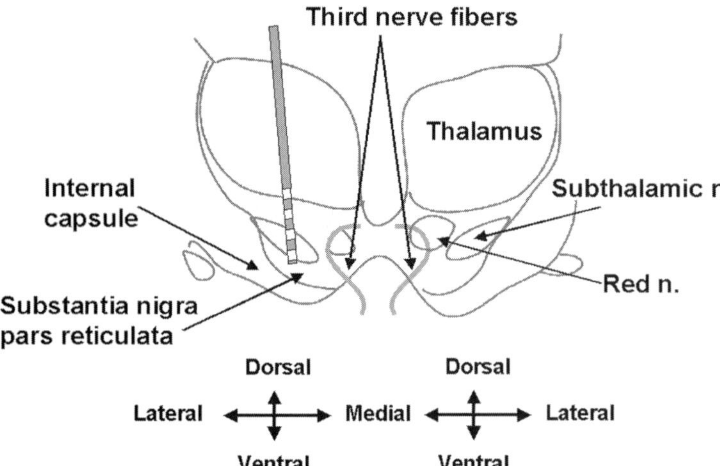

Fig. 13.20 Schematic representation of the regional anatomy about the subthalamic nucleus in the coronal plane.

the STN is bordered medially by the nerve roots of the third nerve nucleus in planes more caudal than are shown in the figure and the hypothalamus in planes more rostral. The internal capsule is lateral and ventral to the STN. Also, the STN is divided into three components (not shown) with the dorsolateral portion representing the sensorimotor region, which is the primary target of the DBS. The medial and ventral regions project to the regions involved in cognitive and emotional behavior. Unintended stimulation of these regions can produce profound mood changes, either depression or hypomania.

Although the therapeutic mechanisms of action of STN DBS are unknown, generally stimulation of axons passing to, from, or in the vicinity of the STN is required. The therapeutic effect may depend on activation of sufficient numbers of these neuronal elements. Thus monopolar or far bipolar DBS configurations with higher voltage and wider pulse widths would excite a larger volume of brain tissue and a greater percentage of the neural elements within the volume. The common side effects are related to activation of adjacent unintended structures. Such side effects may be mitigated by using close bipolar, low-voltage, and short pulse width DBS. Most of the difficulties with STN DBS are due to side effects. The more common side effects are discussed in the next sections, which describe the regional anatomy involved and suggest diagnostic and therapeutic measures.

Paresthesias

If the medial lemniscus fibers are activated, the patient will note paresthesias on the contralateral side of the body. Often this occurs when the DBS lead is placed too posteriorly (**Fig. 13.21**). There are several therapeutic options. First, the electrical field can be reduced in size by first going to far bipolar DBS contact configuration. If this fails to prevent paresthesias, a close bipolar configuration can be used. Also note that sometimes moving the electrical field

more ventrally, such as by using contacts 1 or 0 in monopolar configuration or bipolar between contacts 0 and 1 can help reduce paresthesias. This is because the medial lemniscus curves anteriorly over the top of the STN and, therefore, is closest to the more dorsal contacts. By moving the electrical field more ventrally, the electrical field moves further away from the medical lemniscus. Note that the angle of the DBS lead in the sagittal plane will influence whether there is a difference in the distance, and therefore, thresholds between the dorsal and ventral contacts and the medial lemniscus. If the angle in the sagittal plane is less vertical, then there will be less difference between the thresholds to paresthesias between the dorsal and ventral contacts. Note that transient paresthesias are generally not a concern.

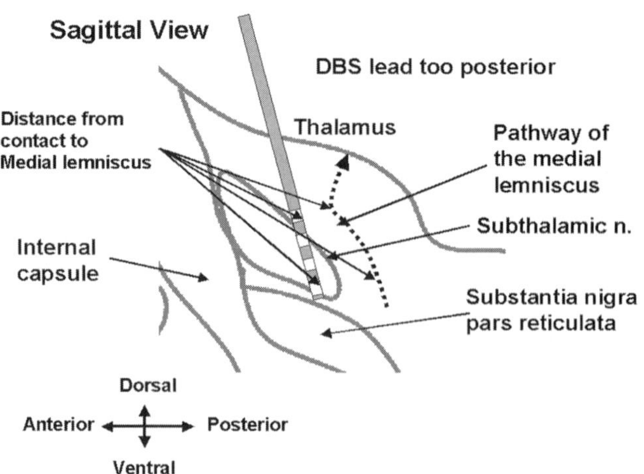

Fig. 13.21 Schematic representation of the regional anatomy of a subthalamic nucleus deep brain stimulation lead placed too posteriorly.

Skewed Deviation of the Eyes Causing Double Vision

If the STN DBS lead is placed too medially, the electrical field can activate nerve fibers of the oculomotor (third) cranial nerve causing muscle contraction of the extraocular muscles and producing skewed deviation (**Fig. 13.22**). Although the oculomotor nucleus is near the midline of the mesencephalon, its fibers course laterally, even to the lateral border of the red nucleus, before turning medially to exit in the interpeduncular fossa. Note that the distance between the dorsal contacts and the third nerve fibers is greater than the distance between the ventral contacts and the third nerve fibers. This distance translates to a greater threshold for activation. Therefore, monopolar stimulation through the dorsal contacts or bipolar between the more dorsal contacts can pull the electrical field away from the third nerve fibers thereby avoiding skewed eye deviation.

Conjugate Deviation of the Eyes

This is less common than skewed deviation of the eyes. The exact mechanisms are unknown. It is possible that the electrical field of a DBS lead placed too laterally could activate the frontopontine tract in the internal capsule en route to brainstem nuclei for conjugate horizontal eye movements. However, in our experience this would be rare. If this were to be the case, increasing the voltage should affect other corticobulbar and corticospinal fibers with the generation of tonic contractions of the contralateral face and body. A more likely explanation is that fibers from the substantia nigra pars reticulata course through the medial STN en route to the superior colliculus, which is involved in saccadic eye movements. In our experience, conjugate deviation of the eyes is associated with an STN DBS lead placed too medi-

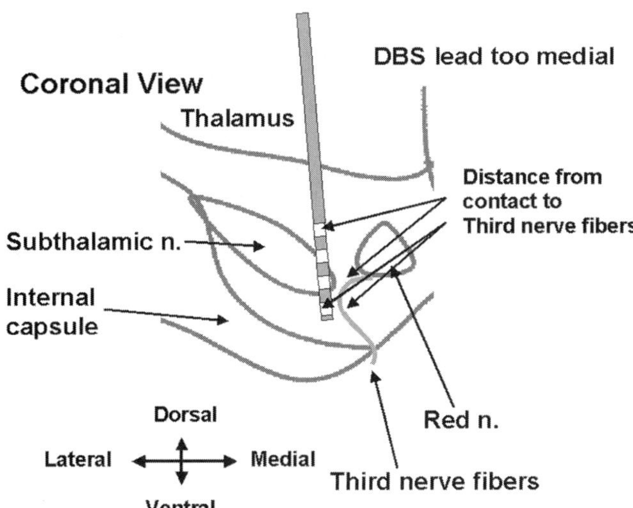

Fig. 13.22 Schematic representation of the regional anatomy of a subthalamic nucleus deep brain stimulation lead placed too medially.

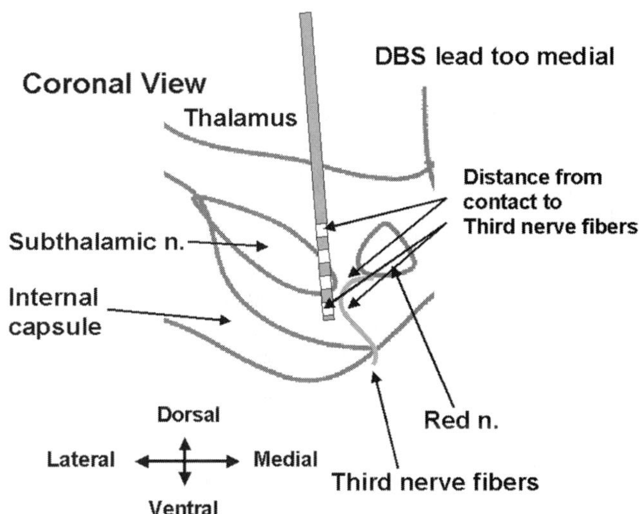

Fig. 13.23 Schematic representation of the regional anatomy of a subthalamic nucleus deep brain stimulation lead placed too medially.

ally. Therapeutic actions similar to that described above for skewed eye deviation can help.

Tonic Muscle Contractions

Activation of the corticobulbar and/or corticospinal tracts coursing in the internal capsule can produce tonic muscle contractions in the contralateral face and/or body. The internal capsule borders the STN laterally, anteriorly, and ventrally. Whether the cause is an STN DBS lead being placed too anteriorly, laterally, or ventrally can be determined by the threshold voltage necessary to produce the tonic contraction at the different DBS contacts, each tested in monopolar configuration. For example, an STN DBS lead placed too anteriorly will bring all the contacts to nearly the same distance to the internal capsule and there will be little difference in the thresholds to produce tonic contraction (**Fig. 13.23**). However, for STN DBS leads placed too laterally or too ventrally, the distance between the dorsal contacts and the internal capsule will be greater than the distance for the ventral contacts (**Figs. 13.24** and **13.25**). Note that an STN DBS lead placed too laterally can often be distinguished from a lead placed too ventrally. The threshold for tonic contraction through the ventral contact will be very low in an STN DBS lead placed too ventrally compared with one place too laterally.

The therapeutic response to an STN DBS lead placed too anteriorly is limited. Any monopolar configuration is liable to produce tonic contractions. Moving the electrical field in the dorsoventral direction by different bipolar configurations is not likely to be helpful. The only effective response would be to shrink the size of the electrical field by close bipolar or tripolar configuration and attempt to maintain high current density, high frequency, and/or large pulse

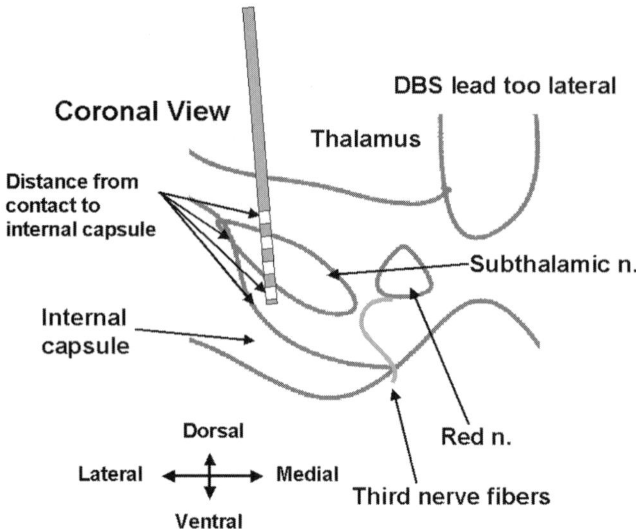

Fig. 13.24 Schematic representation of the regional anatomy of a subthalamic nucleus deep brain stimulation lead placed too laterally.

widths to compensate for the smaller volume to tissue that can be activated.

If the STN DBS lead is too ventral, the electrical field can be moved dorsally, away from the internal capsule, by using monopolar stimulation through the dorsal contacts or bipolar through contacts 1 and 2 or 2 and 3. If this not sufficient, it may be possible to surgically revise the STN DBS lead without removing the entire lead. We have been successful in pulling back an STN DBS lead that is too ventral under fluoroscopic control. For STN DBS leads that are too lateral, STN DBS configurations similar to those for a lead that is too ventral may be attempted.

Gait Ataxia

Occasionally, patients with bilateral STN DBS may experience increased difficulty with gait. Often, the gait problem appears as an ataxia. It can be difficult to differentiate gait abnormalities that are part of the patient's disease that required DBS surgery or from the stimulation itself. Often, observing the patient with the stimulators off and on can help. When gait ataxia is due to the stimulation, the STN DBS lead may be too medial and may thus affect the cerebellar outflow path to the thalamus through the brachium conjunctivum. This pathway projects through and around the red nucleus, which is just medial to the STN (**Fig. 13.22**). The therapeutic approach is similar to that already described for skewed eye deviation.

Dyskinesia

Acutely, STN DBS can produce or exacerbate medication-induced dyskinesia. These effects are probably produced by the same mechanisms that relate to the therapeutic benefit, although this is speculative. However, dyskinesia is not associated to spread of DBS activation to unintended structures. The appearance of dyskinesia with STN DBS should be addressed by medication changes and not reduction in STN DBS parameters. We have seen patients where chronic STN DBS appears to suppress dyskinesia.

Mood

STN DBS can produce profound mood changes in both PD and nonparkinsonian epilepsy patients. The mood changes range from depression to hypomania. Most often, these symptoms are resolved by moving the electrical field more dorsally by using the more dorsal contacts in either monopolar or multipolar configurations.

Ventral Intermediate Thalamus DBS Effects

Patients with essential tremor and other forms of cerebellar outflow tremor often benefit from Vim DBS. As described earlier, knowing the regional anatomy around the DBS target can be very helpful in the postoperative management. The regional anatomy of the Vim in the sagittal and coronal planes is schematically represented in **Figs. 13.26** and **13.27**. The key structures clinically important in DBS management are the sensory relay nuclei in the ventral caudal nucleus of the thalamus (Vc), the basal ganglia relay nucleus ventro-oralis posterior (Vop), and the internal capsule. The Vc lies posterior to the Vim, whereas the Vop lies anterior to the Vim. DBS activation of the Vc can produce paresthesias, which may limit the ability to achieve control of tremor. DBS of the Vop may be less effective than that of the Vim. Lateral and ventral to the Vim lie the corticospinal and cortical bulbar fibers in the internal capsule.

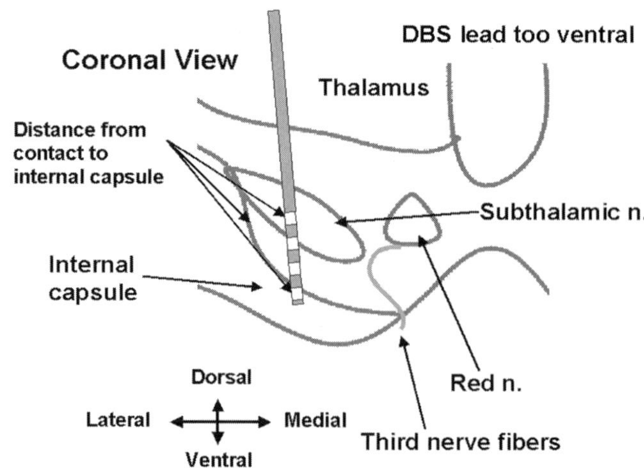

Fig. 13.25 Schematic representation of the regional anatomy of a subthalamic nucleus deep brain stimulation lead placed too ventrally.

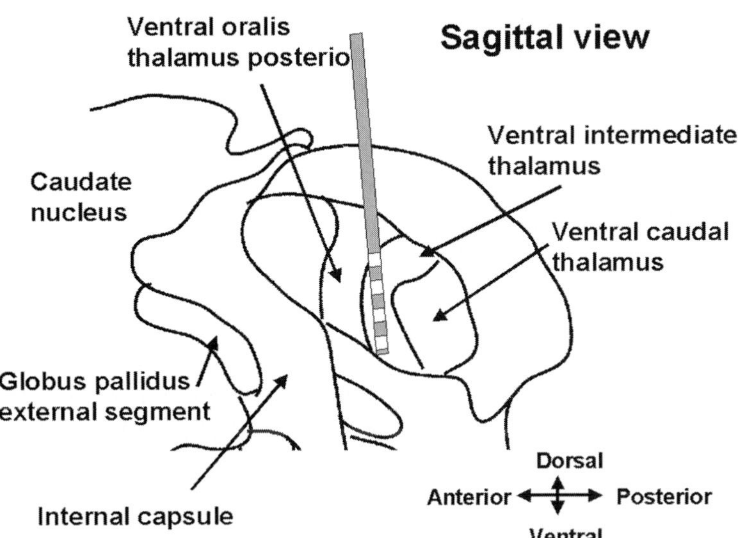

Fig. 13.26 Schematic representation of the regional anatomy around the ventral intermediate thalamus in the sagittal plane.

Insufficient Efficacy in the Absence of Side Effects

Often, Vim DBS requires activation of larger volumes of brain tissue. We had a patient with two DBS leads implanted in a single Vim because the first DBS lead produced some, but insufficient, tremor control with intraoperative DBS testing. A second DBS lead was place just posterior to the first. Postoperatively, the patient had much better control with stimulation through both leads than with either alone. Monopolar or multiple cathodes may be required to activate larger volumes of brain. In addition, long pulse widths can activate more neuronal elements without changing the size or strength of the electrical voltage field (**Fig. 13.3**).

Paresthesias

This side effect is most likely related to the spread of the DBS electrical field posteriorly to the Vc nucleus (particularly the posterior portion that mediates light touch and

pinprick sensation). In this case the orientation of the DBS lead to the long, vertical axis of the Vim is important. If the DBS lead is placed at too great an angle from the vertical, it is possible that the lower contacts may be too close to the Vc, whereas the upper contacts may not be in the Vim (**Fig. 13.28**). Moving the electrical field dorsally by using the upper contacts may activate the Vop and not be very effective. Consequently, it may be necessary to use very focused electrical fields in close bipolar configuration and reverse the more usual polarity. For example, contact 0 could be made anodal (positive) and contact 1 cathodal (negative). This would still result in focal stimulation of the Vim but the current would be pulled away from the Vc. If the DBS lead is not placed at too great an angle from the vertical, moving the electrical field by using more dorsal contacts can still move the field away from the Vc yet still effectively stimulate the Vim. Note that transient paresthesias are generally not a concern.

Tonic Muscle Contraction

A DBS lead placed too laterally or ventrally can place the DBS electrical field too close to the internal capsule. In both cases, the more ventral contacts will have low voltage thresholds for tonic contraction. This difference in thresholds can be exploited to avoid tonic contraction by moving the electrical field more dorsal by using the more dorsal contacts. It is difficult to distinguish a DBS lead that activates the corticobulbar and corticospinal fibers either laterally or ventrally. Sometimes the presence of paresthesias with DBS through the more ventral contacts would suggest a DBS lead that is placed to ventrally because the trajectory often makes the ventral contacts closer to the Vc than the dorsal contacts. If the DBS lead is placed too ventrally and subsequent changes in the DBS active contact configurations still cannot provide sufficient tremor control with reasonable side effects, the DBS lead can be revised under fluoroscopic control as described earlier.

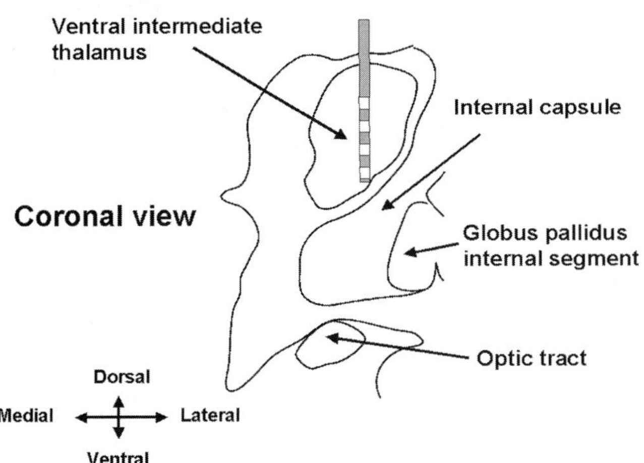

Fig. 13.27 Schematic representation of the regional anatomy around the ventral intermediate thalamus in the coronal plane.

Sagittal view

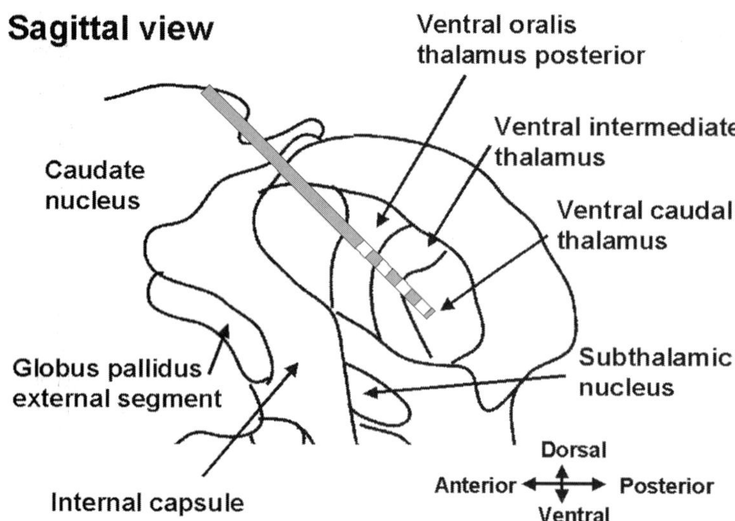

Fig. 13.28 Schematic representation of the regional anatomy around the ventral intermediate thalamus in the sagittal plane with the deep brain stimulation at too great an angle from the vertical.

Speech Impairment

This is a frequent complication of Vim DBS, particularly if done bilaterally. Fortunately, most patients have sufficient improved function with unilateral dominant Vim DBS, and it is usually not necessary to increase risks to speech with bilateral Vim DBS. The exact mechanisms producing speech problems are unclear. There are several possibilities, including (1) Vim DBS producing a subcortical type of aphasia manifesting primarily as word-finding difficulties and disfluency, (2) involvement of cerebellar output to the cortex, and (3) spread to the corticobulbar fibers. The latter can be determined by stimulating at higher voltages to produce frank and observable muscle contraction. In this case, the therapeutic response is similar to that described earlier for tonic contraction; however, this is seldom the case.

In the past, the use of the Itrel II impulse generator allowed patients to choose between two voltage settings. Often, a lower voltage could be found that did not produce significant speech problems although at the sacrifice of some tremor control. Thus, when the patient needed to speak clearly, the patient could change to the lower voltage. When the patient needed greater tremor control, the patient could switch to a higher voltage. This feature is not available in the currently commercially available single-channel impulse generator (Soletra) but is available in the dual-channel impulse generator (Kinetra). The dual channel impulse generator requires that the patient have the hand-held controller (Access Patient Controller, Medtronic, Inc., Minneapolis, MN). However, the added expense of a wasted DBS channel with only unilateral DBS leads needs to be considered. Our approach is that, if intraoperative DBS testing suggests that speech may be a problem postoperatively, we favor the implantation of the patient adjustable impulse generator.

Vim DBS is effective for cerebellar outflow tremor such as occurs in patients with multiple sclerosis[3] and post-anoxic and posttraumatic tremor. Unfortunately, several papers have been published showing no benefit using outcomes measures such as the Extended Disability Status Scale (EDSS).[15] However, these scales are heavily weighted to ambulation, and significant improvements in unilateral upper extremity function are washed out. Given reasonable expectations and selection criteria, Vim DBS can be very helpful in patients with multiple sclerosis.[3]

Globus Pallidus Internal Segment Deep Brain Stimulation Effects

Figs. 13.29 and **13.30** schematically represent the regional anatomy about the GPi in the sagittal and coronal plane. Structures particularly relevant to DBS programming include the posterior limb of the internal capsule containing corticobulbar and corticospinal fibers and the optic tract. DBS activation of the internal capsule can cause tonic

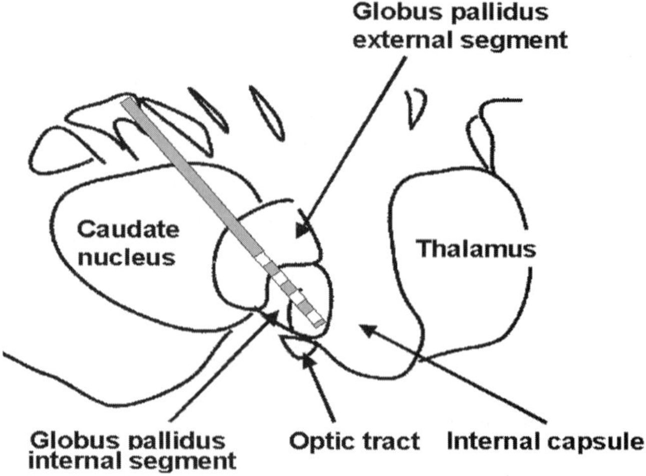

Fig. 13.29 Schematic representation of the regional anatomy around the globus pallidus internal segment in the sagittal plane.

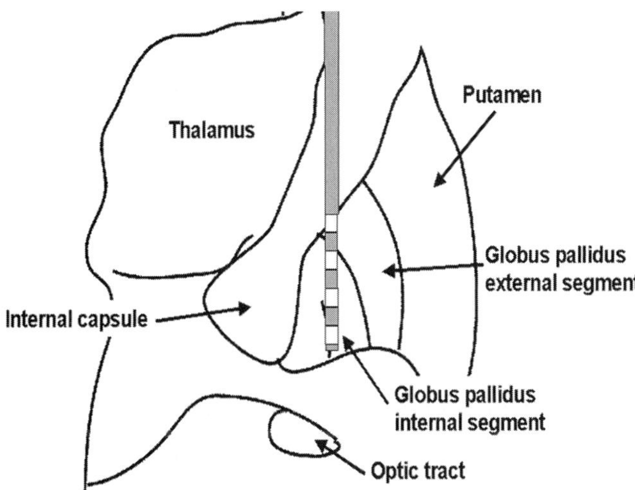

Fig. 13.30 Schematic representation of the regional anatomy around the globus pallidus internal segment in the coronal plane.

contraction. DBS activation of the optic tract can produce phosphenes and other visual disturbances.

Insufficient Efficacy in the Absence of Side Effects

Often, GPi DBS requires activation of larger volumes of brain tissue, which may be related to the fact that the GPi is a large structure. Consequently, monopolar or multiple cathodes may be required. In addition, long pulse widths can activate more neuronal elements without changing the size or strength of the electrical voltage field (**Fig. 13.3**). There has been some discussion in the literature that DBS of the more dorsal regions of the GPi or even of the globus pallidus external segment (GPe) may be better for bradykinesia and akinesia, whereas DBS of the more ventral region of the GPi may actually worsen bradykinesia and akinesia. However, the methods and inferences of these papers are suspect and cogent criticisms have been raised. Interestingly, GPe DBS is effective in humans.[16]

Tonic Contraction

If the DBS electrical field spreads too posteriorly, it can cause tonic contraction. Again, the response depends on the orientation of the DBS lead to the posterior limb of the internal capsule. The usual angle in the sagittal plane is such that the more ventral contacts are closer to the internal capsule. Moving the electrical field more dorsally can move the electrical field more anteriorly away from the internal capsule.

Phosphenes and Visual Disturbance

The optic tract lies just ventral to the GPi, and DBS leads placed too ventrally can cause phosphenes (described as bright lights or scintillating visual illusions) or other visual

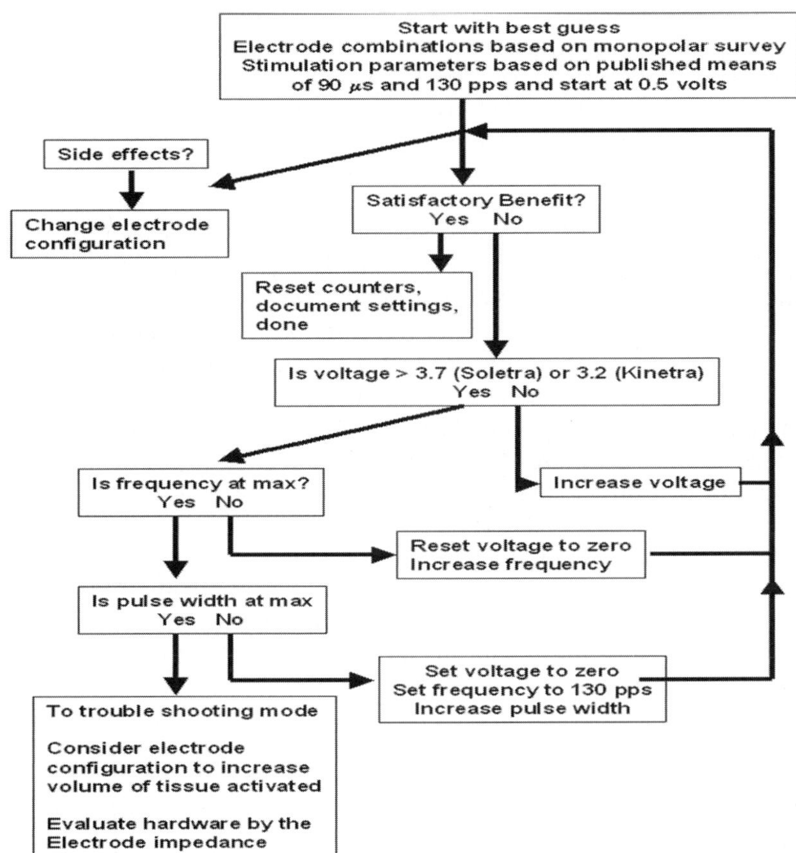

Fig. 13.31 Flow diagram for deep brain stimulation titration.

disturbances such as distortions. Therapeutic responses include moving the DBS electrical field more dorsally by using the dorsal contacts in monopolar or bipolar configurations. If DBS adjustments are insufficient, it may be possible to surgically revise the DBS lead under fluoroscopy.

■ Strategies of Deep Brain Stimulation Management

There is no way to determine ahead of time which DBS configuration and stimulation parameter sets are going to be optimal for any individual patient. DBS management is also challenging because there are literally thousands of possible combinations of DBS active contact configurations and stimulation parameters. One of the most common errors in DBS management is the lack of persistence.

Monopolar Survey

With initiation of DBS, we perform a monopolar survey to establish the regional anatomy and the orientation of the DBS to the patient's unique regional anatomy. Each contact is studied in the monopolar configuration with DBS parameters of pulse width = 90 microsec (μs) and frequency of 130 pps. The voltage is progressively increased until the patient experiences a significant side effect or reaches 5 V. If the effect is unclear, such as a speech disturbance not clearly related to tonic contraction, the voltage is increased further to clarify the response. The programmer should be prepared to stop the stimulation immediately. Based on the patterns of response the DBS active contact configuration most likely to provide the optimal therapy can be selected as described earlier.

Therapeutic Adjustments of Deep Brain Stimulation Parameter Sets

The first goal is maximal relief of symptoms with no or at least, tolerable side effects within established safety limits. Battery life is a secondary consideration. However, if two sets of DBS active contact configurations and stimulation parameter sets are equally effective, then the DBS active contact configuration and stimulation parameter set that have the least drain on the impulse generator battery should be used. The factors contributing to battery life include, in order from most draining to least, (1) multiple active contacts, (2) wide pulse widths, (3) voltages over the impulse generator battery voltage, (4) frequency, and (5) voltage below the impulse generator battery voltage.

The battery voltage is an important consideration in battery life. To achieve stimulation voltages greater than the battery voltage, a separate circuit in the impulse generator is engaged. This results in greater current drainage from the battery. The single-channel Soletra has a battery voltage of 3.7 V. The dual-channel Kinetra has a battery voltage of 3.2 V.

Therapeutic adjustments usually start with the DBS active contact configuration that will be tolerated and will activate the greatest volume of tissue. Generally, we start with monopolar configurations and if they are not tolerated, we move to far bipolar. Also, we start with the average stimulation parameters reported in clinical studies. These are pulse width 90 microsecondsec and a frequency of 130 pps. We start at 0.5 V and then increase in increments of 0.5 V, assessing the patient each time. The voltage is increased up to the impulse generator battery voltage. If the patient experiences a limiting side effect, the DBS active contact configuration is reevaluated and changed. If the patient does not achieve sufficient symptomatic relief but does not experience any limiting side effects, the voltage is set to 0 and the frequency is increased. The voltage again is titrated upward. If the maximum frequency is reached without sufficient benefit, but without limiting side effects, the voltage is set to 0, the frequency is reset to 130 pps, and the pulse width is increased. Voltages and frequencies are increased as described earlier with each new pulse width. If the patient has not experienced sufficient symptomatic relief but has not experienced any limiting side effects, it may be that sufficient volumes of brain tissue have not been activated. At this point, the DBS active contact configuration is reassessed. It may be necessary to use far bipolar configurations or multiple active cathodal (negative) contacts. This strategy is shown in **Fig. 13.31**.

If the patient does not achieve satisfactory control, then there may be a hardware failure or the DBS lead is malpositioned. The electrode impedance function can be used to look at all the possible pairwise configurations and determine impedance and current flow. If the impedances are high (greater than 2000 ohm) and there is little or no current, there may be an electrical discontinuity in the hardware. It should be possible by looking at different pairs of contact configurations to determine the one or more contacts that are associated with the high impedance and decreased current. If there is very low impedance with large current, then there may be a short circuit in the hardware.

Therapeutic failure may also be due to DBS lead migration or fracture. Generally, we obtain anteroposterior (AP) and lateral skull X-rays shortly after surgery. Although the skull X-rays will not show whether the DBS lead is properly positioned, the skull X-rays serve as a baseline. If in the future there is concern about possible lead migration or fracture, a quick skull X-ray could confirm the lead migration or fracture without having to subject the patient to an MRI scan, which, though unlikely, exposes the patient to risks. Malpositioning of the DBS leads can be assessed by MRI scan.

Occasionally, a patient may achieve a very satisfactory response in the physician's office, only to do poorly at home. There may be several reasons, including (1) physiological changes in the brain in response to ongoing stimulation, (2) changes in medications, or (3) inadvertent inactivation of the DBS impulse generators. There are any number of electrical devices that create electromagnetic fields that can interfere with the DBS impulse generator. Some, like metal detectors, are well known; however, we are constantly being surprised by new sources of electromagnetic interference, such as electric dog fences. One clue to such inadvertent impulse generator inactivations is high numbers of activation counts that can be determined by the programming device. The patient and caregivers need to be aware of potential adverse electrical environments and particularly avoid diathermy. If there is any question about electrical safety, the equipment manufacturer should be consulted.

Importance of Patient Ability to Assess Impulse Generator Status

Optional equipment available to patients implanted with currently commercially available impulse generators allow patients to turn the impulse generators on and off to determine whether the impulse generator is on or off and to check the battery status (Access Review Patient Controller for the Soletra impulse generator and Access Patient Controller for the Kinetra impulse generator). In our opinion, this is not optional but necessary for PD patients. Occasionally, patients become confused as to whether the impulse generator is on or off. This is particularly likely early in the course of DBS adjustments when medications are being adjusted simultaneously. Thus there can be a question as to whether the patient's worsening symptoms are related to pharmacological factors or DBS failure. Further, there have been case reports of serious complications from impulse generators suddenly being turned off.[17] The patient or caregiver must be able to determine whether the impulse generator is on or off and act accordingly.

Medication Adjustments

Although some physicians and other health care providers will arbitrarily reduce medications for PD patients after having STN DBS activated, in our experience, this has led to significant problems. The exact medication needs can vary greatly postsurgery and cannot be predicted. Often, there is a "microsubthalamotomy" effect that has required holding subsequent medications for hours and days. Some patients will not have a microsubthalamotomy effect and will need their medications as soon as they are able to take medications by mouth. Even after the initial DBS adjustments, it cannot be determined ahead of time how much and when the patient's medications can be reduced.

For PD patients, the issue often comes up as to which medications to reduce first. We determine which are the most clinically significant medication-related complications. If dyskinesia is the major issue, we first reduce those medications with the highest probability of producing dyskinesia. In order from most to least risk of dyskinesia are (1)

entacapone, (2) immediate release carbidopa/levodopa, (3) controlled-release carbidopa/levodopa, (4) pramipexole and ropinirole, and (5) anticholinergics and amantadine. If cognitive side effects are the most disabling, then medications most likely to cause cognitive effects are reduced first. These in order from most to least likely are (1) anticholinergics, (2) amantadine, (3) pramipexole, (4) ropinirole, (5) controlled-release carbidopa/levodopa, and (6) immediate-release carbidopa/levodopa.

Timing of Medication Adjustments Relative to Deep Brain Stimulation Adjustments

Particularly in PD patients, the DBS can have synergistic effects with the patient's medications. Therefore, the programmer needs to be cognizant of where the patient is in the medication cycle when the DBS is adjusted. We use the STN DBS to improve parkinsonian symptoms and adjust the medications to treat medication-related side effects such as dyskinesia. Occasionally, a programmer will increase the STN DBS and produce marked dyskinesia. The immediate temptation is to reduce the STN DBS. However, we argue that the medications should be reduced and not the STN DBS.

Because we are interested in optimizing the parkinsonian symptoms, it is important to titrate the STN DBS at a time when the patient's symptoms are maximal. Typically, this is in the morning following an overnight fast from medications. We often ask patients to hold their first morning dose of medications until after their DBS adjustment session. However, we ask them what their condition usually is in the morning and whether they can safely hold their medications. An alternative time when the medications may be at the minimal effect is at the time the next medication is due.

After the stimulation adjustment, the patient needs to be observed during a drug maximal state to ensure that the patient does not have an exacerbation of dyskinesia that would require medication adjustments. Typically, the drug maximal state is ~1 hour after the dose of medications.

Strategies for GPi DBS in PD fall into two schools. One uses GPi to optimize PD disability and follows a scheme similar to that described earlier for STN DBS. An alternative is to use GPi DBS to suppress dyskinesia thereby allowing more aggressive medication therapy. In this case, the DBS adjustments should be done at the time when the dyskinesia is at its maximum. This is usually about 1 hour after the patient's medication dose (although this timing may be delayed with controlled-release carbidopa/levodopa or in the case of diphasic dyskinesia). In this case the patient also needs to be observed at a drug minimal state.

Effects of the Time Course of Deep Brain Stimulation Response

The titration of DBS depends on how quickly the symptoms respond. For example, tremor responds almost immediately to STN, GPi, or Vim DBS. Bradykinesia in PD may take seconds to minutes. Gait and balance may take up to 30 minutes or more. We generally evaluate and then change stimulation parameters within a minute or two of changing a stimulation parameter rather than waiting for gait or balance to improve. However, at the end of the session we evaluate the gait and balance.

Dystonia is a special case. The improvement may take weeks to months. Thus one cannot wait weeks to months to make individual changes in the stimulation parameters. Consequently, we initially set the stimulation parameters typically reported in the literature: pulse width = 120 microsecondsec, frequency = 145 pulses per second (pps) and monopolar stimulation through the most ventral contacts tolerated. We then increase the voltage up to the battery voltage as tolerated. If this is not tolerated, we reduce the voltage to just below that which produced side effects. If there is no improvement within 4 weeks, we then increase the voltage to zero, increase the frequency, and again raise the voltage to the battery voltage or whatever is tolerated. If we have raised the frequency to the maximum, we then turn to adjusting the pulse width.

When the patient achieves satisfactory control, it cannot be determined with confidence whether it was the most recent adjustment that resulted in improvement or some previous adjustment with a delayed response. One option would then be to reverse the process to determine the minimal stimulation parameter necessary, thereby prolonging battery life. However, some programmers and patients want to stay at the last setting that provided improvement, and this is not unreasonable.

■ Future of Deep Brain Stimulation

DBS represents a paradigm shift in therapeutics for chronic neurological and psychiatric disorders, which is particularly significant in this era of molecular biology (see Chapter 17). DBS provides remarkable improvement in the lives of patients, and it is initially surprising to the novice. But the brain is basically an electronic device. It transmits and processes information electronically. The brain has more in common with a computer than it does a stew of chemicals. The future of DBS is limited only by the imagination and the willingness of physicians to embrace this technology.

Editor's Comments

In a review of North American practices, initial programming was performed on an average of 18 days after electrode placement but ranged from 1 to 90 days.[18] The most common programmers are the neurologists. Occasionally, medications are reduced during the initial activation of the DBS. Most centers will wait until an effective stimulation can be established. Dose reduction occurs in over 80% of patients, with ~47% having greater than 50% reduction in parkinsonian medications. There is no longer any need for externalization and lead testing prior to implantation for the implantable pulse generator (IPG) for movement disorders.[19] In general, it is the rigidity symptoms that are monitored during STN stimulation trials because these are the most reliable to suggest the appropriate area is being affected. Similar effectiveness is also sought in GPi DBS initial programming. The optimal electrode is evaluated by clinical assessment of the acute effect on rigidity (activate with Froment sign if necessary) for both STN and GPi leads. For Vim leads, tremor is the primary assessment symptom and is activated if needed with mental calculations if necessary. When programming, meticulous notes should be taken on standardized forms to be clear about the effects and save time both immediately and in the future. Be fastidious about the initial programming because it will set the stage for subsequent changes and will save confusion and time later. Many programmers will program several patients simultaneously to maximize efficiency and reimbursement. An assistant can be extremely helpful to rapidly screen patients and still allow time for observation long enough to ensure optimal programming. Work systematically through each parameter and do not skip steps or assume effects. Many parkinsonian patients are believed to be quite stable following initial programming; however, recent reevaluation of this concept suggests that reprogramming may be beneficial in a majority of patients and suggests the continued need for hands-on involvement by a neurologist with expertise in both movement disorders and DBS programming.[20] Programming sessions should be restricted to 1 to 2 hours to prevent fatigue. In difficult cases, the patient should be allowed to rest or go to lunch and return for additional evaluation if necessary the same day.

Programming has to be individualized. There are literally thousands of combinations that can be used in programming a DBS lead. To optimize these in a reasonable logical manner, a systematic approach such as described in this chapter is necessary. Other approaches have been published.[21–24] Most programming will be done with either the Itrel II impulse generator (Medtronic, Inc., Minneapolis, MN) (outdated but still in service) or the Soletra (www.medtronic.com/physician/activa/techmanuals.html). Programming is essentially the same on both, the only difference is that the Itrel II has two different settings, which can be alternately employed using a magnet to switch into a "magnetic amplitude" mode that allows flexibility in the voltage parameters. We have used this very successfully in patients who accept minor, short-term side effects, such as paresthesia, that occur at the higher voltages required to achieve maximum control before a presentation, or meal, or some other short-term interactive activity. The problem has been that it is too complex for most patients to handle and is minimally useful for those that are able to master the ability to switch back and forth. Another problem is that if the "magnetic amplitude" mode is set at zero, patients may have difficulty getting out of this mode without help.

Another IPG is the Kinetra (Medtronic 7428, www.medtronic.com/physician/activa/surg_components), which was approved by the U.S. Food and Drug Administration (FDA) on January 22, 2004, for use in patients with PD or essential tremor. It is used far more commonly in Europe, where it was introduced. The Kinetra allows for two quadripolar leads to be connected to a single unit. This unit unfortunately is more than twice as large (51 cm³) as the Soletra (22 mm³) and as such presents difficulties in terms of implantation in children, thin-skinned patients, and the occasional patients in whom aesthetics are very important. The advantages of the Kinetra are listed in **Table 13.2**. The Kinetra allows many more settings and has three distinct advantages. The first is that the patients themselves can adjust voltage and frequency within a limit prescribed by the treating physician. This is optional and does not have to be provided to patients who are unable to manage it, which is more flexible than the Itrel II. This feature allows the patient to optimize settings for daytime activity and minimize them at night to save battery life. Second, it can be set so that the magnetic switch can be turned off, and therefore not be affected by extraneous magnetic forces. Finally, the battery is reportedly configured so that it is not as adversely affected by voltages greater than 3.6 V. The power consumption is linear, and therefore, there is not the same power drain with settings greater than 3.6 V. Both the Soletra and the Itrel II power consumption dramatically increases above 3.6 to 3.7 V due to a "double circuit" in which the second capacitor is switched into the system. This reduces the battery life. What many programmers are unaware of is that there is a second jump at 7.3 V ("triple circuit"), which will further significantly limit the battery life. Any stimulation requiring this high voltage strongly suggests the need for a different electrode placement closer or more optimally placed within the target.

The Kinetra in theory should be highly beneficial in the treatment of dystonic patients. In general, stimulation of GPi DBS requires higher voltages and the Kinetra is especially useful in its ability to extend battery life. The high amplitudes, frequencies, and pulse widths are the reason that Soletra replacements may be required every year for certain dystonic patients. Kinetra offers extended battery life with these same settings. Unfortunately, the Kinetra is not FDA-approved for dystonia; thus reimbursement is not available for this use in most instances. As a result, there is little interest in using it in the United States. Similarly, the Kinetra is reimbursed at a level less than that for bilateral IPG placements, and as such this will discourage its use. Also, many programmers prefer two separate units because of the ability to alter frequencies independently, which is not available on the Kinetra. Finally, many neurosurgeons approach the problem pragmatically. The IPG waveform differ from theoretical and are different from the Soletra and Kinetra, so parameters must be individualized for each patient.[25] If the Kinetra gets infected, the entire system may be lost bilaterally, whereas if you have two separate units, infection on one side does not necessarily require removal of the device on the other side.

The focus is primarily to maximize beneficial effects and minimize adverse effects. However, the effect on battery life must also be considered because replacements are not without complications. Tricks to increase the battery life include turning the stimulator off at night for patients with essential tremor or rare tremor predominant PD in whom bradykinesia and rigidity are not significant problems. This would be true for either Vim or STN DBS. Although there are some dystonic patients who can keep the stimulator off overnight, these are the exceptions. At least for tremor, there appears to be a plateau of improvement in which stimulation frequency above 130 Hz does not improve tremor control to any significant degree. Although higher frequencies are occasionally required, in general, these will provide marginal benefit and increase the power drainage. It may therefore be better to increase pulse width or amplitude to increase current spread, rather than increasing frequency, which will not increase current spread. Pulse width in STN is clearly less effective for other symptoms.[24] The contacts that are active will also alter the power drainage. Monopolar stimulation is used most commonly in the vast majority of patients. If there are side effects, then bipolar stimulation allows the current spread to be concentrated and narrowed. Because cathodic stimulation is most effective, it is possible to use the best electrode as the cathode.[24] At other times because of the irregularities current spread, a reversed polarity may help. Side effects are frequently from either lateral or ventral stimulation

Table 13.2 Comparison of Soletra and Kinetra*

Feature	Soletra	Kinetra	Potential Kinetra Benefit
Neurostimulator	Single port	Dual port	One neurostimulator but bulky
Amplitude	0–10.5; by 0.1 V	0–10.5; by 0.05 V up to 6.5 V	Finer amplitude adjustments 0–6.5 V
Frequency (range)	2–185 Hz; 28 settings	3–250 Hz; 66 settings	Ability to better titrate therapy but unable to individually program each side
Battery drain	3.6 V double capacitor 7.3 V triple capacitor	Gradual; no double capacitor	Extended battery life with patients requiring greater than 3.6 V
Battery deplete near end of life	Fast	Moderate/slow	Greater predictability; ease with patient management and patient self-management
Battery capacity indication	Not available	Available	Improved prediction for replacement planning
Magnet switch	Always "on"	Disable option	Reduced inadvertent shutoff (electromagnetic interference)
Patient control-adjust stimulation	Not available	Available; physician-prescribed only	Controlled adjustment for more patient control when needed and/or nocturnal battery sparing
Soft start amplitude ramp	One option	Four options	Smoother transitions to maximal amplitude

* Data from Medtronic, Inc., Minneapolis, MN.

of the electrode, and using a more dorsal electrode is an alternative strategy. Whether monopolar or bipolar is used, excellent results can be achieved. The disadvantage of the bipolar is that it will produce a smaller current spread at the same relative voltage. Activating more than two contacts for bipolar stimulation results in an extremely complex field of spread that is usually quite narrow and long (the tripolar stimulation). This is rarely used but can be the only effective stimulation parameter in certain cases. It is certainly worth trying in some circumstances. Regardless of the setting, for Soletra, the voltage should be below 3.6 V to allow battery sparing. If there are only marginal differences between 3.5 V and 3.7 V, the low setting will dramatically prolong the battery life. If the differences are substantial, then consider repositioning the lead. Consider repositioning the lead anytime there is suboptimal performance in a patient who otherwise should do well, especially if the magnetic resonance imaging (MRI) study also suggests suboptimal placement.

It is generally unwise to allow the batteries to be completely drained, and periodic evaluation should allow the programmer to detect when the end of life will occur.[26,27] Patients also may notice increasing symptomatology, which should be a forewarning that the batteries are close to the end of life. Acute return of symptomatology can be quite disturbing to the patient and on occasion can produce severe adverse affects. Although there is the theoretical possibility of development of a neuroleptic malignant syndrome or status dystonicus–like syndrome, these have not yet been documented. Acute loss of power has many potential etiologies (see **Table 13.3**). The easiest and most obvious is a loss of power of the IPG. This can be tested with simple diagnostics. The far more unusual cause would be that of a "twiddler syndrome" in which the IPG has been manipulated voluntarily or involuntarily such that it no longer is oriented properly and interrogation becomes impossible or wires are damaged. It is rare to have a failure of the IPG electronics, but this has occurred, especially with the Kinetra.[28] Interrogation of the IPG should reveal whether there is a fracture that would require replacement of the damaged lead or a short circuit that may require exploration for repair or replacement of loose or damaged connections. Movement or migration of the lead usually occurs in the immediate perioperative period and almost always requires reoperation to correct. Migration of the DBS lead is unusual as a late complication but can oc-

cur especially if the connector is not secured properly. Essential tremor is one of the few diseases in which there is a population of patients who lose effectiveness long term. This can occasionally be rescued by a stimulation holiday and reprogramming. Tolerance is also lessened by turning the stimulator off overnight. Nonetheless, additional therapy may be required for this particular set of patients (see Chapter 11).

Programming of STN presents its own special problems. Here there is a need to balance L-dopa reduction with increased intensity of stimulation. The appearance of dyskinesia is not uncommon during placement of an STN DBS lead. The dyskinesia frequently disappears during chronic STN stimulation.[29–31] Because of the similar effects of STN stimulation and medication, reduction of dopaminergic medication is generally regarded as an important goal of STN DBS management. Some authors have recommended immediate replacement of the controlled released L-dopa and dopamine agonist with monotherapy with L-dopa. We have not found this to be necessary to obtain slow and gradual control of the dyskinesia during DBS programming. Initial programming is performed during the off stage to monitor effects on parkinsonian symptomatology, and as such, the dyskinesia is not a problem. The presence of dyskinesia on medication is treated by slowly decreasing the dopaminergic medication. All of this might take several weeks to perform. The greater the difficulty with dyskinesia from low-dose L-dopa preoperatively, the more problems there will be adjusting stimulation and medication postoperatively. There are rare cases when the optimal electrode is no longer used because of the induction of dyskinesia but rather an adjacent electrode is used so the effects on dyskinesia can be minimized. Care should be taken in reducing dopaminergic medications with STN stimulation in that some symptomatologies such as depression or nonmotor symptoms may be suddenly unmasked. This is also relatively typical with restless leg syndrome where increase in stimulation may sometimes resolve this syndrome; more often it requires additional dopamine medication, although on occasion benzodiazepines or opiates may be of significant benefit without inducing dyskinesia. Similarly, the sudden presence of abulia and anhedonia or depression may represent unintended stimulation of the substantia nigra pars reticulata (SNr) or could be the limbic area of the STN and suggests the need for a more proximal contact to be employed. In postoperative hypomania or ma-

Table 13.3 Loss of Efficacy from Deep Brain Stimulation

Problem	Finding	Diagnostic	Solution
IPG OFF	IPG signal indicates off	None	Turn on
IPG EOL	No signal	Past EOL expectancy	Replace IPG
IPG inverted	No signal	Not past EOL inverted on X-ray occasional electrical shocks feeling in chest	Reposition IPG manually or surgically and warn patient about moving IPG
IPG Hardware failure	No signal or "power on reset"	No values or parameters return to default values	IPG replacement
Wire fracture open circuit	Signal present impedance > 2000 Ω	Head to chest X-rays*	Lead replacement
Wire fracture short circuit	Signal present impedance < 50 Ω	Head to chest X-rays*	Lead replacement
Lead migration	Signal present	Lead moved on skull X-ray or MRI*	Lead replacement

* MRI only after fracture or short circuit ruled-out.
Abbreviations: EOL, end of life; IPG, internal pulse generator; MRI, magnetic resonance imaging.

nia, symptoms may be improved by decreased dopaminergic therapy, but on occasion stimulation will also have to be decreased. There is, in general, the need to keep patients on a small amount of dopaminergic medication for its effects in areas outside of those areas being directly affected by the stimulation. Although we have had patients entirely off medication, in general most return to some degree of medication for optimal improvement. As stated in this chapter, we approach medication adjustments of the many anti-PD medications the patient is taking by increasing or decreasing as needed. If the major problem is dyskinesia, we begin to reduce those medications most likely to cause dyskinesia (entacapone, immediate release dopa, controlled release L-dopa, pergolide, etc.). If the major problem is cognitive side effects from the medications, then we begin to reduce and eliminate those most likely to cause cognitive problems (anticholinergics, amatadine, pergolide, ropinirole, etc.).

In addition to careful adjustment of stimulation parameters for dyskinesia, sometimes the axial symptomatology may also be worsened by stimulation, and this similarly suggests the need for different stimulation parameters or different lead configuration. Induced axial problems, especially when combined with postural disturbance, may suggest a lead placement that is too close to the red nucleus in prerubral fields; replacement of the lead should be considered if stimulation cannot be appropriately adjusted. DBS effects on speech are generally small and beneficial but can be detrimental when close to the corticospinal tract. Thus adjustments may have to be a compromise between effective symptomatic treatment and effective speech. This is usually dysarthria, and careful evaluation should be made to determine whether there is a pseudobulbar dysarthria, which if not correctable by switching to a bipolar configuration or different stimulation parameters may require a lead revision. Speech problems not altered by STN programming should be tested with a L-dopa challenge to be sure it is not the result of too little medication. Tonic corticospinal effects need to be distinguished from dystonia and if therapeutically limiting may require lead revision for resolution.[32] Ocular deviation presents a more complex problem. Monocular eye movements suggest stimulation too medial and are not likely to habituate. Conjugate eye movements are more likely to be due to corticospinal problems; however, there are times where this could be due to oculomotor-basal ganglia loop stimulation.[24] Eyelid apraxia is not uncommon immediately postoperatively but usually completely resolves on its own. This frequently occurs in relationship to blepharospasm, and treatment with botulinum toxin has sometimes been required. Combinations with sweating and mydriasis suggest a too posterior and too medial location. Very late deterioration (greater than 3 years following DBS lead placement) may not be due to improper lead location or stimulation parameters as much as to continued deterioration from the underlying disease. An assessment of clinical deterioration should not be made with leads placed within 6 months or even a year.

Both neuropsychiatric and cognitive problems appear to be much more common with DBS STN lead placement than with other placements. Transient confusion is also more common but should resolve within several days to several months. Persistent hypomania, suicide ideation, apathy, and cognitive disturbances, especially in relation to verbal memory, may be the results of lead placement, especially with leads into the SNr. Treatment of these problems, other than using a higher contact, is extremely difficult and a fixed deficit may result

from lead placement. Postoperative MRI can be most helpful in this evaluation.

Specific problems related to GPi lead placement seem to be less common. Current studies seem to suggest that the GPi STN stimulation can be equally effective in treating Parkinson's disease (see Chapter 15). Concerns about increased dyskinesia during stimulation are less evident with GPi leads, especially the ventral electrodes. There has been a suggestion of a need to balance the effects of stimulation ventral in GPi (decreased dyskinesia but less effective for bradykinesia and gait) versus dorsal (greater anti-Parkinson effect but can produce dyskinesia) to achieve both optimal anti-Parkinson effects and dyskinesia effects.[30,31,33] Others, including Dr. Montgomery, doubt this dichotomy. The need to balance medication and stimulation in GPi is not the same for STN. The ability to diminish drugs with GPi stimulation seems to be less than that with STN. Transient problems with GPi lead placement can include increased freezing, balance difficulties, falls, and gait akinesia. Most studies demonstrate improvements in these symptoms.[1,30,31,34,35] Just as with STN DBS, chronic deterioration of axial and postural stability seems to continue in relationship to the underlying disease.

Although speech difficulties can occur with GPi DBS, these are infrequently reported. Such difficulties usually respond to adjustment of parameters, suggesting that this is a much more limited problem than that with STN DBS. Lead repositioning is therefore less common. Again, although oculomotor difficulties can occur with GPi DBS, these are from current spread into the internal capsule and in most cases can be corrected with programming without the need for DBS lead readjustment. A somewhat unique problem is that of visual disturbance, which does not occur with leads in other locations and suggests that the most ventral contact is being used and that a more dorsal contact should resolve the problem. Again, cognitive, behavioral, and psychiatric problems are reported far less frequently in DBS placements in GPi. Similar to STN DBS, reprogramming rarely affects these problems. However, loss of efficacy may develop with the GPi DBS after a year following the placement of the lead. In those few instances, reprogramming can produce significant benefit and rarely is repositioning of the electrode necessary. With loss of effectiveness of the DBS lead in GPi, many investigators will elect to place the stimulator in STN rather than reimplant it in the GPi if replacement is required. Although most programming is done in the off stage, there are occasional needs with pallidal DBS in PD to program the patients in the on period where dyskinesia can be monitored and the intended clinical response gauged more appropriately. In some cases with effective antidyskinetic effect from GPi stimulation, higher doses of L-dopa may actually be useful. Some programmers suggest that the discontinuation of the parkinsonian medication for GPi DBS is different from that for STN DBS because of its marked effects on dyskinesia. They have recommended starting with the catechol-o-methyltransferase (COMT) inhibitors followed by anticholinergic drugs or amantadine and finally L-dopa and dopamine agonists. We and others would use the same plan as for STN described above.

Programming the GPi lead for dystonia is another special problem. The dystonic changes do not appear to be acute but rather occur over a long period of time (see Chapter 12). As such, adjustments during a clinic visit even over several days may not adequately reflect the ultimate results of the particular parameters being studied. Patients are frequently required to come back and be reevaluated in this situation. Small parameter changes can have dramatic effects that are not apparent at the time of programming. This creates a special difficulty in evaluating and managing these patients. DBS GPi stimulation for dystonia has its unique characteristics requiring greater amplitude and wide pulse widths to stimulate a larger volume as compared with the other nuclei. This results in a very rapid deterioration of the IPG re-quiring frequent battery replacements. Recent studies suggest that, at least in some patients, low-frequency stimulation may be of value and in this setting would dramatically prolong IPG life (personal experience and communications). Improvements in dystonia with DBS GPi frequently allow reduction or discontinuation of antidystonia medication, especially the anticholinergic drugs. Acute discontinuation of stimulation can cause a rebound dystonia which can be very severe.

References

1. Deep-Brain Stimulation for Parkinson's Disease Study Group. Deep-brain stimulation of the subthalamic nucleus or the pars interna of the globus pallidus in Parkinson's disease. N Engl J Med 2001;345:956–963

2. Koller W, Pahwa R, Busenbark K, et al. High-frequency unilateral thalamic stimulation in the treatment of essential and parkinsonian tremor. Ann Neurol 1997;42:292–299

3. Montgomery EB Jr, Baker KB, Kinkel RP, Barnett G. Chronic thalamic stimulation of the tremor of multiple sclerosis. Neurology 1999;53:625–628

4. Bereznai B, Steude U, Seelos K, Botzel K. Chronic high-frequency globus pallidus internus stimulation in different types of dystonia: a clinical, video, and MRI report of six patients presenting with segmental, cervical, and generalized dystonia. Mov Disord 2002;17:138–144

5. Olanow CW, Goetz CG, Kordower JH, et al. A double-blind controlled trial of bilateral fetal nigral transplantation in Parkinson's disease. Ann Neurol 2003;54:403–414

6. Anderson ME, Postupna N, Ruffo M. Effects of high-frequency stimulation in the internal globus pallidus on the activity of thalamic neurons in the awake monkey. J Neurophysiol 2003;89:1150–1160

7. Hashimoto T, Elder CM, Okun MS, Patrick SK, Vitek JL. Stimulation of the subthalamic nucleus changes the firing pattern of pallidal neurons. J Neurosci 2003;23:1916–1923

8. Ranck JB Jr. Which elements are excited in electrical stimulation of mammalian central nervous system: a review. Brain Res 1975;98:417–440

9. Scott A. Neuroscience: A Mathematical Primer. New York: Springer-Verlag; 2002

10. Montgomery EB Jr. Dynamically coupled, high-frequency reentrant, non-linear oscillators embedded in scale-free basal ganglia-thalamic-cortical networks mediating function and deep brain stimulation effects. Nonlinear Studies 2004;11:385–421

11. Baker KB, Montgomery EB Jr, Rezai AR, Burgess R, Lüders HO. Subthalamic nucleus deep brain stimulus evoked potentials: physiology and therapeutic implications. Mov Disord 2002;17:969–983

12. Voges J, Volkmann J, Allert N, et al. Bilateral high-frequency stimulation in the subthalamic nucleus for the treatment of Parkinson disease: correlation of therapeutic effect with anatomical electrode position. J Neurosurg 2002;96:269–279

13. Yokoyama T, Sugiyama K, Nishizawa S, et al. The optimal stimulation site for chronic stimulation of the subthalamic nucleus in Parkinson's disease. Stereotact Funct Neurosurg 2001;77:61–67

14. Lanotte MM, Rizzone M, Begamasco B, Faccani G, Melcarne A, Lopiano L. Deep brain stimulation of the subthalamic nucleus: anatomical, neurophysiological, and outcome correlations with the effects of stimulation. J Neurol Neurosurg Psychiatry 2002;72:53–58

15. Schulder M, Sernas TJ, Karimi R. Thalamic stimulation in patients with multiple sclerosis: long-term follow-up. Stereotact Funct Neurosurg 2003;80:48–55

16. Vitek JL, Hashimoto T, Peoples J, DeLong MR, Bakay AE. Acute stimulation in the external segment of the globus pallidus improves Parkinsonian motor signs. Mov Disord 2004;19:907–915

17. Hariz MI, Johansson F. Hardware failure in Parkinsonian patients with chronic subthalamic nucleus stimulation is a medical emergency. Mov Disord 2001;16:166–168

18. Hamel W, Fietzek U, Morsnowski A, et al. Deep brain stimulation of the subthalamic nucleus in Parkinson's disease: evaluation of active electrode contacts. J Neurol Neurosurg Psychiatry 2003;74:1036–1046

19. Ondo WG, Bronte-Stewart H. The North North American survey of placement and adjustment strategies for deep brain stimulation. Stereotact Funct Neurosurg 2005;83:142–147

20. Moro E, Poon YY, Lozano AM, Saint-Cyr JA, Lang AE. Subthalamic nucleus stimulation: improvements in outcome with reprogramming. Arch Neurol 2006;63:1266–1272

21. Krack P, Fraix V, Mendes A, Benabid AL, Pollak P. Postoperative management of subthalamic nucleus stimulation for Parkinson's disease. Mov Disord 2002;17(Suppl 3):S188–S197

22. Kumar R. Methods for programming and patient management with deep brain stimulation of the globus pallidus for the treatment of advanced Parkinson's disease and dystonia. Mov Disord 2002;17(Suppl 3):S198–S207

23. Dowsey-Limousin P. Postoperative management of Vim DBS for tremor. Mov Disord 2002;17(Suppl. 3):S208–S211

24. Volkmann J, Moro E, Pahwa R. Basic algorithms for the programming of deep brain stimulation in Parkinson's disease. Mov Disord 2006;21(Suppl 14):S284–S289

25. Butson CR, McIntyre CC. Differences among implanted pulse generator waveforms cause viriations in the neural response to deep brain stimulation. Clin Neurophysiol 2007;118:1889–1894

26. Chou KL, Siderowf AD, Jaggi JL, Liang GS, Baltuch GH. Unilateral battery depletion in Parkinson's disease patients treated with bilateral subthalamic nucleus deep brain stimulation may require urgent surgical replacement. Stereotact Funct Neurosurg 2004;82:153–155

27. Anheim M, Fraix V, Chabardes S, Krack P, Benabid AL, and Pollak P. Lifetime of Itrel II pulse generators for subthalamic nucleus stimulation in Parkinson's disease. Mov Disord 2007;22:2436–2439

28. Alesch F. Sudden failure of dual channel pulse generators. Mov Disord 2005;20:64–66

29. Krack P, Pollak P, Limousin P, Benazzouz A, Deuschl G, Benabid A. From off-period dystonia to peak-dose chorea: the clinical spectrum of varying subthalamic nucleus activity. Brain 1999;122:1133–1146

30. Deuschl G, Herzog J, Kleiner-Fisman G, Kubu C, Lozano AM, Lyons KE, Rodrigues-Oroz MC, et al. Deep brain stimulation: postoperative issues. Mov Disord 2006;21:S219–S237

31. Kleiner-Fisman G, Herzog J, Fisman DN, Tamma F, Lyons KE, Pahwa R, et al. Subthalamic nucleus deep brain stimulation: summary and meta-analysis of outcomes. Mov Disord 2006;21:S290–S304

32. Pahwa R, Wilkinson SB, Overman J, Lyons KE. Bilateral subthalamic stimulation in patients with Parkinson's disease: long-term follow up. J Neurosurg 2003;99:71–77

33. Bejjani B, Damier P, Arnulf I, et al. Pallidal stimulation for Parkinson's disease: two targets? Neurology 1997;49:1564–1569

34. Krack P, Pollak P, Limousin P, et al. Opposite motor effects of pallidal stimulation in Parkinson's disease. Ann Neurol 1998;43:180–192

35. Defebvre LJ, Krystkowiak P, Blatt JL, et al. Influence of pallidal stimulation and levodopa on gait and preparatory postural adjustments in Parkinson's disease. Mov Disord 2002;17:76–83

14 Avoiding Complications and Correcting Errors

Philip A. Starr

Several recent publications have reviewed complications of deep brain stimulation (DBS)[1–8] and lesioning surgery[4,9–12] for movement disorders. A summary of our group's perioperative and device-related complications in 405 DBS implants for movement disorders is provided in **Table 14.1**. Procedures were performed with frame-based stereotaxy using magnetic resonance imaging (MRI) and microelectrode recording (MER). Medtronic Activa (Medtronic, Inc., Minneapolis, MN) DBS hardware was used in all cases. The total incidence of unexpected returns to the operating room for management of a complication was 38 cases, or 9.6% of implanted leads.

This chapter describes our current methods for complication avoidance and management. These methods continue to evolve. Although this discussion is oriented primarily toward DBS, many of the principles apply to other stereotactic procedures. Complications uniquely associated with stereotactic lesioning procedures are discussed briefly at the end of the chapter.

■ Operative Complications

Stroke

Stroke is the most serious potential complication of movement disorders surgery. Stroke is defined as a new neurological deficit of vascular origin, lasting longer than 24 hours. Using this definition, our DBS series includes seven strokes, for an incidence of 1.7% per lead and 3.0% per patient. Six of these were hemorrhagic strokes. **Fig. 14.1** shows postoperative brain imaging for representative hematomas. **Table 14.2** provides details of presumed etiologic factors.

Ischemic infarction is very infrequent following DBS surgery, occurring only once in our series (**Fig. 14.2**). In contrast, delayed ischemic capsular infarction has been well described following pallidotomy[10,13] and is probably a more frequent complication of stereotactic lesioning surgery than of DBS.

Asymptomatic hemorrhage is more common than symptomatic hemorrhage but is only detected if postoperative imaging is performed systematically. Our rate of asymptomatic hemorrhage, detected on routine postoperative magnetic resonance imaging (MRI) was 2.2% per lead. A typical asymptomatic hematoma is shown in **Fig. 14.1D**. Most of the asymptomatic hematomas occurred subcortically, 25 to 35 mm superior to the target, corresponding to the location where the guide tube for the microelectrode terminated.

Avoidance of Stroke

Based on our experience, we recommend the following measures to reduce the incidence of stroke:

1. Maintain systolic pressure under 140 and mean arterial pressure (MAP) under 90. In any patient with preexisting hypertension, we place an arterial line and control blood pressure with a continuous intravenous drip (esmolol, nitroglycerine, or nitroprusside).
2. Avoid damage to, or coagulation of, venous structures. We perform surgeries through burr holes where the surface vessels may be directly visualized, rather than a twist drill hole. In addition, subsequent to the two venous infarctions in our series, our stereotactic MRI protocol has included a contrast-enhanced T1-weighted image set to visualize cortical veins as well as arteries. Surgical planning software is then used to plan a trajectory to the target that avoids MRI-visible blood vessels, sulci, and the ventricles.
3. During pallidal surgery, avoid passing instruments deep to the optic tract (OT), into the choroidal fissure. One of our worst DBS complications (**Fig. 14.1A**) was associated with bleeding from a presumed choroidal vessel as we attempted to localize the optic tract. Currently, if we do not locate OT within 2 mm of the base of pallidum, we do not continue more inferiorly.
4. Any sudden Valsalva during or immediately after surgery carries a risk of hemorrhage. If a patient has an upper respiratory infection or any other reversible source of coughing, surgery should be postponed. Smokers with a chronic cough must be advised that their risk of perioperative hemorrhage may be increased.
5. Avoid rapid insertion or withdrawal (> 0.5 mm/s) of instruments into or out of the brain.
6. During and at the end of the procedure, cover the cortical entry with Gelfoam (Pfizer Inc., New York, NY) and fibrin glue, to avoid subdural blood accumulation.

Management of Stroke

Should a new neurological deficit occur during the procedure, surgery is immediately stopped. The anesthesiolo-

Table 14.1 Complications in 405 Deep Brain Stimulus Implants in 228 Patients Implanted 1998–2003 *

Complication	# of cases	% of leads	% of patients	Comments
Hemorrhagic stroke	6	1.5	2.6	Details in Table 14.2
Ischemic stroke	1	0.2	0.4	Capsular infarction with contralateral hemiparesis 1 week postsurgery
Asymptomatic hemorrhage[†]	9	2.2	4.0	All occurred within 3 cm of the anatomical target
Chronic subdural hematoma	1	0.2	0.4	Symptom was headache, treated with burr hole drainage
Delayed lead fracture	2	0.5	0.9	Associated with connector in cervical position $N = 1$; or with use of a titanium miniplate for lead anchoring $N = 1$
Poor lead position resulting in reoperation	9	2.2	3.9	By target: STN $N = 3$, GPi $N = 4$, thalamus $N = 2$
Poor lead position, not reoperated	1	0.2	0.4	Lead placed into nonmotor (anteromedial) STN with little benefit
Lead migration resulting in reoperation	2	0.5	0.9	Associated with use of methylmethacrylate alone for anchoring lead
Infection requiring hardware removal and IV antibiotics	8	2.0	3.5	All ipsilateral hardware removed $N = 4$; only IPG and lead extender removed $N = 4$
Infection requiring IV antibiotics without hardware removal	2	0.5	0.9	Both occurred at scalp wound
Return to operating room for other exploration/repair of subcutaneous hardware	17	4.3	7.5	Problems included: sterile seroma around IPG $N = 1$; hematoma around IPG $N = 1$; hardware disconnection $N = 2$; failure of wound to heal $N = 1$; suspected IPG malfunction $N = 1$; lead extender malfunction $N = 3$; elective repositioning of connector from cervical to cranial position $N = 4$; lead extender replacement to address patient discomfort $N = 1$; connector repositioning for threatened erosion $N = 3$
Intraoperative seizure	1	0.2	0.4	Seizure was focal
Postoperative seizures	3	0.7	1.3	Seizures were generalized ($N = 2$) or focal ($N = 1$)
Tense cerebrospinal fluid collection around IPG	4	1.0	1.8	One case surgically explored; others disappeared with no treatment
Postoperative aspiration pneumonia	2	0.5	0.9	Both patients > 75 years old
Suicide attempt or psychiatric admission hospitalization within 6 months of surgery	3	0.7	1.3	By target: STN $N = 2$; GPi $N = 1$ (all unilateral implants)
Persistent new cognitive impairment	3	0.7	1.3	Two of three patients were > 80 years old; target was STN
Total unplanned reoperations	38	9.6	16.2	

* The mean follow-up time was 35 months.

† Threshold of detection was volume > 0.2 mL.

Abbreviations: IV, intravenous; STN, subthalamic nucleus; GPi, globus pallidus internus; IPG, implantable pulse generator.

gists are asked to redouble efforts at blood pressure control and ensure appropriate oxygenation. All instruments are removed from the brain and the cortex is inspected. Superficial bleeding sources are coagulated and surgery continues. If no surface bleeding is seen and no bleeding is seen from the cortical entry, the scalp is rapidly closed, the headframe is removed, and the patient is taken for a computed tomographic (CT) scan.

Short of a neurological deficit, there may be other more subtle signs of intraparenchymal hemorrhage that is initially asymptomatic and may remain so depending on its final size and location. When we have observed blood coming from the subcortical guide tube after withdrawal of a stylet or microelectrode, a small hematoma is almost always observed on postoperative imaging at a depth corresponding to the termination of the guide tube. During MER,

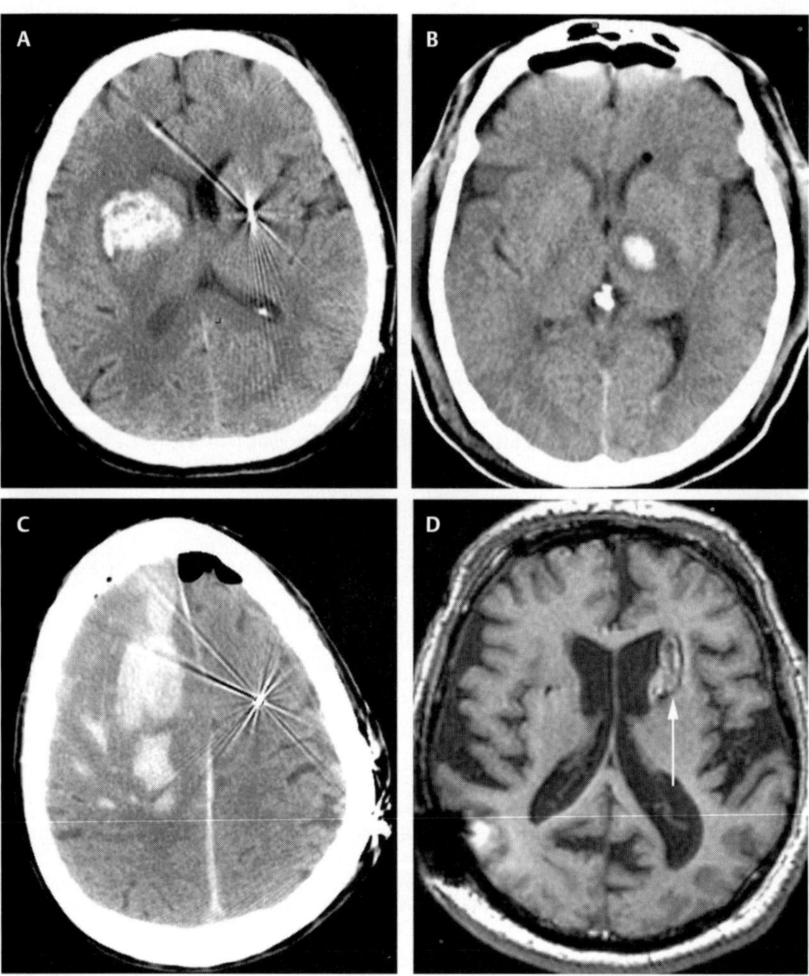

Fig. 14.1 Postoperative axial computed tomographic (CT) scans **(A–C)** or magnetic resonance imaging (MRI) **(D)** of hemorrhages complicating stereotactic deep brain stimulation (DBS) surgery in our series. **(A)** Hematoma that occurred during penetration of a microelectrode into the choroidal fissure, lateral to the optic tract, during microelectrode mapping of globus pallidus internus (GPi). **(B)** Hematoma that occurred during rapid withdrawal (> 1 mm/s) from the subthalamic nucleus (STN). **(C)** Hemorrhagic venous infarct that occurred following inadvertent interruption and coagulation of a bridging dural vein. **(D)** An asymptomatic hematoma in the left caudate nucleus (*white arrow*), immediately anterior to the DBS lead. (The hyperintensity in the right parietal cortex is artifact from the overlying connector of the lead extender).

if a significant region of electrical silence is observed at a depth where neuronal tissue is predicted based on prior adjacent MER tracks, the cause may be a small hematoma. If either of these signs of potential hematoma formation is observed, we halt the procedure and closely observe the patient for subtle new neurological deficit while reconfirming strict blood pressure control. If no deficit occurs in 5 to 10 minutes we proceed with surgery.

Table 14.2 Hemorrhagic Stroke in 405 Deep Brain Stimulation Electrode Implants: Presumed Precipitating Factors

Description of Stroke	Surgical Target	Time of Occurrence	Presumed Etiologic Factors	Outcome
Rapidly evolving large basal ganglia hematoma	GPi	Intraoperative	Crossing choroidal fissure during microelectrode recording, lateral to optic tract	Permanent hemiparesis
Frontal venous infarction	GPi	Intraoperative	Coagulation of a bridging vein	Permanent hemiparesis, aspiration pneumonia, death at 3 months postsurgery
Frontal venous infarction	GPi	2 days postsurgery	Coagulation of a bridging vein	Full recovery
Thalamic hematoma	STN	3 days postsurgery	Fit of severe coughing associated with a URI	Permanent worsening of gait and balance
Capsular hematoma	STN	Intraoperative	Rapid withdrawal of a microelectrode	Full recovery
Capsular hematoma	STN	Intraoperative	Unknown	Full recovery

Abbreviations: GPi, globus pallidus internus; STN, subthalamic nucleus; URI, upper respiratory infection.

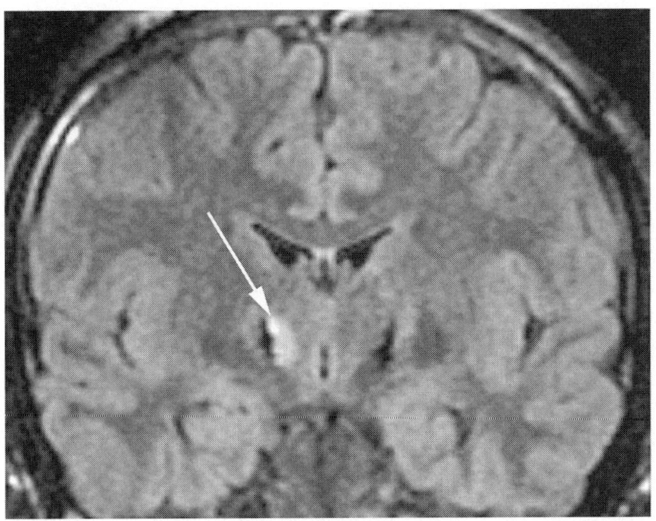

Fig. 14.2 Coronal magnetic resonance imaging (MRI) (FLAIR sequence) showing a delayed ischemic capsular infarction that occurred 1 week after bilateral subthalamic nucleus deep brain stimulation (DBS). The infarcted area (*white arrow*) is adjacent to the right DBS lead.

Infection

In our series, the incidence of serious infection, defined as infection requiring a return to the operating room for removal of all or part of the DBS hardware, was eight cases, or 2.0% per lead and 3.5% per patient (**Table 14.1**). All of these infections have occurred subcutaneously, starting at the lead extender or the implantable pulse generator (IPG). The major offending organisms were *Staphylococcus* (staph) *aureus* and *Staph epidermidis*. We have had no infections in the brain, and in fact cerebral abscess or cerebritis complicating DBS has not been reported in most recent series. Most of our infections presented with some combination of swelling, redness, pain, or drainage over the connector of the lead extender, or over the IPG. Most presented within 1 to 8 weeks of surgery, although one presented as a stitch abscess over an anchoring suture on the connector 2 years after implantation.

Infection Avoidance

Our approach to avoidance of infection, in addition to the obvious meticulous attention to sterile technique, is as follows:

1. Preoperative prophylaxis with an antistaphylococcal cephalosporin at least 30 minutes prior to skin incision, followed by a second dose given 3 hours later, and three postoperative doses.
2. Utilization of the lowest-profile hardware available, with recessing of larger components into a drilled bone trough in patients with thin skin.

3. Emphasis on performing surgery efficiently to reduce operative time.
4. Copious irrigation of all incisions with bacitracin solution prior to closure.

Infection Management

The management of hardware infections has not been standardized. In the report of Oh et al,[6] infections of any part of the device were ultimately treated with removal of all hardware, despite initial attempts at more localized treatment. Our approach is as follows:

1. For superficial infections at incision sites where hardware does not appear to be in direct contact with pus or necrotic tissue, the patient is treated with antibiotics and local wound care without hardware removal, followed weekly with clinical examination until wounds are completely healed.
2. For infections where the lead extender or IPG is in direct contact with pus or necrotic tissue, the affected components are removed immediately on presentation, and then the patient is treated with the appropriate intravenous (IV) antibiotics. If a localized infection around the pulse generator or lead extender is discovered early in its course, this strategy may result in salvage of the brain electrode.
3. An infection in direct contact with the brain lead or an infection along the extender or IPG that has been incubating for many weeks will usually necessitate removal of the DBS lead as well as other involved hardware.
4. In cases where lead removal was necessary, we have been able to reimplant another DBS lead 2 to 3 months after full wound healing, without further infectious sequelae.

Sterile Fluid Collections

Four of our patients have presented within 1 month postsurgery with tense swellings around the IPG, which were fluctuant but painless and without redness or warmth. Surgical exploration of one of these revealed a sterile clear fluid collection consistent with cerebrospinal fluid (CSF). This appears to occur more frequently with burr hole-based anchoring methods that are not watertight (such as the Stimloc system from Medtronic, Inc., www.medtronic.com/physician/activa) because CSF can track down the hardware to accumulate in the pectoral cavity. Sealing the burr hole with Gelfoam and fibrin glue prior to closure has reduced the incidence of these sterile collections. If a swelling around an IPG is not red, tender, or warm, and the incision is healed, our practice is to observe it. Sterile fluid collections typically resolve spontaneously.

Editor's Comments

Prevention of complications starts with the initial patient evaluation (Chapters 4 and 5) and continues through to intraoperative technique (Chapters 7 through 12). Nevertheless, complications will occur. The most common and most severe operative complication is that of hemorrhage. Subdural hematomas are uncommon but can occur in any intracranial procedure. To avoid this complication, anything that can raise intracranial pressure and tear diploic veins such as coughing or bucking must be avoided. In addition, probes should enter through a gyrus in which the pia-arachnoid has been opened to prevent distortion of the cortex and potential tearing of intracranial vessels. This is especially true of the DBS lead, and we recommend direct visualization of the probe into the brain. Operations close to the sinus can result in injury to the sinus or major bridging veins resulting in venous infarction. Scanning to the top of the head, using contrast to visualize these vessels directly, and placing the burr hole in a position that would not put them at risk can minimize the risk of this complication. Although rectilinear approaches are essential for mapping, a slight lateral to medial approach of 1 to 4 degrees is insignificant in its distortion of the map but may provide additional distance from the midline to enhance safety. The more common and more severe problems occur with intraparenchymal hemorrhages. The StealthStation (Medtronic Navigation, Louisville, CO) is especially useful in planning trajectories that will avoid not only cortical veins but also deep sulci that may curve back into the trajectory or deep venous structures such as the veins within the lateral ventricle. Slow, smooth descent of the probe is essential to minimize trauma. Absolutely critical is control of blood pressure during these procedures because even a normally hypotensive patient can become hypertensive during the stress of awake surgery.

The most common immediately postoperative problem is that of infection. "Pickers" cannot leave the wound alone and will consciously or unconsciously pick at it. This behavior puts the implant at risk of infection. Pickers are frequently children and cognitively impaired patients and use of subcuticular sutures combined with tissue adhesive and careful monitoring can help decrease the risk. Beware of a history of self-mutilation, obsessive compulsion, and psychosis. We use antibiotics before, during, and after surgery in an attempt to keep the infection rate to an absolute minimum. This aggressive approach has resulted in a very low infection rate of 2%. Intraoperative antibiotics are generally vancomycin for its intracranial penetration and all instruments that enter the brain are wiped down with antibiotic-containing solution. Postoperatively, the IV antibiotics are used as long as the patient is in the hospital. On discharge, the patients are converted to oral antibiotics, and cephalosporins are used because the main concern is extracranial staph infections. Infections usually occur in a regional manner and can be treated as such. We have had to remove only one entire DBS system. Infections at the burr hole can be minimized using surgical techniques as described in Chapter 7. Since using low-profile caps and pericranial coverage in over 200 DBS lead placements, we have not had a single infection at the burr hole cover. The most common place where we encounter infections at this time is at the connector.

The skin here is relatively thin and the device relatively large. These patients frequently have head trauma, and any laceration should be treated aggressively with antibiotic coverage if it is anywhere near the lead, connector, or extension wire. The use of lower-profile connectors, placing the connector above the incision, and covering the extension lead with an additional layer of temporalis fascia will, it is hoped, reduce this complication. It should also be emphasized to the patient to keep pressure off of this area whether from caps, wigs, or lying on hard surfaces in an attempt to encourage wound healing and diminish tissue necrosis. Operative removal and antibiotic treatment of erosions are the same as for overt infections. Any skin erosion should be treated as an infection even if the skin appears intact over it (**Fig. 14.3**).

Stitch abscesses and any potential superficial infections in the scalp are aggressively treated with antibiotics. Failure to resolve this after a course of antibiotics requires intraoperative evaluation, debridement, and removal of the contaminated equipment, while attempting to preserve the lead. The burr hole cover usually requires placement with a metal plate to ensure security of the lead while removing as much of the contaminated plastic as possible. Long-term IV antibiotic with staph coverage and the addition of rifampin, which frequently acts synergistically, has been successful in cleaning up these types of infections. In the area of the connector, the con-

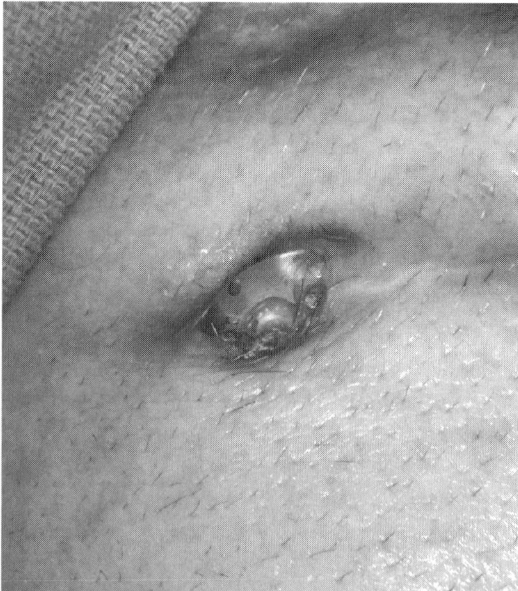

Fig. 14.3 The implantable pulse generator (IPG) is visible below a paper-thin layer of skin that fell apart during skin preparation for surgery. The clavicle is superior and the patient slept on top of the IPG, which pressed against the skin and caused necrosis. Even though there were no organisms isolated, this was treated by IPG and extension lead removal and a 10-day course of antibiotics. The IPG and extension lead were successfully replaced 1 month later in a more inferior position under the pectoral muscle fascia.

nector boot is removed and a new boot placed, if this is the only area that has been contaminated. If there is wider contamination, then the extension lead must be removed in addition. First disconnecting it in the chest and leaving IPG in the chest and then pulling the remaining wire to the contaminated surface perform this. The contaminated area is opened last to prevent cross-contamination of the chest area. Vigorous antibiotic irrigation and the use of dilute hydrogen peroxide are recommended. A new connector can be attached to the lead to facilitate its identification at a later time. This connection should be displaced away from the area that is infected. Again, long-term IV antibiotics are recommended using a cephalosporin and rifampin. Infection in the chest usually requires examination of the connector first, and if this area is not infected then the extension lead is cut below the connector. Attention is then drawn to the chest, which is opened, and the entire IPG and extension lead are then removed. Vigorous intraoperative antibiotic irrigation and postoperative IV antibiotics are similar to those described earlier, but the final choice is based on culture and sensitivity results. Drains are not necessary.

Beware of the swollen subclavicular pocket that is not red, erythematous, and tender. There are a small number of such noninfected fluid collections that require only observation. These should be aspirated to ensure that there is not an infectious component. The fluid is usually straw colored but can be quite foul smelling and full of particulate matter, yet not infected. Although many feel this is a CSF collection, it is much more likely a lymph disruption and with time will resolve spontaneously.

■ Long-Term Hardware-Related Complications

With currently available DBS hardware, the incidence of long-term hardware-related complications is regrettably high,[6,14] and appears to increase during the lifetime of the device. The major hardware complications are those associated with lead fracture, lead migration, and device erosion. Our experience with these complications is detailed in **Table 14.1**.

Lead Fractures

In our series, there have been two lead fractures, one in the neck associated with a low-lying lead extender (occurring 10 months postsurgery), the other under a titanium miniplate used to anchor the DBS electrode (occurring 2 years postsurgery). A lead fracture associated with a low-lying lead extender is shown in **Fig. 14.4**.

Avoidance of Lead Fractures

The most important step in avoiding delayed lead fracture is to place the proximal part of the lead extender (the connector) under the scalp, not in the cervical area where mobility at the junction between the lead and the connector predisposes to fracture. We place the connector posterior and slightly superior to the pinna of the ear. The connector may be anchored with a silk suture to the underlying fascia, or by drilling a small trough in the skull to recess the connector. If a patient is noted on follow-up to have a connector in the cervical area, either from migration or from improper initial placement, we offer elective repositioning to a more rostral level to reduce the risk of delayed fracture. This usually requires retunneling the connector from a parietal incision. Finally, although we initially used titanium miniplates to anchor DBS leads, we have abandoned this method due to our own and others' observation of delayed fractures under the plate.

Management of Lead Fractures

To replace a fractured lead, we perform a new stereotactic procedure and use fluoroscopy to visualize the initial lead and confirm placement of a new one at the same site. MER is not used. It may be possible to slide a new lead "freehand" down the prior gliotic lead track, after visualizing the initial lead on fluoroscopy and removing it, but we do not have experience with this.

Lead Migration

We have observed delayed lead migration in two early cases where the lead was anchored only with methylmeth-

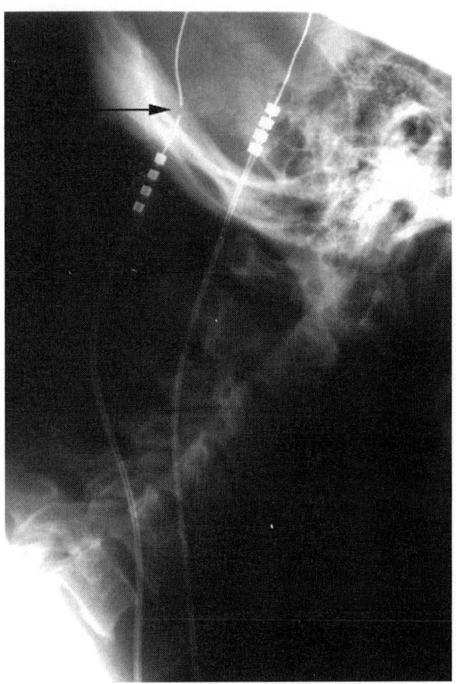

Fig. 14.4 Lateral radiograph showing a lead fracture (*black arrow*) associated with a relatively low-lying connection to the lead extender.

acrylate. Migration has not been observed following use of a titanium miniplate (100 cases) or use of the Stimloc system (300 cases). The most important steps to avoid delayed lead migration are as follows:

1. Do not depend on methylmethacrylate alone to anchor the lead.
2. Leave redundant coils of lead under the frontoparietal scalp so that tension on the connector is not transmitted directly to the lead at the anchoring system. Some redundant coils are normally necessary if the connector is placed under the parietal scalp and the 28 or 40 cm DBS leads are used.

Normally, a lead migration will require a new stereotactic procedure to reinsert the lead.

Hardware Erosion

Avoidance of Hardware Erosion

Erosion of part of the device can occur insidiously and will never be eliminated with current DBS device designs. To minimize the long-term erosion risk, we recommend the following:

1. Use the lowest-profile hardware available. With regard to the Medtronic DBS system, avoid the original Medtronic burr hole cap because this has a profile that is both high and sharp, and avoid the use of the older Medtronic high-profile connectors in favor of the low-profile connector.
2. In patients who are extremely thin, drill a trough in the skull to recess the lead anchoring devices and the connector.
3. At the level of the pulse generator, any excess lead extender wire should be coiled underneath the IPG rather than above it.
4. Erosion may sometimes be prevented by prophylactic surgery. If, on a follow-up visit the skin over the connector is noted to be very thin and avascular, we electively reposition the connector to a new location where a trough is drilled in the parietal bone.

Management of Hardware Erosion

If erosion has just occurred, transposition without device removal may be attempted, but the most conservative treatment is to remove the part of the device that has eroded and replace it later after the skin has completely healed. If an erosion of a pulse generator occurs in a very thin individual, we replace the IPG in the abdomen rather than in the chest.

Editor's Comments

Hardware problems will continue throughout the life of the DBS system. Migrations can occur at any time but are most common early in the postoperative period. An unusual type of migration can occur with severe Valsalva where the lead can be extruded from the thalamus into the lateral ventricles. More common is the migration of the lead during the process of securing it to the burr hole cover. We recommend intraoperative fluoroscopy to directly observe the lead and ensure that migration does not take place. In addition, downward pressure on the connector and extension lead can cause migration of these devices into the neck if they are not secured. The result is that a lead that was well placed can become elevated out of the target area. This requires replacement usually of the entire lead. We do not advise attempts at free-hand lead replacements.

More common are the fractures that can occur anywhere along the system but are most common at the proximal end of the lead near the connector. The lower-profile connectors have helped diminish this, as has the placement below the scalp rather than in the neck. I have never observed a fracture at the burr hole cover except in those situations where the lead was not in the groove but pinched between the cap and base plate or where there has been a metal plate used to hold the lead in place. There apparently is enough movement of the scalp that fatigue and disconnection of the wire can occur below the metal plate. Care must be taken that the contacts of the connector and the IPG are firmly established but are not overtightened where damage to the lead or connector can occur. An excellent method for evaluating potential short circuits and disconnections is discussed in Chapter 13. Care must be taken to secure the lead firmly to the burr hole cover, to secure the connector to the temporalis fascia to prevent its migration, and to secure the IPG to the fascia to ensure that it does not turn or twist and result in migration or lead fracture (**Fig. 14.5**). Conscious or unconscious manipulation of the hardware (twiddler syndrome) is a rare but well-known complication of implanted devices and should be suspected in such cases.

Frontal release signs frequently occur as the result of bilateral penetration of the frontal white matter. Most of these are transient and secondary to edema, but with major hemorrhage or venous infarction they can become permanent. Cognitive problems frequently occur from penetrations near the midline according to Dr. Benabid (Chapter 9). The occasional patient with severe postoperative cognitive disruption may result from penetrations too close to midline structures, even without hemorrhage or infarction. We recommend avoiding midline structures by coming in more lateral to medial by several degrees, which will not interfere with mapping but will avoid middle thalamic nuclei on the approaches to the subthalamic nucleus (STN). Even in the more lateral ventral intermediate (Vim) thalamus, we will start laterally to insure we avoid significant medial injury. Emotional responses of elation and depression have been seen with stimulation of the substantia nigra, and we now avoid putting the lead into the nigra to help decrease the possibility of this complication.

MRI observation of the lead positioning is really quite essential for evaluating surgical placement. The 1.5 tesla MRI has proved

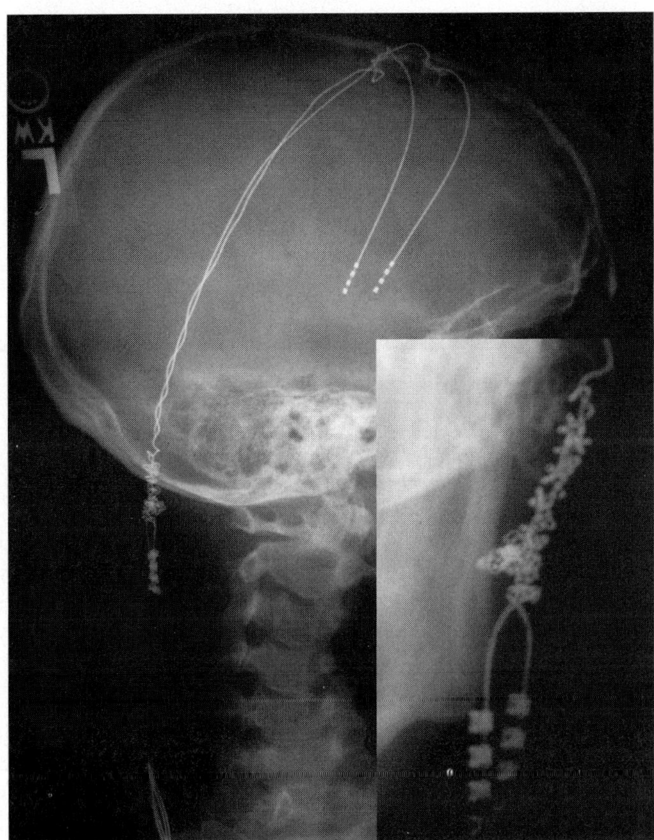

Fig. 14.5 In this patient with dystonia, both deep brain stimulation (DBS) leads were directed to the left and connected to a Kinetra (Medtronic, Inc., Minneapolis, MN) in the abdomen. Apparently, neither extension leads nor the Kinetra were secured to the underlying fascia. The Kinetra rotated and twisted the extension leads, pulling them down into the neck, where they broke.

extremely safe and effective in determining lead location. There have been rare instances of complications, usually with the use of body coils. Ways of preventing this are outlined in detail in **Table 14.3**. The concern relates to the potential for thermal injury. We know from long-term experience that the DBS lead does not move and the IPG does not change parameters. The induction of thermal energy, especially at the tip or at a fracture, may be a source of problems. The heat that is generated can be trivial to potentially deadly.[15] Although the specific absorption rate (SAR) is a good parameter to follow, it is clear that the SARs will vary with the particular MRI system being used; therefore, the recommendations must be applied carefully. Temperatures tend to increase linearly in relation to the SAR value. Keeping the SAR below 0.4 W/kg in the head is a reasonable valve. The 1.5 tesla Siemens Magnetom Vision,

Picker Edge, and GE Echospeed have all been tested, and if proper precautions are applied can be used safely. Experience with 3 tesla is not extensive enough to make any clear recommendations. We do know that the 3 tesla MRI is extremely good for identifying the preoperative anatomical structures. Safety concerns are also present for diathermy, which should be contraindicated following DBS placement and cardioversion, which if an emergency arises must be performed with care and minimal watts. See also the Medtronic physician's manual, available on the company Web site.

In attempting to correct misplaced leads, one should clearly differentiate one's own work from that of others.[16] With appropriate intervention (reprogramming, medication changes, or DBS lead replacement), 51% of patients who complained of "failed" DBS procedures ultimately had good outcomes. Thirty-four percent of these

Table 14.3 Recommendations for Postoperative Magnetic Resonance Imaging of Deep Brain Stimulation Systems

1. Do not assume 1.5 tesla magnetic resonance imaging will always be safe
2. Inform the patient of the potential risks and be sure the study is necessary
3. Perform studies only where there is expertise in imaging deep brain stimulation systems
4. Program the system(s) to 0 V and mode to bipolar before entering the magnetic resonance suite
5. Use only a transmit and receive type radiofrequency head coil
6. Select imaging parameters that do not exceed a specific absorption rate of < 0.1 W/kg in the head if not pretested
7. Continuously monitor the patient throughout the procedure and stop if there are any changes in response or patient complaints

patients had persistently poor outcomes despite maximal intervention. When one is trying to correct someone else's work, the lead may simply be misplaced, but there is also the chance that the patient was inappropriately selected in the first place. Careful reevaluation of the patient should be made and there should be clear clinical justification for proceeding so as not to compound a bad surgical situation. Although in many cases the lead can be replaced without MER, in most cases we do use MER to help establish the optimum placement. In these situations, we leave the misplaced lead in place both to prevent edema, which would interfere with MER, but also to serve as a guide to location on fluoroscopic examination. We have been able to penetrate around a previously placed lead without difficulty, especially when using the StealthStation to plan the trajectories. It should be remembered that the MRI scan of the lead is magnified two to three times, and even trajectories very close to the MRI lead defect have a margin of safety. There is a small current leakage around the lead, even at 0 V, that can interfere with recordings adjacent to an electrode, so it is best to set the 0 contact to negative and case positive to minimize this effect along most of the length of the lead.

■ Rare but Spectacular Complications

Inadvertent Thermal Lesioning

Inadvertent thermal lesioning around a DBS electrode has been reported following cardioversion[17] and diathermy.[18] Diathermy is a treatment of undocumented utility that involves the application of rapidly alternating electromagnetic current to produce "deep tissue heating." When applied near a DBS device, large radio frequency lesions around the DBS contacts in the brain may occur, producing permanent brain damage. Exposure to diathermy is absolutely contra-indicated in patients with deep brain electrodes.

Electrolysis and Gas Production

Normally the current transmitted through a DBS contact is alternating current so that there is no net charge buildup on a contact. A malfunction of a pulse generator that produces a net direct current may result in electrolysis and the production of an intraparenchymal gas bubble presenting as an expanding mass lesion. This has been reported in the context of a malfunction of an external pulse generator that was used for several days of testing through an externalized lead.[19] The authors recommended that the duration of external test stimulation, if done at all, should be kept to a minimum.

Damage to Lead or Lead Extender Due to Patient Manipulation of the Implantable Pulse Generator

If the IPG is not tacked to the underlying pectoralis fascia, it may be possible for a patient to manually rotate the device within its subcutaneous pocket. One of our patients presented with a short circuit between three contacts of the DBS lead, and a new protuberance under the parietal scalp immediately superior to the connector of the lead extender. An X-ray showed a highly unusual coiling of the distal lead near its insertion into the connector. At surgical exploration, extensive twisting of both the lead extender and the lead was found, apparently due to the patient's repeated rotation of the IPG under the skin.

■ Deep Brain Stimulation and Magnetic Resonance Imaging

Because an alternating magnetic field induces a current in a loop of wire, exposure of a DBS lead to MRI can theoretically produce heating of the lead. In several experimental studies in 1.5 T magnets,[20,21] the degree of heating has not been biologically significant. Clinical studies of MRI at 1.5 T of implanted DBS systems (including the pulse generators) have not revealed permanent adverse effects.[22-26] A single case of transient neurological dysfunction in a DBS patient, occurring immediately after MRI in a 1.5 T unit, was recently reported.[27] This may have been due to heating of the lead. Given that thousands of patients with DBS systems have undergone MRI in 1.5 T systems and this is the first report of a clinically noticeable effect, the incidence of this type of event at 1.5 T is probably quite low. The exact degree of heating that occurs in a given situation depends on many factors, including the magnetic field strength, the sequence protocols, the type of transmitting coil used (head coil or body coil), and the configuration and orientation of loops of wire in the implanted system. Exposure to higher field magnets (3 T or higher) is likely to be associated with more significant heating.[28] At this time, we routinely perform MRI of DBS systems at 1.5 T but not at higher field strengths.

■ Troubleshooting the Lead that Doesn't Work

In a busy movement disorders surgery clinic, a frequent request for consultation is for a patient who has an implanted DBS system and is not getting the expected or desired benefit. **Fig. 14.6** provides a summary of our troubleshooting algorithm for nonworking systems. In general, there are five broad reasons for "device failure":

1. There is an electrical malfunction.
2. The electrode is poorly located in the brain.
3. The patient has a diagnosis that will not respond to DBS.

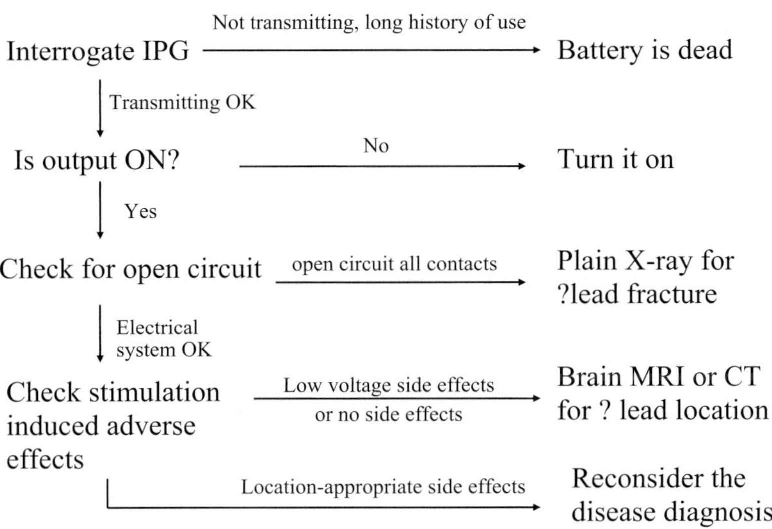

Fig. 14.6 Summary of a troubleshooting algorithm for workup of a deep brain stimulation (DBS) system that is not producing the expected results. CT, computed tomography; IPG, internal pulse generator; MRI, magnetic resonance imaging.

4. The patient has become tolerant to the therapeutic effect of DBS.
5. The patient is poorly programmed.

First, electrical malfunction should be ruled out by interrogating the battery, determining if the battery is generating adequate voltage, verifying that the system is in fact turned on, and checking the current and impedance at each contact to rule out an open circuit. If all four contacts have

developed an open circuit in a system that had previously been working, it is likely that the lead or lead extender is fractured. AP and lateral X-rays of the skull and neck can confirm this in many but not all cases.

If the electrical system checks out well, location-specific stimulation-induced adverse effects are sought. The most common of these are dysarthria and paresthesia for thalamic or subthalamic nucleus DBS, and dysarthria or visual phenomena for globus pallidus internus (GPi) DBS. If these

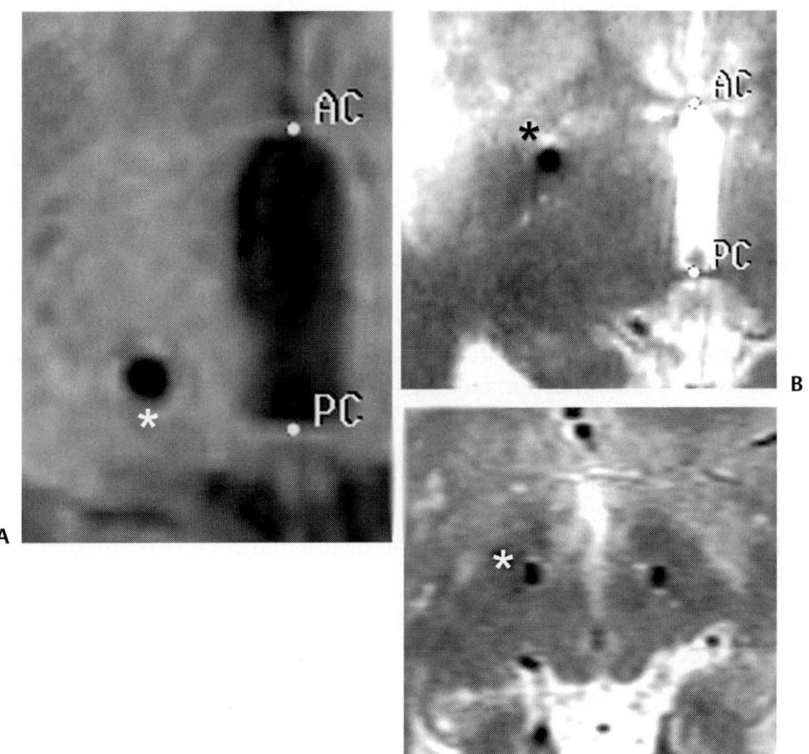

Fig. 14.7 Postoperative axial magnetic resonance images (MRIs) showing leads that have been repositioned due to suboptimal initial location. **(A)** Thalamic deep brain stimulation (DBS) for essential tremor (ET). **(B)** Pallidal DBS for Parkinson disease (PD). **(C)** Subthalamic nucleus (STN) DBS for PD. The asterisk marks the location of the initial suboptimal lead. The hypointense circle is the artifact generated by the repositioned, correctly located lead. AC, anterior commissure; PC, posterior commissure.

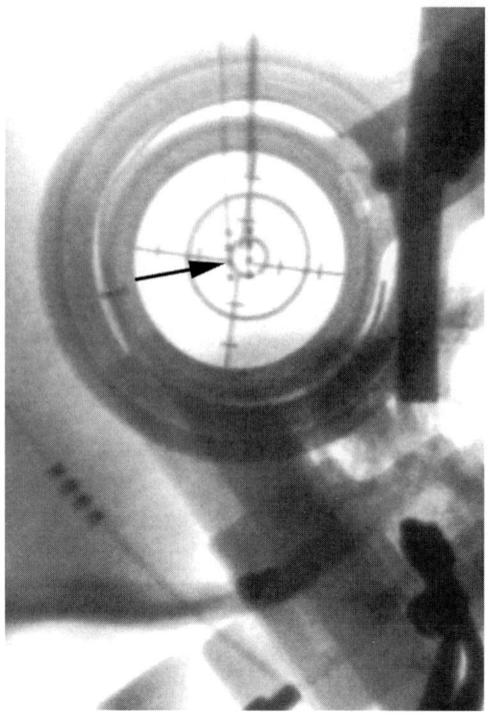

Fig. 14.8 Lateral radiograph illustrating the fluoroscopy technique for repositioning a poorly positioned deep brain stimulation electrode. The arrow points to the original lead, which was 3 mm too posterior in the thalamus. The new lead is shown with contact 1 at the stereotactic target, verified by the radiopaque markers attached to the rings of the Leksell Stereotactic System (Elekta Inc., Norcross, GA).

are not produced at high voltage or are produced at voltages lower than typical therapeutic parameters for each target, the brain should be imaged to check for a misplaced DBS electrode.

Examples of misplaced electrodes, and their subsequent proper positioning, are shown in **Fig. 14.7**. At this time there are no clear guidelines for what constitutes acceptable lead locations, other than that the electrode should be in a position to affect the motor territories of the relevant nuclei (e.g., the dorsolateral STN, posterolateral internal pallidum, or ventrolateral thalamus). If an electrode is malpositioned, we perform stereotactic insertion of a new lead under fluoroscopy, using the initial, malpositioned lead as an internal reference marker (**Fig. 14.8**). MER is not used in this setting. MER is very difficult to interpret if a nearby lead has just been removed because the resulting tissue edema alters neuronal discharge characteristics.

If stimulation-induced adverse effects or imaging indicates appropriate electrode location, then the patient's diagnosis should be revisited. Although DBS has been attempted in atypical parkinsonism and secondary dystonias, it is only marginally effective. Some types of tremor that have been treated by DBS, such as posttraumatic tremor or multiple sclerosis–associated tremor, are less likely to be responsive to DBS than parkinsonian tremor and essential tremor (ET).

Even for patients with an "on-label" indication for DBS therapy, a possibility for long-term failure is physiological tolerance to the therapeutic effect of stimulation. This problem arises primarily in thalamic DBS for ET, for which the incidence of tolerance has been reported at 10 to 30%.[29–31] At least some of these cases are probably due to true physiological tolerance to a well-located electrode, rather than suboptimal electrode positioning. These cases are potentially treatable by lesioning through the DBS elecrode.[32,33] Some have argued that GPi DBS in PD also may manifest tolerance after several years,[34] but this may relate to suboptimal electrode placement rather than true tolerance to GPi DBS. Tolerance to the therapeutic effect of STN DBS in PD with respect to symptoms responsive to Sinemet (Merck & Co., Inc., Whitehouse Station, NJ) has not been reported with follow-up of 5 years.[35] However, as PD progresses, more Sinemet-nonresponsive symptoms such as postural instability, hypophonia, or cognitive impairment may manifest, resulting in a partial loss of benefit to the patient over time.[35] With regard to pallidal stimulation for idiopathic dystonia, length of follow-up is too short in published series to determine if long-term tolerance will be a problem.

Finally, improper programming may be a source of long-term failure, particularly in PD. This can be avoided if the programming is performed by a movement disorders neurologist with expertise in DBS programming (Chapter 13). Published guidelines for DBS programming in PD are also available.[36]

■ Cognitive Decline in Parkinson Disease Patients

Even in the absence of stroke, patients with advanced PD may be at risk for permanent cognitive decline following bilateral STN DBS.[37] The presence of significant cognitive impairment preoperatively or advanced age increases the risk of this complication. It is not yet clear if bilateral GPI DBS carries the same risk. We have had three cases of STN-DBS for PD where postoperative cognitive changes produced persistent new disability by the report of the patients' families (**Table 14.1**). In two of these, the patients were over 80 years old. Our current measures to avoid this complication include the following:

1. PD patients with significant cognitive dysfunction (Mini Mental Status score < 24) are not offered surgery.
2. PD patients over 80 are very rarely accepted for surgery, unless their physical health and cognitive function are unusually good.
3. PD patients over 70, or patients under 70 who have mild cognitive dysfunction, are offered staged implants rather than simultaneous bilateral implants. Formal neuropsychological testing is done before and after the first implant. The second implant is not performed until full neuropsychological recovery from the first implant is documented.

Complications Unique to Lesioning Surgery

In stereotactic radio frequency lesioning for movement disorders, the profile of potential complications is related but not identical to that for DBS implantation. The risk of hemorrhagic stroke is probably similar in both types of procedure. Lesioning surgery does not entail any hardware-related complications and has a much lower rate of infection because there is no indwelling device. Lesioning, however, carries certain risks that are not present with DBS surgery:

1. It is possible to create inadvertent thermal lesions to critical structures surrounding the intended target, such as the corticobulbar/cortisospinal tracts, optic tract, or sensory thalamus.
2. Bilateral lesioning of the thalamus and GPi carries a high risk of permanent speech or cognitive dysfunction, even when lesions are correctly placed.[9,12] It is not yet clear if bilateral lesioning of the STN carries the same risks.
3. Delayed ischemic subcortical infarction appears to be more common in lesioning surgery (principally pallidotomy) than in DBS surgery.[10,13] This may relate to thermal damage to neighboring perforating vessels that occurs at the time of radiofrequency lesioning.

References

1. Hariz MI. Complications of deep brain stimulation surgery. Mov Disord 2002;17(Suppl 3):S162–S166
2. Kondziolka D, Whiting D, Germanwala A, Oh M. Hardware-related complications after placement of thalamic deep brain stimulator systems. Stereotact Funct Neurosurg 2002;79:228–233
3. Beric A, Kelly PJ, Rezai A, et al. Complications of deep brain stimulation surgery. Stereotact Funct Neurosurg 2001;77:73–78
4. Terao T, Takahashi H, Yokochi F, Taniguchi M, Okiyama R, Hamada I. Hemorrhagic complications of stereotactic surgery in patients with movement disorders. J Neurosurg 2003;98:1241–1246
5. Umemura A, Jaggi JL, Hurtig HI, et al. Deep brain stimulation for movement disorders: morbidity and mortality in 109 patients. J Neurosurg 2003;98:779–784
6. Oh MY, Abosch A, Kim SH, Lang AE, Lozano AM. Long-term hardware-related complications of deep brain stimulation. Neurosurgery 2002;50:1268–1274
7. Schwalb JM, Riina HA, Skolnick B, Jaggi JL, Simuni T, Baltuch GH. Revision of deep brain stimulator for tremor: technical note. J Neurosurg 2001;94:1010–1012
8. Joint C, Nandi D, Parkin S, Gregory R, Aziz T. Hardware-related problems of deep brain stimulation. Mov Disord 2002;17(Suppl 3): S175–S180
9. Higuchi Y, Iacono RP. Surgical complications in patients with Parkinson's disease after posteroventral pallidotomy. Neurosurgery 2003;52:558–571
10. Lim JY, DeSalles AAF, Bronstein J, Masterman DL, Saver JL. Delayed internal capsule infarctions following radiofrequency pallidotomy. J Neurosurg 1997;87:955–960
11. Hua Z, Guodong G, Qinchuan L, Yaqun Z, Qinfen W, Xuelian W. Analysis of complications of radiofrequency pallidotomy. Neurosurgery 2003;52:89–99
12. Merello M, Starkstein S, Nouzeilles MI, Kuzis G, Leiguarda R. Bilateral pallidotomy for treatment of Parkinson's disease induced corticobulbar syndrome and psychic akinesia avoidable by globus pallidus lesion combined with contralateral stimulation. J Neurol Neurosurg Psychiatry 2001;71:611–614
13. Baron MS, Vitek JL, Bakay RAE, et al. Treatment of advanced Parkinson's disease by posterior GPi pallidotomy: 1-year results of a pilot study. Ann Neurol 1996;40:355–366
14. Lyons KE, Koller WC, Wilkinson SB, Pahwa R. Surgical and device-related events with deep brain stimulation. Neurology 2001; 56(Suppl 3):A147
15. Rezai AR, Phillips M, Baker K, et al. Neurostimulation systems used for deep brain stimulation (DBS): MR safety issues and implications for failing to follow guidelines. Invest Radiol 2004;39:300–303
16. Okun MS, Tagliati M, Pourfar M, et al. Management of referred deep brain stimulation failures: a retrospective analysis from 2 movement disorders centers. Arch Neurol 2005;62:1250–1255
17. Yamamoto T, Katayama Y, Fukaya C, Kurihara J, Oshima H, Kasai M. Thalamotomy caused by cardioversion in a patient treated with brain stimulation. Stereotact Funct Neurosurg 2000;74:73–82
18. Nutt JG, Anderson VC, Peacock JH, Hammerstad JP, Burchiel KJ. DBS and diathermy interaction induces severe CNS damage. Neurology 2001;56:1384–1386
19. Radbauer C, Volc D, Standhardt H, Alesch F. Pneumocephalus in a patient with deep brain stimulation (DBS): a case report. Mov Disord 2000;15(Suppl 3):58
20. Golombeck MA, Thiele J, Dossel O. Magnetic resonance imaging with implanted neurostimulators: numerical calculation of the induced heating. Biomed Tech (Berl) 2002;47(Suppl 1):660–663
21. Rezai AR, Finelli D, Nyenhuis JA, et al. Neurostimulation systems for deep brain stimulation: in vitro evaluation of MRI-related heating at 1.5-tesla. J Magn Reson Imaging 2002;15:241–250
22. Uitti RJ, Tsuboi Y, Pooley RA, et al. Magnetic resonance imaging and deep brain stimulation. Neurosurgery 2002;51:1423–1431
23. Starr PA, Christine C, Theodosopoulos PV, et al. Implantation of deep brain stimulator electrodes into the subthalamic nucleus: technical approach and magnetic resonance imaging-verified electrode locations. J Neurosurg 2002;97:370–387
24. Schrader B, Hamel W, Weinert D, Mehdorn HM. Documentation of electrode localization. Mov Disord 2002;17(Suppl 3):S167–S174
25. Saint-Cyr JA, Hoque T, Pereira LCM, et al. Localization of clinically effective stimulating electrodes in the human subthalamic nucleus on magnetic resonance imaging. J Neurosurg 2002;97: 1152–1166
26. Yelnik J, Damier P, Demeret S, et al. Localization of stimulating electrodes in patients with Parkinson disease by using a three dimensional atlas-magnetic resonance imaging coregistration method. J Neurosurg 2003;99:89–99
27. Spiegel J, Fuss G, Backens M, et al. Transient dystonia following magnetic resonance imaging in a patient with deep brain stimulation electrodes for the treatment of Parkinson's disease: case report. J Neurosurg 2003;99:772–774
28. Finelli DA, Rezai AR, Ruggieri PM, et al. MR-related heating of deep brain stimulation electrodes: an in-vivo study of clinical imaging sequences. AJNR Am J Neuroradiol 2002;23:1795–1802

29. Hariz MI, Shamsgovara P, Johansson F, Hariz G, Fodstad H. Tolerance and tremor rebound following long-term chronic thalamic stimulation of Parkinsonian and essential tremor. Stereotact Funct Neurosurg 1999;72:208–218

30. Benabid AL, Benazzouz A, Hoffman D, Limousin P, Krack P, Pollak P. Long-term electrical inhibition of deep brain targets in movement disorders. Mov Disord 1998;13:119–125

31. Koller WC, Lyons KE, Wilkinson SB, Troster AI, Pahwa R. Long-term safety and efficacy of unilateral deep brain stimulation of the thalamus in essential tremor. Mov Disord 2001;16:464–468

32. Oh MY, Hodaie M, Kim SH, Alkhani A, Lang AE, Lozano AM. Deep brain stimulator electrodes used for lesioning: proof of principle. Neurosurgery 2001;49:363–367

33. Raoul S, Faighel M, Rivier I, Verin M, Lajat Y, Damier P. Staged lesions through implanted deep brain stimulating electrodes: a new surgical procedure for treating tremor or dyskinesias. Mov Disord 2003;18:933–938

34. Houeto JL, Bejjani PB, Damier P, et al. Failure of long-term pallidal stimulation corrected by subthalamic stimulation in PD. Neurology 2000;55:728–730

35. Krack P, Batir A, Blercom NV, et al. Five year follow-up of bilateral stimulation of the subthalamic nucleus in advanced Parkinson's disease. N Engl J Med 2003;349:1925–1934

36. Krack P, Fraix V, Mendes A, Benabid AL, Pollak P. Postoperative management of subthalamic nucleus stimulation for Parkinson's disease. Mov Disord 2002;17(Suppl 3):S188–S197

37. Saint-Cyr JA, Trepanier LL, Kumar R, Lozano AM, Lang AE. Neuropsychological consequences of chronic bilateral stimulation of the subthalamic nucleus in Parkinson's disease. Brain 2000;123:2091–2108

15 Efficacy and Complications of Deep Brain Stimulation for Movement Disorders

Erich O. Richter, Clement Hamani, and Andres M. Lozano

Chronic electrical stimulation has now become a mainstay of treatment for patients with movement disorders. In fact, due to its effectiveness and potential reversibility, deep brain stimulation (DBS) has gradually replaced lesioning procedures for the treatment of Parkinson disease (PD),[1] dystonia,[2] and essential tremor (ET)[3] in many centers around the world. The three primary targets for DBS in movement disorders surgery are the thalamus, globus pallidus, and subthalamic nucleus (STN). As for lesions, different outcomes might be expected according to the disease and chosen target. We discuss the efficacy and adverse effects of DBS according to target in each of the three major disorders most commonly treated (PD, ET, and dystonia).

■ Efficacy

Thalamus

The motor thalamus is composed of several nuclei that receive afferents from the cerebellum and basal ganglia and send projections to the motor and premotor cortices. Several units in the motor thalamus in humans respond passively or actively to movement,[4,5] and stimulation of the motor thalamus in nonhuman primates elicits motor responses.[6] Stimulation of the thalamus may be efficacious through activation of the cerebellothalamocortical pathway rather than inhibition,[7,8] although the precise method of action remains controversial.

Diverse classifications have been proposed to subdivide the motor thalamus. Due to its extensive use among surgeons, the one created by Hassler is the most commonly employed in clinical practice.[9] According to Hassler, the motor thalamus may be subdivided into oral, caudal, intermediate, and lateropolar segments. The ventral intermediate (Vim) nucleus of the thalamus is the most effective thalamic target for the treatment of tremor in various conditions.[10] The most common disorder that presents with tremor is ET.[3] Tremor is also a cardinal manifestation of PD and frequently presents as a disabling component of conditions such as multiple sclerosis (MS) or cerebellar disorders.

The mere introduction of an electrode to the Vim may result in a decrease in tremor. The duration of this "microthalamotomy effect" is variable, but typically ranges from days to weeks. Nevertheless, in a few patients the effect can persist for years, making stimulation unnecessary.[11] Different components of a patient's tremor may respond differently to stimulation, though this has not been consistently demonstrated in all studies. As a rule, it appears that distal tremor is better controlled than proximal, and rest tremor better than kinetic tremor.

Essential Tremor

Surgical therapy for ET is considered when standard medications (primidone, β-blockers, gabapentin) fail and the patients continue to be disabled. Contralateral arm tremor control is observed in 68 to 79% of the patients treated with thalamic stimulation at 1 year.[12-17] The effects on postural tremor are less dramatic, with a 46 to 56% benefit at 3 months.[12,16] The benefits achieved with thalamic stimulation for ET are still significant at 6 years, although slightly lower than the ones observed at 1 year.[17]

Patients with ET can show the phenomenon of tolerance; that is, patients may require higher stimulation settings to capture tremor benefit.[17,18] At 6 years, the mean stimulation amplitude increased from 2.0 to 2.6 V, mean rate from 156 Hz to 173 Hz, and pulse width from 103 μs to 89 μs.[17] This gradual increase in stimulation may be problematic because it may lead to side effects, such as speech difficulty or paresthesias, as well as premature battery failure. Some have recommended turning the stimulation off at night and attempting to minimize parameters in the hopes of avoiding this. Alternatively, some patients have gone on to have thalamotomy lesions made through their DBS electrodes with good results.[19] The discontinuation of stimulation may induce a rebound effect in which the severity of tremor becomes worse than it was before stimulation commenced. Response of ET to stimulation is graded and diminishes with increasing frequency from 45 to 100 Hz. The optimal stimulation frequency is 100 to 130 Hz for most patients.[20]

Tremor of Parkinson Disease

Contralateral arm tremor improves in 71 to 92% of patients with PD treated with thalamic stimulation at 3 months.[12] This appears to be well sustained, with other series reporting 74% of patients well controlled at 1 year.[13] Contralateral foot tremor can be improved in 55 to 90% of the patients at 3 months.[21]

Although tremor is very well treated with Vim stimulation,[22] this procedure does not treat akinesia, rigidity, gait disturbance, and postural instability.[12,23] For this reason the Vim is rarely the preferred target for patients with PD.[1] Certain patients who have predominantly unilateral tremor may benefit from thalamic surgery,[24] but most patients will progress with time and eventually be disabled by other symptoms. Therefore, thalamic surgery for PD is rarely performed in most centers.

Dystonia

Due to the effectiveness of pallidal DBS in dystonia, thalamic stimulation has not been thoroughly explored in recent years. In a series of 12 patients with primary and secondary dystonia treated with thalamic stimulation in the ventrolateral posterior nucleus, improvements in global functional outcome were noted in 67% of the patients. Yet no improvements in dystonia scores were reported.[25] Individual reports of patients responding well to chronic stimulation of thalamic targets (e.g., ventralis oralis anterior nucleus) have also been published.[26,27]

Other Tremor Disorders

The benefits of thalamic procedures for patients with other disorders, such as posttraumatic tremor, tremor associated with MS, and cerebellar disorders are less predictable, being of lesser magnitude or transient.[28,29] Patients with MS may expect a 60% reduction in their tremor scores with thalamic DBS at 1 year.[30] Nevertheless, this may have a low impact on the quality of life of these patients in the long term due to the associated pyramidal, cerebellar, or sensory symptoms that often develop in these patients postoperatively.[30]

Globus Pallidus

The globus pallidus internus (GPi) is one of the main signal outflow channels of the basal ganglia. It receives afferents from the striatum, globus pallidus externus (GPe), STN, and substantia nigra compacta. It sends efferent projections to the thalamus, habenula, and brain stem tegmental structures, such as the pedunculopontine nucleus. Motor, associative, and limbic territories have been identified in the GPi, with the former comprising the ventrolateral two thirds of the nucleus. In fact, the posteroventral portion of the GPi is considered the preferred target for stereotactic lesioning.

The GPi is a large structure, which provides an opportunity for variations in the site of implantation of DBS electrodes, leading to great variability in surgical outcomes. In PD, this was one of the reasons for the recent inclination toward the use of the STN as a target. For dystonia, the GPi continues to be the most frequently chosen surgical target.

Parkinson Disease

In contrast to Vim surgery, the GPi and STN have emerged as effective targets not only to control tremor but also to ameliorate rigidity, bradykinesia, and gait disturbances.[2,31–49] In addition, motor side effects of dopa-replacement therapy such as dyskinesias, freezing, and on–off fluctuations are effectively reduced with stimulation of these targets.

In general, surgery improves parkinsonism to the level achieved with L-dopa, and the response to surgery can be predicted by the improvement obtained after L-dopa administration. In fact, symptoms that are resistant to L-dopa, such as bladder dysfunction, constipation, speech difficulties, sexual dysfunction, psychological difficulties, seborrhea, and cognitive dysfunction, are also resistant to surgery.[38,50] To date there is little effective medical or surgical therapy for these problems.

The range of reported motor outcomes with chronic stimulation of the GPi for PD is considerable,[47,51] with the best series reporting a 67% improvement[47] in the Unified Parkinson's Disease Rating Scale (UPDRS) motor scores in the off-medication state. Most studies, however, have shown improvements in the range of 30 to 55% with bilateral GPi stimulation[32,52–57] in the off-medication state. Benefits from unilateral stimulation are more modest (around 30 to 40%) and predominantly on the contralateral side, although mild ipsilateral improvements may also be noted.[56,58,59] The reduction in tremor with GPi surgery approximates 80%. The rigidity and akinesia scores improve approximately by 60%, whereas improvement in gait and posture is on the order of 40%. Involuntary movements induced by L-dopa improve on the order of 80 to 90%.[32,52–56,60]

Dystonia

The clinical response to surgery is dependent on the etiology of the dystonia. Although data remain preliminary, it is becoming clear that the primary generalized forms respond better to GPi DBS than do the secondary forms.[25,61–64]

Although the effects of pallidal DBS in PD can be immediate, patients with dystonia may not realize benefit for several days, weeks, or even longer.[65–67] The reasons why the benefits of pallidal stimulation are delayed and often progressive with ongoing stimulation for dystonia patients are not fully understood.

Within the primary generalized dystonias, the genetically identified DYT-1 mutation type is perhaps the most responsive, with early reports demonstrating a 90% decrease in the Burke-Fahn-Marsden Dystonia Rating Scale (BFMDRS) after a 12-month follow-up.[68] This is in agreement with our observations of improvement greater than 80% in DYT-1 dystonia.[61] Other forms of primary generalized dystonia may be slightly less responsive, on the order of 48 to 84%.[69–72]

Cervical dystonia seems to benefit from pallidal DBS as well, with treated patients obtaining a reduction of ~60%[73] in all three components (motor symptoms, pain, and disability) of the Toronto Western Spasmodic Torticollis Rating Scale (TWSTRS). It has been noted by several authors that the time course of response for each of these areas is different. Although pain often responds very quickly, motor symptoms and disability often respond more slowly and progressively.

For secondary dystonias, the average improvement on the Abnormal Involuntary Movement Scale (AIMS) is ~40%.[73] However, the range of responses is quite variable (from 0% to 75%), indicating that this group of heterogeneous conditions needs further investigation to determine the appropriate indications and realistic outcomes. There is evidence that some of these patients may derive benefit from thalamic procedures; the choice of the most appropriate target remains unresolved.[73,74]

Subthalamic Nucleus

The STN has been regarded as an important modulator of basal ganglia output. It receives its major afferents from the cerebral cortex, thalamus, GPe, and brain stem. It projects mainly to both segments of the globus pallidus, substantia nigra, striatum, and brain stem. The STN is primarily composed of projection glutamatergic neurons. Lesions of the STN can induce choreiform movements and ballism on the contralateral side of the body.[75]

Due to the uniformity of the clinical results and the compact size of the nucleus, the STN is currently the most popular target for stimulation in patients with PD.[1,2,32,33,37–47] Overall, STN DBS yields greater than 50% improvement in UPDRS motor scores at 12 months in the off-medication condition in well-selected patients. Tremor, rigidity, and bradykinesia improve 80, 60, and 55%, respectively, on average, at 12 months. With STN surgery, L-dopa–induced dyskinesias improve ~80 to 90%. This is, in part, due to the reduction in dopaminergic drugs that is often achieved after these procedures.[1,2,31,40,45]

The Best Target for Parkinson Disease

The issue of whether the GPi or the STN is a better target for the treatment of advanced PD is still debated.[1,31,32,38,52,57,76,77] The globus pallidus is a larger structure, and there is more heterogeneity in the response to surgery.[78] As previously stated, this may be due to the variation in the position of the electrodes within the pallidal complex.[79,80] By comparison, the STN is smaller and provides more consistent results.[2,31–33,36,38,39,41,42,44,46,47,49] However, there are regions within the STN with limbic and associative connections, which are closely apposed to the motor region of the nucleus. Spillover of electrical stimulation into these territories might explain the higher incidence of cognitive and emotional side effects seen after STN surgery compared with GPi surgery.[76] STN stimulation appears to be more likely to improve bradykinesia.[76] Stimulation of both targets reduces dyskinesias.[76] Of note, STN DBS was also found to improve cervical dystonia and ET.[23,81,82]

Complications of Deep Brain Stimulation Surgery

General Complications

The most fearsome complications of stereotactic procedures are intracranial hemorrhages. With an incidence of ~2 to 3%, most hemorrhages are intraparenchymal, but subdural or intraventricular hemorrhages are occasionally seen as well. Most hemorrhages are asymptomatic, observed only on postoperative brain imaging.[83,84] However, in some patients the effects of a bleed can be serious, leading to permanent sequelae.

There is some debate in the literature as to whether the use of multiple passes of microelectrodes for mapping, while presumably decreasing the adverse effects associated with targeting inaccuracy, may in fact increase the risk of hemorrhage. In a series of 481 lead implantations, 0.6% were associated with hematomas causing permanent deficit.[84] Patients who developed hematomas had a slightly greater, but not significant, number of microelectrode recording penetrations than patients who did not have hematomas.[84] In addition, some neurosurgeons feel that the increased operative time for microelectrode mapping may increase the infection risk. These questions are important but cannot be definitively addressed with the currently available data.

Other acute complications include postoperative nausea in ~3 to 5%, headaches in 1.9 to 5%, seizures in 1.6 to 5.5%, and perioperative confusion in up to 15% of patients.[2,31–33,36,38–45,47,49] Some unusual complications such as venous air embolisms have also been reported.[85,86]

Stimulation-Related Complications

Thalamus

Specific adverse effects encountered with DBS in the Vim include speech problems, corticospinal symptoms, and ataxia, as well as paresthesias related to stimulation of the adjacent tactile ventrocaudal (Vc) nucleus and the medial lemniscus. Because these effects are related to the spread of current to adjacent structures, in many cases stimulation parameters can be adjusted to reduce their incidence.[87]

Paresthesias have been reported in 9 to 100% of these patients, in whom symptoms ceased when stimulation was discontinued.[12,13,16,21] Cerebellar complaints have been reported in less than 10% of the patients. Weakness (from spread of current to the internal capsule) has been reported in less than 12% of the patients. Dysarthria has been reported in less than 8% of the patients following unilateral stimulation. It is significantly more common after bilateral procedures (higher than 45% in most studies).[12,13,16,21]

Globus Pallidus

During globus pallidus surgery, it is important to identify the sensorimotor territory of the GPi (populated by neurons that respond to movements of the limbs), as well as the optic tract and the corticospinal tract. Intraoperative electrical stimulation in the optic tract produces phosphenes, whereas stimulation of the corticospinal tract produces motor contractions.[80,88] During the programming of the patients, increasing stimulation current beyond a given patient's threshold may result in transient paresthesias, tonic contractions of the contralateral side of the body, dysarthria, and photopsia. Decrease in stimulation parameters usually improves these adverse effects. Patients with dystonia may experience a rebound effect when stimulation is discontinued, which may be extremely severe and potentially life threatening.[73,89]

Subthalamic Nucleus

The objectives during surgery on the STN are to identify the sensorimotor territory in the STN and to avoid adverse side affects related to important adjacent structures, such as the fibers of the third cranial nerve (medial to the STN), the corticospinal tract (anterior and lateral), and fibers of the medial lemniscus (posterior). Yet, dyskinesias, paresthesias, diplopia, dystonia, and motor contractions are relatively common side effects with STN stimulation.[57] In addition, hypophonia, eyelid apraxia, increased libido, sialorrhea, hypomania, and decreased memory have also been reported.[90] Depression and weight gain occur in ~5 to 15% of patients.[2,31–33,36,38–40,43–47,49,57,64] There are probably multiple mechanisms underlying these events.

Hardware-Related Complications

There are long-term risks associated with the implantation of any device. These appear to be associated with all applications of DBS. A review of 124 electrodes implanted in 79 patients over a 6-year period[91] showed that 20 patients (25.3%) had hardware-related complications. These involved 23 (18.5%) of the electrodes. Of the 23, there were four lead fractures, four lead migrations, three short or open circuits, 12 infection/erosions, two allergic reactions, and one cerebrospinal fluid (CSF) leak. Although these were not related to the selected target, lead fractures occurred more commonly in patients with prominent cervical dystonia or dyskinesia. The hardware-related complication rate was 8.4% per electrode-year. Importantly, 19.2% of the patients developed complications within the first month, 42.3% between the first and twelfth months, and 38.5% 12 months after the procedure. Thus the possibility of complications persists for the life of the device. Replacement of the implantable pulse generator (IPG) for battery depletion was needed in 12 of the patients ranging from 7 to 70 months after implantation, averaging 45 months.[92]

Certain authors have also noted that lead fracture appears more common in patients with dystonia, likely due to extreme movements of the neck. This complication appears to be more frequent when the connector to the extension cable is low in the neck, below the mastoid process.[70] In another study[2] for PD, the overall rate of hardware infections was 2.9% (33% with removal of at least part of the system), and the incidence of lead problems was 2.9%. Incidence of lead infection appears to be increased by periods of externalization for lead testing.[93]

■ Conclusion

The use of DBS in movement and other neurological disorders is rapidly expanding. This summary of currently available data on the efficacy and complications of DBS will undoubtedly be replaced as further investigations lead to changes in target, improved efficacy, and decreased complications.

Editor's Comments

As the number of patients that have been implanted with DBS systems has increased and the duration of follow-up has lengthened, there has been a virtual explosion of studies examining various outcomes following DBS for movement disorders. Critical for increasing acceptance of DBS in the medical community has been a prospective randomized-pairs trial published in the *New England Journal of Medicine*, which found DBS to be significantly more effective than medical management of patients with PD at 6-month follow-up.[94] In this study, a randomized-pairs trial of 156 patients with advanced PD and severe motor symptoms demonstrated significant improvements in both the quality of life measure Parkinson Disease Questionnaire (PDQ)-39 ($p = .02$) and motor UPDRS III ($p<.001$). Serious adverse events were more common in the DBS group ($p<.04$), but total adverse events were higher in the medication group ($p < .08$). A separate randomized trial with 20 PD patients with mild to moderate disease (mean off-medication UPDRS III of 29 and mean disease duration of 6.8 years) demonstrated significantly greater benefit in motor signs off medication, less L-dopa–induced complications, and lower L-dopa dosage in the DBS surgical patients ($N = 10$) compared with patients receiving medical therapy ($N = 10$).[95] This suggests that DBS could be considered an early therapeutic option in PD.

Other contributions provided additional class III and IV evidence to the literature and interesting perspectives on the impact of DBS on various PD symptomatologies. Very long-term (4- to 5-year postoperative) data following DBS for PD showed similar results to previous 1-year follow-up publications in terms of motor improvements.[96–99] Improvements in tremor, rigidity, and dyskinesias were sustained after 5 years, but there were significant declines in akinesia, speech, postural stability, freezing of gait, and axial symptoms, which is consistent with progression of the natural history of PD. It is more likely that DBS masks the symptoms rather than slowing the progression of the disease.[100] Although the value of meta-analysis is questionable when the data are of poor quality,[101] there are now several meta-analyses, all of which suggest the beneficial effects of DBS on motor activity and activities of daily living.[102,103] One such multivariate analysis of those data revealed that preoperative UPDRS scores and L-dopa responsiveness were independent predictors of motor improvement following bilateral STN DBS.[102]

The role of bilateral versus unilateral surgery was explored in STN DBS for PD. Motor improvements with unilateral STN DBS were found not to be as robust as with bilateral stimulation.[104] Improvement in gait and balance control requires bilateral surgery.[105–111] However, patients received sufficient benefit and did not require additional surgery as of a 12-month follow-up.[109] The advantages are simpler surgery, lower complication rate, and the potential that the technology may dramatically improve before the second-side surgery is required. A prospective study of nine PD patients who underwent unilateral STN DBS found an ipsilateral improvement in UPDRS III of 20% and a reduction in dosage of L-dopa by 15%; most notably these patients did report an improvement in activities of daily living on UPDRS II of 50%.[110] We studied 25 PD patients with unilateral STN DBS and found 31% improvement in UPDRS III.[111] Most of these patients required a second-side surgery in 1 to 2 years, but a few did well for over 4 years. We now only perform unilateral STN DBS surgery on clearly asymmetric or very old and debilitated patients. Similarly, it was observed that unilateral GPi DBS for PD results in unsatisfactory long-term results.[112] Again, patient selection plays an important role.

Also increasingly reported are the motor improvements observed following STN DBS in patients with previous movement disorders surgery. In a series of 15 patients who had previously undergone thalamic surgery, STN DBS resulted in significant improvements in UPDRS motor score, tremor score, activities of daily living, and L-dopa equivalent doses.[113] However, 10 patients who underwent STN DBS after unilateral pallidotomy showed only a 16% improvement in UPDRS scores.[114] Care needs to be taken if gait or freezing problems exist and bilateral STN DBS may be required.[115] A case presentation of a patient treated with DBS after previous thalamotomy as well as adrenal grafting showed 46% improvement in the UPDRS motor section and medication reduction of 81% at 1-year follow-up.[116] Although the actual benefit of STN DBS for patients who had previous procedures ranged from series to series, these studies do provide evidence that the procedure can be performed safely in patients with previous movement disorders surgeries. We have utilized DBS to augment effectiveness as well as correct problems created by other movement disorder surgery, including thalamotomies, pallidotomies, adrenal transplants, fetal transplants, and porcine transplants.

The efficacy of DBS in the treatment of nonmotor complications of PD is being assessed.[117] Continued evidence for improvement in gait, balance control, and sleep patterns has been shown.[118–119] Examination of 14 patients with bilateral STN DBS improved orthostatic hypotension in these patients, thereby improving autonomic regulation.[120] However, in another study bilateral STN DBS did not improve cardiovascular autonomic reflex function in 11 PD patients.[121] Bladder control also seemed to improve, potentially

secondary to modulation of the frontal cortex.[122,123] Weight gains of 10 to 20 lbs was frequently observed following DBS surgery, suggesting the need to monitor and manage patients' weight postoperatively.[124,125]

Old lesion targets and new DBS targets for treatment of PD are being explored.[126,127,129,130] In one study, 27 leads were implanted into the caudal zona incerta, and the 6-month outcomes of those patients compared with outcomes in 17 patients with STN leads.[127] The group reported a greater improvement in contralateral UPDRS motor score, tremor, and rigidity and no complications in the zona incerta patients. Of note, however, four patients who had bilateral implants located dorsomedial to the STN developed reversible hypophonic slurred speech and disequilibrium. The pedunculopontine nucleus (PPN) was also explored as a target as a result of nonhuman primate work, which showed that PPN low-frequency stimulation improved akinesia.[128] Patients who underwent placement of PPN DBS electrodes had significant improvement in gait and postural instability also at low frequencies (20 to 25 Hz).[129,130] This finding was of particular interest because neither STN nor GPi DBS typically have as dramatic effect on these symptoms and the low-frequency stimulation is unquestionably stimulating these neurons. Target selection for DBS in the treatment of movement disorders as well as for emerging applications will no doubt be a major focus of study in the future.

Two controlled trials demonstrated significant improvement in dystonia following DBS. A prospective, blinded assessment trial of pallidal DBS in 22 patients with primary generalized dystonia showed a mean decrease of 51% in the BFMDRS at 1-year follow-up as compared with preoperative score.[71] In a blinded, randomized trial, bilateral pallidal DBS was performed for primary generalized and segmental dystonia in 40 patients, and 3-month outcomes in patients who received actual stimulation were compared with sham stimulation patients.[132] There was a significantly greater improvement in the movement subscore of the BFMDRS in the actual stimulated patients compared with sham. And when all patients were stimulated, substantial improvements were reported in quality of life, level of disability, and all motor symptoms except speech and swallowing compared with baseline. In fact, the most frequent adverse event was dysarthria.

Factors that may affect efficacy in dystonia patients undergoing DBS need further examination (see Chapter 12). One group revealed that patients with the greatest improvements (i.e., > 70% decrease in BFMDRS score), had electrodes located near the intercommissural plane, at a mean distance from the pallidocapsular border of 3.6 mm.[133] Another group published their results in 12 patients with childhood-onset dystonia. Of note, only one of these patients had DYT-1–positive dystonia, and stimulation was effective in all but one patient.[134] Furthermore, they found that three patients with status dystonicus responded to GPi DBS. Clearly, primary generalized or segmental dystonia improves with pallidal DBS and we have long advocated this target.[135] Other than DYT-1 patients, the key will be to be able to screen heterogeneous dystonic patient populations to know who will respond. The use of preoperative surface electromyography to predict clinical response has been suggested.[136]

Groups studying Vim stimulation for ET also evaluated the results on typically difficult-to-treat symptomatology with bilateral or unilateral DBS (see Chapter 11). A prospective study of 22 staged procedures revealed significant improvement in midline tremor from baseline with unilateral stimulation and even greater improvement with bilateral stimulation.[137] Another group examined complication rates following bilateral Vim stimulation and found a 75% incidence of dysarthria and 56% incidence of balance difficulties and thus provided further evidence that bilateral procedures in these patients should be embarked upon with great care.[138] Although we do not have this high complication rate with bilateral Vim for ET patients, as a rule we perform unilateral Vim DBS for the dominant hand of ET patients and do not routinely perform bilateral procedures except for severe midline tremors.

As the acceptance and applications for DBS continue to expand, the number of patients with implantable devices has increased exponentially. As we developed techniques to minimize strokes and infections, it became increasingly clear that long-term hardware problems are a potential limiting factor. The revision rates for DBS surgeries remain significantly higher than in other functional neurosurgical procedures, and widespread use of these devices will mandate optimization of these devices to minimize reoperation rates and overall cost of implantation (see Chapter 14). Hardware complications range in incidence from 11 to 30%.[139–142] Specifically, one group showed that in 100 patients over 2 years, 3.1% of brain electrodes needed revision, and battery failures occurred in 8.4% of patients.[139] Another found that during a 3-year follow-up, hardware-related problems occurred in 13.9% of patients and partial or complete removal was necessary in 4.6% of patients.[140] In a 44-month follow-up of 96 leads at a single institution, there were complications in 28 leads.[141] Of note, the group observed a trend that PD patients were subject more to early complications, whereas patients with dystonia had complications more frequently greater than 6 months postoperatively. There is a learning curve.[142] A study reviewing the existing literature found that in 922 DBS patients, infections occurred in 6.1% of patients, migration in 5.1%, lead fractures in 5%, and skin erosion in 1.3%.[143] The rates will continue to change over time because there will be a certain rate-per-year baseline, but also as techniques evolve and equipment improves we can hope that the high point has been reached and the rates will fall to a minimal level.

Reports of interactions between DBS and other medical devices, namely, cardiac pacemakers and magnetic resonance imaging (MRI), are another problem that must be addressed (see Chapter 14). Case series of patients who have safely been implanted with both DBS systems and pacemakers were reported.[144,145] But are these patients at greater risk if they need cardioversion? Concern over the use of MRI in patients with implanted DBS has increased since Henderson et al[146] published a case report of a PD patient with bilateral STN DBS electrodes who underwent an MRI of the lumbar spine and developed hemiplegia immediately thereafter, presumably secondary to heating of the electrode. Body MRI is currently not advised in patients implanted with current DBS technology. Cranial MRI can be performed but should only be performed in equipment configured to safety specifications determined by the manufacturer (www.medtronic.com/ neuro/et/techmanual.html). However care must be taken with all MRI studies because an additional study found that temperature changes normalized for specific absorption rate (SAR) values may vary significantly from scanner to scanner. When two 1.5 tesla/64 MHz MR systems using a transmit/receive head coil were compared, one scanner had an SAR that was 3.5 to 5.5 times higher than the other.[147] As more and more patients are implanted with DBS devices, both MRI technology and DBS systems will need to be adapted so that these procedures can be performed safely and routinely, even in smaller hospitals or MRI centers.

There are many reports of neurocognitive sequelae following bilateral STN DBS. Although some of these can be corrected with programming (see Chapter 13), there are some that are permanent. One controlled study compared the neuropsychological impact of bilateral STN stimulation of 99 patients 6 months after surgery to 36 PD control patients.[148] They reported psychiatric complications in 9% of STN patients versus 3% of controls. The STN group also showed greater decline in verbal fluency, color naming, selective attention, verbal memory, and overall affect.[149,149] A study of the mental aspects of the quality of life assessment revealed no improvement in emotional well-being, social support, cognition, and communication following bilateral STN DBS.[150] The reported improvements in quality of life that do occur seem to be correlated with relief of bradykinesia.[151] Suicide attempts and permanent apathy were also reported.[99,152,153] A case study of an STN DBS patient who had reproducible mania and corresponding positron emission tomography (PET) changes in the limbic system with stimulation of lower contacts near/in the substantia nigra was reported.[152]

Changes in mood or cognition were generally absent following Vim DBS and GPi DBS.[103,153,154] The continued recognition of the changes in mood and cognition after STN, but not following GPi DBS, sparked further debate on the role of both types of stimulation for PD. A randomized study that prospectively compared STN stimulation patients to GPi patients demonstrated no motoric difference but a 38% reduction in L-dopa in STN versus 3% in GPi patients.[155] In a prospective multicenter study of 69 PD patients treated with bilateral DBS of the STN ($n = 49$) or GPi ($n = 20$), stimulation of the STN or GPi induced a significant improvement (50 and 39%; $p < .0001$) of the off-medication UPDRS-III score at 3 to 4 years with respect to baseline.[156] Stimulation also improved the cardinal features of PD and activities of daily living (ADL) and prolonged the on time spent without dyskinesias. Comparison of the improvement induced by stimulation at 1 year with that at 3 to 4 years showed a significant worsening in the on-medication motor states of the UPDRS-III, ADL, and gait in both STN and GPi groups, and speech and postural stability in the STN-treated group. Although not statistically different in motor improvement, the tendency to improve more with STN DBS than with GPi DBS and the greater decrease in need for L-dopa had suggested the advantage for STN DBS; however, GPi stimulation is associated with far less cognitive and psychiatric postoperative problems and thus needs reevaluation in large, randomized, blinded studies.

As the use of DBS in neurological disorders continues to expand, its future success is dependent on refinement of target and patient selection. Much more effort needs to be focused on developing techniques and devices with lower complication rates and that are safe in patients undergoing other medical procedures. Studies reporting outcomes in terms of both efficacy and complications are essential for optimization of patient care.

References

1. Pollak P, Fraix V, Krack P, et al. Treatment results: Parkinson's disease. Mov Disord 2002;17(Suppl 3):S75–S83
2. Benabid AL, Koudsie A, Benazzouz A, et al. Deep brain stimulation of the corpus luysi (subthalamic nucleus) and other targets in Parkinson's disease: extension to new indications such as dystonia and epilepsy. J Neurol 2001;248(Suppl 3):Iii37–Iii47
3. Pahwa R, Lyons KE, Wilkinson SB, et al. Comparison of thalamotomy to deep brain stimulation of the thalamus in essential tremor. Mov Disord 2001;16:140–143
4. Lenz FA, Dostrovsky JO, Tasker RR, et al. Single-unit analysis of the human ventral thalamic nuclear group: somatosensory responses. J Neurophysiol 1988;59:299–316
5. Lenz FA, Kwan HC, Dostrovsky JO, et al. Single unit analysis of the human ventral thalamic nuclear group: activity correlated with movement. Brain 1990;113(Pt 6):1795–1821
6. Vitek JL, Ashe J, DeLong MR, et al. Microstimulation of primate motor thalamus: somatotopic organization and differential distribution of evoked motor responses among subnuclei. J Neurophysiol 1996;75:2486–2495
7. Molnar GF, Sailer A, Gunraj CA, et al. Changes in cortical excitability with thalamic deep brain stimulation. Neurology 2005;64:1913–1919
8. Molnar GF, Sailer A, Gunraj CA, et al. Thalamic deep brain stimulation activates the cerebellothalamocortical pathway. Neurology 2004;63:907–909
9. Hassler R. Architectonic organization of the thalamic nuclei. In: Schaltenbrand G, Walker AE, eds. Stereotaxy of the Human Brain: Anatomical, Physiological and Clinical Applications. Stuttgart; New York: Georg Thieme Verlag; 1982:140–180.
10. Lozano AM. Vim thalamic stimulation for tremor. Arch Med Res 2000;31:266–269
11. Kondziolka D, Lee JY. Long-lasting microthalamotomy effect after temporary placement of a thalamic stimulating electrode. Stereotact Funct Neurosurg 2004;82:127–130
12. Benabid AL, Pollak P, Gao D, et al. Chronic electrical stimulation of the ventralis intermedius nucleus of the thalamus as a treatment of movement disorders. J Neurosurg 1996;84:203–214
13. Koller W, Pahwa R, Busenbark K, et al. High-frequency unilateral thalamic stimulation in the treatment of essential and parkinsonian tremor. Ann Neurol 1997;42:292–299
14. Lee JY, Kondziolka D. Thalamic deep brain stimulation for management of essential tremor. J Neurosurg 2005;103:400–403
15. Pahwa R, Lyons KE, Wilkinson SB, et al. Long-term evaluation of deep brain stimulation of the thalamus. J Neurosurg 2006;104:506–512
16. Pahwa R, Lyons KL, Wilkinson SB, et al. Bilateral thalamic stimulation for the treatment of essential tremor. Neurology 1999;53:1447–1450
17. Sydow O, Thobois S, Alesch F, et al. Multicentre European study of thalamic stimulation in essential tremor: a six year follow up. J Neurol Neurosurg Psychiatry 2003;74:1387–1391
18. Yamamoto T, Katayama Y, Kano T, et al. Deep brain stimulation for the treatment of parkinsonian, essential, and poststroke tremor: a suitable stimulation method and changes in effective stimulation intensity. J Neurosurg 2004;101:201–209
19. Oh MY, Hodaie M, Kim SH, et al. Deep brain stimulator electrodes used for lesioning: proof of principle. Neurosurgery 2001;49:363–367
20. Ushe M, Mink JW, Revilla FJ, et al. Effect of stimulation frequency on tremor suppression in essential tremor. Mov Disord 2004;19:1163–1168
21. Ondo W, Jankovic J, Schwartz K, et al. Unilateral thalamic deep brain stimulation for refractory essential tremor and Parkinson's disease tremor. Neurology 1998;51:1063–1069
22. Laitinen L. Surgical treatment, past and present, in Parkinson's disease. Acta Neurol Scand Suppl 1972;51:43–58
23. Plaha P, Patel NK, Gill SS. Stimulation of the subthalamic region for essential tremor. J Neurosurg 2004;101:48–54
24. Gray A, McNamara I, Aziz T, et al. Quality of life outcomes following surgical treatment of Parkinson's disease. Mov Disord 2002;17:68–75
25. Vercueil L, Pollak P, Fraix V, et al. Deep brain stimulation in the treatment of severe dystonia. J Neurol 2001;248:695–700
26. Ghika J, Villemure JG, Miklossy J, et al. Postanoxic generalized dystonia improved by bilateral Voa thalamic deep brain stimulation. Neurology 2002;58:311–313
27. Krauss JK, Yianni J, Loher TJ, et al. Deep brain stimulation for dystonia. J Clin Neurophysiol 2004;21:18–30
28. Piette T, Mescola P, Henriet M, et al. A surgical approach to Holmes' tremor associated with high-frequency synchronous bursts. Rev Neurol (Paris) 2004;160:707–711
29. Shahzadi S, Tasker RR, Lozano A. Thalamotomy for essential and cerebellar tremor. Stereotact Funct Neurosurg 1995;65:11–17
30. Berk C, Carr J, Sinden M, et al. Thalamic deep brain stimulation for the treatment of tremor due to multiple sclerosis: a prospective study of tremor and quality of life. J Neurosurg 2002;97:815–820
31. Benabid A, Benazzous A, Piallat B, et al. Subthalamic nucleus deep brain stimulation. In: Lozano A, ed. Movement Disorder Surgery. Vol 15. Basel: Karger; 2000:196–226
32. Burchiel KJ, Anderson VC, Favre J, et al. Comparison of pallidal and subthalamic nucleus deep brain stimulation for advanced Parkinson's disease: results of a randomized, blinded pilot study. Neurosurgery 1999;45:1375–1382
33. Fraix V, Pollak P, Van Blercom N, et al. Effect of subthalamic nucleus stimulation on levodopa-induced dyskinesia in Parkinson's disease. Neurology 2000;55:1921–1923
34. Galvez Jimenez N, Lozano A, Tasker R, et al. Pallidal stimulation in Parkinson's disease patients with a prior unilateral pallidotomy. Can J Neurol Sci 1998;25:300–305
35. Hodaie M, Wennberg RA, Dostrovsky JO, et al. Chronic anterior thalamus stimulation for intractable epilepsy. Epilepsia 2002;43:603–608
36. Houeto JL, Damier P, Bejjani PB, et al. Subthalamic stimulation in Parkinson disease: a multidisciplinary approach. Arch Neurol 2000;57:461–465
37. Krack P, Batir A, Van Blercom N, et al. Five-year follow-up of bilateral stimulation of the subthalamic nucleus in advanced Parkinson's disease. N Engl J Med 2003;349:1925–1934
38. Krack P, Pollak P, Limousin P, et al. Subthalamic nucleus or internal pallidal stimulation in young onset Parkinson's disease. Brain 1998;121:451–457
39. Kumar R, Lozano AM, Kim YJ, et al. Double-blind evaluation of subthalamic nucleus deep brain stimulation in advanced Parkinson's disease. Neurology 1998;51:850–855
40. Limousin P, Krack P, Pollak P, et al. Electrical stimulation of the subthalamic nucleus in advanced Parkinson's disease. N Engl J Med 1998;339:1105–1111
41. Lozano AM. Deep brain stimulation for Parkinson's disease. Parkinsonism Relat Disord 2001;7:199–203
42. Molinuevo JL, Valldeoriola F, Tolosa E, et al. Levodopa withdrawal

after bilateral subthalamic nucleus stimulation in advanced Parkinson disease. Arch Neurol 2000;57:983–988

43. Simuni T, Jaggi JL, Mulholland H, et al. Bilateral stimulation of the subthalamic nucleus in patients with Parkinson disease: a study of efficacy and safety. J Neurosurg 2002;96:666–672

44. Thobois S, Mertens P, Guenot M, et al. Subthalamic nucleus stimulation in Parkinson's disease: clinical evaluation of 18 patients. J Neurol 2002;249:529–534

45. Vingerhoets FJG, Villemure JG, Temperli P, et al. Subthalamic DBS replaces levodopa in Parkinson's disease: two-year follow-up. Neurology 2002;58:396–401

46. Voges J, Volkmann J, Allert N, et al. Bilateral high-frequency stimulation in the subthalamic nucleus for the treatment of Parkinson disease: correlation of therapeutic effect with anatomical electrode position. J Neurosurg 2002;96:269–279

47. Volkmann J, Allert N, Voges J, et al. Safety and efficacy of pallidal or subthalamic nucleus stimulation in advanced PD. Neurology 2001;56:548–551

48. Volkmann J, Sturm V, Weiss P, et al. Bilateral high-frequency stimulation of the internal globus pallidus in advanced Parkinson's disease. Ann Neurol 1998;44:953–961

49. Yokoyama T, Sugiyama K, Nishizawa S, et al. Subthalamic nucleus stimulation for gait disturbance in Parkinson's disease. Neurosurgery 1999;45:41–47

50. Lang AE, Widner H. Deep brain stimulation for Parkinson's disease: patient selection and evaluation. Mov Disord 2002;17 (Suppl 3):S94–S101

51. Tronnier VM, Fogel W, Kronenbuerger M, et al. Pallidal stimulation: an alternative to pallidotomy? J Neurosurg 1997;87: 700–705

52. Deep Brain Stimulation for Parkinson's Disease Study Group. Deep-brain stimulation of the subthalamic nucleus or the pars interna of the globus pallidus in Parkinson's disease. N Engl J Med 2001;345:956–963

53. Brown RG, Dowsey PL, Brown P, et al. Impact of deep brain stimulation on upper limb akinesia in Parkinson's disease. Ann Neurol 1999;45:473–488

54. Durif F, Lemaire JJ, Debilly B, et al. Long-term follow-up of globus pallidus chronic stimulation in advanced Parkinson's disease. Mov Disord 2002;17:803–807

55. Ghika J, Villemure JG, Fankhauser H, et al. Efficiency and safety of bilateral contemporaneous pallidal stimulation (deep brain stimulation) in levodopa-responsive patients with Parkinson's disease with severe motor fluctuations: a 2-year follow-up review. J Neurosurg 1998;89:713–718

56. Marks WJ, Clay HD, Heath S, et al. Unilateral and bilateral deep brain stimulation of the globus pallidus or subthalamic nucleus in patients with medically refractory Parkinson's disease: short-term results from a randomized trial. Mov Disord 2000;15:366

57. Rodriguez-Oroz MC, Obeso JA, Lang AE, et al. Bilateral deep brain stimulation in Parkinson's disease: a multicentre study with 4 years follow-up. Brain 2005;128:2240–2249

58. Gross C, Rougier A, Guehl D, et al. High-frequency stimulation of the globus pallidus internalis in Parkinson's disease: a study of seven cases. J Neurosurg 1997;87:491–498

59. Merello M, Nouzeilles MI, Kuzis G, et al. Unilateral radiofrequency lesion versus electrostimulation of posteroventral pallidum: a prospective randomized comparison. Mov Disord 1999;14:50–56

60. Krack P, Pollak P, Limousin P, et al. Opposite motor effects of pallidal stimulation in Parkinson's disease. Ann Neurol 1998;43: 180–192

61. Eltahawy HA, Saint-Cyr J, Giladi N, Lang AE, Lozano AM. Primary dystonia is more responsive than secondary dystonia to pallidal interventions: outcome after pallidotomy or pallidal deep brain stimulation. Neurosurgery 2004;54:613–619

62. Islekel S, Zileli M, Zileli B. Unilateral pallidal stimulation in cervical dystonia. Stereotact Funct Neurosurg 1999;72:248–252

63. Krauss JK, Loher TJ, Pohle T, et al. Pallidal deep brain stimulation in patients with cervical dystonia and severe cervical dyskinesias with cervical myelopathy. J Neurol Neurosurg Psychiatry 2002;72:249–256

64. Loher TJ, Hasdemir MG, Burgunder JM, et al. Long-term follow-up study of chronic globus pallidus internus stimulation for posttraumatic hemidystonia. J Neurosurg 2000;92:457–460

65. Kumar R, Dagher A, Hutchison WD, et al. Globus pallidus deep brain stimulation for generalized dystonia: clinical and PET investigation. Neurology 1999;53:871–874

66. Tronnier VM, Fogel W. Pallidal stimulation for generalized dystonia: report of three cases. J Neurosurg 2000;92:453–456

67. Volkmann J, Benecke R. Deep brain stimulation for dystonia: patient selection and evaluation. Mov Disord 2002;17(Suppl 3): S112–S115

68. Coubes P, Roubertie A, Vayssiere N, et al. Treatment of DYT1-generalised dystonia by stimulation of the internal globus pallidus. Lancet 2000;355:2220–2221

69. Coubes P, Vayssiere N, El Fertit H, et al. Deep brain stimulation for dystonia: surgical technique. Stereotact Funct Neurosurg 2002;78: 183–191

70. Krauss JK. Deep brain stimulation for dystonia in adults: overview and developments. Stereotact Funct Neurosurg 2002;78:168–182

71. Vidailhet M, Vercueil L, Houeto JL, et al; French Stimulation du Pallidum Interne dans la Dystonie (SPIDY) Study Group. Bilateral deep-brain stimulation of the globus pallidus in primary generalized dystonia. N Engl J Med 2005;352:459–467

72. Zorzi G, Marras C, Nardocci N, et al. Stimulation of the globus pallidus internus for childhood-onset dystonia. Mov Disord 2005;20: 1194–1200

73. Yianni J, Bain P, Giladi N, et al. Globus pallidus internus deep brain stimulation for dystonic conditions: a prospective audit. Mov Disord 2003;18:436–442

74. Chuang C, Fahn S, Frucht SJ. The natural history and treatment of acquired hemidystonia: report of 33 cases and review of the literature. J Neurol Neurosurg Psychiatry 2002;72:59–67

75. Hamani C, Saint-Cyr JA, Fraser J, et al. The subthalamic nucleus in the context of movement disorders. Brain 2004;127:4–20

76. Anderson VC, Burchiel KJ, Hogarth P, et al. Pallidal vs subthalamic nucleus deep brain stimulation in Parkinson disease. Arch Neurol 2005;62:554–560

77. Miyawaki E, Perlmutter JS, Troster AI, et al. The behavioral complications of pallidal stimulation: a case report. Brain Cogn 2000;42: 417–434

78. Bakay RAE. Rational basis for pallidotomy in the treatment of Parkinson's disease. In: Lozano AM, ed. Movement Disorder Surgery. Vol 15. Basel: Karger; 2000:118–131

79. Gross RE, Lombardi WJ, Lang AE, et al. Relationship of lesion location to clinical outcome following microelectrode-guided pallidotomy for Parkinson's disease. Brain 1999;122:405–416

80. Lozano A, Hutchison W, Kiss Z, et al. Methods for microelectrode-guided posteroventral pallidotomy. J Neurosurg 1996;84:194–202

81. Chou KL, Hurtig HI, Jaggi JL, et al. Bilateral subthalamic nucleus deep brain stimulation in a patient with cervical dystonia and essential tremor. Mov Disord 2005;20:377–380

82. Stover NP, Okun MS, Evatt ML, et al. Stimulation of the subthalamic nucleus in a patient with Parkinson disease and essential tremor. Arch Neurol 2005;62:141–143

83. Terao T, Takahashi H, Yokochi F, et al. Hemorrhagic complication of stereotactic surgery in patients with movement disorders. J Neurosurg 2003;98:1241–1246

84. Binder DK, Rau GM, Starr PA. Risk factors for hemorrhage during microelectrode-guided deep brain stimulator implantation for movement disorders. Neurosurgery 2005;56:722–732

85. Deogaonkar A, Avitsian R, Henderson JM, et al. Venous air embolism during deep brain stimulation surgery in an awake supine patient. Stereotact Funct Neurosurg 2005;83:32–35

86. Goodman RR, Kim B, McClelland S, et al. Operative techniques and morbidity with subthalamic nucleus deep brain stimulation in 100 consecutive patients with advanced Parkinson's disease. J Neurol Neurosurg Psychiatry 2006;77:12–17

87. Tasker RR, Munz M, Junn FS, et al. Deep brain stimulation and thalamotomy for tremor compared. Acta Neurochir Suppl (Wien) 1997;68:49–53

88. Kirschman DL, Milligan B, Wilkinson S, et al. Pallidotomy microelectrode targeting: neurophysiology-based target refinement. Neurosurgery 2000;46:613–622

89. Muta D, Goto S, Nishikawa S, et al. Bilateral pallidal stimulation for idiopathic segmental axial dystonia advanced from Meige syndrome refractory to bilateral thalamotomy. Mov Disord 2001;16:774–777

90. Visser-Vandewalle V, van der Linden C, Temel Y, et al. Long-term effects of bilateral subthalamic nucleus stimulation in advanced Parkinson disease: a four year follow-up study. Parkinsonism Relat Disord 2005;11:157–165

91. Oh MY, Abosch A, Kim SH, et al. Long-term hardware-related complications of deep brain stimulation. Neurosurgery 2002;50:1268–1274

92. Bin-Mahfoodh M, Hamani C, Sime E, et al. Longevity of batteries in internal pulse generators used for deep brain stimulation. Stereotact Funct Neurosurg 2003;80:56–60

93. Constantoyannis C, Berk C, Honey CR, et al. Reducing hardware-related complications of deep brain stimulation. Can J Neurol Sci 2005;32:194–200

94. Deuschl G, Schade-Brittinger C, Krack P, et al. A randomized trial of deep-brain stimulation for Parkinson's disease. N Engl J Med 2006;355:896–908

95. Schupbach WM, Maltete D, Houeto JL, et al. Neurosurgery at an earlier stage of Parkinson disease: a randomized, controlled trial. Neurology 2007;68:267–271

96. Schupbach WM, Chastan N, Welter ML, et al. Stimulation of the subthalamic nucleus in Parkinson's disease: a 5 year follow-up. J Neurol Neurosurg Psychiatry 2005;76:1640–1644

97. Rodriguez-Oroz OMC, Zamarbide I, Guridi J, et al. Efficacy of deep brain stimulation of the subthalamic nucleus in Parkinson's disease 4 years after surgery: double blind and open label evaluation. J Neurol Neurosurg Psychiatry 2004;75:1382–1385

98. Visser-Vandewalle V, van der Linden C, Temel Y, et al. Long-term effects of bilateral subthalamic nucleus stimulation in advanced Parkinson disease: a four year follow-up study. Parkinsonism Relat Disord 2005;11:157–165

99. Krack P, Batir A, Van Blercom N, et al. Five year follow-up of bilateral stimulation of the subthalamic nucleus in advanced Parkinson's disease. N Engl J Med 2003;349:1925–1934

100. Hilker R, Portman AT, Voges J, et al. DBS does not slow PD progression. J Neurol Neurosurg Psychiatry 2005;76:1217–1221

101. Bakay RA. Metaanalysis, pallidotomy, and microelectrodes. J Neurosurg 2002;97:1253–1256

102. Kleiner-Fisman G, Herzog J, Fisman DN, et al. Subthalamic nucleus deep brain stimulation: summary and meta-analysis of outcomes. Mov Disord 2006;21:S290–S304

103. Weaver F, Follett K, Hur K, Ippolito D, Stern M. Deep brain stimulation in Parkinson disease: a metaanalysis of patient outcomes. J Neurosurg 2005;103:956–967

104. Esselink RA, de Bie RM, de Haan RJ, et al. Unilateral pallidotomy versus bilateral subthalamic nucleus stimulation in PD: a randomized trial. Neurology 2004;62:201–207

105. Bakker M, Esselink RA, Munneke M, Limousin-Dowsey P, Speelman HD, Bloem R. Effects of stereotactic neurosurgery on postural instability and gait in Parkinson's disease. Mov Disord 2004;19:1092–1099

106. Bastian AJ, Kelly VE, Revilla FJ, Perlmutter JS, Min JW. Different effects of unilateral versus bilateral subthalamic nucleus stimulation on walking and reaching in Parkinson's disease. Mov Disord 2003;18:1000–1007

107. Colnat-Coulbois S, Gauchard GC, Maillard L, et al. Bilateral subthalamic nucleus stimulation improves balance control in Parkinson's disease. J Neurol Neurosurg Psychiatry 2005;76:780–787

108. Nilsson MH, Tornqvist AL, Rehncrona S. Deep-brain stimulation in the subthalamic nuclei improves balance performance in patients with Parkinson's disease, when tested without anti-parkinsonian medication. Acta Neurol Scand 2005;111:301–308

109. Germano IM, Gracies JM, Weisz D, et al. Unilateral stimulation of the subthalamic nucleus in Parkinson disease: a double-blind 12-month evaluation study. J Neurosurg 2004;101:36–42

110. Chung SJ, Jeon SR, Kim SR, et al. Bilateral effects of unilateral subthalamic nucleus deep brain stimulation in advanced Parkinson's disease. Eur Neurol 2006;56:127–132

111. Verhagen L, Arzbaecher J, Sierens D, et al. Unilateral deep brain stimulation of the subthalamic nucleus: a valuable alternative? Neurology 2003;160:A119

112. Visser-Vandewalle V, van der Linden C, Temel Y, et al. Long-term motor effect of unilateral pallidal stimulation is 26 patients with advanced Parkinson disease. J Neurosurg 2003;99:701–707

113. Fraix V, Pollak P, Moro E, et al. Subthalamic nucleus stimulation in tremor dominant parkinsonian patients with previous thalamic surgery. J Neurol Neurosurg Psychiatry 2005;76:246–248

114. Ondo WG, Silay Y, Almaguer M, Jankovic J. Subthalamic deep brain stimulation in patients with a previous pallidotomy. Mov Disord 2006;21:1252–1254

115. Su PC, Tseng H. Gait freezing and falling related to subthalamic stimulation in patients with a previous pallidotomy. Letter to the Editor. Mov Disord 2001;16:376–377

116. Vergani F, Landi A, Antonini A, Sganzerla EP. Bilateral subthalamic deep brain stimulation in a patient with Parkinson's disease who had previously undergone thalamotomy and autologous adrenal grafting in the caudate nucleus: case report. Neurosurgery 2006;59:E1140 (discussion E1140)

117. Kaphan E, Règis J, Witjas T, et al. Effects of chronic subthalamic stimulation on nonmotor fluctuations in Parkinson's disease. Mov Disord 2007;22:1194–1200

118. Cicolin A, Lopiano L, Zibetti M, et al. Effects of deep brain stimulation of the subthalamic nucleus on sleep architecture in parkinsonian patients. Sleep Med 2004;5:207–210

119. Lyons KE, Pahwa R. Effects of bilateral subthalamic nucleus stimulation on sleep, daytime sleepiness, and early morning dystonia in patients with Parkinson disease. J Neurosurg 2006;104:502–505

120. Stemper B, Beric A, Welsch G, et al. Deep brain stimulation improves orthostatic regulation of patients with Parkinson disease. Neurology 2006;67:1781–1785

121. Holmberg B, Corneliusson O, Elam M. Bilateral stimulation of nucleus subthalamicus in advanced Parkinson's disease: no effects on, and of, autonomic dysfunction. Mov Disord 2005;20:976–981

122. Herzog J, Weiss PH, Assmus A, et al. Subthalamic stimulation modulates cortical control of urinary bladder in Parkinson's disease. Brain 2006;129:3366–3375

123. Winge K, Nielsen KK, Stimpel H, Lokkegaard A, Jensen SR, Werdelin L. Lower urinary tract symptoms and bladder control in advanced Parkinson's disease: effects of deep brain stimulation in the subthalamic nucleus. Mov Disord 2007;22:220–225

124. Tuite PJ, Maxwell RE, Ikramuddin S, et al. Weight and body mass index in Parkinson's disease patients after deep brain stimulation surgery. Parkinsonism Relat Disord 2005;11:247–252

125. Macia F, Perlemoine C, Coman I, et al. Parkinson's disease patients with bilateral subthalamic deep brain stimulation gain weight. Mov Disord 2004;19:206–212

126. Velasco F, Jimenez F, Perez ML, et al. Electrical stimulation of the prelemniscal radiation in the treatment of Parkinson's disease: an old target revised with new techniques. Neurosurgery 2001;49:293–308

127. Plaha P, Ben-Shlomo Y, Patel NK, et al. Stimulation of the caudal zona incerta is superior to stimulation of the subthalamic nucleus in improving contralateral parkinsonism. Brain 2006;129:1732–1747

128. Jenkinson N, Nandi D, Miall RC, et al. Pedunculopontine nucleus stimulation improves akinesia in a Parkinsonian monkey. Neuroreport 2004;15:2621–2624

129. Mazzone P, Lozano A, Stanzione P, et al. Implantation of human pedunculopontine nucleus: a safe and clinically relevant target in Parkinson's disease. Neuroreport 2005;16:1877–1881

130. Plaha P, Gill SS. Bilateral deep brain stimulation of the pedunculopontine nucleus for Parkinson's disease. Neuroreport 2005;16:1883–1887

131. Peppe A, Gasbarra A, Stefanie A, et al. Deep brain stimulation of the thalamus could be the elective target for tremor in Parkinson's disease?. Parkinsonism Relat Disord 2008;S1353–8020

132. Kupsch A, Benecke R, Muller J. Pallidal deep-brain stimulation in primary generalized or segmental dystonia. N Engl J Med 2006;355:1978–1990

133. Starr PA, Turner RS, Rau G, et al. Microelectrode-guided implantation of deep brain stimulators into the globus pallidus internus for dystonia: techniques, electrode locations, and outcomes. J Neurosurg 2006;104:488–501

134. Zorzi G, Marras C, Nardocci N, et al. Stimulation of the globus pallidus internus for childhood-onset dystonia. Mov Disord 2005;20:1194–1200

135. Vitek JL, Bakay RA. The role of pallidotomy in Parkinson's disease and dystonia. Curr Opin Neurol 1997;10:332–339

136. Wang S, Xugang L, Yianni J, et al. Use of surface electromyography to assess and select patients with idiopathic dystonia for bilateral pallidal stimulation. J Neurosurg 2006;105:21–25

137. Putzke JD, Uitti RJ, Obwegeser AA, et al. Bilateral thalamic deep brain stimulation: midline tremor control. J Neurol Neurosurg Psychiatry 2005;76:684–690

138. Pahwa R, Lyons KE, Wilkinson SB, et al. Long-term evaluation of deep brain stimulation of the thalamus. J Neurosurg 2006;104:506–512

139. Goodman RR, Kim B, McClelland S, et al. Operative techniques and morbidity with subthalamic nucleus deep brain stimulation in 100 consecutive patients with advanced Parkinson's disease. J Neurol Neurosurg Psychiatry 2006;77:12–17

140. Voges J, Waerzeggers Y, Maarouf M, et al. Deep-brain stimulation: long-term analysis of complications caused by hardware and surgery: experiences from a single centre. J Neurol Neurosurg Psychiatry 2006;77:868–872

141. Paluzzi A, Belli A, Bain P, et al. Operative and hardware complications of deep brain stimulation for movement disorders. Br J Neurosurg 2006;20:290–295

142. Blomstedt P, Hairz MI. Hardware-related complications of deep brain stimulation: a ten year experience (In process citation). Acta Neurochir (Wien) 2005;147:1061–1064

143. Hamani C, Lozano AM. Hardware-related complications of deep brain stimulation: a review of the published literature. Stereotact Funct Neurosurg 2006;84:248–251

144. Capelle HH, Simpson RK Jr, Kronenbuerger M, et al. Long-term deep brain stimulation in elderly patients with cardiac pacemakers. J Neurosurg 2005;102:53–59

145. Ozben B, Bilge AK, Yilmaz E, Adalet K. Implantation of a permanent pacemaker in a patient with severe Parkinson's disease and a preexisting bilateral deep brain stimulator. Int Heart J 2006;47:803–810

146. Henderson JM, Tkach J, Phillips M, et al. Permanent neurological deficit related to magnetic resonance imaging in a patient with implanted deep brain stimulation electrodes for Parkinson's disease: case report. Neurosurgery 2005;57:E1063

147. Baker KB, Tkach JA, Phillips MD, Rezai AR. Variability in RF-induced heating of a deep brain stimulation implant across MR systems. J Magn Reson Imaging 2006;24:1236–1242

148. Smeding HM, Speelman JD, Koning-Haanstra M, et al. Neuropsychological effects of bilateral STN stimulation in Parkinson disease: a controlled study. Neurology 2006;66:1830–1836

149. Funkiewiez A, Ardouin C, Caputo E, et al. Long-term effects of bilateral subthalamic nucleus stimulation on cognitive function, mood, and behaviour in Parkinson's disease. J Neurol Neurosurg Psychiatry 2004;75:834–839

150. Drapier S, Raoul S, Drapier D, et al. Only physical aspects of quality of life are significantly improved by bilateral subthalamic stimulation in Parkinson's disease. J Neurol 2005;252:583–588

151. Lyons KE, Pahwa R. Long-term benefits in quality of life provided by bilateral subthalamic stimulation in patients with Parkinson disease. J Neurosurg 2005;103:252–255

152. Ulla M, Thobois S, Lemaire JJ, et al. Manic behaviour induced by deep brain stimulation in Parkinson's disease: evidence of substantia nigra implication? J Neurol Neurosurg Psychiatry 2006;77:1363–1366

153. Deuschl G, Herzog J, Kleiner-Fisman G, et al. Deep brain stimulation: postoperative issues. Mov Disord 2006;21:S219–S237

154. Pillon B, Ardouin C, Dujardin K, et al. French SPIDY Study Group: Preservation of cognitive function in dystonia treated by pallidal stimulation. Neurology 2006;66:1556–1558

155. Anderson VC, Burchiel KJ, Hogarth P, et al. Pallidal vs subthalamic nucleus deep brain stimulation in Parkinson disease. Arch Neurol 2005;62:554–560

156. Rodriguez-Oroz MC, Obeso JA, Lang AE, et al. Bilateral deep brain stimulation in Parkinson's disease: a multicentre study with 4 years follow-up. Brain 2005;128:2240–2249

Gamma Knife

Ronald F. Young

■ Indications and Controversies

A Brief History of Radiosurgery for Movement Disorders

Lars Leksell developed the idea of radiosurgery specifically for the performance of functional neurosurgical procedures. He sought a less-invasive technique to create lesions within the brain to treat a variety of neurological disorders, including chronic pain, Parkinson disease, and trigeminal neuralgia. In his seminal report in 1951, in which he coined the term *radiosurgery*, he specifically referred to the performance of thalamotomy using a radiosurgical technique.[1] His search for the ideal instrument—which was simple, accurate, reliable, and could be used as a neurosurgical tool—led him through a series of prototypical instruments that employed a variety of radiation sources. He eventually settled on the multisource, fixed position, cobalt-60 gamma unit called the Gamma Knife (Elekta, Inc., Norcross, GA). Several early publications documented the experience of Leksell and his colleagues with functional neurosurgical procedures with the Gamma Knife. With the development of Gamma Knife radiosurgery in the United States in the late 1980s, the emphasis was primarily on the treatment of vascular malformations and brain tumors.

Beginning in the early 1990s, there was a resurgence of interest in functional neurosurgery with the Gamma Knife to treat a variety of disorders, including chronic pain, Parkinson disease and other movement disorders, trigeminal neuralgia, epilepsy, and certain psychoneuroses. This author's personal experience includes more than 500 patients who have undergone Gamma Knife lesioning procedures for the treatment of movement disorders in addition to over 500 more who have undergone radio frequency lesioning procedures, deep brain stimulation (DBS), and, for a time, neurotransplantation, in addition to radiosurgical lesioning. The Gamma Knife procedures were performed at two centers, one located at the Northwest Hospital in Seattle, Washington, and the other at Good Samaritan Hospital in Los Angeles, California. At both centers, multidisciplinary interventional techniques are available for the treatment of movement disorders.

Our selection criteria for radiosurgical lesioning are identical to those for open surgical procedures except as outlined subsequently under "Specific Indications." Preoperative mental status examination is performed in all patients, and dementia is considered a contraindication to any form of surgical intervention. The lesions, in our experience, were made initially with the Model U, 201 Source Gamma Unit and more recently with the Model C. The unit consists of a sealed "central body," which contains 201 Co 60 sources in a hemispheric array. A set of primary collimators within the central body forms the gamma rays into beams. To perform radiosurgical lesioning procedures for treatment of movement disorders, the patient's head is fixed in a Leksell stereotactic frame (Model G, Elekta Inc.), which is positioned within a secondary collimator helmet. The secondary collimator helmet forms the 201 gamma rays into beams 4 mm in diameter, such that all beams are focused on the same fixed point. The target for lesioning is placed at the focal point by application of the calculated x, y, and z stereotactic coordinates of the planned lesions. The theory of the Gamma Knife is that the radiation dose along any single gamma ray beam is too low to produce neural injury, but at the focal point the radiosurgical dose represents the summed dosage of all 201 beams. The beam profile of the 4 mm secondary collimator helmet is such that the 10% isodose line (14 Gy for radiosurgical lesioning) encompasses a volume of only ~500 mm³. Thus the radiation exposure of tissue outside the intended lesion is minimal.

Specific Indications

Radiosurgical lesioning has frequently been proposed only for patients who do not meet the criteria for any form of open surgical procedures for the treatment of movement disorders (e.g., lesioning or DBS). Such conditions include chronic anticoagulation, coagulopathies, cerebral atrophy, inability to understand or follow commands that might be given during surgery, and advanced age. Based on our experience, however, we believe that radiosurgical lesioning can be discussed as an alternative for any patient with a movement disorder who is a candidate for a surgical procedure for treatment of movement disorders.

There are two specific indications for radiosurgical lesioning. These are tremor and levodopa-induced dyskinesias. Patients with parkinsonian, essential, or familial tremor or tremor due to conditions such as multiple sclerosis, cerebral infarction, cerebral infections, and cerebral trauma are considered possible candidates for radiosurgical thalamotomy. Parkinsonian patients who exhibit a major difficulty with levodopa-induced dyskinesias, but who do not have significant difficulties with motor fluctuations and gait and balance disturbances, may be considered candidates for radiosurgical pallidotomy. For patients whose primary problems include motor fluctuations, bradykinesia, rigidity, and particularly gait and balance problems, we believe that currently DBS in the subthalamic nucleus is a better form of surgical treatment than is lesioning, regardless of whether one uses the radiofrequency technique or radiosurgery with the Gamma Knife.

As with the radiofrequency thalamotomy, we perform unilateral thalamotomy with the Gamma Knife as an initial procedure. Although bilateral radiofrequency thalamotomy has been associated with a high incidence of complications, including speech and swallowing difficulties, cognitive disorders, and akinesia, we have not seen these complications with bilateral radiosurgical thalamotomy in a series of 22 patients (six with Parkinson disease and 16 with essential tremor). This is conditional on the interval between the two procedures being at least 1 year apart and that no complications or side effects present after the unilateral procedure. In addition, the MRI scan must demonstrate a lesion of the expected size that is properly located anatomically and without significant surrounding perilesional changes. We have performed bilateral pallidotomy in 12 patients with Parkinson disease; in four patients the lesions were performed on the same day, and in the others with intervals of 1 year or more. Currently, we would not recommend that bilateral pallidotomy be performed on the same day and, as with bilateral thalamotomy, we recommend an interval of at least 1 year between bilateral lesions and MRI confirmation that the first lesion is as normally expected before proceeding to a contralateral pallidotomy. Overall, the mean length of follow-up for patients who underwent bilateral lesioning (thalamotomy and pallidotomy) is 45 months from the second procedure.

Controversies

The primary criticism of Gamma Knife lesioning for treatment of movement disorders is the lack of any method to electrophysiologically corroborate the correct targeting. Typically, in open stereotactic procedures for the treatment of movement disorders, a combination of electrophysiological procedures, including microelectrode recording, microstimulation, and/or macrostimulation, have been employed. In addition, with radio frequency lesioning it is possible to gradually enlarge the size of the lesion and examine the patient as the procedure moves forward to ascertain an end point that includes maximum resolution of preoperative symptoms and minimal or no side effects. This type of monitoring is impossible with radiosurgical lesioning in which the procedure is closed and the targeting is based strictly on anatomical localization.

For many years, a controversy has existed regarding whether the target for lesioning for the treatment of movement disorders is an anatomical or physiological target. Even if the target is agreed to be anatomical, there has been additional controversy regarding the ability of MRI stereotactic localization to accurately identify the target. Concerns about MRI distortion have been expressed because it relates to purely anatomical target localization. We have reviewed and discussed this point in previous publications.[2-4] We believe that, with detailed attention to the stereotactic MRI technique, imaging distortion can either be eliminated or corrected for, so that anatomical target localization is sufficient to accurately locate an intended target for radiosurgical lesioning

In addition, Gamma Knife lesioning does not allow for the lesion to be gradually made and the patients' responses, either positive or negative, assessed. Once the radiosurgical dose is delivered and the response set into motion, there are no external means to control the lesion. The primary cause of complications following radiosurgical lesioning for treatment of movement disorders has been due to lesions that develop larger than expected.[5] Complications or side effects due to mistargeting have not been seen in our experience, although when radiosurgical lesioning fails to improve the symptoms it certainly suggests mistargeting. In most situations when symptoms are not improved, however, radiosurgical lesions develop considerably smaller than expected, and this problem seems to account for the majority of instances in which there is a failure to improve symptoms. We usually do not recommend a repeat radiosurgical procedure to enlarge a small lesion, due to the unpredictable consequences in terms of lesion size for superimposed or closely spaced lesions. Instead, for patients who fail a radiosurgical procedure, we recommend either enlarging the lesion by radio frequency methods or employing a DBS procedure instead.

Finally, there has been considerable concern about long-term radiation complications following radiosurgical lesioning. The Gamma Knife dose profile is extremely steep, however, and the dose of radiation delivered to the majority of the brain is extremely small. Generally, any complications of a radiosurgical lesioning procedure for the treatment of movement disorders appear ~6 to 12 months following the procedure. However, occasionally symptoms may develop earlier, or in some cases substantially later, than this interval.

■ Target Selection and Identification

Thalamotomy

We have attempted to place our radiosurgical lesions for the treatment of tremor in the ventral intermediate thalamic nucleus, and we have utilized the Schaltenbrand and Wahren atlas as a guide to target localization.[6] The procedure begins by application of the Leksell model G stereotactic frame (Electa, Inc., Norcross, GA). We apply the frame with the patient in the sitting position. Mild intravenous sedation (midazolam 1 to 2 mg and fentanyl 50 to 100 µg) is usually employed for patient comfort. Five milliliters of 1% Xylocaine solution (AstraZeneca Pharmaceuticals LP, Wilmington, DE) is injected into the scalp at each of the four pin placement sites to provide local anesthesia. We attempt to place the stereotactic frame as accurately as possible, to avoid errors due to pitch, roll, and yaw. We place the base of the frame parallel to the line extending from the external auditory canal to the floor of the orbit. This line generally corresponds to the trajectory of the anterior commissure (AC)–posterior commissure (PC) line.

In our current protocol, we employ a Siemens MAGNETOM Symphony 1.5 tesla magnetic resonance imaging (MRI) scanner (Siemens Medical Solutions USA, Inc., Malvern, PA). A series of axial scans is performed utilizing the protocol, as described in **Table 16.1**. The axial magnetization prepared rapid gradient echo (MPRAGE) scan is used to localize the AC and PC, aided by sagittal reconstruction images. Two series of short tau inversion recovery (STIR) images are obtained through the area of interest only. Slice thickness for these two sequences is 2 mm with a 2 mm gap. The two series of images are then interleaved to give a contiguous set of scans without any interslice gap.

The images are transported via Ethernet to the Leksell Gamma Plan (Elekta Inc., Norcross, GA) UNIX-based computer workstation for Gamma Knife target planning. A mathematical formula is then used to correct the images for pitch, roll, and yaw errors. To develop our computer algorithm to correct for errors in frame placement, we assumed that the correlation between Leksell stereotactic coordinates and the reference system of the AC–PC plane as utilized in the Schaltenbrand and Wahren Stereotactic atlas could be viewed as the relationship between two orthogonal coordinate systems. This relationship is mathematically defined by the distance between the origins in each dimension and the relative rotation about each axis. The origin of the Leksell coordinate system is taken at the intersection of the diagonals of the fiducial markers in the axial, coronal, and sagittal planes. The origin of the AC–PC reference system is the midpoint of the AC–PC line in the midsagittal plane. The rotation of the coordinate systems makes use of the Euler angles used in classical physics for the orientation of a rigid body. We developed an in-house computer program, which calculates the target localization independent of the frame position. From the Leksell Gamma Plan, we input the stereotactic coordinates of AC, PC, the target, and the axial, coronal, and sagittal angles of rotation. The output is the AC–PC line length, the distance of the target lateral to the AC–PC line (x coordinate), posterior to the mid-AC–PC point (y coordinate), and above the AC–PC plane (z coordinate). The calculations are verified by comparing the AC–PC length between the Leksell Gamma Plan and our program. The accuracy of this method has been repeatedly demonstrated by two methods. The first being the clinical outcomes, which, in terms of safety and effectiveness, are comparable to open stereotactic techniques that employ intraoperative electrophysiological target corroboration. The second is repeated comparisons of the target coordinates and locations of actual lesions demonstrated on postoperative MRI scans and the coordinates used in planning the procedures. These comparisons have been made by obtaining the postoperative MRI scans with the patient's head within the Leksell stereotactic frame and the attached fiducial box, but without skeletal fixation. We have also studied the reproducibility of the same observer making repeated calculations of lesion localizations on the same postoperative MRI scan. The difference between pre- and postoperative target coordinates is nearly always within the same range as the interobservation differences on repeated observations of postoperative lesion coordinates (~0.5 to 1.0 mm).

The position of the AC and PC is identified on the axial MPRAGE images. The anteroposterior (or y) coordinate is determined empirically. For an average intercommissural distance of 26 mm, we select a y coordinate ~5 to 6 mm posterior to the intercommissural point. A reconstructed coronal MRI scan image at that point is then observed. Utilizing the Gamma Plan computer functions, we place the simulated target in the inferolateral corner of the thalamic mass. The target is placed such that the 50% isodose line of the simulated lesion, utilizing the 4 mm secondary collimator helmet of the Gamma Knife, is exactly at the inferolateral border of the thalamus (**Fig. 16.1A,B**). The y and z coordinates for the center of the target are then displayed on the Gamma Plan computer.

Pallidotomy

The target for Gamma Knife pallidotomy is the ventral posteromedial (GPi) segment of the globus pallidus. The protocol for stereotactic frame application and MRI scanning

Table 16.1 Magnetic Resonance Imaging Protocol for Gamma Knife Thalamotomy or Pallidotomy

Siemens MAGNETOM Symphony 1.5 Tesla Magnetic Resonance Imaging Scanner		
	MPRAGE Axial	**STIR Axial and Coronal**
No. of slices	48	12
Slice thickness	1 mm	2 mm
Field of view (FOV)	256 × 256	256 × 256
T_1 (inversion time)	1100	140
T_4 (repetition time)	1500	3190
T_E (echo time)	4.1	33
Nex (No. of excitations)	1	2
Resolution	256 × 256	256 × 256
Time for scan	6 minute 26 second	4 minute 0.1 second

Abbreviations: MPRAGE, magnetization prepared rapid gradient echo; STIR, short tau inversion recovery.

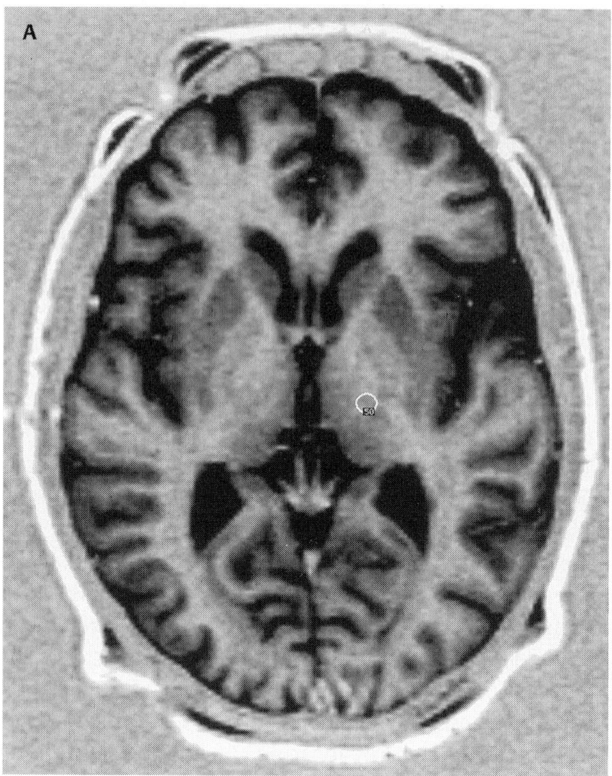

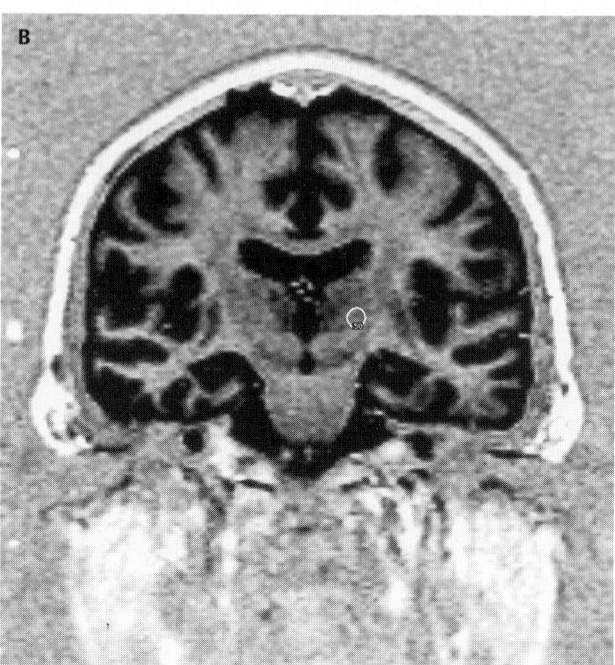

Fig. 16.1 (**A**) Axial and (**B**) coronal magnetic resonance imaging scans obtained from the Gamma Plan computer for preoperative planning for a left ventral intermediate nucleus thalamotomy with the Gamma Knife (Elekta Inc., Norcross, GA).

is identical to that for thalamotomy. The intercommissural distance is determined utilizing the Gamma Plan as for thalamotomy. The anteroposterior coordinate (or y coordinate) for pallidotomy is selected empirically ~3 mm anterior to the intercommissural point. A coronal image is reconstructed at that point utilizing the Gamma Plan computer, and the target is placed in the internal segment of the globus pallidus, such that the 50% isodose line of the simulated lesion, utilizing the 4 mm secondary collimator helmet of the Gamma Knife is immediately superior to the optic tract and immediately inferolateral to the internal capsule (**Fig. 16.2**). The x and z coordinates for the center of the simulated lesion are then displayed by the Gamma Plan computer. The same algorithm previously described for thalamotomy is used to correct for errors of pitch, roll, and yaw in stereotactic frame placement.

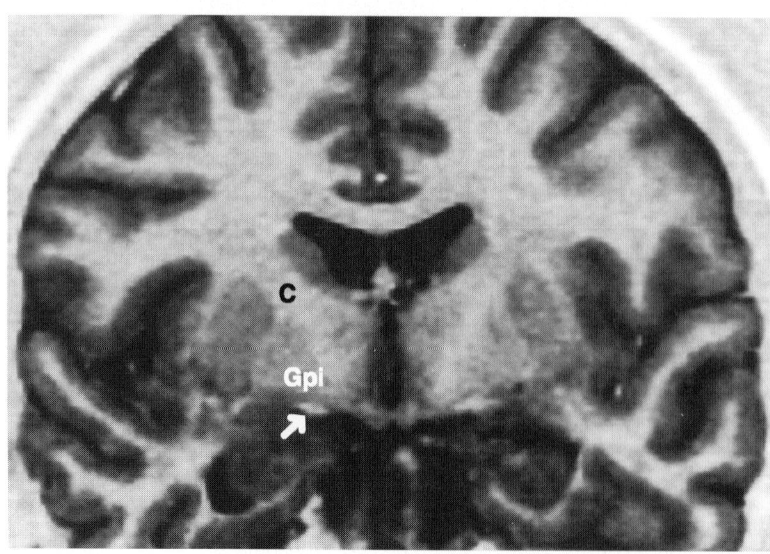

Fig. 16.2 Coronal magnetic resonance imaging scan for planning a pallidotomy. The lesion is centered at the globus pallidus internus (Gpi). The 50% isodose line should be above the optic tract (*arrow*) and tangential to the internal capsule (C).

Editor's Comments

Radiosurgery was invented by Dr. Lars Leksell specifically for the purpose of performing functional neurosurgery. He abandoned that effort early on and began using radiosurgery for other types of disorders for which it is now predominantly known. There are very few functional neurosurgeons who recommend stereotactic radiosurgery for movement disorders. In fact, there are few radiosurgery centers that perform thalamotomy and even fewer that perform pallidotomy. Historically, attempts to use radiosurgery for the treatment of movement disorders has resulted in mixed success. Most believe that the treatment of movement disorders by radiosurgery should be restricted to neurosurgeons familiar with the manifestation of the different movement disorders and their treatment.

Dr. Young is an exception being both an accomplished stereotactic and functional neurosurgeon as well a practicing radiosurgical expert. He has far greater enthusiasm than most anyone else for the use of radiosurgery in the treatment of movement disorders, primarily because of his low complication rate. I believe that his low complication rate is a result of his experience as an accomplished functional neurosurgeon, and he is therefore far more familiar with the target than most neurosurgeons who simply use radiosurgery for functional stereotactic radiosurgery on an occasional basis. He also has extensive experience with radiosurgery thalamotomy for pain.[7] This has not always been the case in other radiosurgery centers.[8–20] There have been deaths, dementias, psychosis, paresthesias, visual field losses, dysarthrias, hypophonias, aphasias, and bizarre movements. With the exception of Dr. Young's series (2 to 3%) these complications were reported to range from 9 to 50% of cases. Complications should include the failure to adequately treat the disorder, which then frequently requires further surgery. The use of steroids to control edema is not uncommon and carries additional risks. For some, the wait until the effects occur months later may have adverse consequences. Complications from functional radiosurgery are not rare but they are not commonly reported by radiosurgeons. Too frequently they are reported by those who have to deal with the problem after the fact.[15]

It is most interesting that functional neurosurgeons will vigorously argue as to whether microelectrode recordings are necessary (see Chapters 7 and 8), but both camps will agree that electrophysiological confirmation of the target is necessary. It is the rare neurosurgeon who would argue that anatomy alone without electrophysiological confirmation is sufficient to demarcate the appropriate functional targets. MRI distortion is a problem[21,22] that image fusion may not solve because it involves a linear correction for a nonlinear problem. This suggests that anatomical registration alone is insufficient. The commonly used target in radiosurgery is the thalamus, which is not a target that can be directly viewed but rather is calculated. Experience undoubtedly helps in accurate targeting. Most functional neurosurgeons believe the target is electrophysiological and not strictly anatomical. When simultaneously performing multiple penetrations, Benabid et al[23] find that, when the target is chosen based on extensive direct anatomical studies using both MRI and intraoperative ventriculography, the ultimate best target for symptomatic benefit is in a different location in over 60% of the cases. Acceptable targets (± 2 mm) result in 70% of cases, but for 30% of cases an unsatisfactory result occurs. Also, Ohye et al[12] found that in failed radiosurgery cases, a clear electrophysiological target could be found. Of equal concern is the reliability of the size of the lesion regardless of where it is placed. The results are not very impressive as reported by most centers.[8–20]

Despite these cautionary remarks, I am enthusiastic about the use of stereotactic radiosurgery in a very limited number of cases. The patient population for which radiosurgery is most useful includes those that are medically debilitated but still require interventional treatment for disabling tremor and are not appropriate candidates for DBS. These should be primarily patients with essential tremor because thalamic lesioning does very little for other symptoms of Parkinson disease. There is, in general, no objection to use stereotactic radiosurgery in patients who are of advanced age, are unable to be taken off anticoagulants, have advanced malignancy, or have severe disabilities caused by cardiac or pulmonary disease such that they are unable to undergo the rigors of surgery. It is a very rare patient who refuses surgery but will accept radiosurgery when the risks and the procedure are carefully discussed. In some cases, patients on anticoagulants can have these stopped for short periods of time. The most stressful part of the procedure is putting on the frame, which is the same for a radiofrequency lesion as a radiosurgical lesion. Unilateral radiosurgery thalamotomy is a reasonably safe and effective means of treating tremor. Bilateral lesioning, even when performed years apart, carries increased risks. The clear preference by both patients and the neurology community is to get away from lesioning all together. DBS is the overwhelming procedure of choice by both neurologist and neurosurgeons. The DBS procedure of course is not without its problems as is evident in Chapter 15.

The key to successful radiosurgery is using a 4 mm collimator with a single isocenter and a dose of 120 to 140 Gy. Ideally, a 5 to 6 mm lesion (40 to 50% isodose line) placed in the appropriate target will result. The investigative work with monkeys suggests that this will produce radiation necrosis at the target.[24] Complications are significantly increased with higher doses (180 to 200 Gy), bigger collimators (8 mm), and multiple isocenters. Missing the target is of concern even if the appropriate dose is prescribed.

Radiosurgery has been used to lesion the globus pallidus, subthalamic nucleus, and striatum. Lesioning of the globus pallidus or subthalamic nucleus is hazardous and is avoided by most stereotactic radiosurgery experts. The pallidal lesions from radiosurgery have a much higher complication rate than those of the thalamus. Strokes have been reported.[11,15,18] Whether this relates to the fact that the blood supply is through end arteries or whether it is due to differences in sensitivity to radiation necrosis, pallidal lesions with radiosurgery have unpredictable final volumes. Several centers that previously performed Gamma Knife pallidotomies have stopped.[9,16] There is even less enthusiasm for lesioning the subthalamic nucleus. A study reported accurately lesioning the subthalamic nucleus with a linear accelerator in the vervet monkey,[25] but careful review suggests this monkey's lesion extended into the substantia nigra. There is little rationale for lesioning the basal ganglia, and there is the potential for creating serious and potentially life-threatening problems.[11,15,26]

■ Dose and Distribution

All radiosurgical lesions for the treatment of movement disorders are made using a single exposure with the 4 mm secondary collimator helmet. Earlier attempts by others to use the 8 mm collimator helmet resulted in lesions, which were too large, resulting in complications. Early attempts to use two closely spaced lesions made with the 4 mm collimator helmet also led to an unacceptably high complication rate. The 4 mm secondary collimator helmet is the smallest available with the Gamma Knife, and utilizing our standard treatment dose of 140 Gy, this combination produces a lesion ~6 mm in diameter or 110 mm³ in volume. It is important to note that 140 Gy represents the maximum—or 100%—radiosurgical dose recommendation and is calculated using the 0.87 output factor for the Gamma Knife. Because of the difficulty in measuring the radiosurgical dose of a collimator as small as 4 mm, the dose is estimated. Therefore, the dose for the 4 mm collimator is determined utilizing an output factor in reference to the 18 mm collimator helmet. In past years, an output factor of 0.8 had been recommended by the Gamma Knife manufacturer. However, in recent years this output factor has been increased to 0.87. In comparing previously published reports on Gamma Knife radiosurgery with the 4 mm collimator, it is important to know whether the radiosurgical doses have been calculated using the 0.8 or 0.87 output factors because this represents a difference of ~9% in the total calculated dose. We have utilized doses as high as 196 Gy and as low as 120 Gy. Based on experience, we do not recommend doses above 140 Gy. Higher doses result in lesions that develop more quickly but are considerably more variable in size and result in a significantly higher number of excessively large lesions associated with complications. Doses below 120 Gy do not reliably produce lesions. At these lower doses, lesions are often too small to produce the desired radiosurgical effect, and at times no anatomically identifiable lesion is produced at all. We have never seen improvements in movement disorders after radiosurgical lesioning unless an identifiable lesion is seen on postoperative MRI scans. Based on our experience in utilizing a variety of doses, we believe that a 140 Gy maximum radiosurgical dose represents the best combination of safety and effectiveness.

■ Results and Complications

Latency of Lesion Development

The reader is referred to several publications that document our experience with Gamma Knife lesioning for movement disorders.[27–32] Unlike the situation with radio frequency lesioning, when lesions are made with the Gamma Knife, the lesions develop gradually. Typically, a low-density lesion can be identified on an unenhanced MRI scan performed about 2 months after the procedure. At this time interval, the lesion usually does not enhance with intravenous gadolinium. By 3 to 6 months, the lesion is identifiable as a clear-cut low-density area on unenhanced T1-weighted images and demonstrates a donut or ringlike appearance with the administration of intravenous gadolinium contrast (**Fig. 16.3**). Lesions typically reach maximum size

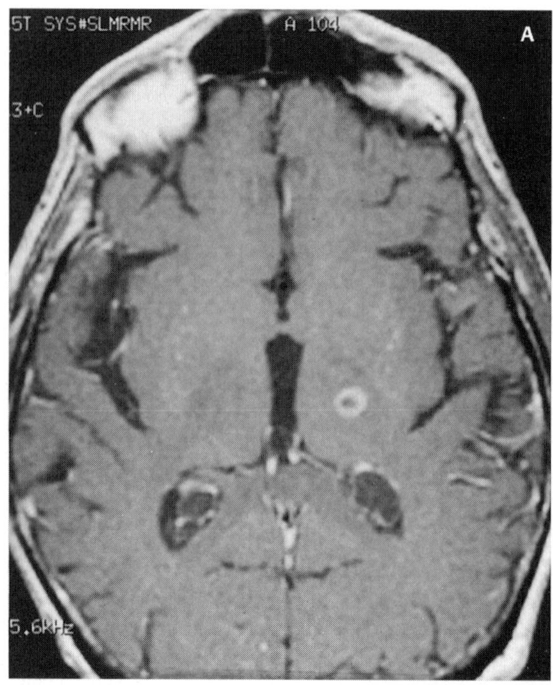
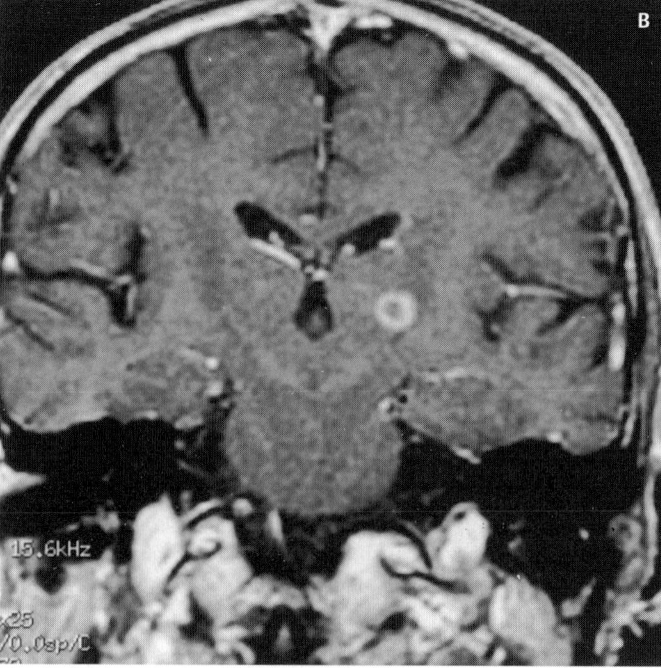

Fig. 16.3 **(A)** Axial and **(B)** coronal gadolinium-enhanced magnetic resonance imaging scans obtained 6 months after left ventral intermediate thalamotomy with the Gamma Knife (Elekta Inc., Norcross, GA).

between ~6 and 9 months after the procedure. It is not uncommon to see an area of perilesional abnormality on T2-weighted postoperative images (**Fig. 16.4**); however, this imaging abnormality is usually not associated with any clinical symptoms and gradually disappears on subsequent follow-up images. Lesions typically remain relatively stable over a period of 1 to 3 years following the procedure and then may gradually decrease in their uptake of intravenous contrast material, so that by 3 to 5 years after the procedure the lesions tend to demonstrate a sharply demarcated low-density border, which enhances minimally or not at all with gadolinium contrast (**Fig. 16.5**).

Onset of Clinical Benefit

Improvement in symptoms generally has its onset ~2 to 4 months after the procedure; coincident with the early development of the lesion on postoperative MRI scans. Clinical benefit typically increases slowly and gradually until ~6 to 9 months after the procedure, when the clinical benefit tends to stabilize. Uncharacteristically, but occasionally, benefits may be delayed as long as 12 to 18 months after the procedure, but this is unusual. For patients with either essential tremor or parkinsonian tremor, between 80 and 85% of patients will become tremor free or nearly tremor free within 1 year of a radiosurgical thalamotomy. Long-

term follow-up (median 48 months) indicates that parkinsonian tremor control remains constant, whereas for essential tremor, delayed recurrences reduce the long-term tremor control to ~80% (**Table 16.2**). Parkinsonian tremor patients showed a decrease in Unified Parkinson's Disease Rating Scale (UPDRS) resting tremor scores from 3.4 ± 0.6 preoperatively to 0.4 ± 0.3 ($p < .0001$) postoperatively. Essential tremor patients also showed marked improvement in tremors, motor performance, and functional disability (**Table 16.3**). For patients who undergo staged bilateral thalamotomy procedures, complete or nearly complete bilateral control of tremor will be realized in between 80 and 85% of patients (**Fig. 16.6** and **Table 16.4**). For levodopa-induced dyskinesias, between 85 and 90% of patients will become either totally or nearly totally free of contralateral dyskinesias within 1 year of radiosurgical pallidotomy (**Table 16.5**). Improvements in UPDRS dyskinesias scores are comparable to those reported by Fine et al[33] in a long-term follow-up study of radiofrequency pallidotomy (**Table 16.5**). In addition, patients who undergo radiosurgical pallidotomy experience an average improvement in off-medication UPDRS scores of ~35 to 40% for bradykinesia, rigidity, activities of daily living, and total UPDRS score. Similar benefits are seen in the early follow-up period for on-medication UPDRS scores; however, these benefits tend to decrease over follow-up periods of 5 to 10 years. For patients who

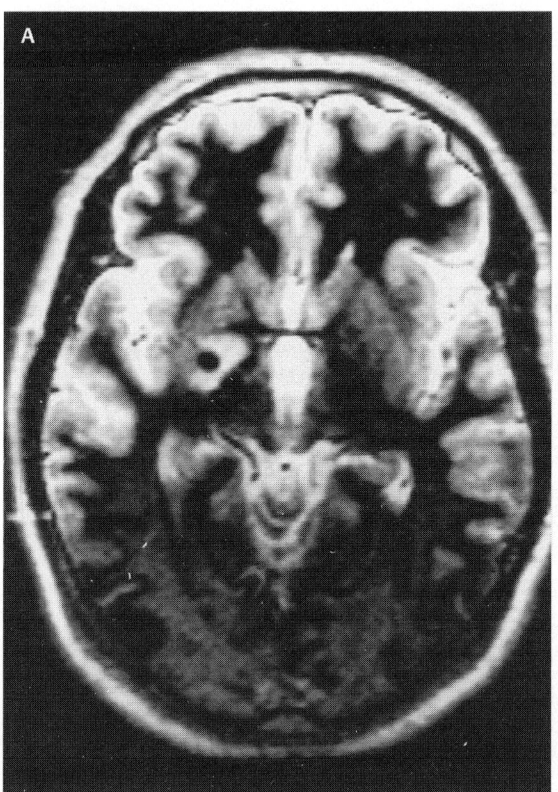
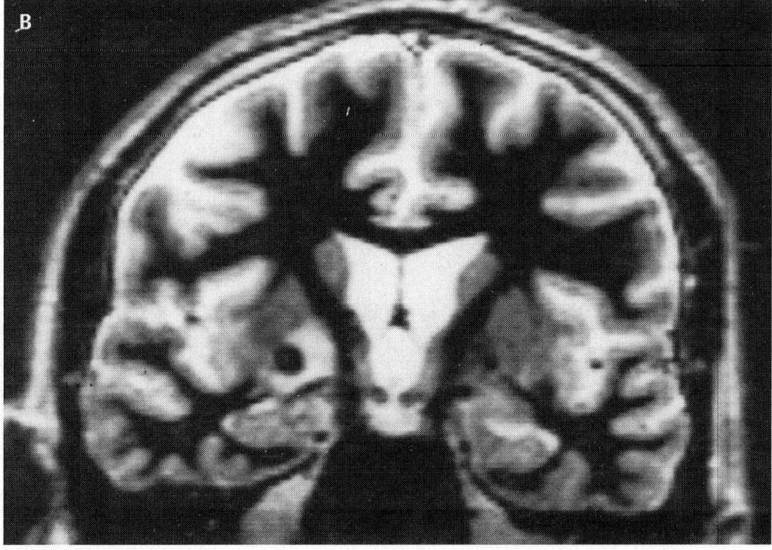

Fig. 16.4 (A) Axial and **(B)** coronal magnetic resonance imaging scan obtained 9 months after right pallidotomy with the Gamma Knife (Elekta Inc., Norcross, GA). The abnormal perilesional signal was not associated with any side effects and resolved by 18 months. (From Young RF. J Neurosurg 1998;89:183–193. Reprinted with permission.)

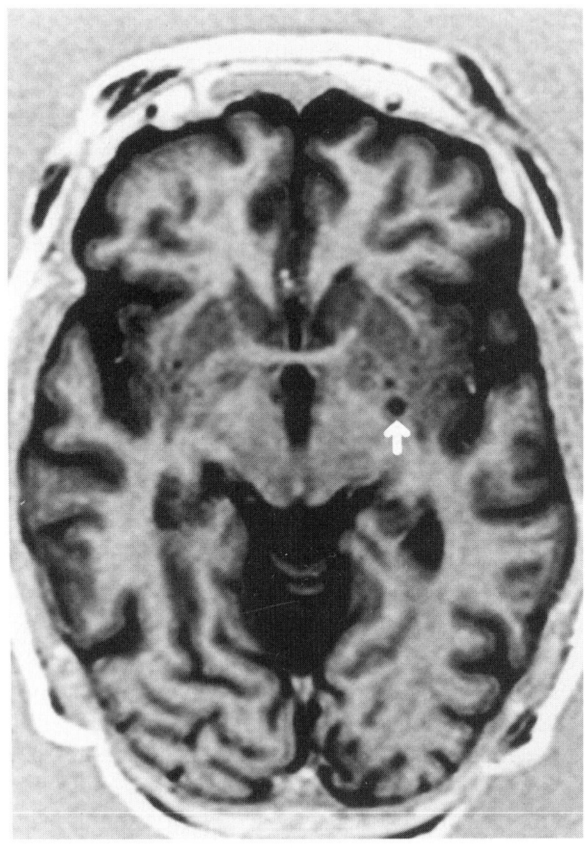

Fig. 16.5 Axial magnetic resonance imaging scan that demonstrates the sharp demarcation between the left pallidotomy lesion made with the Gamma Knife (Elekta Inc., Norcross, GA) 2 years previously and the normal surrounding brain tissue.

Table 16.2 Results: Thalamotomy for Tremor

Etiology	No. of Patients	Tremor Free after Gamma Knife
Parkinson	61	54 (88.5%)
Essential tremor	102	82 (80.4%)
Other	6	4 (67%)
Total	169	140 (82.8%)

Table 16.3 Essential Tremor: Clinical Tremor Rating Scale

	Preop	6 Months	Last Follow-Up
Part A Tremor Location/severity Max 88	64 (72%)	28 (28%)	13 (15%)
Part B Specific motor tasks Max 36	27 (75%)	11 (30%)	7 (19%)
Part C Functional disability	17 (53%)	9 (28%)	6 (18%)

undergo bilateral pallidotomy, levodopa-induced dyskinesias will be abolished bilaterally for nearly 75% of patients, with an average improvement of 38% in UPDRS scores for bradykinesia, rigidity, and activities of daily living.

Delayed Onset of Complications and Time Course

As mentioned earlier, complications of radiosurgical lesioning procedures for the treatment of movement disorders

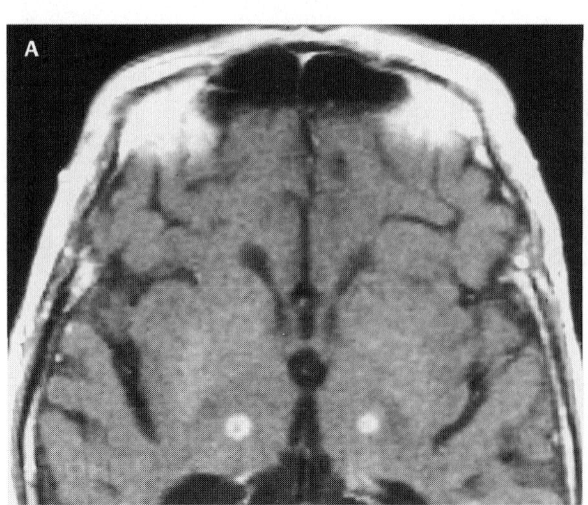

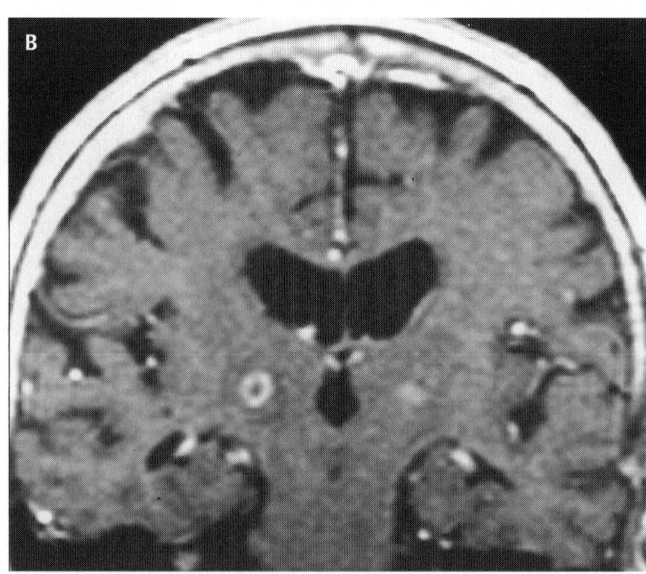

Fig. 16.6 (A) Axial and **(B)** coronal gadolinium-enhanced magnetic resonance imaging scans that demonstrate bilateral ventral intermediate thalamotomy lesions made with the Gamma Knife (Elekta Inc., Norcross, GA). The lesion on the right is 1 year old, and the one of the left is 4 years old.

Table 16.4 Bilateral Gamma Knife Lesioning. Total N = 34

Procedure	N	Tremor Bilateral	Tremor Free Unilateral	Dyskinesia Bilateral
Thalamotomy for P.D. Tremor	6	*5 (83.3%)	1 (16.6%)	N/A
Thalamotomy for Essential Tremor	16	*12 (75%)	2 (12.5%)	N/A
Pallidotomy	12	N/A	N/A	9 (75%)

*17/22 = 77.3% Tremor free bilateral.
N/A = Not applicable.

Table 16.5 UPDRS Dyskinesia Score After Gamma Knife Pallidotomy Unilateral

	Our Experience	Fine et al[33]
Pre-op	2.5 ± 1.0	2.2
6 Months	0.6 ± 0.5 (76%)*	0.4 (82%)*
Last evaluation	0.8 ± 0.8 (68%)*	0.7 (68%)*

*$P < 0.05$

are virtually always due to lesions that become larger than expected. Typically, side effects or complications of such procedures occur ~9 to 15 months after the procedure; however, they may occur earlier than 6 months and longer than 18 months after such procedures. Complications following Gamma Knife thalamotomy for treatment of tremor include contralateral sensory loss, dyscoordination, weakness, and dysphasia. In our experience, such symptoms are seen on a transient basis in 6% of patients and on a permanent basis in 3% of patients. Complications following pallidotomy include contralateral homonymous hemianopsia, which we have seen in two patients out of a total of more than 68 pallidotomy procedures performed, resulting in a risk of ~3%. In both cases, the visual field defect appeared to be permanent. Contralateral weakness and dyscoordination have been seen in only a single patient following

a radiosurgical pallidotomy, resulting in a risk of slightly greater than 1%. In 2001, Okun et al described complications of lesioning for treatment of movement disorders in eight patients who had undergone Gamma Knife radiosurgical procedures at a different center.[15] In an editorial that accompanied the Okun report, Jankovic,[34] the editor, referred to an unacceptably high "rate" of complications after Gamma Knife lesioning, even though the Okun report gave no indication of the total number of patients or lesions from which the eight complications were derived. Even though the Okun report provides limited information about each reported complication, a review of that publication suggests a variety of errors in technique, including excessively large radiation doses, mistargeting, and performance of bilateral lesions with a short interval between lesions and without determining that the first lesion was as expected before proceeding with the second (contralateral) lesion. We believe that our experience over more than 13 years with large numbers of carefully followed patients documents the safety and effectiveness of radiosurgical lesions made with the Gamma Knife for treatment of movement disorders. In fact, our rate of postoperative complications is considerably lower overall than the vast majority of reports of complications following radio frequency lesioning or DBS. We believe that radiosurgical lesioning with the Gamma Knife could be offered as an alternative option to all patients who are candidates for lesioning procedures for the treatment of movement disorders.

References

1. Leksell L. The stereotaxic method and radiosurgery of the brain. Acta Chir Scand 1951;102:316–319
2. Young RF, Vermeulen S, Grimm P, Posewitz A. Electrophysiological target localization is not required for the treatment of functional disorders. Stereotact Funct Neurosurg 1996;66(Suppl 1):309–319
3. Young RF, Vermeulen S, Posewitz A. Functional neurosurgery with the Leksell Gamma Knife. Radiosurgery 1996;1:218–228.
4. Young RF. Functional neurosurgery with the Leksell Gamma knife. Stereotact Funct Neurosurg 1996;66:19–23
5. Friehs GM, Noren G, Ohye C, et al. Lesion size following Gamma Knife treatment for functional disorders. Stereotact Funct Neurosurg 1996;66(Suppl 1):320–328
6. Schaltenbrand G, Wahren W. Atlas for Stereotaxy of the Human Brain. Stuttgart: Thieme; 1977
7. Young RF, Vermeulen S, Grimm P, et al. Gamma Knife thalamotomy for the treatment of persistent pain. Stereotact Funct Neurosurg 1995;64(Suppl 1):172–181
8. Bonnen JG, Iacono RP, Lulu B, Mohamed AS, Gonzalez A, Schoonenberg T. Gamma Knife pallidotomy: case report. Acta Neurochir (Wien) 1997;139:442–445
9. Friedman JH, Epstein M, Sanes JN, et al. Gamma Knife pallidotomy in advanced Parkinson's disease. Ann Neurol 1996;39:535–538
10. Pan L, Dai JZ, Wang BJ, Xu WM, Zhou LF, Chen XR. Stereotactic gamma thalamotomy for the treatment of Parkinsonism. Stereotact Funct Neurosurg 1996;66(Suppl 1):329–332

11. Friedman DP, Goldman HW, Flanders AE, Gollomp SM, Curran WJ. Stereotactic radiosurgical pallidotomy and thalamotomy with the Gamma Knife: MR imaging findings with clinical correlation—preliminary experience. Radiology 1999;212:143–150

12. Ohye C, Shibazaki J, Ishihara J, Zhang J. Evaluation of gamma thalamotomy for parkinsonian and other tremors: survival of neurons adjacent to the thalamic lesion after gamma thalamotomy. J Neurosurg 2000;93(Suppl 3):120–127

13. Niranjan A, Kondziolka D, Baser S, Heyman R, Lunsford LD. Functional outcomes after Gamma Knife thalamotomy for essential tremor and MS-related tremor. Neurology 2000;55:443–446

14. Siderowf A, Gollump SM, Stern MB, Baltuch GH, Riina HA. Emergence of complex, involuntary movements after Gamma Knife radiosurgery for essential tremor. Mov Disord 2001;16:965–967

15. Okun MS, Stover NP, Subramanian T, et al. Complications of Gamma Knife surgery for Parkinson disease. Arch Neurol 2001;58:1995–2002

16. Duma CM, Jacques D, Kopyov OV. The treatment of movement disorders using Gamma Knife stereotactic radiosurgery. Neurosurg Clin N Am 1999;10:379–389

17. Ohye C, Shibazaki T, Zhang J, Andou Y. Thalamic lesions produced by gamma thalamotomy for movement disorders. J Neurosurg 2002;97(5, Suppl)600–606

18. Friedman JH, Fernandez HH, Sikirica M, Stopa E, Friehs G. Stroke induced by Gamma Knife pallidotomy: autopsy result. Neurology 2002;58:1695–1697

19. Duma CM, Jacques DB, Kopyov OV, Mark RJ, Copcutt B, Farokhi HK. Gamma Knife radiosurgery for thalamotomy in parkinsonian tremor: a five-year experience. J Neurosurg 1998;88:1044–1049

20. Niranjan A, Jawahar A, Kondziolka D, Lundsford LD. A comparison of surgical approaches for the management of tremor: radiofrequency thalamotomy, Gamma Knife thalamotomy and thalamic stimulation. Stereotact Funct Neurosurg 1999;72:178–184

21. Schad L, Lott S, Schmitt F, Sturm V, Lorenz WJ. Correction of spatial distortion in MRI. J Comput Assist Tomogr 1987;11:499–505

22. Sumanaweera TS, Adler JR Jr, Napel S, Glover GH. Characterization of spatial distortion in magnetic resonance imaging and its implications for stereotactic surgery. Neurosurgery 1994;35:696–703 (discussion 703–704)

23. Benabid AL, Lebas JF, Grand S, et al. Deep Brain Stimulation for Movement Disorders. In: Winn HR (ed). Youman's Neurological Surgery. 5th ed. 2004 Vol.3:2803–2827

24. Kondziolka D, Conce M, Niranjan A, Maesawa S, Fellows W. Histology of the 100 Gy-Thalomotomy in the baboon. Radiosurgery 2002;4:279–284

25. De Salles AA, Melega WP, Lacan G, Steele LJ, Solberg TD. Radiosurgery performed with the aid of a 3-mm collimator in the subthalamic nucleus and substantia nigra of the vervet monkey. J Neurosurg 2001;95:990–997

26. Bhatia KP, Marsden CD. The behavioural and motor consequences of focal lesions of the basal ganglia in man. Brain 1994;117(Part 4):859–876

27. Young RF, Shumway-Cook A, Vermeulen S, Grimm P, Blasko J, Posewitz A. Gamma Knife radiosurgery as a lesioning technique in movement disorder surgery. Neurosurg Focus 1997;2:e11

28. Young RF, Vermeulen S, Posewitz A, Shumway-Cook A. Pallidotomy with the Gamma Knife: a positive experience. Stereotact Funct Neurosurg 1998;70(Suppl 1):218–228

29. Young RF, Posewitz A. Noninvasive lesioning: functional neurosurgery. In: Alexander E III and Maciunas RJ, ed. Advanced Neurosurgical Navigation. New York: Thieme 1999:507–517

30. Young RF. The Gamma Knife in movement disorder surgery. In: Lazano, AM, ed. Movement Disorder Surgery. Basal: Karger 2000;15:272–278

31. Young RF, Jacques S, Mark R, et al. Gamma Knife thalamotomy for treatment of tremor: long-term results. J Neurosurg 2000;93(Suppl 3):128–135

32. Young RF. Gamma Knife treatment for movement disorders. Semin Neurosurg 2001;12:128–135

33. Fine J, Duff R, Chen R, et al. Long-term follow-up of unilateral pallidotomy in advanced Parkinson's disease. N Engl J Med 2000;342:1708–1714

34. Jankovic J. Surgery for Parkinson disease and other movement disorders: benefits and limitations of ablation, stimulation, restoration, and radiation. Arch Neurol 2001;58:1970–1972

17 The Future of Treatment for Advanced Parkinson Disease

Shivanand P. Lad, Eleonora M. Lad, Roy A. E. Bakay, and Jeffrey H. Kordower

This chapter provides an overview of our present understanding and some of the future potential for various surgical and/or restorative treatments for advanced Parkinson disease (PD) that have been performed to date and are currently being investigated.

Advances in Deep Brain Stimulation

The continued success of deep brain stimulation (DBS) requires device optimization, advances in lead/stimulation technology, and effective combination of DBS with adjunct techniques.

First, leads must be more durable and less inflammatory and must easily provide stimulation while resisting electromagnetic interference. Further understanding of electrode properties on brain parenchyma, through clinicopathological studies and the Medtronic-sponsored market surveillance "Brain Autopsy Research Program" (www.medtronic.com), will aid in these adaptations.

Next there must be customized lead technology to more precisely deliver targeted stimulation, potentially through alteration of electrode geometries. To date, the use of neural engineering design tools and finite element models have led to a better understanding of how varying the dimensions of electrode contacts affects the volume of tissue activated at stimulation parameters used in clinical settings. One study demonstrated that when the heights and radii of contacts were increased, as compared with standard 3387/3389 electrodes, the volume of tissue activated increased and decreased, respectively.[1] In addition to altering contact dimensions, varying spacing and number of contacts can offer additional customization of stimulation. Another potential modification involves altering the current direction. Potentially, by bisecting or quartering the lead, current could be focally spread toward areas for optimal effect and away from areas that induce side effects.

Development of more sophisticated stimulation technologies, such as closed-loop systems, is also a potential area of growth. Currently, DBS is an open-loop system (i.e., no feedback is present to alter stimulation parameters as needed). The development of sensor technology for the DBS system could improve the efficacy of DBS in the treatment of diseases, such as epilepsy, where seizures occur intermittently and electroencephalographic changes precede ictal events. On-demand use of DBS for essential tremor has been tried with patients performing their own turning on and off of stimulation so that the unit was on only 22% of the time, thus improving battery life.[2] The first true attempt at using DBS in a closed-loop system for the treatment of epilepsy through stimulation of the anterior nucleus of the thalamus resulted in a 40% seizure reduction in a small number of treated patients.[3] Thus the technology is available, though the details and practical aspects will need to be refined. Further in the future, DBS technology may augment brain–computer interface systems (BCIs), which use invasive electrode techniques to obtain recordings from populations of individual neurons.[4-10] Electrodes that simultaneously stimulate and record may facilitate learning and rehabilitation because preliminary studies have shown that electrical stimulation leads to improved motor outcome in impaired individuals.[11-13] Though much work is needed to optimize microelectrodes and three-dimensional control for effective BCI, combining BCI technology with high-frequency stimulation may lead to further neurorehabilitation advances.[14] Competing with the mechanical devices will be the biological therapies.

Biological Therapies for Parkinson Disease

Since its discovery in the 1960s, treatment of Parkinson disease (PD) has focused on dopamine (DA) replacement via the prodrug levodopa (L-dopa), which is converted to dopamine centrally by aromatic amino acid decarboxylase (AADC). To reduce the peripheral metabolism of L-dopa, and side effects such as nausea and vomiting, L-dopa is administered in combination with a peripheral AADC inhibitor such as carbidopa (Sinemet, Merck & Co., Inc., Whitehouse Station, NJ) or benserazide (Madopar, Roche, Switzerland). This is true even though it is now becoming widely appreciated that the nigrostriatal degeneration seen in PD may occur relatively late in the disease process[15] and that PD is a disease of both the central and peripheral nervous system.[16] Still most of the therapeutic interventions for PD focus on modifying cardinal symptoms that are mediated by nigrostriatal degeneration. In this regard L-dopa remains the most widely used and most effective antiparkinsonian agent to date, providing substantial clinical benefit initially for almost all PD patients. However, several limitations prevent its long-term clinical effectiveness.[17] First, motor complications such as dyskinesias and motor fluctuations are common, developing in up to 80% of PD patients treated with L-dopa for > 5 years. Second, PD patients develop symptoms unresponsive to L-dopa therapy, including freezing episodes, postural instability, falls, autonomic dysfunction, constipation, depression, and dementia. Third, despite the early symptomatic value of L-dopa, the underlying neurodegenerative process in PD continues unabated, with most patients experiencing permanent disability. Altogether, chronic treatment with L-dopa coupled with advancing disease eventually results in severe disability for patients. Over time, it becomes increasingly difficult to deliver a dose of L-dopa that both controls parkinsonian motor features and avoids dyskinesias. Patients with advanced PD may cycle between disabling "on" and "off" states for the majority of each day. These problems limit the long-term utility of L-dopa and have resulted in a search for more effective treatment strategies.

Current medical approaches to the treatment of L-dopa–induced motor complications include manipulation of the dose and frequency, addition of dopamine agonists, long-acting formulations of levodopa, catechol-O-methyl transferase (COMT) inhibitors, monoamine oxidase-B (MAO-B) inhibitors, and N-methyl-D-aspartic acid (NMDA) receptor antagonists.[18] These adjuvant treatments can provide benefit to individual patients, particularly when motor complications are mild, but are ineffective for patients with established motor fluctuations and dyskinesias. Over the past decade, insight into basal ganglia circuitry in the normal and disease states has allowed for the development of novel neuroprotective and restorative treatment approaches that have the potential to greatly improve the quality of life for PD patients.

■ Cellular Therapies for Parkinson Disease

One of the many surgical approaches being investigated for the treatment of PD is neurotransplantation, a therapeutic approach with the aim of replacing the neurons that are lost in PD. The advantages of this method are targeted delivery of neurons, which attempts replacement of neurotransmitters and neurotrophic factors at the desired site, regulation of implanted cells by the surrounding brain cells, and long-term function due to incorporation of the implanted cells in the brain.[19]

Neural transplantation was first tested in animal models. As early as 1890, neural grafting started to be performed. These early experiments characterized the embryonic neurons in terms of phenotype and ability to create normal connections within the adult host brain. In the host studies employing transplantation as a treatment for neurological disorders, the types of cells transplanted were either fetal neural tissue or chromaffin cells of the adrenal gland. Optimal neural cells useful for transplantation are cells that have finished their migration in the developing brain, no longer divide, and are at a level of maturity at which they express the neuronal phenotype desired, but have not yet extended neurites that would be damaged during tissue collection and transplantation.[20] Neural tissue collected for grafting by microdissection is transplanted either as a cell suspension or as solid grafts of small pieces of tissue via stereotactic methods. During tissue processing and transplantation within the host brain, fetal neurons are faced with numerous challenges that negatively impact their survival, such as oxidative stress, ischemia, lack of trophic factors, and host immune reaction against the transplanted cells. As a result, only 5 to 20% of transplanted cells survive the grafting procedure, with most of the cell death occurring in the first 4 days after transplantation.[21]

Grafts of neural origin can be (1) autografts, in which tissue is harvested from the host; (2) allografts in which cells are taken from an individual of the same species; or (3) xenografts in which tissue is obtained from a different species. During transplantation, the blood–brain barrier is temporarily opened by the surgical procedure, allowing the immune cells to have access to the brain. Allografts and xenografts present molecules on the cell surface that may be recognized by the immune system as foreign during this time period, causing the rejection of the grafts. Graft rejection can be prevented by the use of immunosuppressive therapy during the few days in which the blood–brain barrier is open. However, in clinical trials employing allogeneic fetal neural tissue, the duration of immunosuppression has varied extensively, from no immunosuppression use[22] to up to 6 months.[23] Transplantation immunology in the central nervous system (CNS) is complicated and rarely studied in primates. The published work suggests that allografts in primates and humans are unlikely to reject.[24]

PD is one of the CNS disorders most amenable to transplantation due to the strong relationship between cardinal symptoms and striatal dopamine insufficiency. Thus the hope is that transplantation of dopamine-secreting cells into the striatum may help reestablish striatal function and restore movement in PD patients. Neural transplantation as a clinical therapy for PD started in 1985 with autologous transplants of chromaffin cells of the adrenal gland.[25] Transplanted chromaffin cells produce dopamine, norepinephrine, and epinephrine. The first clinical trials of chromaffin cell transplants were performed in Sweden and Mexico and were soon followed by trials by U.S. investigators. The results of the surgery were disappointing. The patients experienced a very modest and short-lived (1 to 2 years) improvement in symptoms, and 40% of the 126 patients that underwent surgery in the United States suffered from complications of the procedure.[20] Data from patients that came to autopsy revealed that no DA-producing chromaffin cells had survived. Thus the improvement in symptoms in some patients was likely due to a neurotrophic effect on the host DA neurons.[26,27] Due to the poor success of this surgical approach, chromaffin cell transplantation was halted in the United States in 1991.

In 1988, human fetal ventral mesencephalon (VM) transplants replaced chromaffin cell transplants. During the following decade, more than 200 patients received fetal DA neuron grafts worldwide.[19] The results of these transplantation trials were highly variable in terms of transplantation method, improvement in symptoms, and development of side effects. Although many grafted patients have shown motor improvement, others have experienced significant worsening of levodopa-induced dyskinesias (LIDs). LIDs in nongrafted individuals are involuntary, excessive movements that are due to long-term use of L–dopa, the mainstay pharmacological treatment for PD.[28]

Initial transplantation studies performed in the 1990s were unblinded and employed a small number of patients. Nevertheless, they suggested that fetal DA neurons survived and could generate moderate clinical improvements over 3 to 4 years.[29–39] An important clinical grafting study was the large, double-blinded, placebo-controlled clinical trial performed by Freed and colleagues.[22] Forty patients with severe PD, between the ages of 34 and 75, were randomly assigned to a neuron cell transplant group or to a sham transplant group. Before surgery, the Unified Parkinson's Disease Rating Scale (UPDRS) scores of all 40 patients off medication were an average of 58 to 71, and the UPDRS scores on medication were 12 to 30. Each patient received solid tissue grafts derived from a total of four fetal VMs. The tissue was in the shape of strands that had been cultured for up to 4 weeks and then implanted in the putamen using a frontal approach. In the sham-transplanted patients, holes were drilled through the skull but transplant needles never penetrated the dura. The primary outcome of the study was a subjective global rating of change in disease severity at 1 year after surgery, ranging from –3.0 (maximal aggravation) to 3.0 (maximal improvement). At 1 year after surgical procedure, the transplantation group and sham-treated group did not differ in their mean scores on the global rating scale (0.0 ± 2.1 for the transplant group, and –0.4 ± 1.7 in the sham group, respectively). Fifteen percent of the patients experienced dystonia and dyskinesia during off phases, defined as periods when L–dopa was reduced or even withdrawn. Although these results were disappointing, transplantation was effective in ameliorating parkinsonian symptoms in the younger patients (under 60 years of age), as measured by UPDRS (p = .01), and Schwab and England scales (p = .006).

A second double-blind, controlled transplantation trial was conducted by Olanow and collaborators.[23] Thirty-four patients with severe PD between the ages of 30 and 75 were randomized to receive bilateral grafts with one or four donors VMs per side in the postcommissural putamen or a sham surgery. Transplanted patients had two surgical procedures separated by 1 week. Sham-treated patients received burr holes that only partially penetrated the skull. Unlike the method used by Freed et al,[22] tissue used for transplantation was stored for a maximum of 2 days before transplantation. Patients were treated with cyclosporine for 2 weeks before the surgical procedure and for 6 months thereafter. Transplanted patients exhibited increased stria-

tal fluorodopa uptake, suggestive of surviving DA neurons. The primary end point of the study was a change in the UPDRS scores during off phases. Unfortunately, results of the study revealed no difference in the primary end point measure between placebo and transplant groups. It was found that patients in the four-donor group had a tendency, albeit not statistically significant, to have a greater symptomatic improvement than patients in the one-donor group. Perhaps in a manner analogous to the Freed study, patients with milder disease (although not necessarily younger) had a significant treatment effect compared with sham-treated patients (p = 0.006). After the surgery, a large proportion of grafted patients (56%) developed dyskinesias during practically defined off periods despite amelioration of dyskinesia during on periods in many patients. The mechanisms mediating the postoperative worsening of some aspects of dyskinesias are unclear. There is reason to suspect that several factors are causative: graft-derived patterns of reinnervation, immune response to grafted cells, L–dopa priming, and others. The role of these factors on the development of levodopa and graft-induced dyskinesias is being elucidated in primate and rodent models.[40,41]

Clinical trials have suggested that fetal nigral transplantation is beneficial for a certain population of PD patients. However, many patients do not show symptomatic improvements after surgery, and many develop side-effects such as debilitating dyskinesias. In addition, the survival of implanted neurons on a percentage basis is relatively poor, making it necessary to transplant large amounts of tissue per patient. Fetal dopaminergic tissue is difficult to obtain due to a lack of availability and ethical considerations. Given these problems, it is not likely that fetal nigral grafting is feasible for generalized therapy for PD. However, all research performed in the field of nigral grafting was and continues to be an important learning tool in laying the foundation for future transplantation strategies using other cell-based therapies.

Stem Cell Transplantation

Another exciting alternative source of cells are stem cells for which two principally different ways of grafting in PD are being evaluated.[42–44] In the first method, cells are predifferentiated in vitro to dopaminergic neurons prior to transplantation (**Fig. 17.1**). Thus stem cells could become an almost unlimited source for the generation of DA neurons. The cell preparations could be standardized and quality controlled with respect to viability and purity. The second alternative is that the stem cells or progenitor cells differentiate in vivo to dopaminergic neurons after implantation into the striatum or substantia nigra. These neurons may integrate better as compared with primary fetal DA neurons and, in the ideal scenario, reconstruct the nigrostriatal pathway. However, whether this will be possible remains to be seen. It will require understanding the mechanism(s) needed to instruct the immature stem cells

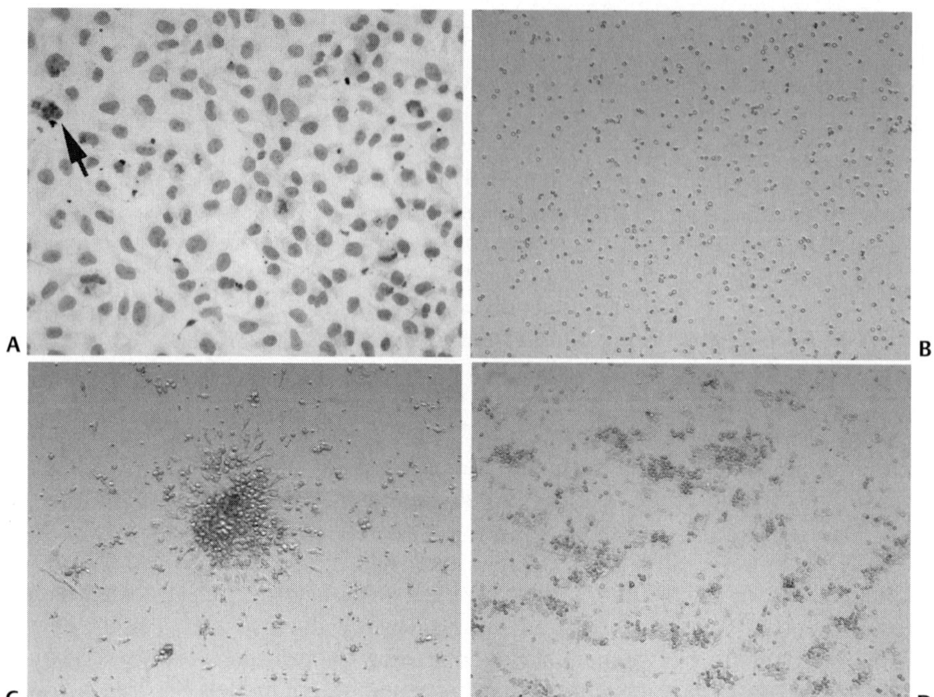

Fig. 17.1 Potential sources of dopaminergic cells are shown. **(A)** Human NT2 progenitor cells in culture for 3 days. Cell lines from tumor are a concern for tumor regression (arrow points to multinucleated cell). **(B)** Rat neural SVZ cells in isolation (division 1) within proliferation media. **(C)** Human neurosphere (conglomeration of neuroblasts) after replating 1 week in differentiation media. **(D)** Rat neural SVZ cells clumping together after three divisions (~21 days) and now 2 days in proliferation media.

to differentiate into the missing DA neurons and function in the PD brain. Hypothetically, DA neurons could be made from stem cells of four different sources: embryonic stem cells from the fertilized egg, embryonic neural cells from the fetal or those of adult brain, or stem cells in other tissues (e.g., the hematopoietic system). Another still unresolved issue is whether nondopaminergic neurons and glial cells, normally present in the mesencephalic grafts used so far in PD patients, are important for the differentiation and function of the DA neurons. If this is the case, an enriched population of predifferentiated DA neurons may not be the optimal preparation.

In general, cell replacement strategies based on stem cells or progenitor cells offer several advantages over fetal VM cells. First, human fetal material may not be needed, reducing both the practical and ethical issues associated with the use of fetal tissue. Second, unlimited numbers of dopaminergic neurons can be produced in vitro, allowing for a detailed characterization and standardization of their properties and quality. Third, these types of cells allow for the generation of stem/progenitor cell banks because the cells can be cryopreserved and expanded according to needs. Thus DA neurons derived from stem/progenitor cells constitute one of the most promising tools for cell replacement therapy in PD. The functional benefits observed in younger[22] or less severe[23] PD patients, even though these effects were observed with secondary end points, suggest that cell-based replacement therapies may be effective with proper patient selection. Thus there is still a future for dopaminergic cell–based therapies in PD if a reliable source of cells can be identified. Stem cells can be that

source. Potentially, stem cells can be propagated in vitro to produce large numbers, if not a limitless number, of cells for grafting and studies are under way to create an environment to drive these cells to both neuronal and dopaminergic phenotypes. It appears that fibroblast growth factor and sonic hedgehog are necessary for the induction of a dopaminergic phenotype. Stem cells can be derived from embryonic, fetal, and adult sources although at the present time, the embryonic stem cells appear the most promising in preclinical studies.

Initial attempts to study embryonic stem cells in models of PD used cells derived from mice. Following grafting into 6-OHDA lesioned rats, robust survival of implanted stem cells, the presence of a neuronal phenotype with dopaminergic properties, and functional recovery on standard tests relevant to this model have been demonstrated.[45–47] As an intermediary step, investigators have grafted stem cells derived from monkeys into cynomolgus monkeys and rodents.[47,49] Modest survival was reported for several months, but, clearly, optimization of the procedure is still required. Recently, Goldman and colleagues[50] reported benefit following grafting of human embryonic stem cells in rats receiving intraventricular 6-OHDA. These cells were grown in vitro on mouse feeder layers and would not be practical for clinical trials. Still the authors found robust survival of grafted cells for up to 8 weeks following transplantation. In vivo, the cells maintained the dopaminergic phenotype that had been demonstrated previously in vitro. Additionally, they reported benefit on a variety of functional tests. Thus stem cells show promise for future therapeutic trials. However, significant challenges still remain. Prior to initiating clinical trials with stem cells, growth control in vivo needs to be demonstrated, long-term survival and maintenance of dopaminergic phenotype needs to be established, and, critically, the origin and mechanism of the off-medication dyskinesias, seen in the fetal transplant trials, need to be eliminated so this severe graft-induced side effect does not recur in future stem cell trials.

Alternative Cell-Based Therapies

A new option for cell transplantation has been explored. Human retinal epithelial pigment cells (hRPE) have long been known to produce a precursor to dopamine, L-dopa, as a step in the formation of neuromelanin.[51] The hRPE cells are placed on a microcarrier consisting of 100 μm cross-linked porcine gelatin particles, and the product is called Spheramine (Titan Pharmaceuticals, Inc., South San Francisco, CA) (**Fig. 17.2**). These particles may enhance survival of transplanted cells in the CNS by providing a physical support structure for epithelial cell growth. These cells release several different trophic factors in addition to L-dopa. Spheramine grafts in rats improved motor function.[52] A sham-controlled study in monkeys rendered hemiparkinsonian with intracarotid 1-methyl-4-phenyl-1,2,3,6-tetrahydropyridine (MPTP) demonstrated significant improvement in the experimental group with respect to monkey UPDRS motor subscore.[53] The Spheramine-grafted monkeys demonstrated lasting dopaminergic activity, verified by positron emission tomography (PET) scan. Based on these favorable results, a pilot study was performed in six patients. All patients in the pilot study showed dramatic initial improvements of nearly 34% from baseline in UPDRS scores when off medication. Total UPDRS scores and multiple other behavioral tests demonstrated improvements at 6 months.[54] At 12 months, three of six patients still showed improvement compared with baseline.[55] This approach is in a pivotal phase II clinical trial (Bayer Scheria, Berlin).

■ Neurotrophic Factor for Parkinson Disease

PD is a chronic neurodegenerative disease with symptoms typically appearing after ~50% of substantia nigra dopamine neurons have degenerated and ~70% of striatal DA is lost.[51] Disease progression results in continued loss of nigral DA neurons and striatal DA at a rate of ~5 to 10% per year.[57] The slow, progressive nature of this disease provides opportunities for therapeutic intervention aimed at blocking nigral cell loss, and possibly promoting regeneration and axonal sprouting of surviving dopaminergic neurons.

Neurotrophic factors represent a family of proteins that play a critical role in controlling neuronal survival, differentiation, growth, and apoptosis and have therefore received considerable interest as therapeutic agents in neurodegenerative disorders. Since the initial discovery of the prototypic neurotrophin, nerve growth factor (NGF), 50 years ago by Levi-Montalcini, numerous additional trophic factors have been discovered.[58–60] Attempts to supply trophic factors clinically have thus far been disappointing due to poor delivery methods. In initial clinical trials, trophic factors were delivered either systemically or into the cerebrospinal fluid (intraventricularly or intrathecally) in patients suffering from amyotrophic lateral sclerosis, peripheral neuropathy, and Alzheimer and PD. In each of these trials, the trophic factor did not reach its target neurons due to either poor penetration across the blood–brain barrier or limited passage of protein from the cerebrospinal fluid into the brain parenchyma. Furthermore, neurotrophic factors, whose receptors are expressed widely throughout the CNS, produce unacceptable side effects when delivered by non-site-specific routes.

From past clinical trials, it is clear that, in addition to identifying a promising trophic factor, it is essential to have a viable delivery mechanism that ensures delivery specifically to those vulnerable neurons in that particular disease state. Dopaminergic nigrostriatal neurons are sensitive to

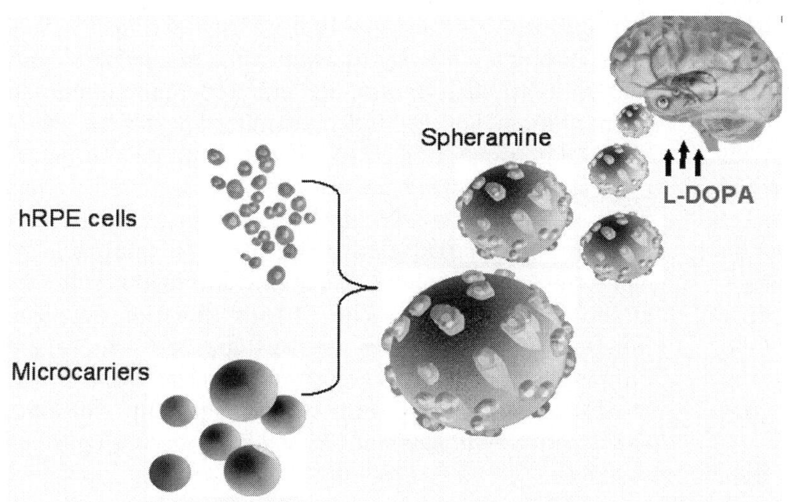

Fig. 17.2 A drawing of the formation of Spheramine (Titan Pharmaceuticals, Inc., South San Francisco, CA) by attaching to retinal pigmented epithelial cells to gelatin microcarrier and injection into the brain.

a variety of trophic factors,[59,60] including members of the fibroblast growth factor family (FGF-1, FGF-2), the glial cell line–derived neurotrophic factor family (GDNF, neurturin, persephin), platelet-derived growth factor (PDGF), insulin growth factors (IGF-1, IGF-2), brain-derived neurotrophic factor (BDNF), and neurotrophin-4 (NT-4). Of these proteins, GDNF seems to be the most potent trophic factor for nigrostriatal dopamine neurons that are affected in PD.

GDNF has been shown to prevent the structural and/or functional consequences seen in virtually every rodent model of PD, including those with lesions induced by 6-hydroxydopamine, methamphetamine, and axotomy as well as the degenerative changes associated with aging. One exception to this rule is the failure of GDNF to prevent the structural and functional consequences engendered by overexpression of α-synuclein. Still, based on the majority of these studies, experiments were performed in MPTR parkinsonian monkeys, with similar GDNF treatment benefits. On the basis of these rodent and primate experiments, Amgen Inc. (Thousand Oaks, CA, www.amgen.com) initiated a clinical trial testing the safety and efficacy of intraventricular monthly bolus injections of GDNF into the cerebral ventricles of patients with idiopathic PD. The clinical trial failed because of poor efficacy and treatment-related side effects. The limited efficacy was likely due to an insufficient concentration of GDNF reaching the striatum.[61] When moving from an animal model to a human, there is a substantial increase in the tissue volume through which this large protein must penetrate. Furthermore, side effects were reported and no restoration of dopaminergic fibers in the striatum was evident in one subject postmortem.[61] The reported side effects were likely due to spread throughout the cerebrospinal fluid, allowing GDNF to act on its receptors all across the CNS and the study was terminated.[62]

Intraparenchymal Glial Cell Line–Derived Neurotrophic Factor Delivery

Other methods for GDNF delivery in humans include direct parenchymal infusion and gene therapy approaches using viral vector delivery. Gill and collaborators recently tested the former method, with local delivery of GDNF via continuous intracerebral infusion into the posterodorsal putamen of advanced PD patients by chronic pump infusion.[63] In this phase I clinical trial, five patients were selected who had idiopathic, L-dopa–responsive Parkinson disease and were poorly controlled despite optimal medical therapy. Sites for catheter implantation into the dorsal putamen were determined using co-localization studies of magnetic resonance imaging (MRI) and PET scans of [^{18}F]dopamine uptake. After implantation, pumps were programmed to deliver a continuous infusion of 14.4 µg of r-metHuGDNF/putamen/day and were refilled monthly with fresh solution.

The clinical side effects due to GDNF infusion itself were limited to Lhermitte phenomenon (tingling from the neck to arms, trunks, and legs, provoked by neck flexion). This event was mild, intermittent, nondistressing, and usually at higher GDNF doses.

In all patients, PD symptoms improved after 3 months, and periods of severe immobility were eliminated after 6 months of GDNF infusion. Overall reductions of 48% and 45% in UPDRS scores during the off and on phases were observed. There was a significant reduction in dyskinetic movements by over 60% on medication and no dyskinetic movements off medication.[63] Similar results were seen in a second open-label trial.[64] One year following the initiation of treatment, patients were reported to improve by 42% and 38% in UPDRS off and on states, respectively. Interestingly, the authors report a loss of benefit within 9 to 12 months of sponsor-mandated cessation of the GDNF treatment. Both of these experiments were phase I safety/toxicity trials with no control group, and these results, like all open-label trials, could be confounded by placebo effects and experimenter bias. Based upon these data, however, Amgen initiated a phase II double-blind trial using moderately advanced patients who received bilateral intraputamenal GDNF (14.4 µg/d) or vehicle via a single point source using nonconvection-enhanced delivery. This trial failed to reach its primary end point (UPDRS off) and ~10% of the patients developed antibodies against GDNF.[65] Furthermore, monkeys receiving intraputamenal GDNF at a high dose, which was then withdrawn, developed severe cerebellar damage. Although technique[66] and statistics[67] may have been the biggest problems, based upon these findings Amgen has abandoned this approach.[68]

Viral Glial Cell Line–Derived Neurotrophic Factor

An alternative method for delivering high titer levels of GDNF to site-specific loci is using viral delivery of the GDNF gene to target sites. Rather than chronic intrastriatal infusion of GDNF protein, a single injection of a virus delivering the GDNF gene would provide long-term expression of this protein to the PD striatum. Methods for viral delivery include either ex vivo or in vivo gene therapy. In the ex vivo approach, retroviral vectors are used to transfect cells (e.g., fibroblasts, astrocytes, stem cells) in a culture dish; these cells are then transplanted into rodent or nonhuman primate models of PD. Indeed, similar approaches using fibroblasts transfected to secrete NGF and ciliary neurotrophic factor (CNTF) have been employed in clinical trials for the treatment of Alzheimer disease[69] and Huntington disease,[70] respectively. Advantages to this approach include the fact that ability to employ autologous cells obtained from the graft recipient thus obviating potential immune responses. However, this approach has severe limitations as well, including substantial transgene downregulation. For a long-term neurodegenerative disease, this approach will likely not be an efficient and efficacious strategy.

In vivo gene therapy is a more clinically relevant approach where engineered replication-deficient viruses are utilized to transfect host brain cells. Efficient long-term expression of GDNF in the nigrostriatal system has been achieved with three different vector systems, specifically recombinant adenovirus (Ad), adeno-associated virus (AAV), and lentiviral (LV) vectors. Each of these vector systems holds promise for gene transfer of therapeutic proteins to nondividing cells of the adult central nervous system.[71]

LV vectors are derived from a group of retroviruses, which includes the HIV viruses. They share the useful properties of the commonly used retroviral vectors, with the additional advantage that the LV vectors can also integrate into nondividing cells. They have a large cloning capacity, at least 9 kb, and are stably integrated into the genome of the target cells (i.e., properties that are highly favorable for long-term expression of transgenes in the nervous system).[72]

Ad vectors are advantageous in that they can accommodate large pieces of DNA (up to 8 kb), can be generated free of contaminant replication-competent virus at very high titers, and can transfect both dividing and nondividing cells. The transferred DNA remains as a nonintegrated episome in the nucleus and is, therefore, most adequate for transient expression of transgenes in nondividing cells. When *Ad-GDNF* injected into the striatum before a unilateral 6-hydroxydopamine (6-OHDA) lesion, both striatal dopamine and nigral perikarya were spared and motor function was sustained.[71] By contrast, if *Ad-GDNF* is injected into the midbrain, nigral perikarya are spared, but dopaminergic striatal innervation is lost and motor function is not sustained. These studies demonstrate that preservation of striatal innervation as well as nigral perikarya is critical for protecting motor function and will guide future gene therapy experiments. However, as a delivery system, Ad vectors are not presently the vector of choice. Historically, they have consistently produced inflammatory and immune responses and their safety profile, even employing later-generation gutless vectors, is inferior to other vector choices.[73]

Thus, although this delivery method provided proof of principle that gene delivery of *GDNF* is possible, less toxic vectors will be necessary before this technology can be used in a clinical trial. Recombinant AAV vectors have 96% of the viral genome removed, leaving only the two short inverted terminal repeats, which are sufficient for packaging and integration of specific transgenes.[74] An advantage of AAV vectors is that they can integrate and stably express their transgene product in nondividing cells, including neurons, and that the absence of viral genes minimizes the expression of foreign proteins and hence decrease the risk of triggering host immune responses. Several different AAV serotypes have been identified with varying degrees of transfection efficiency and specificity. The disadvantage is that the rAAV DNA packaging capacity is small, less than 5 kb, which limits the size of the gene constructs that can be delivered with the rAAV system. Another limiting factor is that the transgene is expressed with a delay of several days and increases gradually over the first 2 to 3 weeks, probably due to the fact that a second strand of DNA needs to be synthesized in the transduced cells before the transgene can be expressed. This is an important parameter to consider for experimental studies but has little impact for clinical trials.

Of the three vector systems discussed, only AAV has been used for testing gene therapy approaches in phase I or phase II clinical trials in patients with PD. Ceregene Inc. in collaboration with Kordower and coworkers has reported consistent gene expression and biological activity following AAV-neurturin delivery to intact, aged, and MPTP-treated monkeys[75-77] with functional benefit seen for up to 10 months in parkinsonian animals (**Fig. 17.3**). In 2006, Ceregene Inc. (San Diego, CA; www.Ceregene.com) initiated a phase II randomized, double-blind clinical trial testing the safety and efficacy of AAV-neurturin, a trophic factor gene that is an endogenous functional analogue of GDNF in patients with PD. Presently, two other phase I clinical trials using AAV are under way. One trial (Genzyme, Cambridge, MA; www.Genzyme.com) delivers the aromatic amino acid decarboxylase in an attempt to maximize the clinical efficacy of levodopa while minimizing dopa-related side effects. A third trial (Neurologix Inc., Fort Lee, NJ; www.Neurologix.net) delivers glutamic acid decarboxylase to the subthalamic nucleus in an attempt to quiet PD-mediated overactivity of this basal ganglia structure. From all available data, it seems that the AAV vector system is safe, even when injected in high titers, and that they induce, at most, a very limited inflammation or cellular immune responses in the brain. Recently, long-term studies performed in parkinsonian nonhuman primates have supported the concept that AAV delivery of therapeutic agents would be safe and effective. Bankiewicz and coworkers[78,79] have nonhuman primate data with the longest follow-up

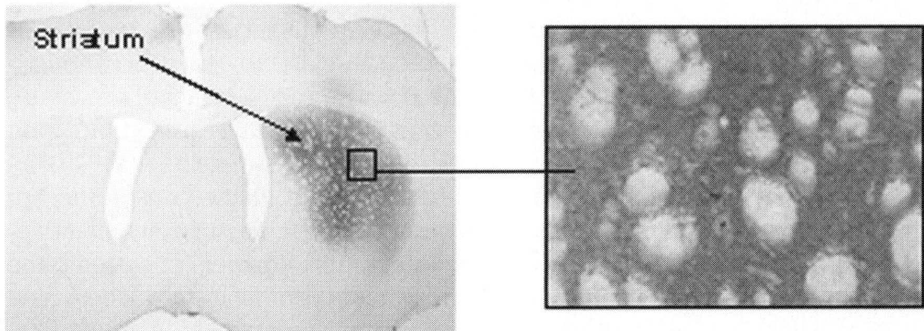

Fig. 17.3 Photographic micrographs of a parkinsonian monkey brain after transfection with adeno-associated virus (AAV)-neurturin (Cere-120) demonstrating immunoreaction to neurturin protein at low and high power.

(5 to 6 years) and use imaging and function status to indicate that transgene expression remains high over this period of time, and functional benefits from AAV-AADC delivery are enduring.

There are several issues being studied in animal models related to the level and site of the expression of the transgene, as well as the possible negative or adverse side effects that might be induced by sustained, high-level expression of this biologically active molecule in the human brain. In addition, direct gene delivery to the CNS raises safety issues including potential risk of contaminating helper virus. The possibility of insertional mutagenesis, or activation of cellular proto-oncogenes, in the cases where the vector is integrated into the genome, is also a concern that needs to be taken seriously. Furthermore, the functional implications of aberrant sprouting as seen in the substantia nigra and putamen after intraparenchymal protein delivery or viral delivery of trophic factors is an issue that remains to be resolved. The amount of aberrant sprouting is dose dependent, and future clinical trials will have to find the lowest therapeutic dose to minimize this response. Since we are only beginning to collect the relevant human data to guide us on these key safety issues, work should continue on the development of vectors that are regulatable. However, existing information points to the safety of the current constitutive promoter approach, the lack of any regulatable promoter that is truly efficient in shutting off transgene expression, coupled with the immune response engendered by regulatable promoters, this aspect of vectorology may not necessarily be a priority, and efforts to build an exhaustive empirical safety profile using a constitutive vector may be a safer approach.

■ Challenges for Future Treatments for Parkinson Disease

Many advancements in viral-based vectors for gene delivery to cells of the central nervous system have been achieved. However, improvements are still needed with respect to safety and efficiency of gene transfer into neurons. The desired features of viral vectors for gene delivery into the brain include the following: (1) a large transgene capacity is often needed within a vector to include a gene(s) of interest and its appropriate regulators; (2) high transduction efficiency is needed to transfer a gene of interest to a population of neural cells, with limited volume delivery; (3) stability of transgene expression is required in many applications and is affected by how the transgene is maintained within the host-cell nucleus (free, episomal, or integrated), long-term regulation of promoters, and immune responses to antigenic proteins encoded in the virus or transgenes; (4) the appropriate dose of transgene product can be critical, and inclusion of sequences within the vector that can regulate the transcription of the transgene will be

required for this control; (5) cell specificity of gene transfer within the nervous system (to neurons versus glia cells, or to more specific phenotypes of each) will depend on cell-specific promoters, expression of viral vector-specific receptors, or route of axonal transport of the vector in the brain, or a combination of all three; (6) effective clinical application of gene therapy approaches will require both a lack of toxicity and inflammatory immune responses.

Future cell replacement therapies for PD will build upon results from clinical trials as well as from studies of animal models. Requirements to be fulfilled by grafts to induce clinically valuable improvement include the following: (1) grafted cells must express the complete machinery for DA synthesis and release, and possess the morphological and electrophysiological properties of fully mature mesencephalic DA neurons (the importance of nondopaminergic cells in influencing the outcome after transplantation needs to be fully explored); (2) the cell number must be adequate to ensure survival long-term in each putamen with grafted DA neurons reestablishing a dense, functional, DA-releasing terminal network homogeneously in the striatum; (3) the grafts should become functionally integrated into host basal ganglia-thalamo-cortical neural circuitries, ideally, reconstructing the nigrostriatal pathway and establishing the appropriate afferent and efferent connections; (4) future successful therapies for PD will require improved criteria for patient selection and assessment as well optimum graft placement and dosage. The distribution, degree, and rate of degeneration of dopaminergic and nondopaminergic neurons in the patient's brain will determine to what extent a dopaminergic graft can restore normal function. Combinations of cell therapy with gene therapy to create an optimal environment for proper growth, attachment, and function may be required.[80] Detailed preoperative imaging techniques (e.g., high-resolution fluorodopa-PET), will be invaluable tools to design the optimum transplantation procedure for individual patients.

In another possible future, DBS systems could be combined with biological delivery systems technology, such as endovascular technologies that have advanced with the advent of drug-eluting stents.[81,82] There are several potential types of adjuvant therapies that may be possible, ranging from drug infusions to gene therapy to stem cells. Microdialysis work in models of DBS have demonstrated that increases in extracellular glutamate and gamma-aminobutyric acid are induced by subthalamic nucleus DBS.[83] Work in gene therapy, growth factors, and neural transplantation has shown further promise. As advances are made in all of these therapies, the potential exists to use them in combination with DBS both because DBS systems of the future may offer a delivery mechanism and because stimulation itself may result in a more responsive cellular milieu.[84,85] Furthermore, closed-loop low-frequency stimulation of transplanted cell populations may augment its effectiveness. Ultimately, the integration of biological systems and electronic close-loop systems will usher in a whole new BCI technology for repair and restoration of function.

The future of DBS has significant possibilities and its successes will be dependent on multiple factors. First, as new applications emerge, refinement of target and patient selection and the development of multidisciplinary teams specific to the diseases being treated will be crucial. Second, devices must be optimized to enable customized stimulation delivery and systems that are more compatible with activities of daily living. Lastly, the potential for adjuncts to DBS are limitless and will no doubt be the focus of research for years to come.

References

1. Butson CR, McIntyre CC. Role of electrode design on the volume of tissue activated during deep brain stimulation. J Neural Eng 2006;3: 1–8
2. Kronenbuerger M, Fromm C, Block F, et al. On-demand deep brain stimulation for essential tremor: a report on four cases. Mov Disord 2006;21:401–405
3. Osorio I, Frei MG, Sunderam S, et al. Automated seizure abatement in humans using electrical stimulation. Ann Neurol 2005;57: 258–268
4. Serruya MD, Hatsopoulos NG, Paninski L, Fellows MR, Donoghue J. Instant neural control of a movement signal. Nature 2002;416: 141–142
5. Taylor DM, Tillery SIH, Schwartz AB. Direct cortical control of 3D neuroprosthetic devices. Science 2002;296:1829–1832
6. Carmena JM, Lebedev MA, Crist RE, et al. Learning to control a brain–machine interface for reaching and grasping by primates. PLoS Biol 2003;1:E42
7. Musallam S, Corneil BD, Greger B, Scherberger H, Andersen RA. Cognitive control signals for neural prosthetics. Science 2004;305: 258–262
8. Kennedy PR, Bakay RA, Moore MM, Adams K, Goldwaithe J. Direct control of a computer from the human central nervous system. IEEE Trans Rehabil Eng 2000;8:198–202
9. Hochberg LR, Serruya MD, Friehs GM, et al. Neuronal ensemble control of prosthetic devices by a human with tetraplegia. Nature 2006;442:164–171
10. Patil PG, Carmena JM, Nicolelis MA, Turner DA. Ensemble recordings of human subcortical neurons as a source of motor control signals for a brain–machine interface. Neurosurgery 2004;55:27–38
11. Hummel FC, Cohen LG. Non-invasive brain stimulation: a new strategy to improve neurorehabilitation after stroke? Lancet Neurol 2006;5:708–712
12. Levy RM, Ruth A, Huang ME, et al. Cortical stimulation for motor recovery after stroke: impact on neuropsychological performance and functional imaging. Neurosurgery 2006;59:480
13. Brown JA, Lutsep HL, Weinand M, Cramer SC. Motor cortex stimulation for the enhancement of recovery from stroke: a prospective, multicenter safety study. Neurosurgery 2006;58:464–473
14. Bakay RAE. Implantable brain-computer interfaces: neurosurgical experience and prospective. In: Dilorenzo DJ, ed. Neural Engineering Text (in press)
15. Braak H, Braak E. Pathoanatomy of Parkinson's disease. J Neurol 2000;247(Suppl 2):II3–II10
16. Langston JW. The Parkinson's complex: parkinsonism is just the tip of the iceberg. Ann Neurol 2006;59:591–596
17. LeWitt PA, Nyholm D. New developments in levodopa therapy. Neurology 2004;62(Suppl 1):S9–S16
18. Olanow CW. The scientific basis for the current treatment of Parkinson's disease. Annu Rev Med 2004;55:41–60
19. Bakay RAE, Kordower JH, Starr PA. Restorative surgical therapies for Parkinson's disease. In: Tuszynski MH, Kordower JH, eds. CNS Regeneration: Basic Science and Clinical Applications. San Diego: Academic Press; 1999:389–418
20. Bakay RAE. Neurotransplantation and protective therapy for movement disorders. Semin Neurosurg 2001;12:245–252
21. Sortwell CE, Pitzer MR, Collier TJ. Time course of apoptotic cell death within mesencephalic cell suspension grafts: implications for improving grafted dopamine neuron survival. Exp Neurol 2000;165:268–277
22. Freed CR, Greene PE, Breeze RE, et al. Transplantation of embryonic dopamine neurons for severe Parkinson's disease. N Engl J Med 2001;344:710–719
23. Olanow CW, Goetz CG, Kordower JH, et al. A double-blind controlled trial of bilateral fetal nigral transplantation in Parkinson's disease. Ann Neurol 2003;54:403–414
24. Freed CR, Breeze RE, Schneck SA, et al. Fetal neural transplantation for Parkinson disease. In: Rich RR, ed. Clinical Immunology: Principles and Practice. New York: Mosby, 1996;1677–1687
25. Backlund EO, Granberg PO, Hamberger B. Transplantation of adrenal medullary tissue to striatum in parkinsonism. First clinical trials. J Neurosurg 1985;62:169–173
26. Freed WJ, Poltorak M, Becker JBL. Intracerebral adrenal medulla grafts: a review. Exp Neurol 1990;110:139–166
27. Kordower JH, Cochran E, Penn RD, et al. Putative chromaffin cell survival and enhanced host-derived TH-fiber innervation following a functional adrenal medulla autograft for Parkinson's disease. Ann Neurol 1991;29:405–412
28. Brotchie JM, Lee H, Venderova K. Levodopa-induced dyskinesia in Parkinson's disease. J Neural Transm 2005;112:359–391
29. Freed CR, Breeze RE, Rosenberg NL, et al. Transplantation of human fetal dopamine cells for Parkinson's disease: results at 1 year. Arch Neurol 1990;47:505–512
30. Lindvall O, Brundin P, Widner H, et al. Grafts of fetal dopamine neurons survive and improve motor function in Parkinson's disease. Science 1990;247:574–577
31. Spencer DD, Robbins RJ, Naftolin F, et al. Unilateral transplantation of human fetal mesencephalic tissue into the caudate nucleus of patients with Parkinson's disease. N Engl J Med 1992;327:1541–1548
32. Lindvall O, Sawle G, Widner H, et al. Evidence for long-term survival and function of dopaminergic grafts in progressive Parkinson's disease. Ann Neurol 1994;35:172–180
33. Freed CR, Breeze RE, Schneck SA. Transplantation of fetal mesencephalic tissue in Parkinson's disease. N Engl J Med 1995;333:730–731
34. Freeman TB, Olanow CW, Hauser RA, et al. Bilateral fetal nigral transplantation into the postcommissural putamen in Parkinson's disease. Ann Neurol 1995;38:379–388
35. Huang S, Pei G, Kang FA, et al. Transplant operation of human fetal substantia nigra tissue to caudate nucleus in Parkinson's disease: first clinical trials. Clin J Neurosurgery 1989;5:210–213
36. Kopyov OV, Jacques D, Lieberman A, et al. Clinical study of fetal mesencephalic intracerebral transplants for the treatment of Parkinson's disease. Cell Transplant 1996;5:327–337

37. Lopez-Lozano JJ, Bravo G, Brera B, et al. Long-term improvement in patients with severe Parkinson's disease after implantation of fetal ventral mesencephalic tissue in a cavity of the caudate nucleus: 5-year follow-up in 10 patients. J Neurosurg 1997;86:931–942

38. Peschanski M, Defer G, N'Guyen JP, et al. Bilateral motor improvement and alteration of L-dopa effect in two patients with Parkinson's disease following intrastriatal transplantation of foetal ventral mesenchephalon. Brain 1994;117:487–499

39. Widner H, Tetrud J, Rehncrona S, et al. Bilateral fetal mesencephalic grafting in two patients with parkinsonism induced by 1-methyl-4-phenyl-1,2,3,6- tetrahydropyridine (MPTP). N Engl J Med 1992;327:1556–1563

40. Steece-Collier K, Collier TJ, Danielson PD, et al. Embryonic mesencephalic grafts increase levodopa-induced forelimb hyperkinesia in parkinsonian rats. Mov Disord 2003;18:1442–1454

41. Lee CS, Cenci MA, Schulzer M, et al. Embryonic ventral mesencephalic grafts improve levodopa-induced dyskinesia in a rat model of Parkinson's disease. Brain 2000;123(Pt 7):1365–1379

42. Arenas E. Engineering a dopaminergic phenotype in stem/precursor cells: role of *Nurr*1, glia-derived signals, and Wnts. Ann N Y Acad Sci 2005;1049:51–66

43. Sonntag KC, Simantov R, Isacson O. Stem cells may reshape the prospect of Parkinson's disease therapy. Brain Res Mol Brain Res 2005;134:34–51

44. Levy YS, Stroomza M, Melamed E, et al. Embryonic and adult stem cells as a source for cell therapy in Parkinson's disease. J Mol Neurosci 2004;24:353–386

45. Bjorklund LM, Sanchez-Pernaute R, Chung S, et al. Embryonic stem cells develop into functional dopaminergic neurons after transplantation in a Parkinson rat model. Proc Natl Acad Sci U S A 2002;99:2344–2349

46. Kim JH, Auerbach JM, Rodriguez-Gomez JA, et al. Dopamine neurons derived from embryonic stem cells function in an animal model of Parkinson's disease. Nature 2002;418:50–56

47. Yang M, Stull ND, Berk MA, et al. Neural stem cells spontaneously express dopaminergic traits after transplantation into the intact or 6-hydroxydopamine-lesioned rat. Exp Neurol 2002;177:50–60

48. Sanchez-Pernaute R, Studer L, Ferrari D, et al. Long-term survival of dopamine neurons derived from parthenogenetic primate embryonic stem cells (cyno-1) after transplantation. Stem Cells 2005;23:914–922

49. Takagi Y, Takahashi J, Saiki H, et al. Dopaminergic neurons generated from monkey embryonic stem cells function in a Parkinson primate model. J Clin Invest 2005;115:102–109

50. Roy NS, Cleren C, Singh SK, et al. Functional engraftment of human ES cell-derived dopaminergic neurons enriched by coculture with telomerase-immortalized midbrain astrocytes. Nat Med 2006; doi:10.1038/nm1495

51. Boulton M. Melanin and the retinal pigment epithelium. In: Marmor MF, Wolfensberger TJ, eds. The Retinal Pigment Epithelium: Function and Disease. New York: Oxford University Press; 1998:68–85

52. Subramanian T, Marchionini D, Potter EM, et al. Striatal xenotransplantation of human retinal pigment epithelial cells attached to microcarriers in hemiparkinsonian rats ameliorates behavioral deficits without provoking a host immune response. Cell Transplant 2002;11:207–214

53. Watts RL, Raiser CD, Stover NP, et al. Stereotaxic intrastriatal implantation of human retinal pigment epithelial (hRPE) cells attached to gelatin microcarriers: a potential new cell therapy for Parkinson's disease. J Neural Transm Suppl 2003;65:215–227

54. Bakay RA, Raiser CD, Stover NP, et al. Implantation of Spheramine in advanced Parkinson's disease (PD). Front Biosci 2004;9:592–602

55. Stover NP, Bakay RAE, Subramanian T, et al. Intrastriatal implantation of human retinal pigment epithelial cells attached to microcarriers in advanced Parkinson disease. Arch Neurol 2005;62:1833–1837

56. Fearnley JM, Lees AJ. Aging and Parkinson's disease: substantia nigra regional selectivity. Brain 1991;114:2283–2301

57. Brooks DJ. The early diagnosis of Parkinson's disease. Ann Neurol 1998;44(Suppl 1):S10–S18

58. Lad SP, Neet KE, Mufson EJ. Nerve growth factor: structure, function and therapeutic implications for Alzheimer's disease. Curr Drug Targets CNS Neurol Disord 2003;2:315–334

59. Collier TJ, Steece-Collier K, McGuire S, et al. Cellular models to study dopaminergic injury responses. Ann N Y Acad Sci 2003;991:140–151

60. Chen S, Le W. Neuroprotective therapy in Parkinson disease. Am J Ther 2006;13:445–457

61. Kordower JH, Palfi S, Chen EY, et al. Clinicopathological findings following intraventricular glial-derived neurotrophic factor treatment in a patient with Parkinson's disease. Ann Neurol 1999;46: 419–424

62. Nutt JG, Burchiel KJ, Comella CL, et al. Randomized, double-blind trial of glial cell line-derived neurotrophic factor (GDNF) in PD. Neurology 2003;60:69–73

63. Gill SS, Patel NK, Hotton GR, et al. Direct brain infusion of glial cell line-derived neurotrophic factor in Parkinson disease. Nat Med 2003;9:589–595

64. Slevin JT, Gerhardt GA, Smith CD. Improvement of bilateral motor functions in patients with Parkinson disease through the unilateral intraputaminal infusion of glial cell line-derived neurotrophic factor. J Neurosurg 2005;102:216–222

65. Lang AE, Gill S, Patel NK, et al. Randomized controlled trial of intraputamenal glial cell line-derived neurotrophic factor infusion in Parkinson disease. Ann Neurol 2006;59:459–466

66. Salvatore MF, Ai Y, Fischer B, et al. Point source concentration of GDNF may explain failure of phase II clinical trial. Exp Neurol 2006;202:497–505

67. Hutchison M, Gurney S, Newson R. GDNF in Parkinson disease: an object lesson in the tyranny of type II. J Neurosci Methods 2006;163:190–192

68. Sherer TB, Fiske BK, Svendsen CN, et al. Crossroads in GDNF therapy for Parkinson's disease. Mov Disord 2006;21:136–141

69. Tuszynski MH, Thal L, Pay M, et al. A phase I clinical trial of nerve growth factor gene therapy for Alzheimer disease. Nat Med 2005;11:551–555

70. Gaura V, Bachoud-Levi AC, Ribeiro MJ, et al. Striatal neural grafting improves cortical metabolism in Huntington's disease patients. Brain 2004;127(Pt 1):65–72

71. Bjorklund A, Kirik D, Rosenblad C, et al. Towards a neuroprotective gene therapy for Parkinson's disease: use of adenovirus, AAV and lentivirus vectors for gene transfer of GDNF to the nigrostriatal system in the rat Parkinson model. Brain Res 2000;886:82–98

72. Kordower JH, Emborg ME, Bloch J, et al. Neurodegeneration prevented by lentiviral vector delivery of GDNF in primate models of Parkinson's disease. Science 2000;290:767–773

73. Bohn MC, Choi-Lundberg DL, Davidson BL, et al. Adenovirus-mediated transgene expression in nonhuman primate brain. Hum Gene Ther 1999;10:1175–1184

74. Wu Z, Asokan A, Samulski RJ. Adeno-associated virus serotypes: vector toolkit for human gene therapy. Mol Ther 2006;14: 316–327

75. Gasmi M, Herzog CD, Brandon EP, et al. Striatal delivery of neurturin by CERE-120, an AAV2 vector for the treatment of dopaminergic neuron degeneration in Parkinson's disease. Mol Ther 2007;15:62–68

76. Kordower JH, Herzog CD, Dass B, et al. Delivery of neurturin by AAV2 (CERE-120)-mediated gene transfer provides structural and functional neuroprotection and neurorestoration in MPTP-treated monkeys. Ann Neurol 2006;60:706–715

77. Dass B, Olanow CW, Kordower JH. Gene transfer of trophic factors and stem cell grafting as treatments for Parkinson's disease. Neurology 2006; 66(10, Suppl 4)S89–S103

78. Forsayeth JR, Eberling JL, Sanftner LM, et al. A dose-ranging study of AAV-hAADC therapy in Parkinsonian monkeys. Mol Ther 2006; 14:571–577

79. Bankiewicz KS, Forsayeth J, Eberling JL, et al. Long-term clinical improvement in MPTP-lesioned primates after gene therapy with AAV-hAADC. Mol Ther 2006;14:564–570

80. Behrstock S, Svendsen CN. Combining growth factors, stem cells, and gene therapy for the aging brain. Ann N Y Acad Sci 2004;1019: 5–14

81. Eisenberg MJ, Konnyu KJ. Review of randomized clinical trials of drug-eluting stents for the prevention of in-stent restenosis. Am J Cardiol 2006;98:375–382

82. Gupta R, Al-Ali F, Thomas AJ, et al. Safety, feasibility, and short-term follow-up of drug-eluting stent placement in the intracranial and extracranial circulation. Stroke 2006;37:2562–2566

83. Windels F, Bruet N, Poupard A, Feuerstein C, Bertrand A, Savasta M. Influence of the frequency parameter on extracellular glutamate and gamma-aminobutyric acid in substantia nigra and globus pallidus during electrical stimulation of subthalamic nucleus in rats. J Neurosci Res 2003;72:259–267

84. Lee PY, Chesnoy S, Huang L. Electroporatic delivery of TGF-beta1 gene works synergistically with electric therapy to enhance diabetic wound healing in db/db mice. J Invest Dermatol 2004;123: 791–798

85. Iida Y, Oda Y, Nakamori S, et al. Transthoracic direct current shock facilitates intramyocardial transfection of naked plasmid DNA infused via coronary vessels in canines. Gene Ther 2006;13: 906–916

Index

Note: Page numbers followed by *f* and *t* indicate figures and tables, respectively. CP indicates Color Plate.

A

Ablative surgery, 13. *See also* Functional neurosurgery
  for dystonia, 170
  historical perspective on, 1, 2, 2*f*
  for Parkinson disease, selection and evaluation of patient for, 58
  therapeutic effects of, mechanism of, 16, 18–21
Action potential(s), 187–188, 188*f*
Activities of Daily Living, 12, 54, 59, 161, 162, 231, 232, 255
Adenoassociated virus (AAV), GDNF gene therapy with, 253–254, 253*f*
Adenovirus (Ad), as vector for gene therapy, 253
Adrenal medulla, autologous, transplantation of, historical perspective on, 7
Adverse effects
  of functional neurosurgery, assessment of, 55
  stimulation-induced, 182–183, 187, 229–230, 232
    troubleshooting for, 223–224, 223*f*
Air embolism, 78–79, 80, 229
  prevention of, 85, 87
Airway
  intraoperative control of, 76, 79
    with intraoperative seizures, 78
  obstruction, intraoperative, 79
  preoperative assessment of, 72–73
Akinesia, 17, 58
  parkinsonian, 155
    treatment of, 155
Albin, R.L., 16
Alcohol injection, historical perspective on, 3–4, 5
Alexander, G.E., 16
Alfentanil, drug interactions with, 72
Allergic reaction, hardware-related, 230
Alpha Omega microguide software, 133, 138
American Parkinson Disease Association Inc., 39
American Society for Stereotactic and Functional Neurosurgery, 40
Anesthesia
  approach to, decision-making about, 72
  complications of, 80
  for deep brain stimulation, 169, 171
  for electrophysiological mapping, 76, 169
  for frameless techniques, 73
  for imaging, 73
  and intraoperative neurophysiology, 76–78, 77*f*, 78*t*, 171
  and postoperative care, 80
  for stereotactic frame placement, 72–73
  for stimulation mapping, 76
Anesthesiologist, 79
Anesthesiology, 36
Anesthetics, drug interactions with, 72
Angel dust. *See* MPTP
Ansa lenticularis
  magnetic resonance imaging of, 93*f*
  surgical approaches to, historical perspective on, 2, 5
Ansotomy, historical perspective on, 2, 3*f*
Anterior choroidal artery, surgical approaches to, historical perspective on, 2*f*, 5, 6
Anterior commissure (AC), 69, 95, 131, 223
Antibiotic prophylaxis, 84, 218
Antibiotics, for postoperative infection, 109
Anticholinergics, adverse effects and side effects of, 72
Anticoagulation
  perioperative management of, 60*t*
  in surgical candidate, 59–60
Anticonvulsants
  for dystonia, 168
  prophylactic, 84
Antihypertensive therapy, perioperative management of, 61, 79–80, 84
Antiplatelet agents, perioperative management of, 60*t*, 61, 84
Anxiety, 34
Apathy, postoperative, 232
Apomorphine, effect on electrophysiology, 83
Aspiration pneumonia, postoperative, 215*t*
Aspirin therapy, perioperative management of, 60*t*, 61
Ataxia, stimulation-induced, 201*f*, 202, 229
Athetosis, treatment of, historical perspective on, 1, 2, 5
Atypical Parkinsonism, 53, 58, 60
Axon Instruments Guideline System 3000A, 88, 88*f*

B

Baclofen
  for dystonia, 168
  intrathecal pump for, number of implantations (1992-2000), 38
Balance, 17
Basal ganglia

Alexander and Delong model of, 16–17
anatomy of, 13–15
in dystonia, 174
electrophysiology of, 17–18
functions of, 1
microcircuitry of, 13, 14*f*
microelectrode recording in, 173–174, 173*f*, 174*f*
output
   direct pathway, 13, 14*f*, 16–17
     in Parkinson disease, 15
   indirect pathway, 13, 14*f*, 16–17
     in Parkinson disease, 15, 16
physiology of, 13–15
surgical approaches to, historical perspective on, 2–3, 167
Basal ganglia–thalamocortical network, 13, 14*f*, 16–17
  neuronal activity, 13–15, 14*f*
    in dystonia, 14*f*
    in normal monkey, 14*f*
    oscillatory, 16, 17
    in Parkinson disease, 14*f*, 15–16
    patterns of, 15, 16
    rate-based model of, 15–16
    somatosensory responsiveness and, 16
    synchrony in, 15, 16
  neurotransmitters in, 13, 14*f*, 15
BCI. *See* Brain–computer interface systems (BCI)
Behavior, effects of surgery on, assessment of, 53
Ben-Gun, 134, 138
Benserazide, 247
Benzodiazepines, for dystonia, 168
Beta-blockers, drug interactions with, 71*t*, 72
BG. *See* Basal ganglia
Bias, 8
Billing. *See* Reimbursement
Bioengineering, 37
Bispectral Index (BIS), 76
Blepharospasm, 166, 211
Blood pressure
  intraoperative control of, 214, 215, 218
  intraoperative monitoring of, 79–80, 84, 214
Botulinum toxin, for dystonia, 168
Bradycardia, drug-induced, 71*t*, 72
Bradykinesia, 17
  treatment of, historical perspective on, 5–6
Brain–computer interface systems (BCI), 247
Brain-derived neurotrophic factor (BDNF), 252
Brain stimulation. *See* Deep brain stimulation (DBS);
    Stimulation
Brion, S., 3*f*
Broca, P., 1
Brodmann area(s), ablation, historical perspective on, 2
Browder, J., 2, 2*f*
Buchanan, D.N., 2
Bucy, P.C., 2, 2*f*
Bulbotomy, historical perspective on, 2*f*
Burdenko, N.N., 2, 2*f*
Burke-Fahn-Marsden Scale (BFMS), 55, 168, 231
Burr hole procedure, 85, 87, 214, 218

conscious sedation for, 76
  in frameless approach, 144
Butyrophenone derivatives, drug interactions with, 72

C
Carbidopa, 247
Cardiovascular status, preoperative evaluation of, 70, 71*t*
Cardioversion, safety considerations in, 222, 232
Cartesian coordinates, stereotaxic use of, 1, 3, 6, 8, 138
Catechol-*O*-methyltransferase (COMT) inhibitors, 248
Caudate nucleus, surgical approaches to, historical
    perspective on, 2
Central median and parafasciculus (CM/PF) thalamic
    complex, 17
Cerebellar cortex, stimulation, historical perspective on, 1
Cerebellar nucleus, stimulation, historical perspective on, 1
Cerebral atrophy, 51. *See also* Multiple system atrophy (MSA)
Cerebral cortex
  ablation, historical perspective on, 2, 2*f*
  in dystonia, 174–175
  stimulation, historical perspective on, 1
Cerebrospinal fluid (CSF)
  leakage
    intraoperative, prevention of, 87, 145
    postoperative, 109, 230
  tense collection around IPG, 215*t*, 217
Cervical collar, for patient immobilization in frameless
    approach, 142, 143*f*, CP 10.6
Cheese effect, 71*t*, 72
Chorea. *See* Huntington disease (HD)
Chromaffin cell transplantation, for Parkinson disease, 248
Clarke, R.H., 4, 6, 138
Clozapine, for dystonia, 168
Cluster headache, 137
CM/PF. *See* Central median and parafasciculus (CM/PF)
    thalamic complex
Cognition
  effects of surgery on, 60, 232
    assessment of, 53
  postoperative defects, 162–163, 211, 215*t*, 220, 232
    in Parkinson disease, 224
    stereotactic lesioning and, 225
  in surgical candidate, 52, 58, 70
COMPASS, 31
Complications
  of deep brain stimulation, 48, 162–163, 214–217, 215*t*,
    216*f*, 217*f*, 222, 229
    hardware-related, 215*t*, 219–222, 230, 232
    neurocognitive, 232
    outcomes with, 221–222
    psychiatric, 210–211, 215*t*, 232
  with Gamma Knife, 238, 241
  hardware-related, 162–163, 215*t*, 219–222, 230, 232
  operative, 80, 214–217, 215*t*
    incidence of, 214
    prevention of, 218
  patient education about, 60
  psychiatric, 210–211, 215*t*, 232

of radiosurgery, 241
  with radiosurgical thalamotomy, 238
  of stereotactic lesioning, 225
Computed tomography (CT). *See also* Image fusion
  postoperative, and detection of hemorrhage, 214, 216*f*
  preoperative, with frameless technology, 142, 143*f*
  sedation for, 73
  for surgical planning, 63, 157
Confusion, perioperative, 229
Consciousness, declining, intraoperative, 79
Cooper, I.S., 2*f*, 3*f*, 4, 5, 6, 167, 170
Coordinator, role of
  intraoperative, 49
  postoperative, 49
  in preoperative care, 49
Cordotomy
  cervical anterolateral, historical perspective on, 2
  extrapyramidal cervical, historical perspective on, 2
  lateral column, surgical approaches to. historical
    perspective on, 2, 2*f*
  posterolateral, historical perspective on, 2
Core Assessment Program for Intracerebral
    Transplantation-PD (CAPIT-PD), 52, 53
Core Assessment Program for Surgical Interventional
    Therapies in Parkinson's Disease (CAPSIT-PD), 53
Corticobasal ganglionic degeneration, 51
Corticospinal tract, somatotopy of, 96
Cosman-Roberts-Wells (CRW) Stereotactic Apparatus,
    26–27, 26*f*, 31, 84, CP 3.2
  advantages of, 31
  components of, 26–27, 26*f*
  costs of, 27
Coumadin, perioperative management of, 60
CPT. *See* Current procedural terminology (CPT) code
Craniotomy
  historical perspective on, 1
  transventricular, historical perspective on, 2
CRW. *See* Cosman-Roberts-Wells (CRW) Stereotactic
    Apparatus
Cryoprobe, 4
Current procedural terminology (CPT) code, 40, 43*t*–44*t*

D
Dandy, W.E., 2
DBS. *See* Deep brain stimulation (DBS)
Deep brain stimulation (DBS), 13
  active contact configuration for, 195–196, 196*f*
  adjuncts to, 254–255
  advances in (future directions for), 55, 110, 208, 231,
    232, 247, 254–255
  advantages of, 18–19
  adverse effects of, 182–183, 187, 229–230, 232
    troubleshooting for, 223–224, 223*f*
  anatomical considerations in, 190–191, 199–206
  asymmetric pulses, 198, 199*f*
  bilateral, 162
  in closed-loop system, 247, 254
  complications of, 48, 162–163, 210–211, 214–217, 215*t*,
    216*f*, 217*f*, 222, 229 (*See also* Complications)
    hardware-related, 182, 215*t*, 219–222, 230, 232
    neurocognitive, 232
    outcomes with, 221–222
    psychiatric, 210–211, 215*t*, 232
  constant voltage *versus* constant current, 192
  devices for, 181, 208–209, 209*t* (*See also* Internal pulse
    generator (IPG))
    failure, troubleshooting, 209–210, 210*t*, 222–224,
      223*f*, 224*f*
    programming, 19, 158, 183, 187–213, 208
      troubleshooting for, 224
  diagnoses unresponsive to, 224
  for dystonia, 50–51, 166–186, 211–212
    anesthesia for, 169, 171
    complications of, 182
    efficacy of, 231
      factors affecting, 231
    equipment for, 182
    headframe placement for, 169
    historical perspective on, 167–168
    indications for, 168
    microelectrode recording in, 172–174
    patient evaluation and selection for, 168
    results, 175–183, 176*t*–178*t*
    Rush exclusion criteria, 170–171
    Rush inclusion criteria, 170
    selection and evaluation of patient for, 54–55
    target acquisition for, 169
    targets for, 168–169
    technical considerations in, 169
  efficacy of, 227–231
    factors affecting, 187
    randomized trials of, 230
  electrode configurations
    advantages and disadvantages of, 193–194, 195*t*
    bipolar, 193, 193*f*, 209–210
      close, 194, 195*t*
      far, 194, 195*t*
    monopolar, 193, 193*f*, 209–210
    and size and strength of electrical fields, 192–195,
      193*f*, 194*f*, 195*f*
    tripolar, 193, 193*f*
  electronics of, 190–199
  for essential tremor, 50, 59, 156, 162
    bilateral *versus* unilateral, 231–232
    complications of, 232
    efficacy of, 231–232
    outcome with, predictors of, 54
    prognostic factors for, 54
    selection and evaluation of patient for, 54
    thalamic, efficacy of, 227
  excitatory effects of, 18
  extraoperative testing, 104
  frameless, equipment for, 27–29, 27*f*, 28*f*, CP 3.4
  GPi (*See* Globus pallidus, internal segment (GPi))
  high-frequency, 190, 191*f*
  historical perspective on, 1, 8, 12

indications for, 13, 50–52
inhibitory effects of, 18
lead(s)
    advances in (future directions for), 247
    anchoring, 158
    fracture, 162, 219, 219*f*, 230
        causes of, 220, 221*f*
        delayed, 215*t*, 219
        management of, 219, 219*f*
        prevention of, 219, 219*f*, 220
        reoperation for, 108, 108*f*
    implantation of, 100–102
    location, magnetic resonance imaging of, 102–103,
        103*f*, 120–121, 121*f*, 169, 220–221, 222
    malfunction, 162
    migration, 162, 219–220, 230
        causes of, 220
        management of, 220
        prevention of, 220
        and reoperation, 215*t*, 220
        reoperation for, 108, 108*f*
    narrow-spaced, and relative voltage distribution,
        194–195, 195*f*
    placement of, 158, 169
    removal, and radiofrequency lesioning, 109, 109*f*
    securing, 102–103, 102*f*, 103*f*
    in suboptimal location
        management of, 200–206, 210–211, 223*f*, 224
        not reoperated, 215*t*
        and reoperation, 215*t*, 221–222, 224, 224*f*
        troubleshooting for, 223–224
    wide-spaced, and relative voltage distribution,
        194–195, 195*f*
and magnetic resonance imaging, 222, 232
management of, strategies for, 206–208
and medication adjustments, 207, 210–211, 211
monopolar survey, 206
neuronal elements excited by
    action potentials generated by, 187–188, 188*f*
    definition of, 187
    frequency (in pulses per second) and, 190, 191*f*
    orientation of electrical field and, 189–190, 190*f*, 191*f*
    pulse width and, 188–189, 189*f*
    voltage and, 188
outcomes with, neurocognitive, 232
pallidal (*See also* Globus pallidus)
    adverse effects of, 182–183, 229–230
    for dystonia, 168–169, 182
        efficacy of, 231–232
    efficacy of, 228–229, 231–232
pallidotomy and, 60, 182
parameter settings for, 19
for Parkinson disease, 50
    bilateral *versus* unilateral, efficacy of, 231
    candidates for, 54
    efficacy of, 230–231
    and medication adjustments, 207, 210–211, 211

optimal target for, 229
    selection and evaluation of patient for, 58
    target for, 54
patient selection for, 52–55
in pedunculopontine nucleus, 17, 231
physiologic tolerance to therapeutic effect of, 224
preoperative evaluation for, 59–61, 70–72
profitability of, 41, 45*t*–46*t*
rationale for, 12
regional anatomy and, 190–191, 199–206
reimbursement for, 35–36, 40, 41, 45*t*–46*t*
and resonance effects, 190, 191*f*
response to, time course of, 207–208
risks of, 48
safety, 196–198, 197*f*, 198*f*
stimulator implantation (*See also* Internal pulse
        generator (IPG))
    under general anesthesia, outcomes with, 74*t*–75*t*, 78
STN (*See* Subthalamic nucleus (STN), stimulation)
surgical center for, selection of, 48–50
target sites for, 13
thalamic, 13
    adverse effects of, 229
    for dystonia, 168–169
        efficacy of, 228
    efficacy of, 227–228
    for essential tremor, efficacy of, 227
    historical perspective on, 8
    for parkinsonian tremor, efficacy of, 227–228
    for pathological tremor, 156
    and thalamotomy, comparison of, 163
    for tremor, 153, 155
thalamotomy and, 60
therapeutic adjustments, 181–182, 205*f*, 206–207
    timing of, 207
therapeutic effects of, mechanism of, 16, 18, 20–21
for tremor, 153–165
    anatomical targeting for, 157
    efficacy of, 162
    indications for, 154
    monitoring during, 160
    physiological targeting for, 158, 159, 161*f*
    potential targets for, 155
    results, 163
    sensory and motor effects of, separation of, 160–161
    stereotactic frame placement for, 157
    surgical exposure and trajectory for, 157–158, 159,
        159*f*, 160*f*
Vim (*See* Ventrointermedius (Vim) nucleus, stimulation)
Delong, M.R., 16
Dementia
    DBS-induced, 183
    Lewy body, 58
    in surgical candidate, 52, 53, 58, 60, 70
Denervation, peripheral, for cervical dystonia, 167
Depolarization blockade, 20–21
Depression, 34, 210

assessment for, 53
  postoperative, 230
  in surgical candidate, 52
Dexmedetomidine (DEX)
  dosage and administration of, 79
  indications for, 79–80, 84, 169
Diathermy, safety considerations in, 221, 222
Diplopia, stimulation-induced, 201, 201*f*, 230
Direct current lesioning, 1, 4
Disability, severity of, documentation of, 52
Disequilibrium, stimulation-induced, 231
L-Dopa, 247
  adverse effects and side effects of, 12, 16
    surgical approaches for, historical perspective on, 7
  for dystonia, 168
  historical perspective on, 1, 5, 6–7, 12
  mechanism of action of, 18
  for Parkinson disease
    complications of, 247–248
    limitations of, 247–248
  responsiveness to
    in Parkinson disease, 59
    in surgical candidate, 53, 58
Dopamine
  in basal ganglia–thalamocortical network, 13, 14*f*
  depletion, in Parkinson disease, 12, 15
Dopamine antagonists, 72
Dopamine receptor(s)
  D1, 13, 15
  D2, 13, 15
Dopaminergic challenge testing, specifications for, 53
Dopaminergic medications, perioperative management of, 61
Double vision. *See* Diplopia
Draping, intraoperative, 76, 84–85
Dysarthria, stimulation-induced, 162, 223–224, 229, 230
Dyskinesia
  after fetal tissue transplantation, 7, 249
  drug-induced, pathophysiology of, 15–16
  levodopa-induced, 6, 248, 249
    pathophysiology of, 17
    radiosurgery for, 237–238
  stimulation-induced, 202, 210, 230
  treatment of, historical perspective on, 5, 8
Dysphonia, spasmodic, 166
Dyspraxia, postoperative, historical perspective on, 1
Dystonia
  adult-onset, 166
  age of onset, prognostic significance of, 166
  anesthetic complications in, 80
  basal ganglia–thalamocortical network neuronal
      activity in, 14*f*
  brachial, 166
  cervical, 166 (*See also* Torticollis)
    DBS for, efficacy of, 228–229
    focal, peripheral denervation procedures for, 167
    intraoperative evaluation of neck movement in,
      frameless technology and, 143, 147

    peripheral denervation procedures for, 167
    rating scale for, 168
    surgery for, historical perspective on, 169–170
  childhood-onset, DBS for, 231
  classification of, 166–167
  clinical characteristics of, 12, 59, 60
  clinical evaluation of, 168
  cranial–cervical, 166
  crural, 166
  deep brain stimulation for (*See* Deep brain stimulation
      (DBS), for dystonia)
  definition of, 166
  L-dopa and, 16, 166–167
    peak dose, 16
  dopa-responsive, 59
  DYT-1 (*See DYT1* gene mutation)
  early-onset, 166
  epidemiology of, 38
  focal, 12, 166
    deep brain stimulation for, results, 175–179
    secondary, 166–167
    treatment of, 54–55, 59, 168
  generalized, 12, 51, 166
    rating scales for, 55
    treatment of, 54
  heredodegenerative, 166
  intraoperative complications in, 80
  laryngeal, 166
  medical treatment of, 12, 59, 166, 167, 168
    efficacy of, 169
  medication interactions in, 71*t*, 72
  multifocal, 166
  neuropathology of, 12
  "off," 16
  pallidal DBS for, efficacy of, 228–229
  pantothenate-kinase-associated neurodegeneration and, 51
  in Parkinson disease, drug-induced, 71*t*, 72
  pathophysiology of, 12, 14*f*, 15–16, 17
    rate hypothesis of, 175
  physiological models of, 174
  posttraumatic, 166–167
  preoperative comorbidity in, 70–72, 71*t*
  primary, 50–51, 59, 166
    genetics of, 12, 51
    rate and pattern model for, 19–20, 19*f*
  primary generalized
    deep brain stimulation for
      efficacy of, 231
      results, 180
    surgical outcomes with, 168
  prognosis for, 166
  rating scales for, 168
  rebound effect, with discontinuation of stimulation, 230
  secondary, 12, 51, 166–167
    deep brain stimulation for, results, 179–180
    pallidal DBS for, efficacy of, 228–229
    treatment of, 55

segmental, 12, 166
 deep brain stimulation for, efficacy of, 231
 treatment of, 54–55
stimulation-induced, 230
surgery for, 60, 119
 historical perspective on, 167, 169–170
 microelectrode recording in, 120
 selection and evaluation of patient for, 54–55, 59, 70–72
thalamic DBS for
 efficacy of, 228
 results, 180
treatment of, 13
 historical perspective on, 6, 12
Dystonia Medical Research Foundation, 39
Dystonia musculorum deformans, 166
Dystonia-plus syndromes, 166
DYT1 gene mutation, 51
 and response to deep brain stimulation, 54, 59, 122, 168, 181, 228
 and response to stereotactic lesioning, 168

E
Elderly
 preoperative screening of, 70, 71*t*
 surgical risk factors in, 70
Electrode(s), 3, 4. *See also* Microelectrode recording
Electrolysis, 1
 with DBS contact, 222
Electrophysiological mapping, 116–120
 anesthesia for, 76, 171
 as quality assurance procedure, 122
Electrophysiology, 187–190
 of basal ganglia, 17–18
Emerging applications, 231
Epilepsy, 6, 13, 19, 137
Error(s), in movement disorder surgery
 correction for, 87
 prevention of, 87
 sources of, 87, 122
Error distribution system, 17–18
Essential tremor (ET)
 anesthetic complications with, 80
 causes of, 153
 clinical characteristics of, 59
 deep brain stimulation for (*See* Deep brain stimulation (DBS), for essential tremor)
 diagnosis of, history in, 59
 differential diagnosis of, 50, 59, 153, 153*t*
 epidemiology of, 12, 38, 59, 153
 familial, 153
 incidence of, 153
 intraoperative complications with, 80
 medical treatment of, 12, 59
 medication interactions in, 71*t*, 72
 preoperative comorbidity in, 70, 71*t*
 preoperative evaluation of, 54
 prevalence of, 59, 153

radiosurgery for, 237–238
 results, 243, 244*t*
surgery for, selection and evaluation of patient for, 54, 59
treatment of, historical perspective on, 5, 12
tremor cells in, 155
ET. *See* Essential tremor (ET)
Evidence-based medicine, 8
Excitation, 1
Extrapyramidal symptoms, in Parkinson disease, drug-induced worsening of, 71*t*, 72
Extrapyramidal system, 16
 surgical approaches to, historical perspective on, 2, 3*f*
 understanding of, historical perspective on, 1–2
Eye(s)
 conjugate deviation, 211
 stimulation-induced, 201
 skewed deviation, 211
 stimulation-induced, causing diplopia, 201, 201*f*
Eyelid apraxia, stimulation-induced, 211, 230

F
Faradic stimulation, 1
Fenelon, F., 3*f*
Fetal tissue transplantation, for Parkinson disease, 7, 248–249
Fibroblast growth factor (FGF), 252
Fiducials
 for frameless target localization, 140, 141–142, 142*f*, 143, 144*f*, 148, CP 10.2, CP 10.3, CP 10.8
 implantation of, anesthesia for, 73
 MRI distortion caused by, 66
Fluoroscope, C-arm, in frameless approach, 143, 144*f*, CP 10.7
Foerster, O., 2
Foramen of Monro, as stereotactic landmark, 3
Forel field(s), 5–6, 104*f*, 155
 magnetic resonance imaging of, 159*f*
Fosphenytoin, for intraoperative seizures, 78
Frame(s). *See* Stereotactic apparatus
Frameless technology, 8, 31, 62, 140, 172. *See also* Nex-frame Frameless Microelectrode Recording Guidance Assembly
 anesthetic approach with, 73
 for stereotactic functional neurosurgery, 140–152
 advantages of, 147
 draping for, 143, 144*f*, CP 10.7
 in dystonia, 169
 electrode depth tracking with, 146, 148
 fiducials for, 140, 141–142, 142*f*, 143, 144*f*, 148, CP 10.2, CP 10.3, CP 10.8
 microrecording with, 146, 148
 operative procedure, 141–147, 142*f*–147*f*, CP 10.9B
 patient positioning for, 142–143, 143*f*, CP 10.6
 pitfalls of, 148–149
 preoperative imaging for, 142, 143*f*, CP 10.5
 results with, 147
 sedation for, 142
 skull fixation for, 144–145, 145*f*
 surgical planning with, 148

system verification, 141, 141*f*
target depth, 145–146
trajectory guide, 144–145, 145*f*, 146*f*
target localization for, 140–143, 141*f*, 142*f*, 143, 144*f*,
    CP 10.2, CP 10.3, CP 10.8
FrameLink Stereotactic Linking System software, 85, 85*f*,
    145, 157
Freezing, 17
Fritsch, G., 1
Frontal release signs, 220
Functional neurosurgery, 8, 12. *See also* Ablative surgery;
        Functional neurosurgery; Robotic surgery;
        Stereotactic surgery
    advances in (future directions for), 55, 110
    adverse events with, assessment of, 55
    anatomical targets for, 19–20
    anesthetic approach for, 72, 74*t*–75*t*
        decision-making about, 72
    bilateral
        procedure for second side, 104, 105*f*
        risks of, 241
    candidates for, 52
        preoperative concomitant conditions in, 70, 71*t*
    center for, selection of, 48
    complications of (*See* Complications)
    contraindications to, 60
    evidence-based criteria for, 55
    historical perspective on, 6, 153
    indications for, 50–51, 58
    infection after, treatment of, 109
    intraoperative care for, multidisciplinary team for, 49
    lesioning, procedure for, 103
    long-term effects of, assessment of, 55
    multidisciplinary approach for, 32
    operating room setup for, 86, 86*f*
    outcomes with
        factors affecting, 60
        patient/family expectations for, preoperative man-
            agement of, 60
    planning for, 85–86, 85*f*
    postoperative care for, multidisciplinary team for, 49–50
    preoperative care for, multidisciplinary team for, 48–49
    preoperative preparation for, 61, 83–84
    preparation for, 58–67
    selection and evaluation of patient for, 52–55, 58–59,
        59–61, 70–72
    therapeutic effects of, mechanism of, 18–21
    training in, 31
Functional neurosurgery practice
    and adjunct medical fields, 36–37
    building up, 32, 37, 41
    business of, 38–40
    capital expenses for, 25–27
    core team in, 32–36, 33*f*, 37
    facilities and support for, assessment of, 41, 42*t*
    neuronal recording systems for, 29–30, 29*t*
    program for, building, 32, 37
    reimbursement in, 40–46
    setting up, 25–45
    staff for, 32
    stereotactic targeting software for, 30–32, 30*t* (*See also*
        Software)
Fusion imaging, 157

G
Gait, 17
    disturbances
        parkinsonian, treatment of, 155
        stimulation-induced, 201*f*, 202
Gamma-aminobutyric acid (GABA), 13
    in basal ganglia–thalamocortical network, 13, 14*f*
    in dystonia, 174–175
Gamma Knife, 7, 237–246. *See also* Radiosurgery
    bilateral lesioning with, results, 243, 245*t*
    clinical applications of, 237
    complications with, 238, 241, 244–245
    controversies about, 238
    historical perspective on, 237
    indications for, 237–238
    mistargeting with, 238
    patient evaluation and selection for, 237
    radiation dose with, 238, 241, 242
    results with, 242–245
    targeting for, 238
        for pallidotomy, 239–240, 240*f*
        for thalamotomy, 238–239, 240*f*
Ganglionectomy, historical perspective on, 2
Gangliosidosis
    GM$_1$, 166
    GM$_2$, 166
Gas, intraparenchymal, production of, by DBS contact
        electrolysis, 222
GDNF. *See* Glial cell line–derived neurotrophic factor (GDNF)
General anesthesia, 70
    complications of, 80
    for deep brain stimulation, 78, 171
        outcomes with, 74*t*–75*t*, 78
    for imaging, 73
    indications for, 70, 72
    for microelectrode mapping, 76–78
    recommendations for, 80
    for surgery, 74*t*–75*t*, 76–78, 84
Gene therapy
    advances in (future directions for), 254
    in vivo
        in Parkinson disease, 252–254
        viral vectors for, 252–253
Gillingham, F.J., 2
Glial cell line–derived neurotrophic factor (GDNF), 252
    therapy with
        for Parkinson disease
            adverse effects and side effects of, 252
            intraparenchymal delivery, 252
            results, 252

in rodent model of Parkinson disease, 252
  viral delivery of, 252–254
Global Dystonia Rating Scale (GDRS), 55, 168
Globus pallidus, 13
  external segment (GPe), 13, 14*f*, 17, 171
    magnetic resonance imaging of, 116
    microelectrode mapping, 92*f*
      effects of sedation/anesthesia, 76–77, 171
    microelectrode recordings, 92–93, 94*f*
      in dystonia, 173–174, 173*f*
    microelectrode trajectory for, 92, 93*f*
  imaging of, 64, 116, 116*f*
  indirect targeting of, 65*t*
  internal segment (GPi), 14*f*, 17
    anatomy of, 92, 92*f*, 93*f*
    lead implantation in, 100–102
    lesioning
      for dystonia, 170
      for Parkinson disease, 170
    magnetic resonance imaging of, 116, 130
    microelectrode mapping, effects of sedation/
      anesthesia, 76–77, 77*f*, 171
    microelectrode recording in, 92–96, 92*f*, 94*f*, 95*f*, 96*t*
      in dystonia, 173–174, 173*f*, 174*f*
    microelectrode trajectory for, 92, 93*f*
    operative complications in, 215*t*, 216*t*
    in Parkinson disease, 17
    regional anatomy of, 204–206, 204*f*, 205*f*
    somatotopy, 171
    stimulation, 13
      bilateral *versus* unilateral, efficacy of, 231
      for dystonia, 168, 170–172
      efficacy of, 228–229
      indications for, 60, 155
      insufficient efficacy, without side effects, 205
      in Parkinson disease, 54
      side effects of, 182
      for tremor, 155
    targeting of, 66
  microelectrode recording in, in dystonia, 173–174,
      173*f*, 174*f*
  stimulation
    adverse effects of, 182–183, 229–230
    for dystonia, efficacy of, 228–229
    for Parkinson disease, efficacy of, 228
  surgical approaches to, historical perspective on, 3*f*, 5, 6
Glutamate, in basal ganglia–thalamocortical network, 13,
      14*f*, 15
GP. *See* Globus pallidus
GPe. *See* Globus pallidus, external segment (GPe)
GPi. *See* Globus pallidus, internal segment (GPi)
Guiot, G., 2, 3*f*

H
Hallucination(s), visual
  in Lewy body dementia, 58
  medication-induced, 58

Halothane, drug interactions with, 72
Hardware erosion, 162–163, 230, 232
  management of, 220
  prevention of, 220
Hardware-related complications, 215*t*, 219–222, 230, 232
Hassler, R., 4, 5, 6
HD. *See* Huntington disease (HD)
Headache, postoperative, 229
Hécaen, H., stereotaxic apparatus used by, 3
Hematoma
  capsular, 216*t*
  as operative complication, 214, 216*f*, 229
    asymptomatic, 214, 215*t*, 216*f*
    chronic subdural, 215*t*
    prevention of, 218
    signs of, 215–216
  subdural, postoperative, 163
  thalamic, 216*t*
    postoperative, 163
Hemiathetosis, postscarlatina, treatment of, historical
      perspective on, 1
Hemiballismus, 162
  pathophysiology of, 15–16, 17
  poststroke, 5
  treatment of, historical perspective on, 2, 5
Hemichorea, pathophysiology of, 17
Hemidystonia, 51, 166
Hemiparkinsonism, treatment of, historical perspective
      on, 2, 3*f*
Hemorrhage
  in deep brain stimulation, 123, 162
  in microelectrode recording, 86, 89, 123
  as operative complication, 162, 229
    asymptomatic, 214, 215*t*
    intraparenchymal, 218
    management of, 214–216
    prevention of, 218
    symptomatic, 214, 215*t*
  in pallidotomy, 123
Hess, W.R., 5
Hitzig, E., 1
HIV-infected (AIDS) patients, 61
Horsley, Victor, 1, 2*f*, 4, 6, 138
hRPE. *See* Human retinal epithelial pigment cells (hRPE)
HSi-BP3 gene, in familial essential tremor, 153
Human retinal epithelial pigment cells (hRPE), 251
Huntington chorea. *See* Huntington disease (HD)
Huntington disease, 166
  treatment of, historical perspective on, 3, 6
Huntington's Disease Society of America, 39
Hydrocephalus, 51
Hyperkinesia
  pathophysiology of, 15–18
  surgical treatment of, historical perspective on, 3*f*
Hypertonus, surgical treatment of, historical perspective
      on, 3*f*
Hypokinesia, pathophysiology of, 15–18

Hypomania, stimulation-induced, 210–211, 230
Hypophonia, stimulation-induced, 230, 231

I

Image fusion, 64, 66, 83, 122–123
    preoperative, with frameless technology, 142, 143*f*, CP
        10.5
Image-guided neuronavigation system, 31–32
Imaging, 18. *See also* Computed tomography (CT);
        Magnetic resonance imaging (MRI)
    advances in (future directions for), 8, 37
    historical perspective on, 7
    postoperative, 80
        for hemorrhage detection, 214
    preoperative, 62
    sedation for, 73
    stereotactic, 62–64, 115–116
Impedance recording, for physiological corroboration of
        anatomical target, 117, 118*f*, 122
Implantable pulse generator. *See* Internal pulse generator (IPG)
Implantable stimulator(s). *See also* Internal pulse
        generator (IPG)
    historical perspective on, 1, 7–9
Infection(s)
    postoperative, 162–163, 217, 230
        hardware-related, 215*t*, 217, 230, 232
        microbiology of, 217
        prevention of, 217, 218
        risk factors for, 229
        superficial, treatment of, 218–219
        treatment of, 109, 217, 218–219
    prevention of, 84
Insulin-like growth factor(s), 252
Intercommissural line, as stereotactic landmark, 3
Intermittent pulse generator. *See* Internal pulse generator (IPG)
Internal capsule
    anatomy of, 202
    magnetic resonance imaging of, 93*f*, 116, 132*f*, 159*f*, CP 9.7
    stimulation, 172
    surgical approaches to, historical perspective on, 2
Internal globus pallidus (GPi), 13–23, 67, 110, 174
Internal pulse generator (IPG)
    battery life, 107–108, 209–210, 230
    complications with, 215*t*, 217, 218, 218*f*
    constant voltage *versus* constant current, 192
    end-of-life replacement (for battery depletion),
        107–108, 209–210, 230
    implantation of, 104–107, 106*f*–108*f*, 158, 172
        costs of, 41
        reimbursement for, 40–41
    patient manipulation of (*See also* Twiddler syndrome)
        damage to lead or lead extender by, 222
    programming, 183 (*See also* Deep brain stimulation
        (DBS), devices for)
    status, patient assessment of, 207
International Essential Tremor Foundation, 39
Internet resources, 39
Intraoperative microelectrode recording (MER)

    for confirmation of lead placement, 169
    historical perspective on, 7
Intubation, 84
    emergent, 80
    with intraoperative seizures, 78
    with stereotactic frame in place, 76
IPG. *See* Internal pulse generator (IPG)

J
Jackson, H., 1

K
Klosovski, B.N., 2*f*

L
Laitinen stereotactic apparatus, 116
Lamina pallidi incompleta. *See* Medullary lamina, accessory
Lamina pallidi lateralis. *See* Medullary lamina, lateral
Lamina pallidi medialis. *See* Medullary lamina, medial
Laminectomy, historical perspective on, 1
Laryngeal mask airway (LMA), 73, 76, 79, 169
    with intraoperative seizures, 78
Laryngospasm, 80
Lead(s). *See* Deep brain stimulation (DBS), lead(s)
Lee, A. St. J., 4
Leksell, L., 167, 237, 241
    stereotaxic apparatus used by, 3, 4*f*
Leksell Model G stereotactic head frame, 61–62, 62*f*, 84
Leksell Stereotactic System, 25–26, 26*f*, 116, 157, 237, CP
        3.1
    advantages of, 31
    components of, 25–26, 26*f*
    cost of, 26
Lentivirus (LV), as vector for gene therapy, 253
Lesioning, therapeutic effects of, mechanism of, 18
Leukotome, 4
Levodopa. *See* L-Dopa
Lewy bodies, 12
Lewy body dementia, 58
LFPs. *See* Local field potentials (LFPs)
Lhermitte syndrome, with GDNF therapy, 252
Libido, increased, stimulation-induced, 230
Local anesthesia
    advantages and disadvantages of, 70
    indications for, 72, 171
    and postoperative care, 80
    for stereotactic frame placement, 72–73, 85
    for surgery, 73–76, 85
Local field potentials (LFPs), in subthalamic nucleus,
        oscillatory frequency bands in, 18

M
Macrostimulation
    advantages and disadvantages of, 120
    multiple electrodes and, 138–139
    for physiological corroboration of anatomical target,
        118–120, 122, 158

Magnetic resonance imaging (MRI), 12. *See also* Image fusion
  after radiosurgery, 242–243, 242*f*, 243*f*, 244*f*
  of DBS lead locations, 102–103, 103*f*
  deep brain stimulation and, 222
  diagnostic, 51
  distortion, 83, 158, 238, 241
    overcoming, 63–64
    sources of, 63, 65–66
  fast spin echo inversion recovery, 64, 64*f*, 64*t*
    for target selection, 64–65, 66
  for Gamma Knife thalamotomy or pallidotomy, 239, 239*t*
  intraoperative, 122
  of lead positioning, 220–221
  magnetization-prepared rapid gradient echo (MPRAGE), 66
  postoperative, 80
    of DBS stimulation systems, 220–221, 221*t*
    and detection of hemorrhage, 214, 216*f*
    for hemorrhage detection, 214
  preoperative, with frameless technology, 142, 143*f*
  for robotic surgery, 129–130, 131*f*, CP 9.6
  safety considerations in, 221, 221*t*
  sedation for, 73
  stereotactic
    postoperative, 120–121, 121*f*
    for target localization, 115–116
    for surgical planning/target localization, 63–64, 64*f*,
      64*t*, 83, 84, 123, 157, 159, 159*f*, 171, 238, 241
    parameters used for, 66, 66*t*
    requirements for, 115–116
  three-dimensional, 63–64
Malignant syndrome, 71*t*, 72
Mania, stimulation-induced, 210–211
Marsden and Obeso paradox, 17–18
Mattis Dementia Rating Scale (MDRS), 53
MEA. *See* Midbrain extrapyramidal area (MEA)
Mechanical introduction effect, for physiological
      corroboration of anatomical target, 118
Medication(s)
  for dystonia, 168
  historical perspective on, 1
  parkinsonism caused by, 59
  perioperative management of, 59, 60*t*, 70, 71*t*, 80, 83
  preoperative evaluation of, 59
  tremor caused by, 59
Medication interactions, risk for, preoperative evaluation
      of, 70, 72
Medtronic, 27–32, 41, 44, 64, 85, 87, 88, 95, 100–108,
      146, 149, 151, 160, 161, 170–172, 181, 195–197,
      208–210, 218, 221, 232, 247
Medulla oblongata, rubrospinal and tegmental tracts in, sur-
      gical approaches to, historical perspective on, 2, 2*f*
Medullary lamina
  accessory, magnetic resonance imaging of, 93*f*
  lateral, magnetic resonance imaging of, 93*f*
  medial, magnetic resonance imaging of, 93*f*
Meige syndrome, 177
Memory problems, stimulation-induced, 230
Meperidine, drug interactions with, 72

MER. *See* Microelectrode recording (MER)
N-Methyl-D-aspartate (NMDA) receptor antagonists, 248
Metoclopramide, drug interactions with, 72
Mexiletine, for dystonia, 168
Meyers, R., 2–3, 2*f*, 3*f*
Microelectrode recording (MER)
  advances in (future directions for), 110, 138–139
  advantages and disadvantages of, 120
  alternatives to, 115
  artifacts, 87, 89, 89*t*, 90*f*
    mechanical, 89, 90*f*
    pulse, 89, 90*f*
  in basal ganglia, 173–174, 173*f*, 174*f*
  clinical applications of, 29
  in deep brain stimulation for dystonia, 172–174
  deep sedation for, 76–78
  depth of recording in, 87
  equipment for, 28–30, 29*t*, 32
  general anesthesia for, 76–78
  globus pallidus internus, 92–96, 92*f*, 94*f*, 95*f*, 96*t*
  hemorrhage in, 86, 89
  historical perspective on, 83
  imaging and, 36–37
  interference with, sources of, 88, 89, 89*t*
  intraoperative
    for confirmation of lead placement, 169
    historical perspective on, 7
  and intraoperative testing, 89–91
  microdrive for, 29–30
  microelectrode guide tube for, 87, 88
  micropositioner system for, 87–88
  multiple simultaneous recordings in, 88–89, 88*f*, 138–139
  neurophysiologist's role in, 34–35
  outcomes with, evaluation of, 123–124
  procedure for, 87–89
  rationale for, 115, 122
  recording equipment for, 30
  sedation effects and, 169
  with stereotactic surgery, 83–114
  subthalamic nucleus, 96–100, 97*f*, 98*f*, 99*t*
  for targeting, 64–65, 115, 122, 158, 171, 241
  in target localization/refinement, 122–123
  thalamic, 91–92, 91*t*
  in thalamus, 174
Microlesioning, 118
Microsubthalamotomy, 207
microTargeting Platform (FHC), 149–151, 150*f*, 151*f*
Midazolam, 79
  indications for, 73
  for intraoperative seizures, 78
Midbrain extrapyramidal area (MEA), 17
Midcommissural point (MCP), 65, 83, 168
Minnesota Multiphasic Personality Inventory (MMPI), 53
Misdiagnosis, 60
Monitoring, intraoperative, with local anesthesia, 73
Monkey
  basal ganglia–thalamocortical network, neuronal
      activity in, 14*f*

MPTP model of Parkinson disease, 16
physiological experiments in, historical perspective on, 1
Monoamine oxidase inhibitors (MAOIs), 248
drug interactions with, 72
Montgomery and Asberg Depression Rating Scale (MADRS), 53
Mood changes
postoperative, 232
stimulation-induced, 202
Mortality rate(s), historical perspective on, 1, 2, 4, 5, 6
Motor cortex
primary, ablation, historical perspective on, 2
surgical approaches to, historical perspective on, 2*f*
Movement disorder neurologist
and preoperative screening of patients, 59
role of, 32–34, 37
intraoperative, 49
postoperative, 49
in preoperative period, 48
Movement disorders, pathophysiology of, 15–18
Movement Disorder Society, 40
Movement disorder surgery. *See* Functional neurosurgery
Movement-related cortical potentials (MRCPs), in dystonia, 174–175
MPTP, parkinsonism caused by, 6–7, 16
monkey model, surgical interventions in, 19–20
pathophysiology of, 15
MSA. *See* Multiple system atrophy (MSA)
Multiple sclerosis (MS), tremor in. *See* Tremor, in multiple sclerosis
Multiple system atrophy (MSA)
clinical course of, 51
clinical presentation of, 51
differential diagnosis of, 50, 51, 60
magnetic resonance imaging in, 51
positron emission tomography in, 58
subgroups of, 51
Muscle contractions, stimulation-induced, 201–202, 201*f*, 202*f*, 203, 205, 230
Muscle relaxants, for dystonia, 168
Myers, R., 167

N
Narabayashi, H., 4, 5
stereotaxic apparatus used by, 3
National Parkinson Foundation, 39
Nausea, postoperative, 229
Nerve growth factor (NGF), 251
Neurological deterioration, intraoperative, 79, 80
Neurologist. *See* Movement disorder neurologist
NeuroMate robotic arm. *See also* Robotic surgery
advantages of, 138
components of, 126–128, 127*f*
computer for, 126–128
robotic arm of, 126, 127*f*, CP 9.2
stereotactic frame for, 128, 128*f*, CP 9.3

Neuronal elements, definition of, 187
Neuronal recording systems, 29, 29*t*
equipment for, 28–30, 29*t*
microdrive for, 29–30
recording equipment for, 30
Neuronavigation systems, 30–32, 30*t*
Neurophysiologist, role of, 34–35
Neuropsychologist, role of, 34
Neuroradiology, 36–37
Neurosurgeon
and preoperative screening of patients, 59
role of, 36, 37
intraoperative, 49
in preoperative period, 48–49
Neurotransmitter(s)
in basal ganglia–thalamocortical network, 13, 14*f*
of striatal spiny neurons, 13
Neurotransplantation, for Parkinson disease, 248
allografts for, 248
autografts for, 248
xenografts for, 248
Neurotrophic factors, 251–255
therapy with
delivery mechanism for, 251–252
historical perspective on, 251
Neurotrophin 4 (NT-4), 252
Neurturin. *See* Glial cell line–derived neurotrophic factor (GDNF)
Neuturin gene therapy, 252
Nexframe Frameless Microelectrode Recording Guidance Assembly, 27–28, 27*f*, CP 3.4
Nexframe Passive Head Rest, 142
Nexframe System, 27–28, 27*f*, 140
advantages of, 148
clinical use of, 145, 145*f*
disadvantages of, 148–149
multilumen adapters for, 146, 147*f*, CP 10.12
offset adapter, 146, 147*f*, CP 10.12
results with, 147
reticules system, 148, 149*f*
trajectory guide, 144–145, 145*f*, 146*f*
Nitrogen, liquid, in cryoprobe, 4
Nonsteroidal anti-inflammatory drugs (NSAIDs), perioperative management of, 60*t*
nRt. *See* Reticular nucleus (nRt)
Nurse practitioner, role of, 35, 37
in preoperative care, 49

O
Obrador, S., 4
Obsessive-compulsive disorder (OCD), 13, 19, 137
Ohm's law, 191–192, 192*f*
Oil–procaine lesioning, 4
Oil–procaine–wax lesioning, 4
Okuma, T., 4, 5
Oliver, L.C., 2, 2*f*
Olivopontocerebellar atrophy (OPCA), 51
OPCA. *See* Olivopontocerebellar atrophy (OPCA)

Opiates, drug interactions with, 72
Oppenheim, H., 166
Optic tract, 93–96, 95*f*, 214
  magnetic resonance imaging of, 93*f*, 116

P
Pacemaker, cardiac, in surgical candidate, 52, 59, 232
Pain control, medications for, perioperative management
    of, 60*t*
Pallidoansotomy, 5
Pallidothalamotomy, 5
Pallidotomy, 13
  bilateral, in Parkinson disease, 238
  complications of, 214
  and DBS, 60
  for dystonia
    efficacy of, 170
    historical perspective on, 167
  gamma knife and, 7
  historical perspective on, 1, 2*f*, 5–6, 7, 8, 167
  indications for, 20
  Marsden and Obeso paradox and, 17
  posteroventral (PVP), 167
  procedure for, 103
  radiosurgical
    complications of, 245
    current status of, 241
    indications for, 237–238
    targeting, 239–240, 240*f*
  response to, predictors of, 58
  target localization for, 122–123
  therapeutic effects of, mechanism of, 16
Pallidum
  magnetic resonance imaging of, 132*f*, CP 9.7
  surgical approaches to, historical perspective on, 5
Pantothenate-kinase-associated neurodegeneration
    (PKAN), dystonia caused by, 51
Paresis, postoperative, historical perspective on, 1
Paresthesia, stimulation-induced, 160, 200, 200*f*, 203,
    204*f*, 223–224, 229, 230
Parkinson disease (PD), 166. *See also* MPTP, parkinsonism
    caused by
  adjuvant therapies for, advances in (future directions
      for), 254
  anesthetic complications in, 80
  basal ganglia–thalamocortical network neuronal
      activity in, 14*f*
  biological therapy, 247–248
  cardinal symptoms of, 12
  cell replacement therapy for, 248–251
    advances in (future directions for), 254
  cellular therapy, 248–251
  clinical course of, 247–248
    before L-dopa, 5
  clinical presentation of, 58
  cognitive decline in, postoperative, 224
  DBS for
    optimal target for, 229
    pallidal, efficacy of, 228
    subthalamic nucleus, efficacy of, 229
  deep brain stimulation for (*See* Deep brain stimulation
      (DBS), for Parkinson disease)
  diagnosis of, 58
    history in, 59
  differential diagnosis of, 50, 51, 59
  disability in, documentation of, 52
  epidemiology of, 38
  globus pallidus internus microelectrode recordings in,
      93, 95*f*
  intraoperative complications in, 80
  juvenile, 51
  medication interactions in, 71*t*, 72
  medications for, deep brain stimulation and, 207
  motor symptoms of, anatomical substrate of, 16
  neuroprotective therapy in, 248
  nonmotor symptoms of
    anatomical substrate of, 16
    DBS for, efficacy of, 231
  off–on evaluation, standardized, 53
  pathology of, 12
  pathophysiology of, 12, 14*f*, 15, 247, 251
  positron emission tomography in, 58
  preoperative comorbidity in, 70, 71*t*
  restorative therapy in, 248
  surgery for
    outcomes, factors affecting, 53
    selection and evaluation of patient for, 53–54, 58, 70
  treatment of, 13
    L-dopa and, 6–7
    goals of, 247
    historical perspective on, 1–2, 5, 6, 8, 12
  tremor cells in, 155
  tremor of, thalamic DBS for, efficacy of, 227–228
  young-onset, 51
Parkinson Disease Questionnaire (PDQ), 230
Parkinsonism
  atypical (*See also* Multiple system atrophy (MSA))
    clinical features of, 58
  drug-induced, 59
  postencephalitic, historical perspective on, 5
Parkinsonism, atypical, 53, 58, 60
Parkinson's Disease Foundation, 39
Parvocellular ventralis caudalis (Vcpc) nucleus, 92
Patient expectations, preoperative management of, 60
Patient liaison, 35–36
Patient referral, 38, 38*f*, 41
PD. *See* Parkinson disease (PD)
Pecker, J., 2
Pedunculopontine nucleus (PPN), 17
  stimulation, 17, 231
Pedunculotomy, historical perspective on, 2*f*
Persephin. *See* Glial cell line–derived neurotrophic factor
    (GDNF)
Phenothiazines, drug interactions with, 72
Phosphenes, 205–206
Photopsia, stimulation-induced, 230

Physician's assistant, role of, 35, 37
  in preoperative care, 49
Physiological experiments, historical perspective on, 1
Pickers, 218
Pineal gland, as stereotactic landmark, 3
PKAN. *See* Pantothenate-kinase-associated neurodegeneration (PKAN)
Placebo effect, 8
Platelet-derived growth factor (PDGF), 252
Pneumocephalus, 79, 80
Polenov, A.L., 2, 2*f*
Positioning, patient, intraoperative, 84–85
  with local anesthesia, 73
Positron emission tomography (PET)
  cortical, in dystonia, 175
  [¹⁸F]fluorodeoxyglucose
    in atypical parkinsonism, 58
    in Parkinson disease, 58
  in tremor, 153
Posterior commissure, 63, 65, 69, 83, 85, 95, 131, 159, 223
Posterior rhizotomy, historical perspective on, 2
Posterior ventromedial (Vmpo) nucleus, 91–92
Posteroventral pallidum
  macrostimulation in, 119
  magnetic resonance imaging of, 116, 116*f*
Postoperative care, providers of, in long term, 60–61
Postural stability, 211, 230, 232
PPN. *See* Pedunculopontine nucleus (PPN)
Practice. *See* Functional neurosurgery practice
Precentral cortex, surgical approach to, historical
    perspective on, 2
Prefrontal lobotomy, 3
Premotor cortex, surgical approaches to, historical
    perspective on, 2*f*
Preoperative care, multidisciplinary team for, 48–49
Preoperative evaluation of patient, 37, 51–55, 59–61, 70–75
Prochlorperazine, drug interactions with, 72
Professional societies, 40
Programming, 19, 32, 35, 37, 38, 40, 44, 49, 52, 100, 138,
    161, 181, 213, 221
Progressive supranuclear palsy (PSP)
  clinical presentation of, 51
  differential diagnosis of, 50, 51
  magnetic resonance imaging in, 51
Propanolol, drug interactions with, 72
Propofol, 79
  drug interactions with, 72
  effect on intraoperative neurophysiology, 76–78, 77*f*, 78*t*, 84
  indications for, 73, 76, 84, 142, 169
PSP. *See* Progressive supranuclear palsy (PSP)
Psychiatric admission hospitalization, postoperative
    (within 6 months), 215*t*
Psychiatric complications, 210–211, 215*t*, 232
Psychiatry, 37
Psychologist, role of
  postoperative, 49–50
  in preoperative care, 49
Psychopathology, 34

Psychosis, in surgical candidate, 52, 53, 60
Publicity, 38–39
Pulvinotomy, historical perspective on, 5, 167
Putamen
  magnetic resonance imaging of, 93*f*, 116
  microelectrode mapping of, 92*f*
  surgical approaches to, historical perspective on, 2
Putnam, T.J., 2, 2*f*
PVP. *See* Pallidotomy, posteroventral (PVP)
Pyramidal system
  ablation, historical perspective on, 2, 2*f*
  surgical approach to, historical perspective on, 2, 2*f*
Pyramidotomy, historical perspective on, 2*f*

Q
Quality of life, DBS and, 232

R
Radiofrequency lesioning
  historical perspective on, 4
  for tremor, 153
Radiosurgery. *See also* Gamma Knife
  advantages of, 237, 241
  clinical benefit of, onset of, 243–244, 244*f*, 244*t*, 245*t*
  complications of, 241
    delayed onset of, 244–245
  for essential tremor, results, 243, 244*t*
  historical perspective on, 241
  indications for, 237–238, 241
  lesion development, latency of, 242–243, 242*f*, 243*f*
  for movement disorders, historical perspective on, 237
  pallidal, complications of, 241, 245
  principles of, 237
  radiation dose for, 238, 241, 242
  results with, 242–245
  of subthalamic nucleus, 241
  thalamotomy
    complications of, 245
    for tremor, results, 243, 244*t*
RBRVS. *See* Resource Based Relative Value System (RBRVS)
Red nucleus, magnetic resonance imaging of, 132*f*, CP 9.7
Reduced Space Electrode, 134
Referrals, 38, 38*f*, 41
Reimbursement, 40–46
  collection tips, 41, 42*t*
  usual and customary billed charges, for physician billing, 41, 43*t*–44*t*
Relative Value Unit (RVU), 40
Remifentanil, indications for, 73, 76, 84
Reoperation
  causes of, 215*t*
  unplanned, causes, 215*t*
Resource Based Relative Value System (RBRVS), 40
Respiratory status, preoperative evaluation of, 70–72, 71*t*
Restless legs syndrome, 210
Reticular nucleus (nRt), 15
Reticule system, 61, 62*f*
Retinal epithelial pigment cells. *See* Human retinal epithelial pigment cells (hRPE)

Rewired for Life Foundation, 39
Rhizotomy, cervical, for dystonia, 169–170
Riechert, T., 4, 5, 6
Riechert/Mundinger (RM) Stereotactic Frame, 27, 27*f*, 31
Rigidity, 17–18
    in Parkinson disease, drug-induced, 71*t*, 72
    parkinsonian, treatment of, 155
    treatment of, historical perspective on, 5–6
Riluzole, for dystonia, 168
Robotic surgery, 126–139. *See also* NeuroMate robotic arm
    advances in (future directions for), 138–139
    advantages and disadvantages of, 136–138
    angiography for, 129, 129*f*
    clinical applications of, 136–138
    complications of, 136
    electrode implantation in
        target planning for, 130–132, 130*f*, 131*t*, 132*f*, CP 9.7
        technique for, 132
    electrophysiologic testing in, 132–135, 133*f*, 134*f*, 135*f*,
        CP 9.8, CP 9.9
    flat digitized detectors for, 127*f*, 128–129, 128*f*, CP 9.3
    image data for, acquisition of, 129–130
    magnetic resonance imaging for, 129–130, 131*f*, CP 9.6
    method for, 129–135
    microrecording and stimulation in, 132–135, 133*f*, 134*f*,
        135*f*, CP 9.8, CP 9.9
    number of cases, 135
    rationale for, 136–138
    results, 135–136
    stereotactic frame for, application of, 129
    ventriculography for, 129, 130*f*
    X-ray acquisition for, 129–130
    X-ray tubes for, 127*f*, 128
RVU. *See* Relative Value Unit (RVU)

S
Scientific method, 8
SDS. *See* Shy-Drager syndrome (SDS)
Secretary, 35–36
Sedation, 79
    conscious, for burr hole procedure, 76
    deep
        electrical stimulation under, 78
        for microelectrode mapping, 76–78
        recommendations for, 80
        for surgery, 74*t*–75*t*, 76–78
    for deep brain stimulation, 169
    effect on intraoperative neurophysiology, 76–78, 77*f*, 78*t*
    for frameless techniques, 73
    for imaging, 73
    for stereotactic frame placement, 72–73, 84
    for surgery, 84
SEEG. *See* Stereoelectroencephalography (SEEG)
Seizures
    intraoperative, 78, 80, 215*t*
    postoperative, 80, 215*t*, 229
Seligiline, drug interactions with, 72
Semimicroelectrodes, 122, 169

Sevofluorane, effect on intraoperative neurophysiology,
    77–78, 77*f*, 78*t*
Shy-Drager syndrome (SDS), 51
Sialorrhea, stimulation-induced, 230
Skull phantom, 141, 141*f*, CP 10.1A
Sleep disturbance, in surgical candidate, 59
SNc. *See* Substantia nigra, pars compacta (SNc)
SND. *See* Striatonigral degeneration (SND)
SNr. *See* Substantia nigra, pars reticulata (SNr)
Software
    Alpha Omega microguide, 133, 138
    FrameLink Stereotactic Linking System, 85, 85*f*, 145, 157
    for microTargeting Platform (FHC), 150, 150*f*
    neuronavigation, 126–128, 137, 137*f*, CP 9.13
    for planning with frameless technology, 141
    stereotactic targeting, 30–32, 30*t*
    targeting, 65
        frame-based, 65
    for trajectory-based aiming, 145, 146*f*, CP 10.10
Spasticity, treatment of, historical perspective on, 5, 6
Specific absorption rate (SAR), 221, 232
Speech dysfunction. *See also* Dysarthria; Dysphonia, spas-
        modic; Hypophonia, stimulation-induced
    stereotactic lesioning and, 225
    stimulation-induced, 204, 211, 229, 231
Spheramine, 251, 251*f*
Spiegel, E.A., 2*f*, 3–4, 5–6
Spiegel/Wycis stereotaxic apparatus, 3, 4*f*
Spiny neurons, striatal, 13
STarFix system, 27, 28–29, 28*f*, 140, 149, 151*f*, CP 3.5
Status dystonicus, DBS for, 231
StealthStation, 31–32, 85, 85*f*, 145, 146*f*, 218, CP 10.10
Stem cell transplantation, for Parkinson disease, 7,
        249–251, 250*f*
Stereoelectroencephalography (SEEG), 127, 129, 135,
        135*f*, 137, 137*f*, CP 9.13
Stereoencephalotomy, 3
Stereotactic apparatus
    application of, 61–62, 62*f*, 84, 157, 169
        accuracy of, 65
        anesthesia for, 72–73
        errors in, prevention of, 87
        precautions with, 87
    capital expense for, 25–27
    components of, 25–27
    costs of, 25–27
    development of, 1, 3, 4*f*, 6
    historical perspective on, 8
    reapplication of, 62
    selection of, 31, 61
    types of, 3, 4*f*
Stereotactic atlas, first, 1, 6
Stereotactic imaging, 62–64
Stereotactic lesioning, complications of, 214, 225. *See also*
        Complications
Stereotactic surgery. *See also* Functional neurosurgery
    ablative, reintroduction of, historical perspective on, 7
    early era of, 3–6

first human procedure, 6
goal of, 1
historical perspective on, 1, 3–6, 8
with microelectrode recording, 83–114
outcomes with, evaluation of, 123–124
procedures, numbers of, trends in, 6
without microelectrode recording, 115–125
outcomes with, evaluation of, 123–124
Stereotactic targeting software, 30–32, 30*t. See also* Software
Sterile fluid collections, as operative complication, 217, 219
Stimloc, 87, 102, 102*f*, 144, 146, 148
Stimulation. *See also* Deep brain stimulation (DBS)
direct current, 1
electrical, 1
faradic, 1
historical perspective on, 7–8
mechanical, 1
therapeutic effects of, 18
unipolar *vs.* bipolar, 1
Stimulation mapping
anesthesia for, 76, 78, 171
deep sedation and, 78
STN. *See* Subthalamic nucleus (STN)
Striatonigral degeneration (SND), 51
Striatum, 13
Stroke
definition of, 214
as operative complication, 214–217, 215*t*, 229
delayed ischemic subcortical, stereotactic lesioning
and, 225
frontal venous, 216*t*
hemorrhagic, 214, 215*t*
precipitating factors/etiology, 214, 216*t*
ischemic, 214, 215*t*, 217*f*
management of, 214–216
prevention of, 214
in stereotactic lesioning, 225
venous, prevention of, 218
tremor caused by (*See* Tremor, in stroke patient)
Substantia nigra, 13
magnetic resonance imaging of, 97*f*
pars compacta (SNc), 13
in Parkinson disease, 14*f*
pars reticulata (SNr), 13, 14*f*, 17
magnetic resonance imaging of, 97*f*
stimulation of, 101*f*
unintended stimulation of, 210, 211
stimulation of, emotional responses caused by, 210, 220
Subthalamic nucleus (STN), 13, 14*f*, 17, 155
anatomy of, 96, 97*f*
gamma activity in, 18
imaging of, 64
indirect targeting of, 65*t*
lead implantation in, 100–102, 101*f*
lesioning, procedure for, 104, 104*f*
local field potentials in, oscillatory frequency bands in, 18
macrostimulation in, 119–120

magnetic resonance imaging of, 116, 117*f*, 130–131,
132*f*, CP 9.7
mechanical stunning effect (microlesion) in, with introduction of stereotactic probe, 118
microelectrode mapping, effects of sedation/anesthesia,
77, 77*f*
microelectrode recordings, 96–100, 97*f*, 98*f*, 99*t*
operative complications in, 215*t*, 216*t*
in Parkinson disease, 17
radiosurgery of, 241
regional anatomy, 199–202, 199*f*, 200*f*
somatotopy of, 99, 100*f*
stimulation, 13, 19–20, 20*f*, 210–211
adverse effects of, 230
bilateral *versus* unilateral, efficacy of, 231
for dystonia, 170
efficacy of, 229
historical perspective on, 8
indications for, 60, 155
for Parkinson disease, 54, 58
and nonmotor symptoms, 231
in patients with previous surgery, efficacy of, 231
for tremor, 54
surgical interventions in, 19–20, 20*f*
historical perspective on, 5, 7
targeting of, 64–65, 66
advances in (future directions for), 109–110
in Parkinson disease, 19–20, 19*f*
Subthalamotomy
historical perspective on, 2*f*
for Parkinson disease, 19–20
procedure for, 104, 104*f*
therapeutic effects of, mechanism of, 16
Sugita apparatus, 31
Suicide attempt, postoperative (within 6 months), 215*t*, 232
Support groups, outreach to, 41
Surgery. *See* Functional neurosurgery; *specific procedure*
SurgiPlan, 31–32
Sympathetic ramisection, historical perspective on, 2
Synaptic inhibition, 20–21

T
Takebayashi, H., 2
Talairach, J., 5
Talairach stereotactic system, 31
Targeting. *See* Target localization
Target localization, 85–86, 85*f*, 159, 159*f*, 160*f. See also*
Macrostimulation; Microelectrode recording (MER)
accuracy of, 66–67
factors affecting, 241
anatomical, 122–123
factors affecting, 241
computer-assisted, 65
direct methods, 64, 66–67, 83
for frameless techniques, 140–143, 141*f*, 142*f*, 143,
144*f*, CP 10.2, CP 10.3, CP 10.8
for Gamma Knife, 238

imaging for, 62–64
indirect methods, 64, 65*t*, 66–67, 83
intraoperative adjustment, 116–120
magnetic resonance imaging for, 63–64, 64*f*, 64*t*
methods, comparison of, 122
physiologic, 122–123, 158
  factors affecting, 241
radiographic, 122–123
for robotic surgery, 130–132, 130*f*, 131*t*, 132*f*, CP 9.7
Target selection. *See* Target localization
Technology, 8
Thalamic deep brain stimulation, 13
  adverse effects of, 229
  for dystonia, 168–169
    efficacy of, 228
  efficacy of, 227–228
  for essential tremor, efficacy of, 227
  historical perspective on, 8
  for parkinsonian tremor, efficacy of, 227–228
  for pathological tremor, 156
  and thalamotomy, comparison of, 163
  for tremor, 153, 155
Thalamic nuclei, 13–15
  Anglo-American classification of, 154*f*
  anterior, 13
  Hassler classification of, 154*f*, 155, 155*t*
  medial, 13
  microelectrode recordings, 91–92, 91*t*
  nomenclature for, 5
  posterior, 13
  terminology for, 154*f*, 155, 155*t*
  ventrolateral, 13–15
    surgical approaches to, historical perspective on, 5
  Walker nomenclature for, 155, 155*t*
Thalamic subnuclei, 155
Thalamotomy
  bilateral, in Parkinson disease, 238
  and DBS, 60
  for dystonia
    efficacy of, 170
    historical perspective on, 167
  with Gamma Knife, 238
  historical perspective on, 167
  Marsden and Obeso paradox and, 17
  procedure for, 103
  radiosurgical, 237
    complications of, 245
    indications for, 237–238
    targeting, 238–239, 240*f*
    for tremor, results, 243, 244*t*
  and thalamic DBS, comparison of, 163
  therapeutic effects of, mechanism of, 16
  for tremor, 153
  ventrolateral, historical perspective on, 2*f*
Thalamus
  anatomy of, 13–15, 91, 155
    relevant to neurosurgery, 154*f*

in dystonia, 174
imaging of, 64
magnetic resonance imaging of, 130–131, 132*f*, CP 9.7
microelectrode mapping of, 91, 155, 157*f*
microelectrode recordings, 91–92, 91*t*, 174
  pitfalls of, 91–92
microelectrode tracts through, 91, 91*t*, 156*f*, 157*f*
neuronal activity in, in Parkinson disease, 15–16
physiology of, 13–15
somatotopic organization of, 91
stimulation (*See* Deep brain stimulation (DBS), thalamic)
surgical approaches to, historical perspective on, 5, 6
ventrolateral
  microelectrode tracts through, 156*f*
  nomenclature/terminology for, 155, 155*t*
Thermal injury
  with deep brain electrodes, 222, 232
  with MRI, 221, 221*t*, 232
  in stereotactic lesioning, 225
Thyroidectomy, historical perspective on, 2
Toronto Western Spasmodic Torticollis Scale (TWSTRS),
    55, 168
Torticollis, 166. *See also* Dystonia, cervical
  spasmodic, treatment of, historical perspective on, 7, 170
Tourette syndrome, 81
Tremor
  action, 153
  asymmetrical, treatment of, 156
  bilateral
    asymmetrical, treatment of, 156
    symmetrical, treatment of, 156
  cerebellar (intention), 50
    deep brain stimulation for, 162, 204
    differential diagnosis of, 153, 153*t*
    etiology of, 156
    treatment of, historical perspective on, 5
    tremor cells in, 155
  in cerebellar disorders, thalamic DBS for, efficacy of, 228
  cerebellar outflow, 153
  deep brain stimulation for (*See* Deep brain stimulation
      (DBS), for tremor)
  definition of, 153
  drug-induced, 59
  dystonic, 153, 166
    differential diagnosis of, 153, 153*t*
  essential (*See* Essential tremor (ET))
  familial
    genetics of, 153
    radiosurgery for, 237–238
  head, 59
  Holmes, 50
    deep brain stimulation for, 162
    differential diagnosis of, 153, 153*t*
    etiology of, 156
    tremor cells in, 155
  kinetic, differential diagnosis of, 153, 153*t*
  in multiple sclerosis, 156

deep brain stimulation for, 162, 204
    complications of, 162
    efficacy of, 228
    radiosurgery for, 237–238
parkinsonian, 17, 54, 59, 153, 155
    radiosurgery for, 237–238
    thalamic DBS for, efficacy of, 227–228
    treatment of, 161–162
        historical perspective on, 2, 5
postanoxic, deep brain stimulation for, 204
posttraumatic, 156
    deep brain stimulation for, 162, 204
    radiosurgery for, 237–238
    thalamic DBS for, efficacy of, 228
postural, differential diagnosis of, 153, 153*t*
psychogenic, 153
radiosurgery for, 237–238
rest, 153
    in Parkinson disease, surgical treatment for, 54
rubral (*See* Tremor, Holmes)
in stroke patient, 156
    deep brain stimulation for, 162
    radiosurgery for, 237–238
surgery for, selection and evaluation of patient for, 54, 59, 70
task-specific, 153
treatment of, historical perspective on, 5–6, 8
unilateral, treatment of, 156
voice, 59
"Tremor" cells, in thalamic nuclei, 91, 153, 154*f*, 155
Trigeminal neuralgia, 6
Twiddler syndrome, 210, 220
Tyramine crisis, 72

U
Uchimura, Y., stereotaxic apparatus used by, 3
Unified Dystonia Rating Scale, 55
United Dystonia Rating Scale (UDRS), 168
United Parkinson Disease Rating Scale (UPDRS), 52, 230–231
    dyskinesia score, after Gamma Knife pallidotomy, 243, 245*t*
    motor subscore, 53

V
Vc. *See* Ventralis caudalis (Vc) nucleus
Vendors, 37
Ventralis caudalis (Vc) nucleus, 156*f*, 159, 159*f*
    anatomy of, 202
    caudal, 91
    microelectrode recordings, 91–92, 91*t*
    neurons
        Vcae, 155
        Vcpe, 155
    "shell," 91
Ventralis oralis anterior (Voa) nucleus, 155, 155*t*, 156*f*
    stimulation, for dystonia, 168
    voluntary cells in, 155
Ventralis oralis posterior (Vop) nucleus, 155, 155*t*, 156*f*
    anatomy of, 202

stimulation, for dystonia, 168
    voluntary cells in, 155
Ventral mesencephalon (VM), fetal, transplantation of, for Parkinson disease, 248–249
Ventricles, enlarged, 51
Ventriculography, for surgical planning, 63
Ventrointermedius (Vim) nucleus, 155, 155*t*, 156*f*, 159*f*
    anatomy of, 153
    indirect targeting of, 65*t*
    lead implantation in, 100–102
    macrostimulation in, 119
    magnetic resonance imaging and, 116
    mechanical stunning effect (microlesion) in, with introduction of stereotactic probe, 118
    microelectrode recordings, 91–92, 91*t*
    in Parkinson disease, 17
    regional anatomy of, 202–204, 203*f*, 204*f*
    stimulation
        adverse effects of, 229
        for dystonia, 168
        for essential tremor, 50, 54, 60, 153, 162
            efficacy of, 231–232
        insufficient efficacy without side effects, 203
        for tremor, 153–154, 159–162
            targeting of, 157
    surgical approaches to, historical perspective on, 5
    targeting, 116
    voluntary cells in, 155
Ventro-oralis posterior (Vop) nucleus
    microelectrode recordings, 91–92, 91*t*
    stimulation, for essential tremor, 50
Vim. *See* Ventrointermedius (Vim) nucleus
Viral vector(s), for gene therapy, 253–254
Visual phenomena, stimulation-induced, 205–206, 211, 223–224
Vitamin E, perioperative management of, 60*t*, 61
Voluntary cells, 155
von Willebrand disease, 61
Vop. *See* Ventro-oralis posterior (Vop) nucleus
VoXim software, 126–128, 137, 137*f*, CP 9.13

W
Walker, A.E., 2, 2*f*, 5
Weakness, stimulation-induced, 229
Weight gain, postoperative, 230, 231
White matter, frontal, penetration of, 220
Wilson disease, 166
Writer's cramp, 166
Wycis, H.T., 2*f*, 3–4, 5–6

X
X-ray, intraoperative, historical perspective on, 3

Z
Zamorano-Dujovny frame, 31
Zona incerta, 92, 104*f*, 155
    stimulation, for Parkinson disease, 231
    surgical approaches to, historical perspective on, 7